# The Hepatobiliary System
Fundamental and Pathological Mechanisms

# NATO ADVANCED STUDY INSTITUTES SERIES

A series of edited volumes comprising multifaceted studies of contemporary scientific issues by some of the best scientific minds in the world, assembled in cooperation with NATO Scientific Affairs Division.

### Series A: Life Sciences

*Volume 1* – Vision in Fishes: New Approaches in Research
edited by M. A. Ali

*Volume 2* – Nematode Vectors of Plant Viruses
edited by F. Lamberti, C.E. Taylor, and J.W. Seinhorst

*Volume 3* – Genetic Manipulations with Plant Material
edited by Lucien Ledoux

*Volume 4* – Phloem Transport
edited by S. Aronoff, J. Dainty, P. R. Gorham, L. M. Srivastava, and C. A. Swanson

*Volume 5* – Tumor Virus–Host Cell Interaction
edited by Alan Kolber

*Volume 6* – Metabolic Compartmentation and Neurotransmission: Relation to Brain Structure and Function
edited by Soll Berl, D.D. Clarke, and Diana Schneider

*Volume 7* – The Hepatobiliary System: Fundamental and Pathological Mechanisms
edited by W. Taylor

*Volume 8* – Meat Animals: Growth and Productivity
edited by D. Lister, D. N. Rhodes, V. R. Fowler and M. F. Fuller

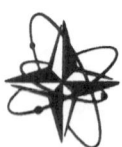

The series is published by an international board of publishers in conjunction with NATO Scientific Affairs Division

| | | |
|---|---|---|
| A | Life Sciences | Plenum Publishing Corporation |
| B | Physics | New York and London |
| C | Mathematical and Physical Sciences | D. Reidel Publishing Company Dordrecht and Boston |
| D | Behavioral and Social Sciences | Sijthoff International Publishing Company Leiden |
| E | Applied Sciences | Noordhoff International Publishing Leiden |

# The Hepatobiliary System

## Fundamental and Pathological Mechanisms

Edited by

## W. Taylor

*The Medical School*
*The University*
*Newcastle upon Tyne, England*

**PLENUM PRESS ● NEW YORK AND LONDON**
Published in cooperation with NATO Scientific Affairs Division

Library of Congress Cataloging in Publication Data

NATO Advanced Study Institute on the Biliary System, 2d, Aalborg, Denmark, 1975.
The hepatobiliary system.

(NATO advanced study institutes series: Series A, Life sciences; v. 7)
Includes bibliographical references and indexes.
1. Biliary tract—Congresses. 2. Biliary tract—Diseases—Congresses. 3. Liver—Congresses. 4. Liver—Diseases—Congresses. I. Taylor, William, 1922-    II. Title. III. Series. [DNLM: 1. Biliary tract—Congresses. W3 N136 1975h/WI700 N108 1975h]
RC849.N37  1975                    612'.35                    76-2486

Proceedings of the Second NATO Advanced Study Institute on the Biliary System, held in Aalborg, Denmark, August 24-30, 1975

© 1976 Plenum Press, New York
Softcover reprint of the hardcover 1st edition 1976

A Division of Plenum Publishing Corporation
227 West 17th Street, New York, N. Y. 10011

United Kingdom edition published by Plenum Press, London
A Division of Plenum Publishing Company, Ltd.
Davis House (4th Floor), 8 Scrubs Lane, Harlesden, London, NW10 6SE, England

ISBN 978-1-4615-8902-0    ISBN 978-1-4615-8900-6 (eBook)
DOI 10.1007/978-1-4615-8900-6

# Foreword

A volume on the biliary system appeared in 1965, based on a symposium of the NATO Advanced Institute held in September, 1963, in Newcastle upon Tyne in England. It soon became an authoritative text on the problems of the biliary tract and, for instance, the discussion on the biliary secretion of organic anions, organic cations and inorganic ions were classic references. The worn pages of the volume in many libraries, including my own, bespeak its usefulness over ten long years. The initiative and energy of the Director of the first Institute have to be admired, even more so since he was able to assemble a Second Institute in Aalborg, Denmark, in 1975. His wisdom is reflected in the selection of the subjects discussed. The comparison between the two volumes tells something about the advancement in the time interval in knowledge about liver and biliary tract diseases, about the turnover of researchers interested in the liver and its diseases, and also about the present philosophy in biologic science. For this comparison, this volume is particularly suited because, in contrast to many other recent conferences, the more leisurely pace of the NATO Institutes permits more comprehensive but still scholarly reviews of the problems.

The foreword of the first volume, written by my colleague, the late Harry Sobotka, expresses his, now dated, astonishment about the progress of knowledge of biology of the bile, so much less accessible to study than urine. He states his satisfaction that the study of morphological observations was being supplemented by graphic presentation of functional data. Ten years later we almost forget that such developments were still surprising.

Taylor, in the opening address to this Second Institute, in a way on which I cannot improve, points out the progress made in these ten years and gives the reason why he selected the topics presented.

Interesting is an account of the degree to which the scholarly predictions of the excellent summaries in the first volume came true.  Almost prophetically, Sherlock raised the ethical problem of transferring animal experimental procedures to man.  Her statement that the mechanism of cholestasis is mysterious is as true today as it was then.  But when she considered gallstones "a dreadful subject to work on," we can look with satisfaction at the past ten years, when the putative mechanism was moved from mechanical processes in the biliary tract to alterations of hepatocytic function.  Her question of whether the biliary tract is a simple conduit or contributes to the constitution of the bile, as the renal tubule does, has been resolved in favor of the latter.  Her emphasis on genetics in both gallstone formation and in adverse drug reactions has been justified.

Brauer, as a physiologist, emphasized two problems:  the mechanism of bile formation, and the hepatocytic injury and its relation to recovery.  The first problem has since been clarified to a measure anybody scarcely hoped for, but the pathogenesis of liver cell injury and particularly of the death of the hepatocyte is a greater problem today than it was ten years ago.  The initial injury caused by biliary retention can be explained by detergent action of bile acids on hepatocellular organelles and possibly by some effects of bilirubin.  By contrast, the mechanism of liver cell death has become more of a riddle in biliary retention as well as in chemical or immunologic or virus induced liver injury.  The common terminal event is cell membrane injury, but how it comes about is not established.  This lack of information interferes with attempts to favor hepatocytic regeneration and to provide a rational therapy for the sick liver cell beyond the removal of the offender.

Andrews emphasized the importance of the blood, biliary, and tissue fluid flow, as well as intracellular transport.  His analysis of the situation sounds almost up-to-date because here the development followed the prediction more clearly than in any other area.

Doisy referred, as would be expected, to the field of bile acids, in which he pioneered, and predicted significant results from Haslewood's comparative studies and hoped, with more justification than one would have then expected, that Bergström's school at the Karolinska would open up the field.  Supported by the Mayo Clinic's additional contributions, this is probably the area in

which greatest progress has been made in biliary tract disease in
these ten years.  We marvel at his wisdom when he regrets the
neglect of lithocholic acid, which is at present a limiting factor
in the chemotherapy of gallstone disease.

The turnover of scientists reflected in speakers and participants is an interesting comment on the sociology of science.  Besides the unfatigable Director, only two scientists spoke at both
Institutes and one then only in the discussion.  Otherwise, only
four of the speakers and participants of the first conference were
also present at the second although four of the key speakers of
the first were invited but regretfully could not attend.

The years between 1963 and 1975 saw a dramatic change in the
intellectual climate of biomedicine in the entire world.  A sociologic revolution altered the values and standards of society as a
whole and the governments' as its arm.  The aspirations of the
youth shifted emphasis from biologic to sociologic problems in
medicine, often with antagonism toward science as a potential
source of environmental disaster.  A revolution in university
governance in many parts of the Western but also of the Eastern
world thus may have caused the fear in many that in this time of
turmoil or crisis, many of the values might be destroyed that had
brought biomedicine to its peak.  It is reassuring that the academic standards of this conference and the intellectual climate of
the assembly remained as solid as they were at the first.  It is
even more reassuring that an essentially political body, as NATO
is, considered it important to assemble biologic scientists by
giving this conference its support when one might have assumed
that NATO would be preoccupied with more mundane problems.  Let us
hope that a Third Institute will be assembled in a similar spirit
of peaceful endeavor.  Besides Dr. Taylor and the splendid hosts
in Aalborg, symbolized by Dr. E.H. Thayson, the NATO organization
deserves the appreciation of the scientific community.

Hans Popper

# Preface

This volume contains the Lectures, Commentaries and Discussions of the Second NATO Advanced Study Institute on 'The Biliary System' held in Aalborg, Denmark in August, 1975. In selecting the topics for presentation at the Institute, which took two years to plan, I did not attempt to cover all aspects of the hepatobiliary system. Indeed, so vast is the information on this system, and so rapid the progress, that it would be difficult to present a comprehensive survey of the subject at a single Institute.

The purpose of the Institute was to bring together workers from as many disciplines of the biomedical sciences as possible, so that fundamental aspects of membrane structure and transport mechanisms could be seen in relation to the indirect methods which are of necessity applied to structure and function in normal and experimentally disturbed hepatobiliary systems, and finally to attempt to relate these to problems facing the clinical hepatologist. I hope it is obvious that multidisciplinary interchanges of ideas, concepts and problems in different fields of research were a salient feature of the discussion sessions.

It is also apparent from the papers and discussions that although a vast amount of data about the hepatobiliary system has been accumulated in the past few years, our real understanding of the normal and abnormal processes in the bile secretory apparatus has been furthered only a little. Mysteries remain, and many of these have been highlighted by the work of the Institute. Differences of opinion about many processes, methods of approach, etc. have been freely discussed, but not necessarily resolved.

It is my hope and expectation that the free interchange of ideas during the formal and informal meetings of the participants will encourage new outlooks, result in greater collaboration and, above all, to stimulate workers in one area to consider their results in the light of results obtained by others using different approaches to the problems.

I am grateful to the members of the Advisory Committee, particularly Drs. Popper and Thaysen, who provided invaluable advice and a great deal of encouragement in my efforts to organise the programme.

The meeting could not have been held without the financial support of the Scientific Affairs Division of NATO, and I am sure that all who attended the Institute would wish me to express their thanks to NATO.   I am particularly indebted to Dr. T. Kester of NATO for his advice and help during the planning of the Institute.

Generous financial support was also provided by Dr. H. Falk and by Drs. R. Preisig and G. Paumgartner.

We are greatly indebted to Dr. Hess Thaysen for his unflagging efforts to assist with the local organisation of the Institute, which created such a pleasant atmosphere at the Institute.   Also we express our thanks to the Civic Authorities of the City of Aalborg, and also to the citizens of Aalborg whose kind and friendly natures made our stay in the city so pleasant.

Most of the material in the discussion sessions is presented without editing by the participants themselves.   Many will regret, and, perhaps justifiably, criticise the lack of references to back up the statements made in these discussions.   However, I feel that the rapid publication of this volume will compensate for the lack of references.   Also, it may be felt that the volume lacks comprehensive coverage and a balanced appraisal of all current problems related to the hepatobiliary system.   Although the Advisory Committee were generous with their suggestions and comments about the programme, the ultimate decisions about the selection of speakers, the form of the programme and the rapid production of this volume are mine.   Therefore, any failure in the wisdom of these decisions is my responsibility alone.

Whatever success the Institute may have had, and the value of this volume, are due to the enthusiastic support of the

contributors and other participants, and I express my gratitude
to them for their efforts.

W. TAYLOR, DIRECTOR.
Newcastle upon Tyne.
November, 1975.


Advisory Committee:        H. Adlercreutz (Finland)
                           G.A.D. Haslewood (U.K.)
                           N.B. Myant (U.K.)
                           F. Orlandi (Italy)
                           H. Popper (U.S.A.)
                           H. Sarles (France)
                           S. Sherlock (U.K.)
                           J. Sjövall (Sweden)
                           E.H. Thaysen (Denmark)
                           N. Tygstrup (Denmark)

Honorary Presidents:       H. Dam (Denmark)
                           G.A.D. Haslewood (U.K.)
                           H. Popper (U.S.A.)

# Contents

SESSION 2

STRUCTURE AND FUNCTION IN THE
HEPATOBILIARY SYSTEM

# CONTENTS

## SESSION 4B
### BILE ACIDS AND LIPIDS II.

## SESSION 5
### CHOLESTASIS

# THE HEPATOBILIARY SYSTEM: RETROSPECT AND PROSPECT. A PERSONAL VIEW

W. Taylor

Director of the Second Nato Advanced Study Institute
Dept. of Physiology, The Medical School, The University
Newcastle upon Tyne, England

In the Preface to the published proceedings of the First NATO Advanced Study Institute on "The Biliary System" of 1963 I wrote: "Increase in knowledge and the ramification of scientific disciplines have inevitably led to a fragmentation of effort in the study of the biliary system. Often a group interested in one aspect of the system may be unaware of, or not in a position to appreciate the work of others concerning another aspect of the system" (Ref. 1). It seems to me that this statement is just as relevant now as it was in 1963; indeed it may be even more valid. Many more people are now working on a wider variety of aspects of the liver and biliary systems, using different approaches and becoming immersed in their own esoteric problems without attempting or being able to relate their work to that of others. This is not intended as a criticism of the workers or the results they obtain; it is simply a fact of scientific life which is forced upon us for the reasons I have already mentioned.

Therefore I felt that the time had arrived for the holding of a Second Institute on various aspects of the hepatobiliary system. I have selected those areas in which rapid progress has been made over the past twelve years, and other areas in which our knowledge and understanding are deficient or are matters of controversy. The style of a NATO Institute, differing as it does from the usual type of international congress, gives us the opportunity and time to pause to reorientate our thinking; to look back to see what has been achieved; to look critically at the current state of knowledge; to look forward to try to define those areas which might be most amenable to solution; to ask ourselves why important fundamental problems remain unsolved and to speculate on how these problems may be attacked.

We are all aware that two areas of biomedical science have
grown enormously in the past decade;  these are the study of
membranes and of transport in biological systems.    Indeed these
two areas are now scientific disciplines in their own right.
They have their own specialist journals and review volumes, and
also their own Societies at national and international level.
Yet I wonder how many of us have the time or inclination or the
necessary background to appreciate the minor revolution which has
occurred in these two disciplines in recent years.    The study of
the plasma membrane has yielded results of great fundamental
importance which are relevant to the hepatobiliary system.  Methods
are now available for the separation of the canalicular and plasma
membranes from each other and from other cellular components, and
Kupffer cells can be isolated in a fairly pure state.    Hepatologists are now taking advantage of these methods to study
fundamental processes in these cellular components of the liver.
However, a number of technical problems remain;  problems which
may prove to be almost as insuperable as that of obtaining a
sample of primary bile.    The study of membrane structure and of
fundamental transport mechanisms has, of necessity, been applied
to relatively simple systems such as red-cell ghosts and various
types of simple epithelia.    However, the hepatocyte can be
considered as having a heterogeneous plasma membrane system;  the
membrane on the sinusoidal side, which is mainly concerned with
transport of substances into the cell, probably has different
structure and fundamental mechanisms from those of the canalicular
membrane, which is primarily a system for transporting substances
out of the cell.    Net fluxes of substances across these membranes
may vary with the functional state of the intracellular components,
which themselves have specialised membranes, and which are being
acted upon by substances entering and leaving the cell across the
sinusoidal or canalicular membranes.    A variety of hormones may
also be exerting influences on the transport processes and metabolic
state of the hepatocytes.    A further complication is the possibility that there may be intercellular relationships between
adjacent hepatocytes across what may well be another type of
membrane.    Furthermore, in pathological conditions the opening
of the tight junction may provide a further complication to
interpretation of transport phenomena.    Therefore, it seems
unlikely that "hepatocyte ghosts" will be of much value in the
study of hepatic transport processes.

At the First Institute we were given an excellent account of
the transport of ions across the gall-bladder membrane by Dr.
Diamond (Ref. 1, p. 233), but the complexities of what we called
"the sodium pump" were not fully appreciated at that time.    Yet
even while the Institute was in progress the concept of the

$Na^+/K^+$-ATPase membrane system was being elucidated by Skou in this, our host, country (Ref. 2) and now the cation-adenine nucleotide membrane system dominates thinking about transport processes in most biological systems. Also in 1963 we had naive ideas about the mechanism of bile secretion. Our simple concept was that bile was secreted by a process which involved active transport of bile salts into the canaliculus to create an osmotic gradient, and other constituents of bile followed by diffusion in the net flow of water across the canalicular membrane. We also had doubts about the possible role of the ductular system in affecting the composition of bile as it flowed down into the main duct system. However, it is now accepted that biliary secretion has at least three major components: a) bile salt independent flow, which may represent a considerable proportion of basal bile flow; b) bile salt dependent flow (it is now being suggested that this element of bile flow may simply be due to activation by bile salts of the cation-adenine nucleotide mechanism involved in bile salt independent flow; c) modification of bile composition, particularly of water and electrolytes by transport mechanisms within the ductules and ducts, and this is probably the site of action of the hormone secretin (Ref. 3).

In 1963 we had no clear ideas about what determines whether or not a particular substance will be excreted in bile. It was accepted that some substances could enter the hepatocyte from the sinusoidal side, traverse the cell, with or without being metabolized en route, and be either "accepted" or "rejected" by the canaliculus for transport into the bile. "Rejected" substances travelled back across the cell to be eliminated on the sinusoidal side back into the blood. This particular problem was aggravated by the wide species differences in the excretion of substances into bile, and further complicated by the choice of the rat as the major experimental animal. Various explanations have been put forward to explain what determines which substances will be excreted in bile. Elsewhere (Ref. 4) I have suggested that the fundamental mechanism of bile secretion must be the same in all higher animals, in the same way that the fundamental processes which occur in the kidney to produce urine are common to all higher animals. I also proposed that the factors which determine the extent of biliary secretion of organic anions depend upon the nature and specificity of proteins in the matrix of the canalicular membrane which can bind and subsequently aid the transport of organic anions into bile. Those animals, such as the rat, which excrete a wide range of substances in bile were considered to have "primitive" proteins of low binding specificity in the canalicular membrane, while other species, including man, which do not excrete such a wide variety of substances in bile have evolved less "primitive" membrane proteins and hence will "accept" only a limited range of substances for biliary excretion. Another

factor which we did not consider at the First Institute was the
possible existence of intracellular substances such as proteins
which might be involved in the control of biliary excretion.
Now there is abundant evidence that such intracellular binding
proteins, of which ligandin has been most studied, do in fact
exist.    Nevertheless the fundamental role of ligandin and related
proteins in the control of hepatic uptake of organic anions is
still a matter to be resolved.

     At the First Institute Dr. Ralph Brauer was one of the most
vociferous and stimulating members;  he had something pertinent
and profound to say on almost every topic.    Some of his comments
are worthy of reconsideration.    He said:  "... we should find
ourselves spending another five or six conferences merely talking
about bile secretion mechanisms without advancing to any significant extent unless we can find a way of sampling the fluid  which
first enters the bile canaliculi.    Only from that vantage point
can we hope to discuss the changes in the composition of bile as
it travels down the biliary tree.    Placing in focus this problem
of sampling of primary bile may well prove in the long run to be
the most important single accomplishment of this conference"
(Ref. 1, p. 680).    This was a formidable but valid challenge;   as
far as I know nobody has even suggested how this sampling of
primary bile might be achieved.    There is no doubt that if it
could be done, the impact would have as much effect on biliary
physiology as micropuncture studies on renal tubules had on
kidney physiology.    Until Brauer's challenge is accepted and
achieved, we must rely on indirect methods, and then extrapolate
back to what we consider might have been the situation in the
canaliculus.    Many ingenious indirect methods have been devised,
but it may be worthwhile adding this note of caution that, whatever the precautions taken, bile as collected does not necessarily
reflect the bile secreted into the canaliculus.    The need for
careful methodology was also stressed by Dr. Brauer:  "All of us,
I feel sure, are well aware of the fact that in the field of liver
physiology, as in other fields of biological research, problem
formulation and the resolution of problems once formulated depend
to a remarkable extent upon the development of competent and
proper methodology......Each one of us who is using one particular
method as his method of choice for the study of bile secretion is
to a certain extent putting "blinders" on himself:  to remove these
he will have to look at his problem through concurrent multiple
experimental approaches.    This pooling of experimental methods
applied to the same test system, together with an increased
awareness of the anatomical realities of our subject, are two of
the major charges that each of us as experimenters should, I
believe, take home with us from this meeting".    It is my
impression that these wise comments were heeded by many, and I

hope that the Second Institute will reinforce the idea of multi-disciplinary approaches to our problem.

As a result of the need for "competent and proper methodology" as stated above, our knowledge of bile acid metabolism has increased enormously since 1963; to such an extent that a two-volume book on bile acids issued recently is now somewhat out of date (Ref. 5). For example the recent introduction of radioimmunoassay methods is not referred to in those volumes. As yet, the radioimmunoassay methods appear to lack the specificity required for many problems, and it may well be that their use will be restricted to clinical problems.

The concentration of effort on research into bile acids tended to turn attention away from other important components of bile, the bile pigments and the other lipids, mainly phospholipids and cholesterol. In 1963 we discussed bilirubin metabolism, but seemed to consider that only free or mono- or diglucuronides of bilirubin were of any importance. The possibility that bilirubin might be excreted as a sulphate was reluctantly conceded. In recent years more attention has been given to bile pigments, and exciting discoveries have been made in this field.

A question raised by myself and others at the First Institute was: "What is the function, if any, of the cholesterol in bile?" As Dr. Doisy pointed out (Ref. 1, p. 685), bile is not an ultra-filtrate of plasma, so the presence of cholesterol in bile cannot be explained in that way. This is an important question because of the role of this sterol in the aetiology of gallstones. The triangular coordinate concept of Small, well documented elsewhere (Ref. 5, p. 249) implicates cholesterol as a primary factor in gallstone formation, but whatever the validity of this concept, it is a major step forward compared with the empirical observations of previous work as exemplified in the report of Burnett in the proceedings of the First Institute (Ref. 1, p. 601). Another advance since 1963 has been the attempt to treat gallstones by giving patients rather large doses of chenodeoxycholic acid. Why this particular bile acid should be more efficacious than other bile acids in dissolving gallstones is still a mystery, and it seems to me that useful fundamental information could be obtained by an investigation of this problem. Many centres have undertaken studies of this form of treatment, but its value as an alternative to surgical treatment of gallstones is still a matter of controversy. Full assessment of its value requires the sort of large controlled survey to be carried out in the United States. The emphasis on cholesterol and bile acids has tended to overshadow the other parameter in the triangular concept theory, viz. the biliary phospholipids, but current research on these substances appears to be redressing the balance.

The biliary excretion of hormones and antibiotics was widely covered at the First Institute, and this topic has been updated elsewhere (Ref. 4).   However, in the last decade the biliary excretion of various drugs and xenobiotics has been extensively studied, and theories about mechanisms of biliary excretion have been proposed on the basis of that work.   This is an area of importance for the clinical pharmacologist and clinician, since it now seems that many drugs in common use may return via the enterohepatic circulation to the peripheral circulation in their original form or as metabolites with residual biological activity. This obviously creates problems in therapeutics, and it seems to me that the possibility that a drug may undergo enterohepatic circulation should form part of any drug screening programme.   It would also be interesting to know if there is any relationship between the potential hepatotoxicity of a drug and its subsequent fate in the biliary tract.   Little attention has been paid to the effects of these substances excreted in bile on the composition, or amount, of bile produced as a result of administering these substances.   Little is known about the basic processes which determine why a particular substance or its metabolites may be preferentially excreted in bile or urine, or how such substances may affect the intestinal microflora and therefore alter the pattern of substances such as the bile acids which are normally returned to the liver via the enterohepatic circulation.   A striking example of the importance of taking this into account is the demonstration that administration of antibiotics has a profound effect on steroid hormone metabolites present in the bile of human subjects treated with ampicillin (Ref. 6).   It is not unreasonable to suppose that similar effects will be exerted on the metabolism of bile acids by the intestinal microflora and so have marked effects on the types and amounts of secondary bile acids returning to the liver.

In a summary of the clinical topics dealt with at the First Institute, Professor Sheila Sherlock said: 'With regard to my own particular clinical problem of cholestasis, I have no idea at the moment how this is going to be tackled.....we are no nearer solving the mechanism by which biliary secretory failure occurs in man'' (Ref. 1, p. 676).   Professor Andrews also commented: ''I have been much impressed by the fact that cholestatic jaundice presents a fairly constant picture although there are a great number of aetiological agents.   There are some variations.   For instance, there is more cell damage in some cases than in others, sometimes the portal tracts are involved, sometimes not.   However, a great variety of stimuli produce cholestasis, and it is fairly obvious that there must be, as it were, a ''final common path''. The path must be reasonably non-specific, because not only are bile salts affected but so also are bile pigments and cholesterol. If we can find the nature of the ''final common path'' it will help

the clinicians and the physiologists" (Ref. 1, p. 684).    Dr.
Brauer took a more fundamental view:   "We have listened to a
great deal of exciting information concerning the effects on
bile secretion of agents.......which are capable of producing
liver injury..... In all cases there was in fact evidence of
liver injury.   In very few, if any of these instances, however,
could anyone be sure at present whether the effects on bile
secretion are the result of cell injury and cell death, or whether
they are the attempts of surviving cells to restore themselves to
an equilibrium which has been disturbed.   It seems quite certain
that, when this kind of injury is inflicted upon cell population,
much more than merely the bile-forming mechanism is disrupted.
The formulation of any conclusions concerning the bile secretory
mechanism therefore requires in each case clarification of the
primary biochemical lesions produced" (Ref. 1, p. 682).

It remains to be seen how valid these comments were, and how
much more we might have learned about cholestasis since 1963.

It was my hope, which I think was at least partially fulfilled,
that the First Institute stimulated research and created new
approaches to the then outstanding problems of the biliary system.
In this paper I have given a personal view of some of the salient
points which were occupying people's minds in 1963, and also to
pose some questions about how these problems have been solved or
put into another form in the expectation that my own views will
precipitate lively discussion and criticism.

My personal contribution to the field of hepatobiliary pathophysiology is minute compared to that of most other workers in the
field.   However, a great English scientist wrote almost 100 years
ago:   "Some may think that the same talents and industry would be
better devoted to original work;   but it must be allowed that to
elucidate and render accessible the labours of others may be a
service as valuable as the addition of new material to the common
store" (Lord Rayleigh, 1874).   That statement provides my excuse,
if one be needed, for undertaking the onerous task of organising
two NATO Advanced Study Institutes and editing the proceedings.


## REFERENCES

1.   The Biliary System.   Proceedings of the First NATO Advanced
Study Institute.   Edited by Taylor, W. Blackwells Scientific
Publications, Oxford, 1965.

2.   Skou, J.C. (1965).   Enzymatic basis for active transport of
$Na^+$ and $K^+$ across cell membranes.   Physiol. Rev. 45, 596-617.

3.    Erlinger S. & Dhumeaux, D. (1974).  Mechanisms and control
of secretion of bile water and electrolytes.  Gastroenterol.
66, 281-304.

4.    Taylor, W. (1971).  The excretion of steroid hormone metabolites in bile and aeces.  Vitamins & Hormones 29, 201-285.

5.    The Bile Acids.  Edited by Nair, P.P. & Kritchevsky, D.
(1972).  Vols. 1 and 2.  Plenum Press, New York.

6.    Martin, F., Peltonen, J., Laatikainen, T., Pulkkinen, M. &
Adlercreutz, H. (1975).  Excretion of progesterone metabolites
and estriol in feces from pregnant women during ampicillin
administration.  J. Steroid Biochem. 6, 1339-1346.

# Membranes and Transport Mechanisms

# MEMBRANE STRUCTURE

J. A. Lucy

Department of Biochemistry and Chemistry, Royal Free
Hospital School of Medicine, University of London,
8 Hunter Street, London WC1N 1BP, U.K.

## INTRODUCTION

The importance of the structure of membranes in relation to
hepatobiliary physiopathology is virtually self-evident. A hepatocyte cannot function correctly if the membranes of its constituent
organelles are in any way abnormal. It is also important that the
turnover and replacement of membranes and of the individual components of membranes proceeds correctly. It has been pointed out
by Siekevitz (1975) that although the lifetime of a human hepatocyte and of its membranes is of some six to twelve months, the
protein and phospholipid molecules of its endoplasmic reticulum
membranes, by contrast, have lifetimes ranging from one to twenty
days. Normal turnover therefore maintains structural continuity
in liver cell membranes, despite the constant replacement of their
constituent molecules. The smooth endoplasmic reticulum is, in
fact, particularly complex in this respect in that, unlike the
organelle in other cells, the smooth endoplasmic reticulum of the
hepatocyte contains "detoxication" proteins that metabolise
foreign compounds including carcinogens, pesticides and drugs.

The plasma membrane of the hepatocyte is also of special
interest in that it is concerned in various ways in the secretion
from the cell of a remarkable range of substances, e.g. albumin,
lipoproteins, retinol-binding protein, and bile. The plasma
membrane of the hepatocyte is of additional importance since it is
highly differentiated, being composed of two surfaces that face
sinusoids and that are concerned with the transport of material to
and from blood, as well as several other surfaces that are in
contact with neighbouring hepatocytes. These latter surfaces not
only possess various kinds of specialized junctions between

adjacent hepatocytes, but also contain the curious regions of
plasma membrane that are capable of secreting bile without their
being significantly damaged by the surfactant molecules.  Present
day techniques are beginning to allow the separation and characterization of laterally-differentiated regions of hepatocyte surface
membrane, as in the recently published work of Wisher and Evans
(1975).  It is interesting to note that the various laterally-
differentiated regions of the plasma membrane of hepatocytes
presumably lose their structural identity, when these cells fuse
into multinucleated giant cells in the unusual cytotoxic response
that has been observed by Grieg et al., (1973) to occur in the
livers of animals treated with the chlorinated aromatic compound
2,3,7,8-tetrachlorodibenzo-p-dioxin (dioxin).

     Within the last few years the general field of membrane
structure has seen a considerable change in approach.  Until
relatively recently, review articles on this subject (e.g. Hendler,
1971) often included a survey of the models for the structure of
membranes put forward by various investigators, and the individual
characteristics of models of membrane structure suggested by
Sjöstrand (1971), Green (Vanderkooi and Green, 1970), Singer
(Lenard and Singer, 1968), Wallach (1969) and Zahler (1969),
Benson (1966), Deamer (1970), and Lucy (1968) were discussed at
some length by Fisher and Lucy (1972).  Today one model receives a
major share of attention, - the fluid mosaic model proposed by
Singer and Nicolson (1972).  That is not to say that all membranes
are now thought to have identical structures.  On the contrary,
although the Singer and Nicolson model embodies some primary
features that appear to apply to the majority of membranes, it is
also possible to add to or modify this model in order to allow for
the special characteristics of individual membranes.  As a result,
controversy over molecular models for the structure of membranes
has receded within the last few years.  At one time, differing
interpretations of membrane structure appeared to be irreconcilable.
Now the majority of investigators would probably agree that,
firstly most membranes are constructed from common classes of
components that are arranged according to a basic structural
pattern, secondly, considerable variations nevertheless occur from
one membrane to another, both regarding analytical composition and
the three-dimensional disposition of the component parts of the
membranes.

     Three years ago it was suggested (Fisher and Lucy, 1972) that,
while the '60's were the decade of membrane models, the '70's will
see the development of intensive, multidisciplinary studies of
membranes.  This may lead to determinations of three-dimensional
sequences of membrane structure in terms of where the proteins are
located, to what extent they project through the membrane, to what
extent the lipid is present in a symmetrical or asymmetrical
bilayer or in a micellar or other organisation, and to what degree

the lipid is closely associated with protein at different sites on
the membrane: this would provide for the three-dimensional
characterization of membrane structure in dynamic terms.  As far
as can be seen, studies on membranes are currently developing in
this way.

## THE SINGER AND NICOLSON MODEL

Before discussing some aspects of the varied facets of
membrane structure and function, many of which are explicitly or
implicitly taken into account in the Singer and Nicolson model, it
will no doubt be helpful to recapitulate the essential features of
the model itself.  These are illustrated in Figure 1.  A lipid
bilayer provides the basic structural framework for the membrane.
This bilayer is responsible for membrane integrity, stability and
impermeability.  The bilayer structure is, however, interrupted by

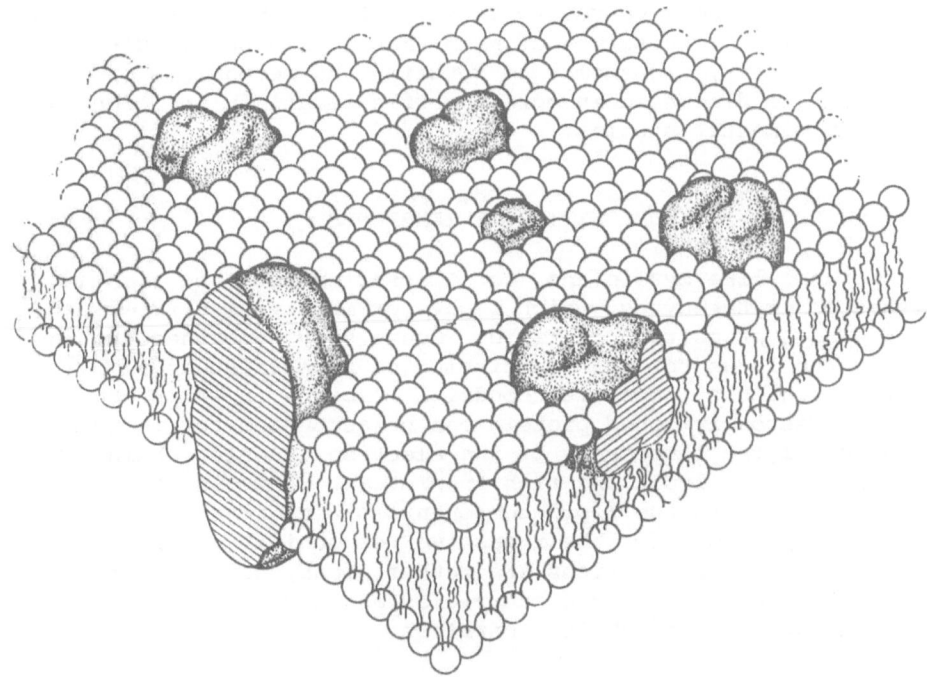

Figure 1.  The fluid mosaic model proposed by Singer and Nicolson.
The solid bodies with stippled surfaces represent the globular
integral proteins which, at long range, are randomly distributed
in the lipid bilayer, within the plane of the membrane.  Reproduced with permission from Singer and Nicolson (1972).

inserted proteins which penetrate to varying degrees into the lipid domain, and many of which are bound to the lipid to a greater or lesser extent by hydrophobic interactions.  The intramembraneous particles that are visualised in the interior of membranes by the technique of freeze fracture correspond to such inserted proteins. Some of the proteins are accessible from one side of the lipid bilayer, others from the other side, while yet others project through from one side of the lipid bilayer to the other.  The proteins of these various kinds are considered to be capable of lateral movement, but not of tumbling or flip-flop motion within the plane of the membrane.  Nevertheless, lateral movement is not unrestricted.  An unrestricted movement would clearly be contrary, for example, to the known lateral differentiation of the plasma membranes of certain cell types, including hepatocytes.  In their original formulation of the fluid mosaic model for membrane structure, Singer and Nicolson therefore suggested that some unknown agent, which was extrinsic to the membrane (either inside or outside the cell), interacts at numerous sites with proteins that are integral with the lipid bilayer, thereby restricting the lateral movement of these proteins.  More recently Singer (1974) has published a comprehensive review in which this, and other aspects of the molecular organisation of membranes (membrane fluidity, membrane asymmetry, transmembrane rotation and mechanisms of transport), are discussed in more specific detail in the light of current experimental studies.


## COMPOSITION OF MEMBRANES

Membranes like myelin and, to a lesser extent, the plasma membranes of erythrocytes, which behave primarily as barriers, contain a high proportion of lipid.  Conversely membranes that are primarily the locus for the functioning of interrelated enzyme complexes, e.g. the inner mitochondrial membrane in which about half of the strongly-bound protein can be accounted for in terms of known catalytic components of the electron transfer chain, are relatively poor in lipid and rich in protein.  This is to be expected since it is the lipid components of membranes that are primarily responsible for their passive permeability characteristics.  These generalisations are rather broad, however, since most membranes exhibit enzyme activities and also behave, at least to some extent, as permeability barriers.

Of greater interest are the variations in lipid and protein composition between normal cells and cancer cells that are currently an interesting field of study.  For example, Bergelson (1968) has reported that the specificity of phospholipid composition usually observed on comparing the composition of the membrane of one type of sub-cellular organelle with the membrane of a different type of organelle does not seem to prevail in

tumour cells.  Cardiolipin, which is normally present only in the
inner mitochondrial membrane, occurred in the microsomal fraction
of Jensen sarcoma cells.  Similarly sphingomyelin was found in the
mitochondria of these cells, whereas it is normally present only
to a limited extent in mitochondria but is high in the plasma
membranes of cells.  Abnormalities of this kind have been found to
apply to a poorly differentiated, fast growing hepatoma but not to
a minimal deviation hepatoma or to regenerating liver (Bergelson
et al., (1974).

In relation to membrane proteins, it has recently been
reported that a significant increase in the density of intramembraneous particles occurs in the freeze-fractured plasma
membranes of BHK 21 hamster cells, after transformation by hamster
sarcoma and polyoma viruses (Torpier et al., 1975).  These workers
have suggested that the newly-appeared particles may represent the
insertion of new proteins in the hydrophobic regions of the plasma
membrane, in response to the action of oncogenic viruses.

A useful review of some of the salient differences in the
behaviour of the surface membranes of normal and tumour cells is
to be found in the recent article by Marx (1974).

## Membrane Lipids

Variations in the polar groups of membrane phospholipids give
rise to different phospholipid classes, e.g. sphingomyelin, phosphatidylcholine, phosphatidylethanolamine.  In addition, wide
variations can occur in the degree to which the hydrocarbon chains
of membrane phospholipids are unsaturated.  As a result, it has
been estimated that an erythrocyte membrane probably contains some
150 - 200 chemically different lipid molecules.  It is therefore
clear that with a complex cell like the hepatocyte a very large
number of different lipid molecules are present in its various
types of membrane.  Hence the inner mitochondrial membrane of
liver is not only peculiarly rich in cardiolipin, it also is more
unsaturated than the outer mitochondrial membrane as well as being
distinguished by containing no cholesterol and little or no phos-
phatidylinositol.  The peculiarities of lipid composition of
individual membranes may possibly be closely related to their
protein composition.  For example it may be significant that it
has been reported that about one third of the phosphatidylserine
in the membranes of human erythrocyte ghosts is apparently closely
associated with membrane proteins, and that this phospholipid does
not mix freely with phosphatidylethanolamine in the lipid bilayer
(Marinetti and Love, 1974).

Among the most recent of ideas concerning the organisation of
membrane lipids in relation to membrane function is that of

asymmetry. It has been known for several years that the glycoproteins of plasma membranes are located on the outer surface of
these membranes and, as will be discussed further below, the
distribution of other membrane proteins is also asymmetric. Lately,
however, it has also become apparent that it is no longer justi-
fiable to assume that membrane lipids are symmetrically distributed, as has been implicit in most thinking since the bimolecular
leaflet was first put forward as a basic structural organisation
for the lipids of biological membranes.

When Bretscher (1972) used radioactively-labelled formyl-
methionyl sulphone methyl phosphate (FMMP) to label intact human
erythrocyte membranes, he found that few phosphatidylethanolamine
molecules reacted. Conversely, after lysis of the cells, this
phospholipid was more effectively labelled, - indicating that only
a few of the molecules of this phospholipid are located in the
outer half of the lipid bilayer of human erythrocyte membranes.
This conclusion has been supported by experiments using isethionyl
acetimidate, a non-penetrating reagent for membranes, and ethyl
acetimidate - which penetrates membranes (Whiteley and Berg, 1974).
However, techniques involving differential labelling of intact and
lysed cells are open to the criticism that it cannot be assumed a
priori that a rearrangement of membrane components does not occur
during lysis (cf., Staros et al., 1974). The general conclusions
obtained with such methods, as applied to erythrocytes, have
nevertheless been supported by experiments using purified phospholipases that are presumed to act only on the exterior of the cell
when haemolysis is absent (Zwaal et al., 1973). From all these
various studies it appears that the outer part of the erythrocyte
plasma membrane consists predominantly of choline-containing
phospholipids (lecithin and sphingomyelin) almost to the exclusion
of other phospholipids. Conversely there appear to be few reactive
phosphatidylserine or phosphatidylethanolamine residues on the
outer surface. Cholesterol may be predominantly in the outer half
of the bilayer, at least in myelin (Caspar and Kirschner, 1971).
Specific allocations of different species of membrane lipid to one
side or to the other of membranes would seem to take us one further
step forward in understanding why membranes contain so many
different kinds of lipid molecules.

At the present time, information on the degree to which
phospholipids are asymmetrically distributed in membranes is
actually available only for erythrocyte membranes. It seems quite
likely, however, that comparable considerations apply to the membranes of other cells, perhaps both to intracellular membranes as
well as to plasma membranes. Conceivably, indeed, the plasma
membranes of all cells may be constructed on a similar asymmetric
basis to that reported for human erythrocytes, in view of the fact
that the overall phospholipid compositions of all plasma membranes
are essentially similar. Emmelot and van Hoeven (1975) have, in

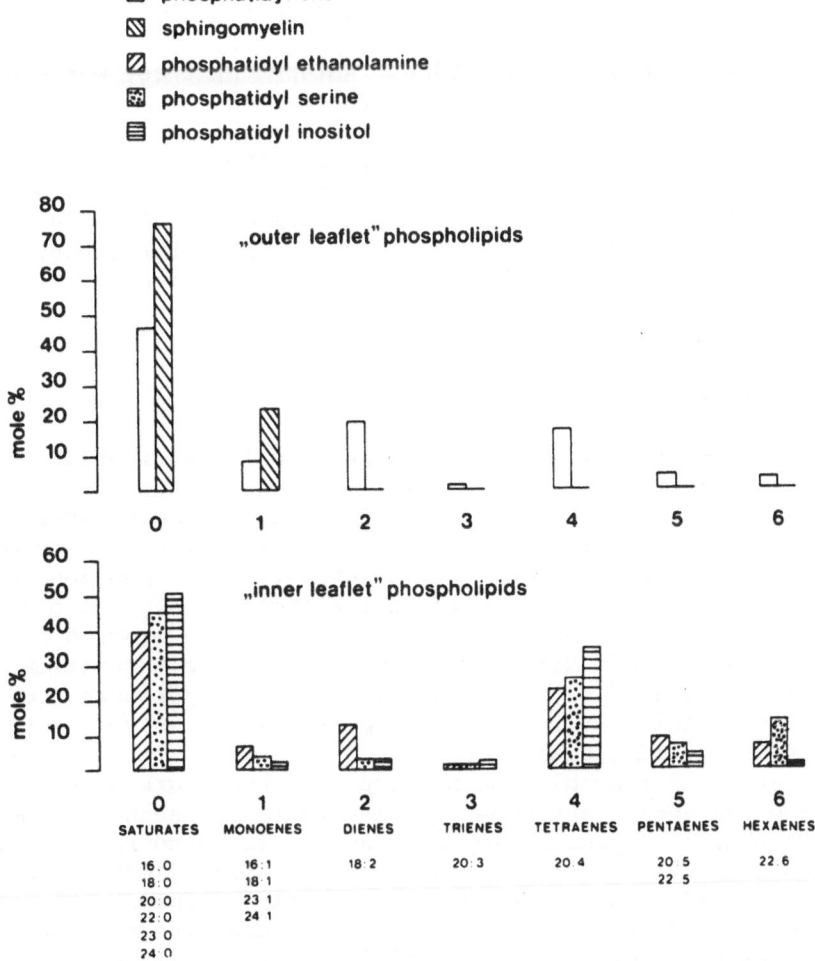

□ phosphatidyl choline
▨ sphingomyelin
▨ phosphatidyl ethanolamine
▨ phosphatidyl serine
▤ phosphatidyl inositol

Figure 2.  Fatty acyl profiles of different phospholipid classes
in plasma membranes isolated from rat liver, showing putative
"outer leaflet" and "inner leaflet" phospholipids.  Reproduced
with permission from Emmelot and van Hoeven (1975).

fact, recently applied such an assumption to the plasma membranes
of rat liver, mouse liver, and a rapidly growing rat hepatoma,
coupled with an analysis of the degree of unsaturation in these
plasma membranes (van Hoeven et al., 1975).  On this basis it
appears that, for all three plasma membranes studied, only about
one third of the double bonds present in the hydrocarbon chains of
the phospholipids occur in sphingomyelin and phosphatidylcholine
(putative "outer leaflet" phospholipids), while the remainder are

found in phosphatidylserine, phosphatidylethanolamine and phos-
phatidylinositol (putative "inner leaflet" phospholipids).  The
detailed breakdown of the fatty acid composition of individual
phospholipids in the plasma membranes isolated by these workers
from rat liver is shown in Figure 2.  The degree to which the
"inner leaflet" phospholipids are polyunsaturated, as compared
with the "outer leaflet" phospholipids, is quite striking.  It
should not be overlooked, however, that the asymmetrical allocation of individual phospholipids shown in Figure 2 is an extrapolation that is based on the analysis of human erythrocytes, and
has not so far been experimentally determined for liver cells.
The reader may be interested in this connection to consult the
comprehensive analysis, by phospholipid class, of the membranes of
the sub-cellular organelles of rat liver that is given in tabular
form by McMurray and Magee (1972).

What will be the effect of an asymmetrical distribution of
phospholipids, and particularly of asymmetrical unsaturation in
the lipid bilayer, on the properties of biological membranes?  To
answer this question, it is necessary to consider the results of
recent physical studies on the thermal properties of phospholipids
and mixtures of phospholipids with cholesterol.  The phospholipids
of biological membranes exhibit transitions from an ordered structural organisation to a disordered structure (phase transitions
from crystal to liquid crystal) on raising the temperature above
the "transition temperature".  The temperatures at which transitions occur in individual phospholipid molecules are dependent
upon the nature of the polar head group, the hydrocarbon chain
length, and the degree and type of unsaturation present (Chapman,
1973).  Molecules of phosphatidylcholine are found to have a lower
transition temperature than molecules of phosphatidylethanolamine.
For the same head group and extent of hydration, lipids with more
unsaturated chains have lower transition temperatures than more
saturated chains, shorter chains exhibit lower transition temperatures than longer ones, and cis-unsaturated chains have lower
transition temperatures than trans-unsaturated chains.  The
transition temperatures of the phospholipids of membranes thus
determine the extent to which the lipids of membranes will be
fluid, and this in turn affects the extent to which the protein
components of membranes may be capable of lateral movement within
membranes.  Asymmetrically-distributed phospholipids may therefore
result in asymmetrical membrane fluidity.  For example, physical
data indicates that the plasma membranes of mouse LM cells may
have two hydrocarbon components, one with upper and lower transition temperatures of 21 and 37°C (attributed to the inner half
of the bilayer), and a second with upper and lower transition
temperatures of 15 and 31°C (attributed to the outer half of the
lipid bilayer).  On this basis, one might expect the outer half of
the plasma membranes of these cells to be more fluid than the
inner half of the leaflet at 21°C (Wisnieski et al., 1974).

The situation is complicated, however, by the possible simultaneous co-existence of fluid and gel regions of lipid (Chapman, 1975). Furthermore cholesterol, which is present in different quantities in different membranes (high in plasma membranes) and may also be asymmetrically distributed across membranes, has a marked effect on membrane fluidity. The effects of cholesterol on membranes depend on whether the membrane phospholipids are above or below their transition temperatures. Below the transition temperature the hydrocarbon chains of the phospholipids will be relatively rigid or gel-like: with such an array of molecules, cholesterol has a disruptive influence that allows increased movement of the acyl chains. With phospholipids that are above their transition temperature, the steroid nucleus prevents flexing of the hydrocarbon chains thus reducing fluidity. Cholesterol may possibly therefore have a dual role in different regions of the same membrane, preventing the formation of crystalline, gel-like areas in some regions, while simultaneously inhibiting the motion of relatively unsaturated phospholipids in more fluid, liquid crystalline regions (Oldfield and Chapman, (1972). These considerations are of particular interest in relation to the cholesterol content and properties of the membranes of tumour cells (Inbar and Shinitzky, 1974; van Hoeven et al., 1975).

It is interesting to note that experiments on phospholipid bilayers, used as an experimental model for biological membranes, have shown that the addition of lipid-soluble drugs not only lowers the transition temperature but also enlarges the temperature range in which two-dimensional domains of fluid and gel phases co-exist. In the presence of the drugs at a given temperature, a greater fraction of membrane is in the fluid phase. It is considered that these results support the conclusion that anaesthetics and related lipid-soluble drugs cause an increase in fluidity, disorder and mobility of the lipid bilayer of membranes, which can modulate the function of membrane proteins (Jain et al., 1975). Morphine compounds and antidepressant molecules also affect the transition temperatures of lecithin-water systems (Cater et al., 1974).

## Membrane Proteins

Some of the proteins of membranes may fulfil a structural role and have no special functional activity, other proteins clearly function as enzymes, others are concerned with transmembrane transport, others as receptors for hormones and other physiologically-active molecules, while yet others - particularly glycoproteins - are involved in cell adhesion, and cell to cell recognition. In passing it is interesting to note that it should not be concluded that all "carrier" molecules involved in transmembrane transport are necessarily proteins. It has recently been reported, for instance, that the movement of chloride ions across lipid bilayers may be mediated by the "flip-flop" movement across the bilayer of molecules of phosphatidylcholine (Toyoshima and Thompson, 1975a, 1975b). While the flux of chloride ions across cell membranes occurring in this way would doubtless be small, as compared with the flux mediated via a protein carrier, it may nevertheless contribute significantly to the overall behaviour of membranes in specific situations.

The proteins of membranes appear to be divisible into two classes, which have been termed peripheral proteins and integral proteins by Singer (1971). Peripheral proteins, like mitochondrial cytochrome C are those proteins that are associated with membranes by weak, non-covalent (mainly electrostatic) bonds. Proteins of this type can be extracted from membranes in a lipid-free form by mild techniques, such as increasing the ionic strength of the medium or by adding chelating agents. By contrast, the integral proteins require quite drastic conditions, e.g., extraction with detergents to remove them from membranes. Even then they are often associated with lipid or, if free from lipid, they are very insoluble and readily aggregate in neutral aqueous buffers. The respective properties of peripheral and integral proteins have recently been summarised in tabular form by Singer (1974), as shown in Table 1.

Probably the best characterised examples of peripheral and integral proteins are to be found in studies on human erythrocytes. Of these, the complex of proteins that is present in human

| Property | Peripheral protein | Integral protein |
|---|---|---|
| Requirements for dissociation from membrane | Mild treatments sufficient: high ionic strength, metal ion chelating agents | Hydrophobic bond-breaking agents required: detergents, organic solvents, chaotropic agents |
| Association with lipids when solubilized | Usually soluble free of lipids | Usually associated with lipids when solubilized |
| Solubility after dissociation from membrane | Soluble and molecularly dispersed in aqueous buffers | Usually insoluble or aggregated in neutral aqueous buffers |

Table 1. Criteria for distinguishing between peripheral and integral membrane proteins. Reproduced with permission from Singer (1974).

erythrocytes and is called spectrin (Marchesi and Steers, 1968), provides an illustration of peripheral proteins.  Spectrin consists primarily of two large polypeptide chains having molecular weights of about 230,000 - 250,000, and a smaller chain of about 43,000, which correspond to components 1, 2 and 5 respectively on poly-acrylamide gel electrophoresis in sodium dodecylsulphate (Steck, 1974).  The entire complex may be regarded as peripheral because it is rapidly released, free from lipids, on treating erythrocyte ghosts with 1 mM EDTA in water.  Spectrin is asymmetrically located in human erythrocyte ghost membranes.  Nicolson et al., (1971), using ferritin-conjugated, anti-spectrin antibody, have demonstrated electron microscopically that ferritin is present on the cytoplasmic surface of these membranes.  Spectrin accounts for about 30% of the total membrane protein in human erythrocytes, and it contains no lipid or carbohydrate.

The major glycoprotein of human erythrocyte membranes, glyco-phorin (Marchesi et al., 1972), provides an interesting example of an integral protein.  It consists of about 60% carbohydrate and 40% protein, with a molecular weight of about 55,000.  The peptide part is apparently a single polypeptide chain with its carboxyl terminal exposed at the cytoplasmic surface of the cell (Segrest et al., 1973).  A sequence of about 23 hydrophobic amino acids (possibly in an $\alpha$-helix) are considered to anchor the glycoprotein hydrophobically to the lipids in the interior of the membrane (Segrest et al., 1972).  Finally, on the exterior surface of the cell, the carbohydrate is present in multiple short oligosaccharide chains attached to the exposed amino-terminal section of the poly-peptide chain.  Glycophorin contains multiple blood-group antigens, the receptors for influenza virus, and receptors for plant lectins.

Another protein of the human erythrocyte membrane, protein E or band 3 which has a sub-unit molecular weight of 93,000 and is the most abundant polypeptide in the membrane (possibly also an anion transport protein, cf., Cabantchik and Rothstein, 1974a, 1974b), has been the subject of a recent investigation by Jenkins and Tanner (1975).  They have reported interesting evidence that the protein has an S-shaped structure which traverses the membrane twice and contains a duplicated set of sites.

Following upon the initial experimental studies on the move-ment of surface antigens in heterokaryons (Frye and Edidin, 1970), an essential feature of the original Singer-Nicolson model for membrane structure, was the movement of membrane proteins.  The mobility of membrane proteins has subsequently been amply substantiated in recent years by the results of studies on the redistribution of membrane receptors on lymphocyte surfaces, and by studies on the influence of the redistributions of receptor molecules on the agglutinability of normal and transformed cells by lectins (cf., Singer, 1974).  However, as indicated above, the

movement of integral proteins in membranes is not unrestricted.
Thus a protein that is antigenically similar to the myosin of
human smooth muscle appears to regulate the translational movement
of integral proteins in the membranes of human fibroblasts
(Painter et al., 1975). Also, unless the ghosts of human erythrocytes are pre-treated to remove spectrin, the translational movement of intramembraneous particles (integral proteins) is
restricted in these cells (Elgsaeter and Branton, 1974). In the
ghost membranes of human erythrocytes, it appears that the intramembraneous particles that are visualised by freeze etching may
contain both glycophorin and band 3 protein (Pinto da Silva and
Nicolson, 1974), and that an antibody-induced aggregation of
peripheral spectrin can result in a collateral aggregation of
integral glycophorin (Nicolson and Painter, 1973).


                        Membrane Fusion

     At first sight it may appear that membrane fusion is of little
relevance to the liver since, under normal circumstances, liver
cells do not fuse into multinucleated cells. Instead they form
specialized junctions between cells that allow intercellular
communication without complete cell fusion (cf., Pappas, 1975;
Loewenstein, 1975). Intracellular membrane fusion is nevertheless
very important. Thus lysosomes could not fulfil their functions
if lysosomal membranes did not undergo membrane fusion. In addition, the release of secreted materials from hepatocytes by
exocytosis involves membrane fusion. The phenomenon of membrane
fusion depends on a temporary loss of membrane stability, and it
is therefore apparent that the incipient structural instability of
biological membranes, and the control of this instability, are
aspects of membrane structure that have an important influence on
cellular function.

     To conclude this review of membrane structure, it is there-
fore appropriate to consider some of the factors involved in
membrane fusion, as far as they are known from studies on cell
fusion, especially since some of these factors are directly
relevant to the aspects of membrane structure that have already
been considered in this paper. However, although our initial work
on membrane fusion centered on the compound lysolecithin and its
interesting fusogenic properties, our studies on lysolecithin will
not be discussed here as they have recently been reviewed elsewhere
(Lucy, 1975).

     It appears that an increase in membrane fluidity facilitates
membrane fusion. This follows from the fact that addition of free
fatty acids, or of fatty acid esters, with low melting points, to
chicken erythrocytes induces the formation of multinucleated cells
(Ahkong et al., 1973a). Insertion of such molecules into membranes

will presumably increase the proportion of hydrocarbon chains in a
relatively liquid state.  It has also been observed that hen
erythrocytes are fused into multinucleated cells by the application
of heat alone in the absence of exogenous lipids (Ahkong et al.,
1973b).  Other workers have found that vesicles of phospholipid
that are below their transition temperature produce less cell
fusion than similar numbers of vesicles containing lipids at or
above their transition temperature (Papahadjopoulos et al., 1973,
Papahadjopoulos et al., 1974).  Finally, benzyl alcohol which is
not itself fusogenic, but is known to increase membrane fluidity
(Metcalfe et al., 1968), also facilitates cell fusion (Fisher, 1975).

Secondly, the way in which fusogenic agents interact with
membranes may depend upon the asymmetric structure of the membrane
concerned.  It has been observed that fusogenic lipids exhibit
interactions, not shown by non-fusogenic lipids, in mixed monolayers with several species of phospholipid, particularly those
phospholipids containing a choline head group (Maggio and Lucy,
1975).  By contrast, fusogenic lipids show little specific interaction in this model system with natural or synthetic preparations
of phosphatidylethanolamine.  These observations on the importance
of the choline group in the molecular interactions of low-melting
fusogenic lipids with phospholipids may indicate that cell fusion
induced in erythrocytes is mediated by the asymmetrical distribution of choline-containing phospholipids in the outer half of
the lipid bilayer of erythrocyte membranes.

Thirdly, it has been proposed that the lateral movement and
aggregation of integral membrane proteins is important in membrane
fusion, either to allow fusion to occur via interdigitation of
membrane proteins (Poste and Allison, 1973), or to facilitate
fusion by the interaction of the membrane lipids of adjacent cells
(Ahkong et al., 1975).  5M Dimethyl sulphoxide and glycerol, agents
which are known to aggregate the intramembraneous particles of
unfixed lymphocytes, have in fact been found capable of inducing
hen erythrocytes to fuse into multinucleated cells (Ahkong et al.,
1975).

From these studies on cell fusion occurring in erythrocytes,
we see that membrane fluidity, membrane asymmetry, and the movement
of membrane proteins, are emerging as factors of importance in the
control of the fusion of erythrocyte plasma membranes.  If the
behaviour of the intracellular membranes of liver cells is governed
by similar principles to those applying to the plasma membranes of
red cells, we may perhaps expect these three parameters to be
important also in the processes of intracellular membrane fusion
that are essential to the normal functions of liver cells.

REFERENCES

Ahkong, Q.F., Fisher, D., Tampion, W. and Lucy, J.A.   Mechanisms
of cell fusion.   Nature (London) 253, 194-195 (1975).

Ahkong, Q.F., Fisher, D., Tampion, W. and Lucy, J.A.   The fusion
of erythrocytes by fatty acids, esters, retinol and
α-tocopherol.   Biochem. J. 136, 147-155 (1973a).

Ahkong, Q.F., Cramp, F.C., Fisher, D., Howell, J.I., Tampion, W.,
Verrinder M. and Lucy, J.A.   Chemically-induced and thermally-
induced cell fusion: lipid-lipid interactions.   Nature (London)
New Biol. 242, 215-217 (1973b).

Benson, A.A.   On the orientation of lipids in chloroplast and cell
membranes.   J. Am. Oil Chem. Soc. 43, 265-270 (1966).

Bergelson, L.D., Dyatlovitskaya, E.V., Sorokina, I.B. and Gorkova,
N.P.   Phospholipid composition of mitochondria and microsomes
from regenerating rat liver and hepatomas of different growth
rate.   Biochim. Biophys. Acta 360, 361-365 (1974).

Bergelson, L.D., Dyatlovitskaya, E.V., Torkhovskaya, T.I.,
Sorokina, E.B. and Gorkova, N.P.   Dedifferentiation of phospho-
lipid composition in subcellular particles of cancer cells.
FEBS Lett. 2, 87-90 (1968).

Bretscher, M.S.   Asymmetrical lipid bilayer structure for biological membranes.   Nature (London) New Biol. 236, 11-12 (1972).

Cabantchik, Z.I. and Rothstein, A.   Membrane proteins related to
anion permeability of human red blood cells.   1. Localization
of disulfonic stilbene binding sites in proteins involved in
permeation.   J. Membrane Biol. 15, 207-226 (1974a).

Cabantchik, Z.I. and Rothstein, A.   Membrane proteins related to
anion permeability of human red blood cells.   2. Effects of
proteolytic enzymes on disulfonic stilbene sites of surface
proteins.   J. Membrane Biol. 15, 227-248 (1974b).

Caspar, D.L.D. and Kirschner, D.A.   Myelin membrane structure at
10Å resolution.   Nature (London) New Biol. 231, 46-52 (1971).

Cater, B.R., Chapman, D., Hawkes, S.M. and Saville, J.   Lipid
phase transitions and drug interactions.   Biochim. Biophys.
Acta 363, 54-69 (1974).

Chapman, D.   Fluidity, phase transitions and protein rotation in
cell membranes.   In NATO Symposium on lipids, proteins and
receptors.   R.M. Burton and L. Packer, Eds., Bi-Science
Publications Division, In press (1975).

Chapman, D.   Some recent studies of lipids, lipid-cholesterol and
membrane systems.   In Biological Membranes, D. Chapman and
D.F.W. Wallach, Eds., Academic Press, Vol. 2, 91-144 (1973).

Deamer, D.W.   An alternative model for molecular organization in
biological membranes.   Bioenergetics 1, 237-246 (1970).

Elgsaeter, A. and Branton, D.   Intramembrane particle aggregation
in erythrocyte ghosts.   1. The effects of protein removal.
J. Cell Biol. 63, 1018-1030 (1974).

Emmelot, P. and van Hoeven, R.P.   Phospholipid unsaturation and
    plasma membrane organization.   Chem. and Phys. Lipids 14, 236-
    246 (1975).

Fisher, D. Fluidity and cell fusion.   In NATO Symposium on lipids,
    proteins and receptors.   R.M. Burton and L. Packer, Eds.,
    Bi-Science Publications Division, In press (1975).

Fisher, D. and Lucy, J.A.   Membrane Structure.   In Fundamentals of
    Lipid Chemistry, R.M. Burton and F.C. Guerra, Eds., Bi-Science
    Publications Division, 613-656 (1972).

Frye, L.D. and Edidin, M.   The rapid intermixing of cell surface
    antigens after formation of mouse-human heterokaryons.   J. Cell
    Sci. 7, 319-335 (1970).

Grieg, J.B., Jones, G., Butler, W.H. and Barnes, J.M.   Toxic effects
    of 2,3,7,8-tetrachlorodibenzo-p-dioxin.   Fd. Cosmet. Toxicol.
    11, 585-595 (1973).

Hendler, R.W.   Biological membrane ultrastructure.   Physiol.
    Reviews 51, 66-97 (1971).

Inbar, M. and Shinitzky, M.   Cholesterol as a bioregulator in the
    development and inhibition of leukemia.   Proc. Natl. Acad. Sci.
    U.S.A. 71, 4229-4231 (1974).

Jain, M.K., Wu, N.Y-M. and Wray, L.V.   Drug-induced phase change
    in bilayer as possible mode of action of membrane expanding
    drugs.   Nature (London) 255, 494-496 (1975).

Jenkins, R.E. and Tanner, M.J.A.   The major human erythrocyte
    membrane protein.   Biochem. J. 147, 393-399 (1975).

Lenard, J. and Singer, J.S.   Structure of membranes: reaction of
    red blood cell membranes with phospholipase C.   Science 159,
    738-739 (1968).

Loewenstein, W.R.   Cellular communication by permeable membrane
    junctions.   In Cell membranes - biochemistry, cell biology and
    pathology, G.W. Weissmann and R. Claiborne, Eds., H.P. Publish-
    ing Co., 105-114 (1975).

Lucy, J.A.   The fusion of cell membranes.   In Cell membranes -
    biochemistry, cell biology and pathology.   G.W. Weissmann and
    R. Claiborne, Eds., H.P. Publishing Co., 75-83 (1975).

Lucy, J.A.   Ultrastructure of membranes: micellar organization.
    Brit. Med. Bull. 24, 127-129 (1968).

Maggio, B. and Lucy, J.A.   Studies on mixed monolayers of phospho-
    lipids and fusogenic lipids.   Biochem. J. 149, 597-608 (1975).

Marchesi, V.T., Tillack, T.W., Jackson, R.L., Segrest, J.P. and
    Scott, R.E.   Chemical characterization and surface orientation
    of the major glycoprotein of the human erythrocyte membrane.
    Proc. Natl. Acad. Sci. U.S.A. 69, 1445-1449 (1972).

Marchesi, V.T. and Steers, E. Jr.   Selective solubilization of a
    protein component of the red cell membrane.   Science 159, 203-
    204 (1963).

Marinetti, G.V. and Love, R.   Extent of cross-linking of amino-
    phospholipid neighbors in the erythrocyte membrane as influenced
    by the concentration of difluorodinitrobenzene.   Biochem.
    Biophys. Res. Commun. 61, 30-37 (1974).

Marx, J.L.  Biochemistry of cancer cells: focus on the cell
    surface.  Science  183, 1279-1282 (1974).
McMurray, W.C. and Magee, W.L.  Phospholipid metabolism.  Annu.
    Rev. Biochem.  41, 129-160 (1972).
Metcalfe, J.C., Seeman, P. and Burgen, A.S.V.  The protein
    relaxation of benzyl alcohol in erythrocyte membranes.  Molec.
    Pharmac. 4, 87-95 (1968).
Nicolson, G.L. and Painter, R.G.  Anionic sites of human erythro-
    cyte membranes.  II. Antispectrin-induced transmembrane
    aggregation of the binding sites for positively charged
    colloidal particles.  J. Cell Biol. 59, 395-406 (1973).
Nicolson, G.L., Marchesi, V.T. and Singer, S.J.  The localization
    of spectrin on the inner surface of human red blood cell mem-
    branes by ferritin-conjugated antibodies.  J. Cell Biol. 51,
    265-272 (1971).
Oldfield, E. and Chapman, D.  Dynamics of lipids in membranes:
    heterogeneity and the role of cholesterol.  FEBS Lett. 23, 285-
    297 (1972).
Painter, R.G., Sheetz, M. and Singer, S.J.  Detection and ultra-
    structural localization of human smooth muscle myosin-like
    molecules in human non-muscle cells by specific antibodies.
    Proc. Natl. Acad. Sci. U.S.A.  72, 1359-1363 (1975).
Papahadjopoulos, D., Poste, G., Schaeffer, B.E. and Vail, W.J.
    Membrane fusion and molecular segregation in phospholipid
    vesicles.  Biochim. Biophys. Acta 352, 10-28 (1974).
Papahadjopoulos, D., Poste, G. and Schaeffer, B.E.  Fusion of
    mammalian cells by unilamellar lipid vesicles: influence of
    lipid surface charge, fluidity, fluidity and cholesterol.
    Biochim. Biophys. Acta 323, 23-42 (1973).
Pappas, G.  Junctions between cells.  In Cell membranes - bio-
    chemistry, cell biology and pathology.  G.W. Weissman and
    R. Claiborne, Eds., H.P. Publishing Co., 87-94 (1975).
Pinto da Silva, P. and Nicolson, G.  Freeze-etch localization of
    concanavalin A receptors to the membrane intercalated particles
    of human erythrocyte ghost membranes.  Biochim. Biophys. Acta
    36, 311-319 (1974).
Poste, G. and Allison, A.C.  Membrane fusion.  Biochim. Biophys.
    Acta 300, 421-465 (1973).
Segrest, J.P., Kahane, I., Jackson, R.L. and Marchesi, V.T.  Major
    glycoprotein of the human erythrocyte membrane: evidence for an
    amphipathic molecular structure.  Arch. Biochem. Biophys. 155,
    167-183 (1973).
Segrest, J.P., Jackson, R.L., Marchesi, V.T., Guyer, R.B. and
    Terry, W.  Red cell membrane glycoprotein: amino acid sequence
    of an intramembranous region.  Biochem. Biophys. Res. Commun.
    49, 964-969 (1972).
Siekevitz, P.  Dynamics of intracellular membranes.  In Cell memb-
    ranes - biochemistry, cell biology and pathology.  G.W.
    Weissmann and R. Claiborne, Eds., H.P. Publishing Co., 115-122
    (1975).

Singer, S.J. The molecular organization of membranes. Ann. Rev. Biochem. 43, 805-833 (1974).

Singer, S.J. The molecular organization of biological membranes. In Structure and function of biological membranes. L.I. Rothfield, Ed., Acad. Press, 146-222 (1971).

Singer, S.J. and Nicolson, G.L. The fluid mosaic model of the structure of cell membranes. Science 175, 720-731 (1972).

Sjöstrand, F.S. Molecular structure and function of cellular membranes. In Cell membranes - biological and pathological aspects. G.W. Richter and D.G. Scarpelli, Eds., The Williams and Wilkins Co., 1-29 (1971).

Staros, J.V., Haley, B.E. and Richards, F.M. Human erythrocytes and resealed ghosts. J. Biol. Chem. 249, 5004-5007 (1974).

Steck, T.L. The organization of proteins in the human red blood cell membrane. J. Cell Biol. 62, 1-19 (1974).

Torpier, G., Montagnier, L., Biquard, J-M. and Vigier, P. A structural change of the plasma membrane induced by oncogenic viruses: quantitative studies with the freeze-fracture technique. Proc. Natl. Acad. Sci. U.S.A. 21, 1695-1698 (1975).

Toyoshima, Y. and Thompson, T.E. Chloride flux in bilayer membranes: the electrically silent chloride flux in semispherical bilayers. Biochemistry 14, 1518-1524 (1975a).

Toyoshima, Y. and Thompson, T.E. Chloride flux in bilayer membranes: chloride permeability in aqueous dispersions of single-walled, bilayer vesicles. Biochemistry 14, 1525-1531 (1975b).

Vanderkooi, G. and Green, D.E. Biological membrane structure. I. The protein crystal model for membranes. Proc. Natl. Acad. Sci. U.S.A. 66, 615-621 (1970).

Van Hoeven, R.P., Emmelot, P., Krol, J.H. and Oomen-Meulemans, E.P.M. Studies on plasma membranes. XXII. Fatty acid profiles of lipid classes in plasma membranes of rat and mouse livers and hepatomas. Biochim. Biophys. Acta 380, 1-11 (1975).

Wallach, D.F.H. Membrane lipids and the conformations of membrane proteins. J. Gen. Physiol. 54, 3s-36s (1969).

Whiteley, N.M. and Berg, H.C. Amidination of the outer and inner surfaces of the human erythrocyte membrane. J. Mol. Biol. 87, 541-561 (1974).

Wisher, M.H. and Evans, W.H. Function polarity of the rat hepatocyte surface membrane. Isolation and characterization of plasma-membrane subfractions from the blood-sinusoidal, bile-canalicular and contiguous surfaces of the hepatocyte. Biochem. J. 146, 375-388 (1975).

Wisnieski, B.J., Parkes, J.G., Huang, Y.O. and Fox, C.F. Physical and physiological evidence for two phase transitions in cytoplasmic membranes of animal cells. Proc. Natl. Acad. Sci. U.S.A. 71, 4381-4385 (1974).

Zahler, P. New aspects in research on erythrocytes. The structure of the erythrocyte membrane. Experientia 25, 449-456 (1969).

Zwaal, R.F.S., Roelofsen, B. and Colley, C.M.   Localization of
   red cell membrane constituents.   Biochim. Biophys. Acta 300,
   159-182 (1973).

ACKNOWLEDGEMENT

   Work undertaken in this laboratory that is referred to in
this article was supported by the Medical Research Council and
the British Council.

   Fig. 1:  copyright 1972 by the American Association for the
Advancement of Science.

DISCUSSION OF LECTURE BY J.A. LUCY

Popjak:  Apropos of your discussion of cell-membrane fusion, I
am reminded of how common it is to see doubly nucleated cells in
liver sections.   At the same time it is extremely rare to see a
mitotic figure.   It is very probable that such doubly nucleated
cells in the liver do arise by fusion because I recall some of
my very ancient experiments I did sometime in the 1940's with
diphtheria toxin.   Within 24 hours of the administration of an
LD50 dose of toxin to rabbits, 30 to 40 per cent of the liver cells
became doubly nucleated whereas in the normal liver there are only
about 10 per cent.   I wonder what the effect of diphtheria toxin
is and how it produces this.

    You imply that it is the association of the lipid portion of
the membranes which is important in membrane fusion, but I noticed
that in carrying out your experiments with the erythrocytes you
used a pH of 5.6.   This suggests to me that you have interfered
with the proteins by bringing them close to their isoelectric
point.   Would you care to comment on that?

Lucy:  Your comments raise a number of points.   I should say
that we can get fusion at pH 7, but we found that fusion occurred
much more readily at pH 5.6.   This is probably because the
electrostatic charge on the cells is reduced at the lower pH.
This will have two effects.   It will enable the cells to come
closer together because they would not be repelling each other
so much as at pH 7.   It would also allow intramembraneous
proteins to aggregate within the membrane.   So I think that the
effect of pH is on proteins, and that it has these two different
actions.

    The second point concerns the action of diphtheria toxins.
We have in fact been looking at some glycolipids isolated from
diphtheria and related organisms, and we made comparable observations to those I have already mentioned.   Glycolipids from these
organisms will indeed cause red cells to fuse:  the unsaturated
glycolipids being more effective.   Also there seems to be some
correlation between adjuvant activity and fusion activity, because
if you acetylate the glycolipids they become inactive as adjuvants
and as fusogens.   Quite likely, the inflammatory response in

29

which multinucleated cells are produced in tuberculosis and many
other diseases is the result of the action of substances, present
in either the bacterial cell wall or produced by the organism,
acting on the membranes of the cell.

Kuenzle:    I have a question about the synthesis of membranes.
Two hypotheses have been put forward;  one that the individual
lipids and proteins could be incorporated into pre-existing
membranes;  the other that pieces of membrane are formed on the
endoplasmic reticulum and then inserted into the membranes.
What is your view about this?

Lucy:    I think that probably most people support the idea of
membrane flow, which is the kind of thing you mentioned in the
second suggestion.    The endoplasmic reticulum may be a major site
for the synthesis of membranes, including the plasma membrane
which grows by insertion of membrane made in the endoplasmic
reticulum.    A cell that is secreting a great deal by exocytosis
provides a special example of this mechanism.    But such a cell
presumably has a second special mechanism for removing parts of
the membrane continuously.    Otherwise, obviously, the plasma
membrane would get bigger and bigger.

Hofmann:    Is it reasonable to speculate that the outer bilayer or
leaflet of the canalicular membrane contains predominantly
phosphatidyl choline and the inner membrane such things as phosphatidyl serine and phosphatidyl inositol?    What is the phospholipid
and cholesterol composition of the inner and outer membrane of the
hepatocyte canalicular membrane?

Lucy:    Unfortunately, anything that one can say in answer to that
question is only by extrapolation from the data available on other
systems.    The only information that I am aware of is on erythrocytes, because these cells are the easiest to study.    If you can
extrapolate from the data on erythrocytes, then you might say that
the canalicular membrane has more phosphatidyl choline in the
outer half of its bilayer.    Whether one is justified in making
such an extrapolation is a totally open question.

    With regard to cholesterol;  as far as I know there is only
one indication as to where this may be.    In myelin, it has been
suggested that there is more cholesterol in the outer half than
in the inner half of the bilayer.    This was a conclusion based
on X-ray diffraction studies, and as you may know, this technique
produces a lot of results which one tries to reconcile with one
or the other kind of model.    The suggestion that the experimental
data is compatible with a model that shows cholesterol in the
outer half is possibly open to dispute.    Also, if you want to
relate this work to the canalicular membrane, then you have to

make an extrapolation from myelin to the canalicular membrane.

Ostrow:   This is a follow-up to Dr. Hofmann's question.   It has been suggested that the way the phospholipid-cholesterol-bile salt micelles get into bile is that the bile salts dissolve pieces of membrane.   It is interesting that both cholesterol and lecithin constitute the main lipid components of both the micelle and the outer membrane.   Has anyone done any studies with isolated membranes of any type to determine whether the bile acids select-ively pull these two components out of the outer leaf as opposed to the inner leaf of a membrane?

Lucy:   I am not aware of any direct experiments along those lines, but I think it would be very interesting to do.

Popper:   We really have three cell membrane portions in the hepatocyte, not just two.   Doubtlessly there must be a difference between the membrane limiting the inter-cellular cleft and having few or no microvilli and probably permitting an exchange between neighbouring hepatocytes, and the membranes lining the peri-sinusoidal space and the canaliculi.   Is anything known about the crucial constitution of the intercellular cleft membrane, the contractile proteins and the configuration of its constituents? To my knowledge, all that we know about the hepatocyte organelle membranes concerns the smooth endoplasmic reticulum.   My other question deals with the influence of free radicals which are constantly formed and act on the phospholipids and may therefore have an effect on fusion and other processes.   What do you think about this?

Lucy:   I would agree with you that there is probably no structural data available, because it is only fairly recently that the techniques have been available for separating the component membranes.   With regard to the free radicals, Professor Slater might have more pertinent comments than any I can make. I would nevertheless like to say that, if free radicals are involved, it is the unsaturated phospholipids which would be affected.   The inner half of the membrane is therefore likely to be more at risk than the outer half in any changes induced by free radicals.

# TRANSPORT THROUGH BIOLOGICAL MEMBRANES

Hans H. Ussing

Institute of Biological Chemistry A, University of
Copenhagen, 13 Universitetsparken, DK-2100 Copenhagen Ø,
Denmark.

## INTRODUCTION

In the following we shall use the term "membrane" in a purely
pragmatic sense: A sheet of unstirred material, separating two
well stirred solutions. What unifies the concept of membrane is
its physical function as a barrier as well as the methods by which
such structures can be studied (Ussing, Erlij and Lassen, 1974).
Thus a capillary wall or a kidney tubule wall will be considered
to be membranes as well as plasma membranes and basement membranes.

The restriction of the term membrane to the structures seen
as "unit membranes" in the electron microscope is not advisable,
because even membranes of simple appearance may show functional
"sandwich structure", and because, sometimes, the main barrier is
not the plasma membrane.

In the following we shall discuss the different modes of
transport through membranes, both "simple" ones and epithelia.
Most examples will be taken from studies of epithelia, because
they may have a more direct bearing upon the subject of the
present conference.

## MODES OF TRANSPORT THROUGH PLASMA MEMBRANES

a) <u>Simple Fick diffusion</u>. Gases, water and many lipophilic
molecules seem to penetrate in a way that can be described by
simple diffusion. The same often seems to be the case for small
hydrophilic molecules, but from the size of glycerol and upwards,

simple diffusion seems to be too slow for specific requirements, and the cells have developed other devices for transport.

b) <u>Electro-diffusion through specific channels</u>.  It is becoming increasingly clear that electrolytes pass through highly specific channels.  Thus in excitable membranes (muscle, nerve, etc.) the sodium channels are quite specific for that species (and lithium), whereas the potassium channels usually admit only K, Rb and Cs (compare Keynes, 1975).  Similar specificities are seen in the case of alkali metals in epithelia as we shall discuss below.  It is typical of the specific ion channels that it is the combined effect of the concentration difference and the electric potential difference which determines the ionic flux.  The resultant effect can often be approximated satisfactorily by the constant field equation of Goldman (1943).

c) <u>Facilitated diffusion</u>.  One frequently encounters cases where a given substance penetrates the membranes of certain cells much faster than expected from the size and lipid solubility of the substance.  Sometimes the explanation may be that the substance passes a specific electrodiffusion channel.  But far more frequent is a behaviour which can more easily be explained as the result of the presence of a specific membrane carrier. The carrier is assumed to be a molecule or part of a molecule which cannot leave the membrane but which can change place in the membrane so that it makes contact with either the inside or the outside (but not with both sides simultaneously).  Furthermore the carrier must be able to combine with the molecular species which has to be transported and the complex must be able to pass through the membrane faster than the molecule could move by simply diffusing through the membrane.

d) <u>Exchange diffusion</u>.  A special case of carrier-mediated transport is "exchange diffusion" (Ussing, 1947), which is seen when the carrier is saturated on both membrane faces.  Under these conditions a molecular species exchanges against itself, so that with isotopes one can observe rapid exchange, whereas, chemically, there is no net transport.  If the carrier is absolutely specific for one species exchange diffusion has no physiological function.  However, if two or more species can use the same carrier one can get rapid exchange between the two species. The most important case is the chloride-bicarbonate exchange in the red cells which allows rapid anion exchange despite a very low permeability for the individual ions, $Cl^-$ and $HCO_3^-$ (for references see Ussing, Erlij and Lassen, 1974).

e) <u>Coupled (passive) carrier transport</u>.  Some carrier systems are so designed that they can pass the membrane only when they have found, simultaneously, two different specific molecules

or when they have found none.   The classical example is the
passage of glucose from the gut lumen to the cells of the small
intestine which depends on the simultaneous passage of sodium ions
(Crane, 1965).   Sodium-dependent transport systems for sugars and
amino acids are widespread.

   f)  Solvent drag.   If water-filled pores are present in a
membrane, one can predict that the flow of solvent, produced
either by osmosis or by hydrostatic pressure difference, may drag
along dissolved molecules.   It is generally agreed that most
water penetration of cell membranes does not go through well
defined holes or pores.   However, it is known that the polyene
antibiotics, like amphotericin react with cholesterol-containing
membranes to form distinct pores (see Licthenstein and Leaf, 1965).
Even in homogeneous (non-porous) membranes there may be interaction between solute and solvent, but the effects are rarely
significant.

   g)  Active transport.   The term "active transport" is used
for cases where chemical energy from metabolic processes is used
to give a transport process a preferential direction ("vectorial
transport").   Active transport is indicated where transport takes
place against the electrochemical potential (Rosenberg, 1948), or
when the flux ratio as measured with isotopes deviates in a
characteristic manner from the one calculated for simple electrodiffusion (Ussing, 1949).   However, a detailed study of the
system may be necessary before one can decide whether we are
dealing with a case of primary active transport or whether it is
a carrier-mediated passive process coupled with an active transport
or a different molecular species (compare sodium-dependent sugar
transport, see above).   The best known primary active transport
system is the sodium-potassium exchange pump, associated with the
sodium-potassium-magnesium dependent ATPase (Skou, 1957).


## TRANSPORT THROUGH EPITHELIA

   a)  Black box treatment.   The epithelium as a whole may be
treated as the barrier.   If so, one can use the flux ratio test,
mentioned above, to decide whether a given substance can be
assumed to pass by passive processes or whether it is likely to
be subject to active transport.   If one wants to prove the
presence of active transport one may use the short circuiting
technique (Ussing and Zerahn, 1951).   The detailed understanding
of epithelial function requires knowledge of the properties of the
functional units (cell membranes, cell junctions, interspaces).

   b)  The two membrane model of epithelial transport (Koefoed-
Johnsen and Ussing, 1958).   The model was first developed for the

isolated frog skin, but the model with suitable modifications has
been widely used to account for the transport properties of many
epithelia.   The basis for the model is the observation that, in
the presence of a slowly penetrating anion, the potential
difference across the skin varies in a way as if the outward-
facing side of the skin were a sodium electrode and the inward-
facing side a potassium electrode.   The model then makes the
following assumptions:  The outward facing side of the skin is
impermeable to potassium ions but has sodium selective electrodiffusion channels.   The inward-facing side is impermeable to
passively diffusing sodium ions, but possesses selective
electrodiffusion channels for potassium.   The inward-facing
membrane, furthermore, is the seat of an active sodium/potassium
exchange pump, which pumps sodium out of and potassium into the
cells at the expense of the breakdown of ATP.   The pathway for
anions was originally thought to be exclusively cellular.   After
discovery of intercellular leaks via the "tight seals" there has
been a tendency to assume an extracellular pathway for anions.
Recently there has been mounting evidence that both cellular and
extracellular pathways may play a role in the passive anion
transport.   Furthermore, although the sodium-potassium pump
seems to play a dominating role in electrolyte transport, anion
pumps for chloride, bicarbonate and other anions are widespread
just as Ca-pumps, hydrogen ion pumps and specific pumps for
certain organic substances, not handled by the sodium-dependent
carrier systems.   In the following we shall, however, concentrate
on the handling of sodium in epithelia.

    c)  <u>The entry step for sodium</u>.   In the two membrane model of
sodium transport the first step is the entry of sodium into the
cells via a passive but selective sodium channel.   With respect
to the entry step the most important expansion of the hypothesis
is the discovery of coupled carrier transport of sugars, amino
acids etc. where the passive entry of sodium into the cells drags
along specific organic molecules.   By analogy it has been argued
that even in the cases where sodium enters the cells without being
accompanied by organic molecules (frog skin, toad urinary bladder,
large intestine, collecting ducts of the kidney) the entry step
may be mediated by a sodium carrier.   Very recent experiments
(Fuchs, Hviid Larsen and Lindemann, 1975) indicate, however, that
in the frog skin, at least, the sodium entry has all the typical
properties of an electrodiffusion channel.

    d)  <u>Specific, but passive permeability of the inward-facing
cell membrane</u>.   In the case of the frog skin the assumption is
supported by the observation that the cells swell when the
potassium concentration of the inside bathing solution is increased
at the expense of the non-penetrating sodium ion, granted that a

penetrating anion like chloride is used (McRobbie and Ussing, 1961).

e) <u>The localization of the sodium pump</u>.  It is generally assumed that the sodium pumps are located on the baso-lateral surfaces of the transporting cells.  For multilayered epithelia like the frog skin the assumption has been advanced that coupling between the cells of all layers in the Lowenstein sense (Lowenstein and Cannoe, 1964) might contribute to the sodium transport by allowing all cells of the epithelium to act as one transporting unit (Farquhar and Palade, 1964, Ussing and Windhager, 1964).  Recent work has indicated, however (Voute and Ussing, 1970), that most of the transport is performed by one layer only, viz. the first living cell layer under the cornified cells.  There is also some indication that the endoplasmic reticulum of the transporting cell layer may help in ridding the cells of sodium since the endoplasmic system seems to expand pari passu with the rate of sodium transport (Voute, Møllgard and Ussing, 1975).  The system seems to have openings to the inside, but not the outside bathing solution.  The role of the endoplasmic system in active sodium transport is uncertain at this time.

f) <u>The role of the paracellular pathway</u>.  In epithelia like frog skin, toad urinary bladder, large intestine, salivary ducts and collecting ducts of the kidney, the transporting cells are connected by rather tight seals, and the paracellular pathway seems to play a limited role.  In small intestine, proximal tubules, gall bladder and certain other epithelial structures, the situation is different.  The tight junctions in the latter group of organs have a low electric resistance and allow small organic molecules to pass (for references, see Ussing, Erlej and Lassen, 1974).  Such epithelia cannot elaborate an hypertonic secretion.  The ingenious standing gradient of Diamond and Bossert (1967) was advanced primarily to account for the production of isotonic secretions.  Quite recently there has been voiced some doubt whether the hypothesis in its original version can account for the observed facts (see e.g. Hill, 1975a).  The problem is that with the known figures for the length, width and permeability properties of the paracellular pathways, isotonic secretions cannot be produced.  Hill (1975b) therefore proposes electroosmosis as the device used by the cells to transport water. He can show that it is not physically impossible, but he offers no direct evidence for his hypothesis.  If one were allowed to speculate for a moment one might venture the hypothesis that the endoplasmic reticulum would offer a surface sufficiently large for the production of an isotonic secretion.  Apart from the frog skin system we have, however, no evidence for an involvement of the endoplasmic reticulum in sodium and water transport.

## REFERENCES

Crane, R.K. (1965). Fed. Proc. 24, 1000.

Diamond, J.M. and W.H. Bossers (1967). J. Gen. Physiol. 50, 2061.

Farquhar, M.G. and G.E. Palade (1964). Proc. Mat. Acad. Sci. 51, 569.

Fuchs, W., Hviid Larsen, E., and B. Lindemann (1975). Phlügers Arch. Suppl. 355, nr. 141.

Goldman, D.E. (1943). J. Gen. Physiol, 27, 37.

Hill, A.E. (1975a). Proc. Roy. Soc. Lond. B. 190, 99.

Hill, A.E. (1975b). Proc. Roy. Soc. Lond. B. 190, 115.

Keynes, R.D. (1975). Ciba Foundation Symposium 31 (n.s.) p.191, Elsevier, Amsterdam.

Koefod-Johnsen, V. and H.H. Ussing (1958). Acta Physiol. Scand. 42, 298.

Licthenstein, N.S. and A. Leaf (1965). J. Clin. Invest. 44, 1328.

Loewenstein, W.R. and Y. Kanno (1964). J. Cell biol. 22, 565.

MacRobbie, E. and H.H. Ussing (1961). Acta Physiol. Scand. 53, 348.

Rosenberg, T. (1948). Acta Chem. Scandinav. 2, 14.

Skou, J.C. (1957). Biochim. Biophys. Acta. 23, 394.

Ussing, H.H. (1947). Nature 160, 262.

Ussing, H.H. (1949). Acta Physiol. Scand., 19, 43.

Ussing, H.H. and K. Zerahn (1951). Acta Physiol. Scand. 23, 110.

Ussing, H.H. and E. Windhager (1964). Acta Physiol. Scand. 61, 484.

Ussing, H.H., D. Erlij and U. Lassen (1974). Ann. Rev. Physiol. 36, 17.

Voute, C.L., K. Møllgard, and H.H. Ussing (1975). J. Membrane Biol. 21, 273.

Voute, C.L. and H.H. Ussing (1970). Exp. Cell Res. 62, 375.

DISCUSSION OF LECTURE BY H.H. USSING

Taylor:   Professor Ussing, in your work you use such terms as
'pores', 'channels' and 'gates', and I wonder how you relate these
to what Professor Lucy has been telling us about modern concepts
of membrane structure.

Ussing:   One must assume that the diffusion channels about which
I speak are associated with proteins, because lipids probably
would not have the selectivity and permeability necessary for the
rapid movement of ions across membranes.   I think that the type
of protein which extends right across the membrane might be the
pathway for, say, the sodium channel.   In the exchange diffusion
phenomenon, where one can have equilibration with one side of the
membrane but not with both sides at the same time, I think that
this indicates that there must be some kind of molecule which can
be involved in a sort of 'flip-flop' mechanism.   In the general
model it is not assumed that the proteins which are inside the
inner leaflet can flop over and cross into the outer leaflet.
But that type of mechanism is exactly what we need to explain the
chloride-bicarbonate exchange or the sugar-sodium combined transport.   Therefore I think that eventually we will find selective
proteins which can move from one leaflet to the other.

Ritland:   In cirrhosis of the liver there is said to be retention
of sodium even if the plasma level is very low.   How can this
sodium pump operate in cirrhosis, and how does it fit in with the
blocking effects of diuretics?

Ussing:   Does the retention of sodium occur in the liver cells?

Ritland:   No, in the kidney.

Ussing:   Similar mechanisms to those I have described could occur
in the kidney, and inhibitors of the sodium pump could be present
in cirrhosis.   I would not like to speculate further on that
point.

Case:   I would like to raise the question of the possible
connection between the endoplasmic reticulum and the basal
membrane.   Did you say that you can only show the deposition of
lanthanum inside the cells when a hydrostatic pressure was applied?

<u>Ussing</u>:    In the frog skin preparation we have to use hydrostatic
pressure to obtain deposition of lanthanum.    But with the urinary
bladder of the toad penetration of lanthanum occurs even in the
absence of hydrostatic pressure.

<u>Case</u>:    Are these channels open to more traditional markers of
intracellular space such as ferritin or horse-radish peroxidase?

<u>Ussing</u>:    It is very much a question of size.    In the experiments
I am talking about, lanthanum has approximately the same size as a
sodium ion, so the lanthanum will penetrate barriers which would
not allow such large molecules as proteins to pass through.

<u>Lucy</u>:    With respect to the point raised by Dr. Taylor, there is
some evidence that protein 'band III', which is found in erythrocytes and which goes through the membrane more than once, is
associated with anion transport, particularly chloride.

<u>Altmann</u>:    May I make some comments about the vacuoles of liver
cells which are commonly found in animal and human material.
There is no doubt that they are of pinocytotic origin.    By using
a small degree of hydrostatic pressure these vacuoles can be
readily produced.    Inside the vacuoles one finds fibrin and
other blood constituents, so I have some doubts that the endoplasmic reticulum is always involved in the formation of these
vacuoles.

<u>Ussing</u>:    I agree.    We should approach the results of our experi-
ments with caution.    There is the possibility, but certainly no
proof, that there is a normal pathway between the endoplasmic
reticulum and the lateral space.    On the other hand, in the
experiments you describe both the vacuoles and the endoplasmic
reticulum are greatly expanded, but we cannot tell whether this
expansion is the result of biosynthesis or some sort of transport
effect.

<u>Coleman</u>:    Many of the membrane proteins which are involved in
transport certainly do not seem to have the ability to flip over.
For instance, ouabain only affects transport when added to the
outer face of the membrane, but not when added to the inner
surface.    So if a particular protein is involved in transport
across the membrane one would expect it to flip over when ouabain
is added to either side of the membrane.

<u>Ussing</u>:    That may be so, but in the particular case of sodium
transport the protein involved must traverse the whole membrane.

<u>Coleman</u>:    Yes, but I was suggesting that some molecules may go
through the membrane without any flip-over action being involved.

Ussing:    I agree.

Forker:    Would you care to speculate on what appears to many of
us to be a paradoxical situation in liver cells.  They have very
unusual permeability to relatively large water-soluble molecules,
such as mannitol.  At the same time liver cells are very efficient active transporters of such substances as bile salts, and
presumably of sodium, across the epithelium.  Mannitol, for
example, will be in diffusion equilibrium at all rates of bile
flow in some species and certainly in the dog.  So the liver
cell has very high permeability for mannitol which does not cross
other biological membranes very readily.  Is there any easy way
to reconcile these observations?

Ussing:    There could be many reasons for this, but it would seem
that the liver has a selective transport mechanism for mannitol.

Forker:    But this phenomenon is not restricted to mannitol;
erythritol and other substances behave in the same way as mannitol,
so I cannot see how this can be explained by suggesting that there
is a selective and specific transport system involved.

Ussing:    If the cut-off in the cell membrane is slightly higher
than in other membranes, then this could be the important factor.
The order of magnitude of size of substances being transported is
of major importance.

Taylor:    I think that what is concerning a lot of us here who are
involved in hepatic transport processes is that most of the
classical transport mechanism work has been done with inorganic
or small ions and with relatively small molecules such as glucose.
We are interested in fairly large molecules which are equilibrating in the liver and biliary system in what appears to be a
unique way.  I hope this problem will be resolved in our later
discussions.

# MECHANISM OF TRANSPORT OF INORGANIC IONS INTO BILE

J. Graf and M. Peterlik

Dept. of General and Experimental Pathology

University of Vienna, Austria

## 1. INTRODUCTION

The main driving force of bile secretion is, according to Sperber (1965), the active transport of bile salts into the bile canaliculi. But, although diminished, bile flow and bile secretory pressure are maintained without bile salt secretion (e.g. Boyer and Klatskin 1970) and it has been frequently supposed that inorganic ion transport is responsible for this bile salt independent fraction of bile flow. The following studies were designed to learn of the mechanisms by which inorganic ions are transported into the bile canaliculi. It will be shown, that sodium, potassium, and chloride enter the bile canaliculi at least through two different pathways, their properties indicating a transcellular and a paracellular transport mechanism.

## 2. MATERIAL AND METHODS

Animals: male albino rats, wistar strain, weighing between 180 and 250 g. The liver was isolated (Miller, 1973), weighed, and connected either to an erythrocyte containing perfusion system (A), (Schimassek 1963), or to a non recycling, erythrocyte free system (B), (Scholtz et al. 1969). In both systems two perfusion apparatus were used in order to rapidly shift the flow through the liver from control or isotope ($^{24}$Na, $^{36}$Cl, $^{42}$K) containing solution to another solution of either different osmolarity, or altered ionic composition (equimolar replace-

ment of $Na^+$, $K^+$ or $Cl^-$ by other solutes as indicated in
the text), or without the respective isotope. The control
medium contained (mM):

System A: bovine erythrocytes were washed and suspen-
ded in: NaCl 136.9; KCl 5.9; $MgCl_2$ 0.5; $CaCl_2$ 1.8; $NaHCO_3$
19.0; Glucose 4.44; $NaH_2PO_4$ 1.23; Na-lactate 1.29; Na-
pyruvate 0.09; Microcillin(R) 10 mg/l; bovine serum albumin 25 g/l, giving a final hemoglobin concentration of
100 g/l. pH was monitored and kept between 7.25 and 7.35
by gassing with 95% $O_2$-5% $CO_2$ or 100% $O_2$. Constant flow
rate through the liver was between 0.8 and 1.5 ml/g x min.

System B: NaCl 118.4; KCl 4.75; $CaCl_2$ 2.5; $KH_2PO_4$
1.2; $MgSO_4$ 1.2; $NaHCO_3$ 25.0; Glucose 5.0, gassed with
95% $O_2$-5% $CO_2$. Flow rate between 3 and 4 ml/g x min.

Bile flow rate was determined by measuring the frequency and weight (6.8-7.8 mg) of bile drops leaving the
bile duct canula. Bile secretion pressure was measured by
keeping the canula in vertical position. Volume changes
of bile within the biliary tree were calculated from pressure changes by equaling 1 cm to 0.80 ul (I.D. of the
canula 0.32 mm).

Ion concentrations were determined by flame photo-
metry (Beckman KLiNa), atomic absorption spectrophotometry
(Perkin Elmer Model 403) and by electrometric titration
of chloride according to Ramsey et al. (1955). Osmolari-
ties were measured with a Knauer Osmometer Type M. Protein
concentrations were determined in single bile drops according to Wunderly et al. (1954). Radioactivities were measured in a Philips 4003-𝛾-spectrometer and a Beckman liquid scintillation counter (LS 230).


## 3. RESULTS AND DISCUSSION

Rat livers were perfused for at least 30 minutes with
control solution in order to allow the organ to recover
from its anaerobic alteration during the preparation
(Schimassek 1963, Graf et al. 1972) and to be concerned
with bile formation mainly independent of bile salts,
which rapidly decrease in bile to below 5% of in vivo
concentrations after interruption of the enterohepatic
circulation (Boyer and Klatskin 1970, Percy-Robb and Boyd
1970, unpublished observations). Within this time bile
flow rate stabilized, attaining a value of 0.774 $\pm$ 0.130
(SD) mg bile $g_{liver}^{-1}$ $min^{-1}$. Biliary ion concentrations
became close to perfusate values (compare table 1), and

bile was isotonic to perfusate, as it is in vivo (Brauer
1959, 1965; Koss 1964). Under control conditions mean
bile secretion pressure of the preparation was $18.95 \pm$
2.95 (SD) cm bile.

Bile ducts may be regarded as dead space with respect
to the localization of ion transport into bile on the
basis of the following experiment: during continuous
collection of bile a pulse of $^{24}$Na, $^{36}$Cl and sulphobromophthalein was infused into the portal vein canula. The
isotopes and the concentrated dye appeared simultaneously
in the bile duct canula after the washout of a biliary
space of 2.3 ul/g$_{liver}$, which corresponds to the capacity
of the biliary tree (Barber-Riley 1965; Häcki and Paumgartner 1973). This indicates that the ions enter the
lumen of the biliary tree at the site of the canaliculus
and not through the walls of the bile ducts. This is in
agreement with the results of erythritol clearence measurements (Boyer 1971) which showed that bile of the isolated rat liver is canalicular in origin and not markedly
modified during its passage through the bile ducts.

### 3.1. Effects of changes of the osmolarity of the perfusion medium on bile formation

Employing the perfusion system A the osmolarity of
the perfusate passing through the liver was suddenly
changed by reduction or increase of the concentration of
NaCl (Fig. 1). Reduction of NaCl caused a sudden and
transient increase of bile flow rate, until bile attained
the osmolarity of the perfusate. A symmetrical transient
reduction of bile flow occurred when the osmolarity of the
perfusate was increased by shifting back to the control
solution. The additional amount of bile flow produced by
a 1 mosmolar reduction of perfusate osmolarity was $24.8 \pm$
8.4 (SD) nl/g(liver). Regarding the total surplus of bile
flow ($\Delta V$) during its transient increase as consequence of
water flow according to the osmotic gradient from perfusate to bile ($C_1 = 0.295$ osmolar to $C_2 = 0.340$ osmolar, in
figure 1) the volume of bile (V) which is diluted by this
water flow was calculated by $C_1( V + \Delta V) = C_2 V$. The obtained value ($8.4 \pm 3.0$ µl/g(liver) may be a slight underestimate of the capacity of the bile canaliculi because
of movement of solutes in the reverse direction of water
flow (reflexion factor $\sigma$ ($= \Delta P/RT\Delta C_s$) $< 1$).

Measuring bile secretion pressure during changes of
the osmolarity ($\Delta [NaCl]$ ) of the perfusion medium showed,
that a transient increase of pressure occured when the

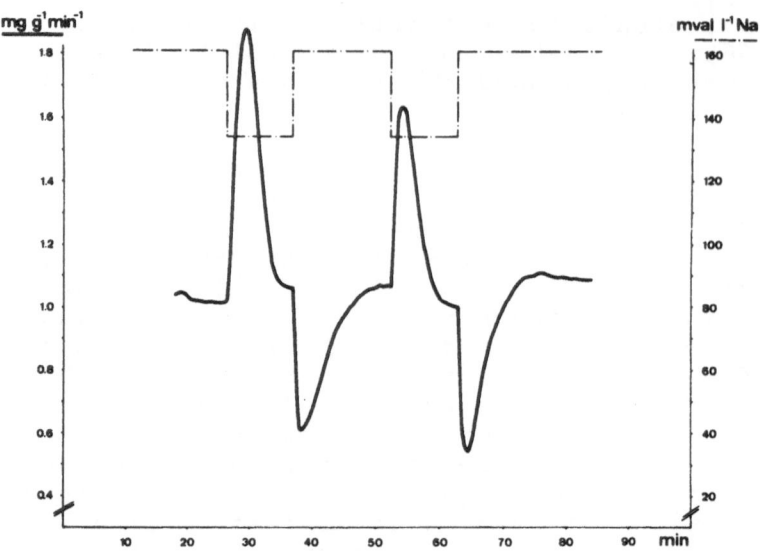

Figure 1: Effects of changes of the osmolarity of the perfusion medium (Δ [NaCl] = 22.5 mM) on bile secretion.

osmolarity of the perfusion medium was reduced and, vice
versa, a transient reduction of pressure was seen when
the osmolarity was increased. The rise of the bile column
within the canula may be regarded as well as an increase
of the volume of bile within the biliary tree, and a calculation of these volume changes showed, that there was a
linear relation between the maximal transient change of
bile volume and the applied change of the perfusate osmolarity of 0.70 ± 0.17 (SD) nl/g(liver)/mM (NaCl) (Fig. 7).

This value is very low compared to the osmotically
induced increase of bile flow rate. A simple explanation
of this discrepancy would be a drastical increase of the
solute permeability between bile and perfusate by the
applied hydrostatic pressure (decrease of $\sigma_i$). This could
be shown indeed by experiments, in which $^{14}$C-cholic acid
uptake from the perfusate and secretion of the conjugated
$^{14}$C-taurocholic acid into bile was measured: as soon as
bile flow ceased by measuring the bile secretion pressure,
regurgitation of $^{14}$C-taurocholic acid into the perfusate
occured, quantitatively equal to the amount secreted into
bile under control conditions. This effect was immediately
reversible after allowing free bile flow (Graf 1975a).
These and the above observations show that a pathway
exists between perfusate and bile which becomes extremely
leaky by application of hydrostatic pressure. This pathway

which has apparently symmetric permeability properties may
be regarded tentatively as paracellular. In the following
experiments the ion transport through this pathway and
through the liver cells was studied.


## 3.2. Effects of changes of the ionic composition of the perfusion medium on bile formation

Bile flow rate showed two characteristic variations
when the ionic composition of the perfusion medium was
suddenly changed. One was an initial steep change of bile
flow rate and then bile flow attained, after 10 to 20 minutes, a stable value, which was different from that during perfusion with the control solution. The slope of the
transient changes was very similar to that seen by changes
of the osmolarity of the perfusate (compare Fig. 1, 2, 3).
A transient increase of bile flow rate was observed when
NaCl was replaced in the perfusion medium by isotonic concentrations of LiCl or $NaNO_3$ (Fig. 2). A transient reduction of bile flow occured after substitution of NaCl by
KCl, Tris(hydroxymethyl)aminomethane-Cl, choline-Cl
(Fig. 3), Na-benzenesulfonate, Na-acetylglycinate, Na-
acetate, $Na_2SO_4$ or sucrose. The amplitude of these changes
was related to the amount of NaCl which has been replaced,
but it also depended on the kind of the substituting ion.
In analogy to the osmotic bile flow changes (3.1.) we may
assume, that these transient effects on bile flow reflect
permeability properties of a paracellular pathway between
bile and perfusate, allowing the passage of sodium, chloride and some substituting ions in both directions but at
different rates. In this case a flow of water would occur
between bile and perfusate when the two fluids have different ionic composition, e.g. bile flow increases when
$NaNO_3$ (+water) moves more rapidly into the canaliculi than
NaCl (+water) moves out of them into the perfusate (Fig.2)
or the bile volume decreases when NaCl (+water) leaves
the canaliculi more rapidly than choline-Cl (+water) enters them. The permeability of such a paracellular pathway
should have symmetrical properties. It could be shown,
that after a time, during which the ion composition of
bile has approached the values of the perfusate, e.g.
after the fast penetrating $NO_3^-$ or the slow penetrating
choline$^+$ have nearly the same concentrations in both
fluids (see below), shifting back to control perfusion
resulted in an transient decrease of bile flow when $NO_3^-$
was the substituting ion for $Cl^-$, or a transient increase
when choline$^+$ was the substituting ion for $Na^+$. On basis
of these findings the following permeability sequence of
this pathway could be estimated: $Li^+ \gtrsim Na^+ > K^+$, $Tris^+ >$ cho-
line$^+$ ; $NO_3^- > Cl^- >$ acetate$^-$, benzenesulfonate$^-$, acetyl-

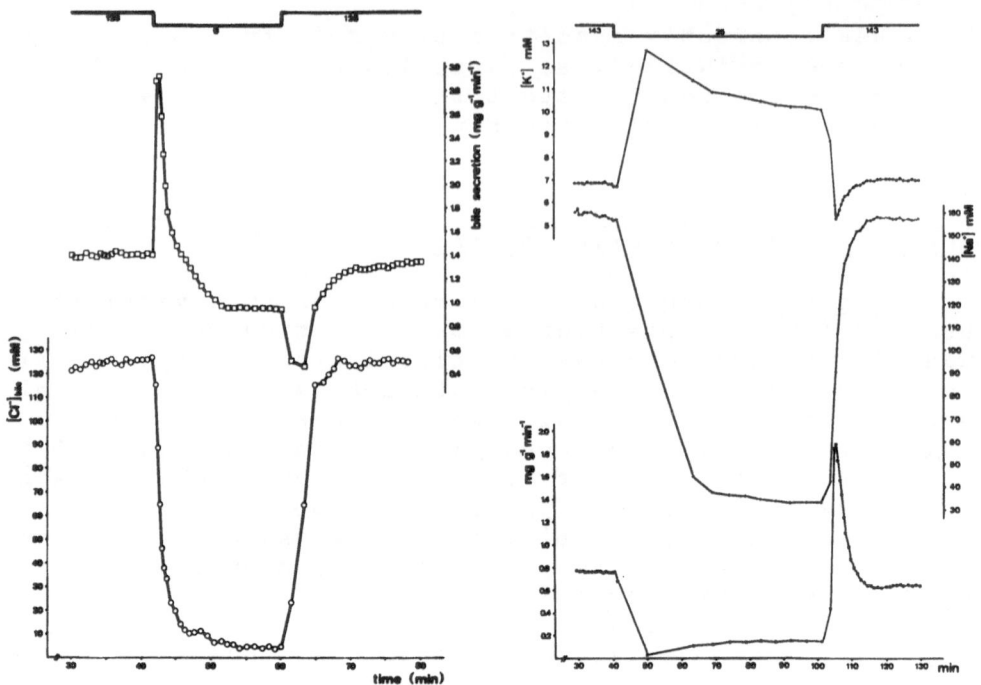

Figure 2 (left): Effect of replacement of Cl⁻ in the perfusion medium by $NO_3^-$ on bile flow (upper trace) and
biliary chloride concentration (lower trace).
Figure 3 (right): Effect of replacement of Na⁺ by choline⁺
on bile flow (lower trace), biliary potassium- (upper
trace) and sodium-concentration (middle).


glycinate⁻ > SO4⁻ ; NaCl > sucrose. Equimolar replacement
of one ion on the right in the sequence by one more left
caused a transient increase of bile flow and, vice versa,
bile flow decreased transiently by replacement from left
to right.

     After these transient changes bile flow attained a
stable value (Fig. 2 and 3) which was again dependent on
both, the amount of  NaCl  that has been replaced and on
the kind of the substituting ion. Fig. 4 shows a plot of
bile flow rate (% of value in control solution) against
the reduction of [Na⁺] and/or [Cl⁻] in the perfusion medium by the respective ions or sucrose (System A). Within
the measured range the relation between  NaCl -reduction
and decrease of bile flow was fairly linear for sucrose,
choline-Cl and KCl as substituents, the other slopes represent mean values, although the individual values may

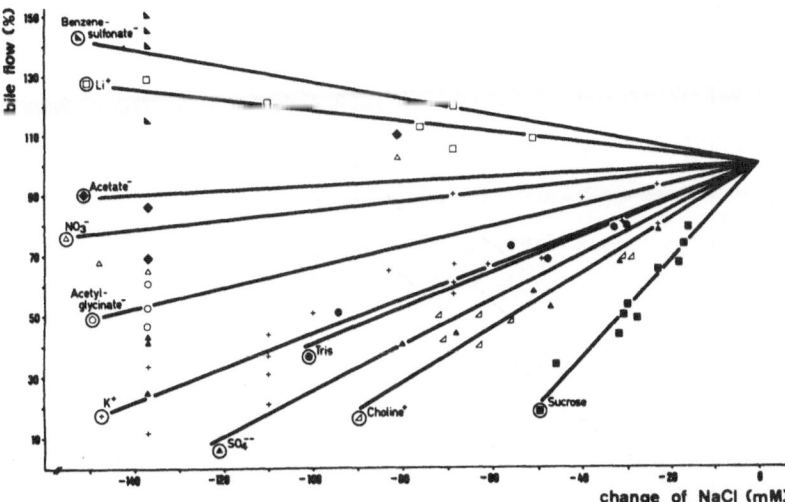

Figure 4: Bile flow rate (% of value during perfusion with
the control solution) after reduction of [NaCl] by the
substituting solutes indicated.

differ from linearity, suggested by the regression lines.
During perfusion with solutions containing $Li^+$, $Tris^+$ or
the organic anions bile flow rate was not entirely stable,
but slowly declined. The values shown are maximum values
measured 10 to 20 minutes after application of the respective solutions. We may assume that these changed bile flow
rates during perfusion with an altered solution result
from interaction of a cellular ion transport mechanism and
a paracellular ion exchange process.

Complete replacement of ions was studied in erythrocyte free perfusions in order to see, whether one of the
investigated ions is essential in maintaining bile secretion. Omission of chloride (replacement by $NO_3^-$ or acetate)
did not abolish bile secretion (Fig. 2). This indicates
that an active transport of chloride through the cells is
not necessary to maintain secretion. Omission of sodium
from the perfusate abolished bile secretion completely
(replacement with choline and Tris). Since it could be
shown, that the substituting ions are able to enter the
bile canaliculus (see below), this observation indicates,
that active (cellular) transport of sodium may be involved
in bile formation. Wether $Li^+$ may substitute for $Na^+$ in
this transport remains unclear (comp. Fig. 4). Shifting
from control to a $K^+$-free medium (replacement by $Na^+$)

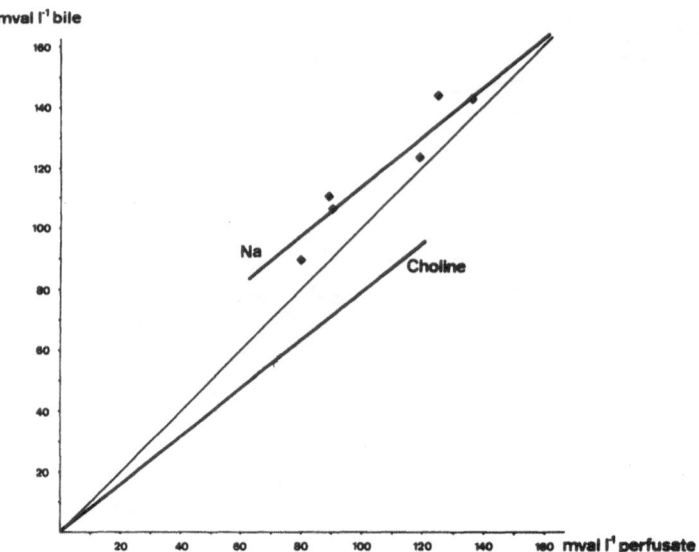

Figure 5: Plot of ion concentration in bile against the respective concentration in perfusate ( :Na$^+$, :choline$^+$) of 12 experiments where sodium was replaced by choline in the perfusion medium ([Na$^+$] + [choline$^+$] = 158.5 mM)

resulted in a small transient increase of bile flow but then it gradually declined. After one hour the flow was reduced to approximately 50% of the control value. By readmission of potassium an initial rapid stimulation of bile secretion was followed by a second phase of gradual recovery to the control value. These effects are related to metabolic changes and activation of sodium pumping as discussed elsewhere (Graf 1975 b).

    Biliary ion concentrations were measured in similar substitution experiments in order to see, whether ions can be transported into bile against a concentration gradient. After a delay, which corresponded to the washout of the dead space of the biliary tree the concentration of that ion which has been replaced in the perfusion medium rapidly fell and the substituting ion appeared in bile, maintaining isotonicity (comp. Fig. 2 and 3). After bile flow had stabilized, following the transitory change, no significant concentration difference between bile and perfusate could be measured in experiments where chloride has been replaced (by $NO_3^-$, acetate, benzenesulfonate). In chloride free perfusions[3](comp. Fig. 2) the chloride concentration in bile decreased towards zero. Sodium concentrations

showed comparable rapid changes in the respective substitution experiments, but it was consistently found, that
the concentration in bile remained finally above the perfusate value. Correspondingly the concentration of the
substituting ion (e.g. $^3$H-choline) remained below the perfusate value (Fig. 5). This indicates that sodium can be
transported into bile against a small concentration gradient. The same was found for potassium which has, even
under control conditions, a higher concentration in bile
than in the perfusion medium. The potassium concentration
also varied when bile flow changed following alterations
of the concentrations of sodium or chloride in the perfusion medium: the concentration decreased when a transient
increase of bile flow was produced by the substitution
experiment, or increased, when the effect was a transient
decrease of bile flow rate (comp. Fig. 3). After shifting
the perfusion from control solution to a potassium free
medium (system B) the potassium concentration in bile
rapidly fell to 1.2 mM but then declined only very slowly,
maintaining an approximate concentration gradient of:
effluent perfusate:bile = 1:10.

The biliary protein secretion remained fairly unchanged in the substitution experiments described. The
biliary protein concentration rose when bile flow rate
was reduced (by replacement of 68.5 mM NaCl by choline-Cl
or KCl), and returned to the control value after shifting
back to the control solution. These effects occurred again
after a delay which corresponded to the washout of the
dead space of the biliary tree. In the choline experiments
a reduction of the bile flow rate by 42.0 $\pm$ 10.3 % corresponded to an increase of biliary protein concentration
from 0.52 $\pm$ 0.07 to 0.92 $\pm$ 0.23 $\mu$g/mg bile. In the potassium experiments bile flow decreased by 30.2 $\pm$ 18.2 % and
protein concentration rose from 0.56 $\pm$ 0.19 to 1.30 $\pm$ 0.25
$\mu$g/mg. Biliary protein output remained fairly constant
(0.4-0.5 $\mu$g/g(liver)/min, control and choline) or slightly
increased (potassium). Beside an unimpaired protein secretion, the delay of changes of the protein concentration
shows again that the observed changes of bile flow rate
can be ascribed to processes occurring at the site of the
bile canaliculus.

Bile secretion pressure varied in accordance to the
transient changes of bile flow rate, produced by replacement of NaCl in the perfusion medium. A transient increase
of bile flow corresponded to a transient increase of pressure, and a reduction of bile flow to a decrease. (By substitution of NaCl with LiCl no significant pressure changes could be observed, by replacement with KCl the expected decrease was preceeded by a short increase, probably

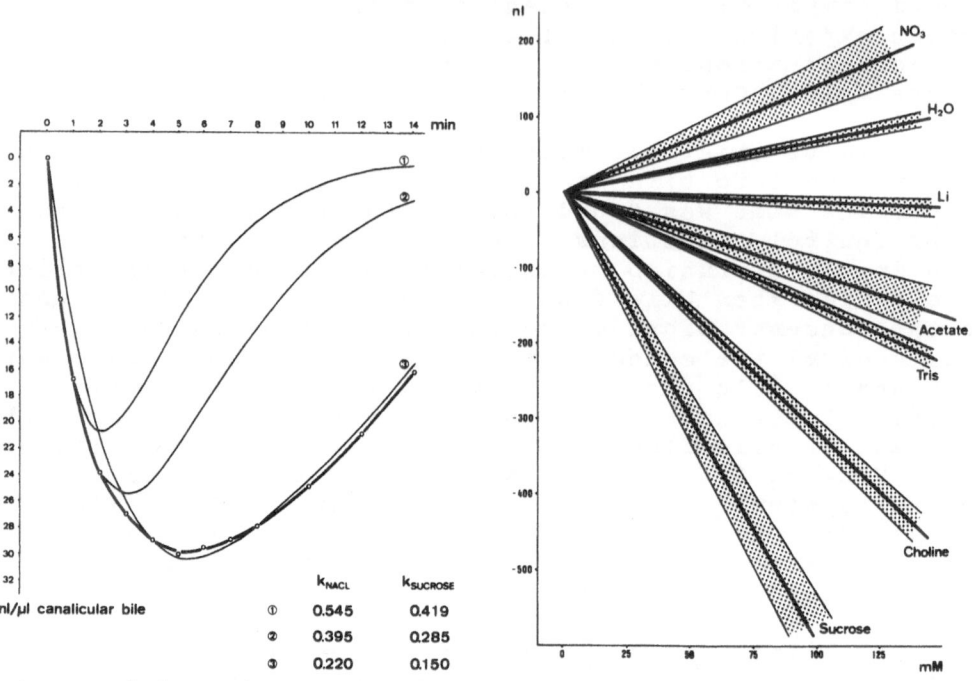

Figure 6 (left): Change of the canalicular bile volume
after replacement of NaCl (37 mM) by sucrose in the perfusion medium, evaluated from the measured pressure changes. The thin lines (1-3) represent theoretical volume
changes, calculated from the rate constants (k, min$^{-1}$)
shown. Compare text.
Figure 7 (right): Correlation of maximal biliary volume
changes, occurring after a shift from control perfusion
to a solution in which different amounts of NaCl (mM)
have been replaced by isotonic concentrations of NaNO$_3$,
LiCl, Na-acetate, Tris-Cl, choline-Cl or sucrose, or to
a solution in which NaCl was reduced without substitution (H$_2$O). Mean slopes $\pm$ SEM.


by K$^+$-induced contraction of the bile ducts). Converting
the measured pressure changes into volume changes of bile
within the biliary tree (see 3.1.) (Fig. 6) revealed a
linear (0.99 > r > 0.92) relation between the change of bile
volume (nl/g liver) and the amount of NaCl reduction by
substitution (Fig. 7). For the individual substituting
solutes the calculated slopes were (nl/g liver/1 mM reduction of NaCl $\pm$ SD): Tris-Cl: -1.50 $\pm$ 0.15; choline-Cl:
-3.16 $\pm$ 0.45; sucrose: -5.95 $\pm$ 1.67; NaNO$_3$: +1.42 $\pm$ 0.85;
Na-acetate: -1.07 $\pm$ 0.33; Na-benzenesulfonate: -1.08 $\pm$

0.29. As already discussed, these transient changes of
bile volume are regarded to be the consequence of solute
and water transport between bile and perfusate according
to their respective concentration gradient, in both directions but at different rates. E.g.: NaCl (+water) leaves
the canalicular lumen more rapidly towards the perfusate
(vascular lumen), than sucrose (+water) moves into the
canalicular lumen, after replacement of NaCl in the perfusion medium by sucrose. On the basis of a canalicular
volume ($V_o$) of 8.4 $\mu$l/g(liver) the rate constants of efflux ($k_1$) (e.g. NaCl) and influx ($k_2$) (e.g. sucrose) according to a symmetric concentration difference of the
respective solutes ($\Delta$C) may be roughly estimated from the
relative change of bile volume ( $V_t/V_o$ ) and the sum of
molar concentrations in bile and perfusate (C) by
$$V_t/V_o = \Delta C \left[\exp(-k_1 t) + 1 - \exp(-k_2 t)\right]/C + \left[C - \Delta C\right]/C.$$
The fit of calculated to measured volume changes is shown
for an experiment where 37 mM NaCl has been replaced by
sucrose (Fig. 6). The calculated changes (lines 1-3) result from pairs of rate constants for NaCl-efflux and
sucrose-influx as indicated. Curves fitting to the maximal
volume changes of other substitution experiments revealed
the mean rate constants k ($min^{-1}$): NaCl: 0.231; Tris-Cl:
0.175; choline-Cl: 0.168; sucrose: 0.147; $NaNO_3$: 0.248.
The reverse changes of the biliary volume occurred, when
the perfusion was shifted back to the control medium.
These changes could be described by the above rate constants as well. E.g.: in experiments where NaCl has been
replaced by sucrose and where the concentration of sucrose
in bile has become close to the concentration of the perfusion medium (measured by $^3$H-sucrose), a transient increase of bile volume was observed, when the perfusion was
shifted back to the control medium. In this case, according to the model, the influx of NaCl into the canaliculi
$-\Delta C$ $(1-\exp(-k_2 t))-$ would proceed more rapidly than the
efflux of sucrose into the perfusate $-\Delta C$ $\exp(-k_1 t)-$
($k_2 > k_1$) and the sum of ions in bile would transiently
increase, explaining the observed increase of bile volume
by equilibration of water to maintain isotonicity. Again
the symmetry of the observed changes is consistent with
the hypothesis, that this transport occurs through a paracellular pathway having the relative permeabilities of
$Na^+ > Tris^+ > choline^+$; $NO_3^- > Cl > acetate$; $NaCl > sucrose$
(compare Fig. 7).

Results of a rather indirect approach were in accordance with this hypothesis: in analogy to measurements of
biionic diffusion potentials in the gall bladder (Wright
and Diamond 1968, Machen and Diamond 1972) variations of
a potential were recorded, measured between 3M-KCl-agar-

bridges inserted into the portal vein and bile duct canula
respectively. By replacement of NaCl (103 mM) in the perfusion medium (system B) by choline-Cl, KCl, Tris-Cl or
sucrose a decrease of the potential of the bile duct lumen
(-1.0 mV, -0.8 mV, -0.8 mV,-0.65 mV respectively, SD =0.2)
was observed, having a time course similar to the transient changes of bile flow or bile pressure, measured in
comparable experiments. The bile duct lumen became more
positive by an equal amount, when the perfusion was shifted back to the control medium. Although these potentials
agree with the proposed relative permeabilities of Na〉K,
Tris〉choline and also Na〉Cl, their amplitude was too
small to exclude errors ( a potential difference arising
at the site of the canaliculus may be severely attenuated
along the bile ducts).

In summary the hitherto presented data revealed the
information, that a pathway exists between the vascular
lumen and the bile canaliculus, which allows rapid, but
selective passage of ions in both directions. Beside support of the view, that this pathway is located between the
liver cells (paracellular) the following isotope flux measurements allowed an evaluation of the parallel, cellular
component of ion transport into bile.

### 3.3. The pattern of isotope efflux into perfusion medium and bile from livers, preloaded with radioactive sodium, potassium or chloride.

Perfused rat livers (system A) were loaded with $^{22}$Na
(or $^{24}$Na), $^{42}$K or $^{36}$Cl during one hour and the efflux of
radioactivity into the perfusion medium and bile was measured during perfusion with an inactive solution for the
following 30 minutes (Dietmaier et al. 1974). After the
rapid washout of the extracellular space (approx. 25 % of
liver volume), the rate constants and specific activities
of the further exponential loss of radioactivity into the
perfusion medium were used to estimate the intracellular
ion concentration and ion flux through the sinusoidal liver cell membrane (compare: Claret and Mazet 1972), using
a value of 2440 $cm^2/cm^3$ liver (Weibel et al. 1969) and
assuming steady state conditions. The mean values obtained
are summarized in table 1. Since $Cl^-$ was found to be passively distributed (Claret and Mazet 1972) the liver cell
membrane potential could be calculated by $E_m = E_{Cl} =
(RT/F) \ln ( [Cl^-]_o / [Cl^-]_i ) = - 40.1$ mV. Applying the con-
stant field assumption (Hodgkin and Katz 1949) the membrane permeability (P) was calculated from flux data, membrane potential and the respective ion concentrations.

Table 1:

Ion transport   a) between liver cells and perfusate,
                b) from liver cells to bile,
                c) from perfusate to bile.


|  |  | $Na^+$ | $K^+$ | $Cl^-$ |
|---|---|---|---|---|
| | 1. Extracellular (perfusate) concentration (mM) | | | |
| | | 158.5 | 5.9 | 147.4 |
| | 2. Intracellular concentration (mM) | | | |
| | | 16.7 | 125 | 33.0 |
| | 3. Biliary concentration | | | |
| | | 162 | 6.7 | 145 |
| a | 4. Rate constant ($min^{-1}$) | | | |
| | | 0.098 | 0.016 | 0.164 |
| | 5. Flux ($x10^{-6}$ mole $g^{-1}$ $min^{-1}$) | | | |
| | | 1.17 | 1.50 | 3.70 |
| | 6. Flux ($x10^{-12}$ mole $cm^{-2}$ $sec^{-1}$) | | | |
| | | 8.38 | 10.3 | 27.4 |
| | 7. Equilibrium potential (mV) | | | |
| | | +60.3 | -81.8 | -40.1 |
| | 8. Permeability ($x10^{-8}$ cm $sec^{-1}$) | | | |
| | | 2.7 | 19.0 | 43.0 |
| b | 9. Rate constant ($min^{-1}$) | | | |
| | | 0.105 | 0.016 | 0.151 |
| | 10. Flux ($x10^{-9}$ mole $g^{-1}$ $min^{-1}$) | | | |
| | | 6.1 | 1.3 | 30.4 |
| c | 11. Rate constant ($min^{-1}$) | | | |
| | | 1.007 | 0.608 | 0.496 |
| | 12. Flux ($x10^{-9}$ mole $g^{-1}$ $min^{-1}$) | | | |
| | | 120 | 3.9 | 82 |


$P_{Na}/P_K$ was 0.144, revealing a membrane potential of -39.8 mV by use of the abbreviated form of the Goldman equation (Hodgkin 1958). Apparent discrepancies to the values obtained by Claret and Mazet (1972) may be explained by the different perfusion methods used.

After one hour perfusion with the radioactive media the specific activities of $Na^+$ and $Cl^-$ were equal in perfusion medium and bile. The exponential decrease of radioactivity in bile during perfusion with the non-radioactive medium showed two components (Fig. 8). After the washout of the dead space of the biliary tree the radioactivity in bile initially rapidly decreased, indicating ready entry of non-radioactive ions from the vascular lumen into

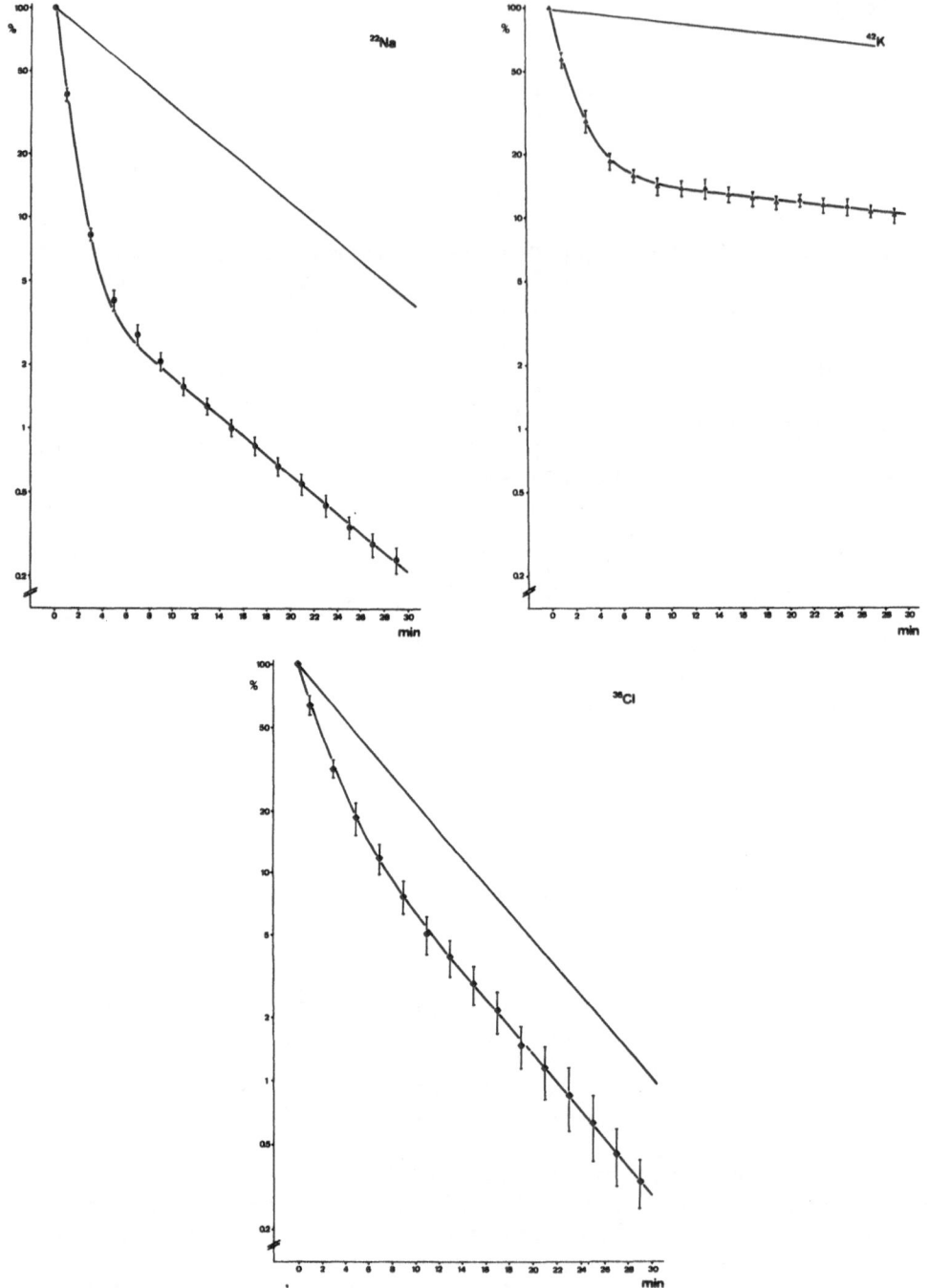

Figure 8: Efflux pattern of $^{22}$Na(left), $^{42}$K(right) and $^{36}$Cl(below) in bile ($\%=A_t/A_o$) compared to the calculated decrease of intracellular specific radioactivity.

the bile canaliculus. The second component was parallel
to the exponential decrease of radioactivity in the perfusion medium, and therefore also parallel to the calculated decrease of intracellular specific activity
(straight lines in figure 8), indicating that a certain
amount of the respective ions derives from the liver cells.
Accordingly it has to be assumed, that ions enter the
biliary lumen at the site of the canaliculus by transport
through the liver cells (slow component) and through a
second pathway, which may be located at the site of leaky
junctions between the liver cells (fast component). To
obtain a quantitative picture the efflux data were submitted to regression analysis and after extrapolation to
time zero the two components of decrease of radioactivity
($A_t$) with time could be described by:
$100\, A_t/A_0 = a\, \exp(-k_1 t) + b\, \exp(-k_2 t)$, where a and b are
the percentual fractions of ion transport into bile by the
cellular and paracellular component respectively. The
corresponding rate constants are shown in table 1, b and
c respectively. The values for potassium were obtained
after making correction for the incomplete equilibration
of specific activities during the loading period. The
fraction of the cellular component, contributing to the
total biliary output of $Na^+$, $K^+$ and $Cl^-$ (4.9%, 25.6 % and
27.1% respectively), is small compared to the amount attributed by the paracellular component. The respective
calculated fluxes from cells to bile and from perfusate
to bile are given in table 1, b and c. We must realize
that these values represent the contribution of the two
transport processes to the final biliary ion output. They
may result from a sum of processes going on at the canalicular level, namely active and passive ion transport
through the canalicular cell membrane and ion transport
or exchange between the vascular and canalicular lumen
through the intercellular space and the "tight" junctions.
The existence of this latter pathway, which has apparently
high, symmetric, but selective permeability properties
(compare the rate constants and 3.2.), makes it likely to
assume that an ionic species, which has been transported
through the liver cells into the canalicular lumen, undergoes exchange with the extracellular space along its
passage through the entire length of the canaliculus.
This implies that only a small fraction of the ions primarily transported through the cells into the canaliculus
appears finally in the effluent bile, the remainder joi-
ning in through the paracellular pathway.

## 4. CONCLUSION

A series of indirect approaches to the problem of inorganic ion transport into bile at the level of the canaliculus was presented. The obtained data are consistent with the existence of a transcellular and paracellular pathway, both having selective but entirely different transport properties. Some data indicated that active transport of sodium may play a role in maintaining bile secretion.

Acknowledgement: This work was supported by the Austrian Fonds zur Förderung der wissenschaftlichen Forschung, Proj. Nr. 2191.

## References

Barber-Riley,G.1965.In:W.Taylor: The Biliary System.
      p 89. Blackwell.
Boyer,J.L.1971.Am.J.Physiol.221,1156
Boyer,J.L.,Klatskin,G.197o.Gastroenterology 59,853
Brauer,R.W.1959.J.Amer.Med.Ass.169,1462
Brauer,R.W.1965.In:W.Taylor:The Biliary System.p 543.
      Blackwell
Claret,M.,Mazet,J.L.1972.J.Physiol.223,279
Dietmaier,A.,Gasser,R.,Graf,J.,Peterlik,M.1974.Digestion
      1o,25
Graf.J.1975.Digestion,in press,abstract,1oth EASL-Meeting
Graf.J.1975.Gastroenterology,in preparation
Graf.J.,Kaschnitz,R.,Peterlik,M.1972.Res.exp.Med.157,12
Häcki,W.,Paumgartner,G.1973.Experientia 29,1o91
Hodgkin,A.L.1958.Proc.Roy.Soc.B.148,1
Hodgkin,A.L.,Katz,B.1949.J.Physiol.1o8,37
Koss.F.W.1964.Arzneimittelforsch.14,69o
Machen,T.E.,Diamond,J.M.1972.J.Membrane Biol.8,63
Miller,L.L.1973.In:I.Bartosek,A.Guaitani,L.L.Miller:Iso-
      lated Liver Perfusion andIts Applications.Raven.N.Y.
Percy-Robb,I.W.,Boyd,G.S.197o.Biochem.J.118,519
Ramsey,J.A.,Brown,R.H.J.,Croghan,P.C.1955.J.exp.Biol32,822
Schimassek,H.1963.Biochem.Zschr.336,46o
Scholz,R.,Thurman,R.G.,Williamson,J.R.,Chance,B.,Bücher,
      Th.1969.J.Biol.Chem.244,2317
Sperber,I.1965.In:W.Taylor:The Biliary System.p457.
Weibel,E.R.,Stäubli,W.,Gnägi,H.R.,Hess,F.A.1969.J.Cell
      Biol.42,68
Wright,E.M.,Diamond,J.M.1968.Biochim.Biophys.Acta 163,57
Wunderly,Ch.,Steiger,R.,Höhringer,H.R.1954.Experientia
      1o,432

DISCUSSION OF COMMENTARY BY J. GRAF

Bradley: If I understand it correctly, your model is consistent with the idea that bile salts are secreted as bile acids, and that sodium exchanges with hydrogen ion in the canaliculus so the bile being secreted is highly acid. Is that right?

Graf: No.

Bradley: But you said that the sodium coming from the cells is such a small percentage of the total sodium in the bile, and that a special fraction of that is associated with bile acid.

Graf: That is so. However, I should mention that all these experiments are done after the liver has been perfused for at least 30 minutes, so the bile salt concentration in the bile is only about 10 per cent of that of normal bile. So here we are concerned essentially with bile salt independent bile secretion.

Bradley: There is another thing that puzzles me. Do you conceive of this movement from the canaliculus of water and salt as an active process that depends upon the quantity of bile present in the canaliculus? You spoke of the decrease in bile flow in terms of back movement of water and salt rather than because of reduction in bile secretion.

Graf: That is related to the volume changes we observe in these pressure experiments.

Bradley: Yes, but this takes place over a long period of time, about 10 to 20 minutes. If this is so, I cannot quite see the volumetric relationships involved.

Graf: I do not know the mechanism by which the substituting ions enter the canaliculus. A slow transport across the liver cells may be involved. For several reasons I would like to suggest that there is some form of vesicular transport through the cells. If this occurred, substituting ions would enter the canaliculus very slowly until there was equal concentration in the bile and the perfusion medium. During this long period, there would be efflux from bile to perfusion medium just as long as there were different concentrations of solutes on both sides.

There are some other points I should mention.    I think that
exchange takes place between the ions in the canaliculus and ions
in the extracellular space.    However, since I cannot measure the
potential within the canaliculus, I cannot calculate how much
active transport takes place within the canaliculus.    The sodium
concentration in bile can be higher than that in the perfusion
medium, which indicates that there is active transport going on.
Also, one can activate the Na/K-ATPase by perfusing the liver with
a potassium-free medium.    During this time, the liver takes up
sodium, but when potassium is added to the perfusion medium bile
flow rapidly increases.    There is indirect evidence that active
sodium transport is involved here, but we have no direct evidence
that there is a sodium pump within the bile canaliculus.

# BIOCHEMICAL STUDIES ON BILE SECRETION

T.F.Slater and M.N.Eakins

Department of Biochemistry
Brunel University
Uxbridge, Middlesex, U.K.

Bile is a complex aqueous fluid produced by the hepatic
parenchymal cells;  the flow rate and composition varies widely
from one species to another.  The major constituents of bile are
water, bile salts and pigments, cholesterol, phospholipids and
inorganic electrolytes.  A mechanism proposed for the secretion of
bile must not only explain the presence in bile of normal constituents, but must also account for the capacity of the biliary system
to excrete and in many cases to concentrate organic anions and
cations with widely  differing physicochemical characteristics.
Furthermore, the overall production of bile is not confined to one
site:  the process begins with some substances that subsequently
appear in the bile (e.g. bilirubin; xenobiotic substances) crossing
the plasma membrane of the parenchymal cell at the sinusoidal aspect;
enzymes present in the endoplasmic reticulum metabolise and conjugate many of these compounds.  Other enzymes conjugate primary
or secondary bile acids with glycine or taurine, while bilirubin
is conjugated, for example, with glucuronide or sulphate.  These
biotransformed compounds must then pass from the endoplasmic
reticulum to the  canalicular site.  Their route is uncertain, but
it has been suggested that it may involve the Golgi apparatus. The
mechanism by which the biliary constituents go to the small
specialisation of the plasma membrane that forms the canaliculus is
unknown.  The production of bile is achieved primarily at the
canalicular site by passage of the components across the membrane
and into the  canalicular lumen.  This fluid may then be modified
as it passes along the bile ductules and ducts and it is not until
it reaches the common bile duct that the fluid is usually sampled
for assay.  Brauer and his co-workers have shown using the isolated
perfused rat liver technique that the driving force for bile
secretion is not the hydrostatic pressure of the blood since bile

can be secreted at a pressure exceeding the perfusion pressure
(Brauer et al.,1954).  Other possible mechanisms are the active
transport of one or more of the biliary constituents or the discharge of 'prepacked' vacuoles into the canaliculus.  Although
water is  the predominent component of bile, there is no evidence
to suggest that water is actively transported in the liver or any
other mammalian cell.  However, water may be moved by an osmotic
gradient  created by the active transport of a solute into a confined region;  such a system would require a large surface area
within a lumen which had one of its ends sealed.  The structure of
the bile canaliculus with the associated numerous microvilli is
consistent with the latter concept.  Sperber (1959; 1965) first
suggested that the active transport of  bile salts into the
canalicular lumen provided a local osmotic  force which caused the
passive transfer of water and electrolytes, thus promoting flow.
This theory has been supported by data indicating a linear relationship between bile flow  and bile salt excretion in the dog (Preisig
et al.,1962), rat (Boyer and Klatskin,1970) and man (Scherstén et
al.,1971).  The demonstration that  taurocholate has a transport
maximum, 357 ±10 $n$mol/min per g of rat liver (Paumgartner et al.,
1974), supports the concept of active transport of bile acids.
More recently evidence has been presented to suggest that the
secretion of bile salts is not the only determinent of bile flow.
A "bile salt-independent" fraction has been described in the rabbit
(Erlinger et al.,1970), rat (Berthelot et al.,1970;  Boyer and
Klatskin,1970) and in man (Boyer and Bloomer,1974).  The exact
nature of this fraction is unclear but Erlinger et al.(1970) have
suggested that sodium may be actively transported across the canalicular membrane and that this process is linked to $Na^+$-$K^+$-ATPase
present in the canalicular membrane.

    Thus both systems, the bile salt-dependent and the bile salt-
independent systems, probably involve the active transport of an
associated component.  With such systems there must be a supply of
"metabolic energy" to drive the active transport process forward.
Experiments with the isolated perfused rat liver and using a variety
of metabolic inhibitors have demonstrated that bile secretion is
dependent upon cellular respiration:  the addition of potassium
cyanide to the perfusate inhibits bile flow (Bizard 1965;
Vanlerenberghe et al.,1970);  inhibitors of glycolysis (e.g.  mono-
iodoacetic acid) and of phosphorylation (e.g. phloridzin) also
inhibit bile flow (Bizard,1965;  Vanlerenberghe et al.,1970) as does
hypothermia (Vanlerenberghe,1965).  From these data and by analogy
with other energy-requiring reactions within the liver cell, it seems
likely that bile  secretion requires the participation of ATP in
the enzyme reactions controlling the transfer of material from  the
liver cell into the canalicular lumen.  This hypothesis is
strengthened by the localisation of ATPases at the canalicular
membrane (Essner et al.,1958;  Novikoff and Essner,1960) and the
relationship between the bile salt-independent fraction and

$Na^+-K^+$-ATPase activity (Frlinger et al 1970).

The possible involvement of ATP in bile secretion has been investigated by examining the relationship between bile flow under a wide variety of conditions and the ATP content of the liver (Slater and Delaney,1970; 1971). The methods and drug treatments used are summarised below.

Carbon tetrachloride: 0.5ml/100g body weight given by stomach intubation under light ether anaesthesia as a mixture 1:3 v/v with liquid paraffin. Control rats given equivalent volume of liquid paraffin.

2,4-Dinitrophenol: 2.5mg or 7.5mg/100g body weight given i.p. dissolved in 0.9% NaCl. Control rats given same volume of 0.9% NaCl.

DL-Ethionine: 100mg/100g body weight given i.p. dissolved in distilled water. Control rats given same volume of distilled water.

Dimethylnitrosamine: 10mg/100g body weight given i.p. from a 2% w/v solution in water. Control rats given water.

M-Sodium malonate and M-Sodium succinate were given i.p. at 1.2ml/100g body weight. Control rats were given the same volume of M-NaCl.

Sodium taurocholate: 50mg/100g body weight in 0.9% NaCl was given i.p.; control rats were given an equivalent volume of saline.

Sodium phenobarbital was given i.p. at 10mg/100g body weight daily for 3 days.

Apart from carbon tetrachloride and sodium phenobarbital, these agents were administered one hour after the externalised biliary fistula operation (see Slater and Delaney,1971) had been completed under pentobarbital anaesthetic. This procedure allowed the collection of bile to give the bile flow rate before the drugs were given. Carbon tetrachloride was given 2 hours before the operation was performed.

One hour following the administration of these agents, a sample of the liver was taken into liquid $N_2$ for subsequent ATP assay by the method described by Slater and Delaney (1970). The necessity for rapid sampling and freezing in such analyses has been emphasised by Faupel et al.(1972). The relationship between the change in the bile flow rate and in the ATP content of the liver was then compiled (Slater and Delaney,1970, Figure 1).

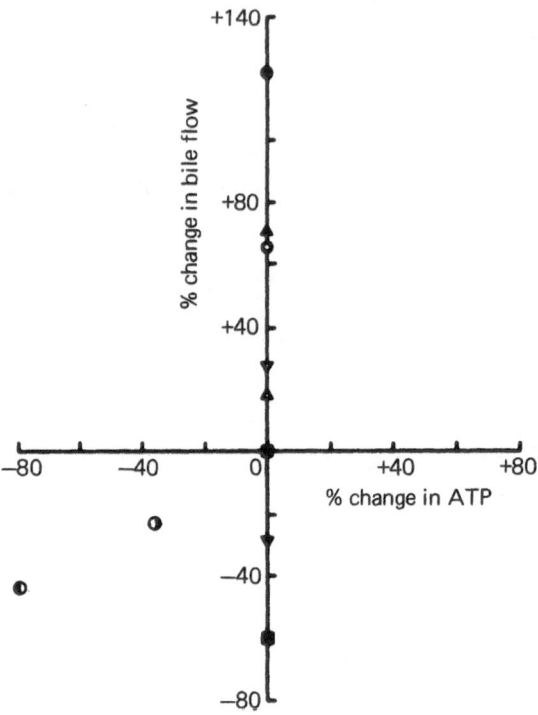

<u>LEGEND FOR FIGURE 1</u>.    Effects of various agents on bile flow rate
                            and total liver ATP in the rat.

Symbols:    ●, sodium taurocholate (15 min); ▲,sodium phenobarbitone
(22 h);  o, sodium salicylate (1 h);  Δ, dimethynitrosamine (1 h);
▽, 2,4-dinitrophenol (30 min);  □ , CCl₄ (2 h); ▼ , sodium succinate
(1 h);  ■ , sodium malonate (1 h);  ◑ , ethionine (90 min);
◑ , ethionine (3 h).   The figures in parenthesis are the times
after dosing.  For further details see Slater and Delaney (1970).


        From Figure 1 it can be seen that only DL-Ethionine produced
a fall in bile flow and in ATP content, the remaining compounds
altering only one of the parameters studied, except carbon tetrachloride which had no effect on either at the time period studied.
The action of 2,4 dinitrophenol was puzzling.  This compound is
known to be an active uncoupler of oxidative phosphorylation in
mitochondria <u>in vitro</u> (Judah,1951) but given at its reported $LD_{50}$
of 7.5mg/100g body weight (Spencer et al.,1948), it produced only
a slight decrease in hepatic ATP levels (Slater and Delaney,1970).
When 2,4 dinitrophenol was added to the perfusate of isolated perfused rat livers, however, there was a fall in the bile flow rate
(Bizard,1965;  Vanlerenberghe et al.1970;  Slater and Delaney,1971).

When administered in vivo a slight increase in bile flow was seen
in rats (Slater and Delaney,1971), whilst dogs showed a considerable
enhancement of the bile flow rate (Stone,1965;  Pugh and Stone,
1968).

A possible explanation of the above observations is that
dinitrophenol is not entering the liver cell in sufficient concentration to uncouple phosphorylation but is retained within extrahepatic compartments;  it is known that dinitrophenol is tightly
bound to serum albumin (Weinbach et al.,1966);  Schimassek,1968).
In the perfused livers, the ratio of uncoupler to perfusate albumin
was higher than under conditions in vivo and consequently more
2,4-dinitrophenol was able to enter the liver.  If this hypothesis
is correct,the displacement of dinitrophenol from its albumin
binding site by an anionic competitor should lead to a fall in the
liver ATP level.

The first agent used as a competitor was CPIB (ethyl α-(4-
chlorophenoxy)-α-methyl proprionate) which is known to bind to
serum albumin (Thorp,1963) and does not enter the rat liver (Platt
and Thorp,1966).  Unfortunately, CPIB was found to be unsuitable
as the concentration range between no effect and rapid death of
the rat was extremely narrow.

The ability of sodium salicylate to displace other anionic
drugs from their albumin binding bile is well known (Anton,1960;
Christensen et al.,1963) and was tried in place of CPIB.

A dose of 20mg/Kg body weight of dinitrophenol given together
with 60mg/Kg sodium salicylate dissolved in 0.9% NaCl with the pH
adjusted to 7.0 and administered i.p. proved to be an effective
combination for decreasing liver ATP (Eakins et al.,1969).  The
change in the bile flow is shown in Figure 2 and the bile salt and
bilirubin excretion given in Figure 3.

Dinitrophenol in the presence of sodium salicylate produced
a decrease in the bile flow rate, salicylate alone giving a
choleresis (Figure 2).  Bile salts measured enzymically using
3α-hydroxy steroid dehydrogenase (Slater and Delaney,1971) were
secreted at a lower rate in the dinitrophenol group than in the
control.  Bilirubin output assayed by the method of Malloy and
Evelyn (1937) was not significantly altered (Figure 3).

To confirm the displacement of the 2,4-dinitrophenol by
salicylate from a binding site in the blood $C^{14}$ labelled 2,4-
dinitrophenol was prepared from 1-chloro-2,4-dinitrobenzene $C^{14}$-
(U) obtained from The Radiochemical Center, Amersham following the
procedure described by Vogel (1970).  The product was recrystallised
twice from ethanol, the yield being 80%.  Purity of the compound
was determined by descending paper chromatography using ethanol-

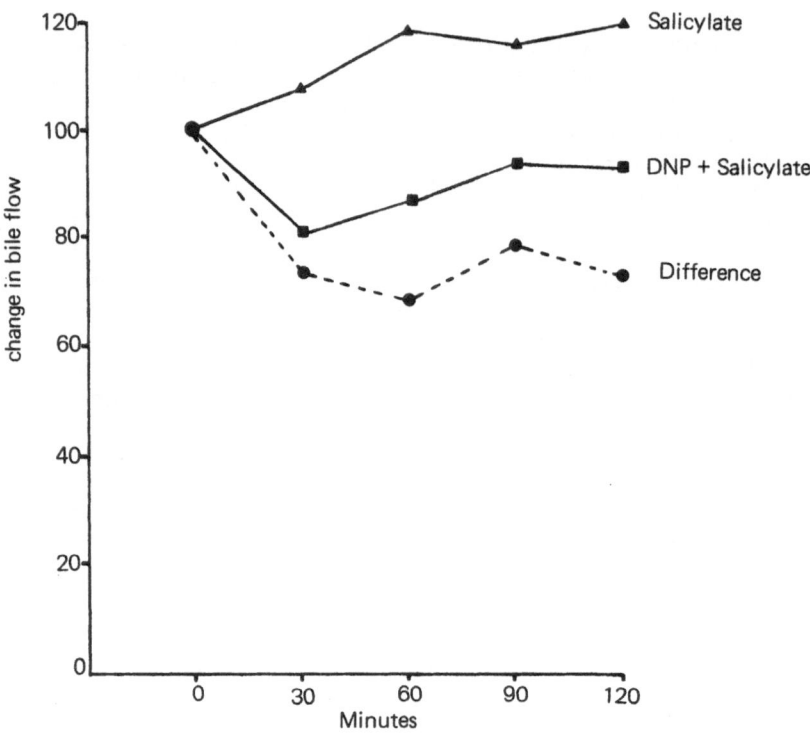

LEGEND FOR FIGURE 2

The percentage change in bile flow following administration of
20mg/kg 2,4-dinitrophenol plus 60mg/kg sodium salicylate or a
salicylate control together with the arithmetic difference between
the two rates.   The results are expressed as the mean of five rats
in the dinitrophenol group and four rats in the salicylate control.

ammonia-water (80-4-16) as solvent. The separated compounds were
visualised using a ferric chloride spray and identities confirmed
by comparison with the Rf value of the pure chemical. Individual
spots were eluted off with hot ethanol and an aliquot added to
scintillation fluid and counted. It was found that 94.4% of the
$C^{14}$ counts were in the 2,4-dinitrophenol spot.

A small amount of the radioactive dinitrophenol was mixed
with the non-radioactive dinitrophenol and injected i.p. into rats
containing an externalised biliary fistula at 20mg/kg alone or
together with 60mg/Kg sodium salicylate. The presence of the
radioactivity in the bile was followed over a period of 2 hours
and at the end of this time liver and blood samples were taken.
These samples were solubilised in strong alkali and then decolour-
ised by the addition of hydrogen peroxide. The results obtained
are shown in Figure 4.

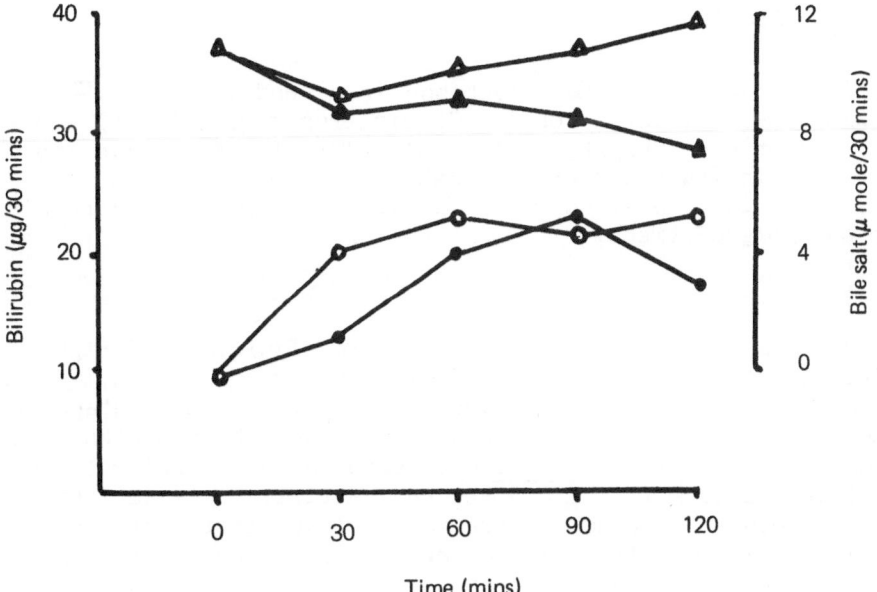

Time (mins)

LEGEND FOR FIGURE 3    The effect of 2,4-dinitrophenol plus
salicylate and salicylate alone on bile sale output and bilirubin
excretion. The results shown are the means of 4 rats in each group.

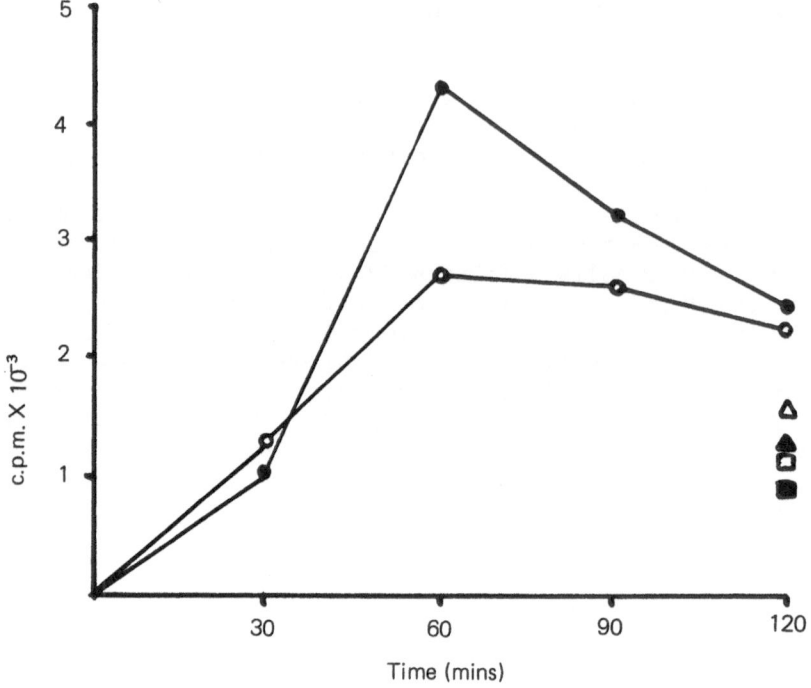

LEGEND FOR FIGURE 4

The C$^{14}$ content of bile (●, o), blood (▲,△) and liver (■ ,□ )
following the administration of $^{14}$C dinitrophenol (20mg/kg alone
(o, △ ,□ ) or with 60mg/kg sodium salicylate (●, ▲,■ ) i.p. to
rats.  The results shown are the mean values of 3 rats in each
group, with bile expressed as cpm/30 minute sample and blood and
liver as cpm/g of tissue.


     The level of C$^{14}$-label in the bile is significantly higher in
the presence of salicylate (Figure 4).  This radioactivity may be
the unchanged dinitrophenol or one or both of the main metabolites,
4-amino-2 nitrophenol or 2-amino-4 nitrophenol which are known to
be produced by the liver in vitro (Eiseman et al.,1972).  These
metabolites would still retain the radioactivity.  Blood radioactivity 2 hours after administration is lower in the presence of
salicylate while the liver levels are higher.  These data would
appear to confirm the belief that salicylate has displaced 2,4-
dinitrophenol from its albumin binding site into the liver, where
it has exerted its effect as an uncoupler of oxidative phosphorylation.  Dinitrophenol plus salicylate could then be used in vivo
in the study of the relationship between ATP and bile flow.

Following the demonstration of the lack of a general correlation between the total ATP content of the liver and bile flow, the possibility was considered that there may be a relationship between an intracellular pool of ATP and the bile flow (Slater and Delaney,1970). A technique was developed which enabled the rapid removal of nuclei and mitochondria from a liver homogenate by passage through Millipore filters (Delaney and Slater,1970). The ATP concentration control could be assayed in this fraction, designated the cell sap fraction (S) and compared to the ATP in the whole liver homogenate. The agents used in the study of the relationship between total ATP and bile flow (see Figure 1) were then used in this new study as were also 2,4-dinitrophenol plus salicylate, and fructose. Intravenous administration of fructose is known to rapidly deplete rat liver adenine nucleotides (Mäenpää et al.,1968), a higher dose given i.p. producing the same effect (Burch et al.,1969). The fall in the nucleotide level is almost solely accounted for by the loss in ATP, with only a small alteration in ADP and AMP levels (Mäenpää et al.,1968; Woods et al.,1970).

The administration of fructose to rats with a biliary fistula produced a very rapid fall in bile flow rate. The fall was maintained over a period of 2 hours with only a slight recovery from the minimum value 30 minutes after administration i.p. (Figure 5). The excretion of bile salt was markedly decreased in this first period but then recovered more towards the control values (Figure 6).

The level of the ATP in the cell sap was measured following fructose or dinitrophenol plus salicylate. These results are given in Table 1.

The results obtained with 2,4-dinitrophenol plus salicylate, fructose and the other agents studied show that in general a relationship between bile flow rate and cell sap ATP exists (Figure 7). There were three exceptions to this general finding : sporidesmin, icterogenin and sodium taurocholate (Slater and Delaney, 1970; Eakins, 1972).

The mode of action of icterogenin and sporidesmin was then subjected to further study. Sporidesmin is a fungal toxin which has been isolated from cultures of Pithomyces chartarum and plays an important role in the pathogenesis of facial eczema in sheep (see Slater et al.,1964). Ingestion of contaminated pastures results in extensive periportal necrosis in the liver and bile duct occlusion (Mortimer,1963). When administered to rats, sporidesmin produced a profound though transient decrease in bile flow (Slater and Griffiths,1963).

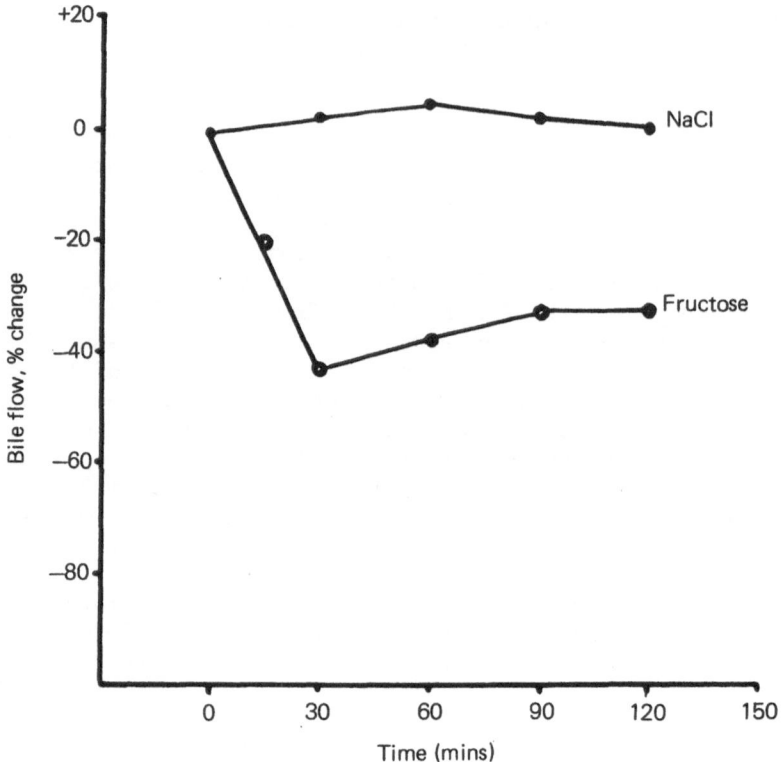

Effect of fructose (40 mmoles/kg body wt.) on bile flow in the
rat.  The controls were injected with an equivalent volume of
saline.  The points shown are the means of 4 animals in each
group.

         In some respects icterogenin, a pentacyclic triterpene acid,
behaves similarly to sporidesmin.  Administration of icterogenin
to herbivorous animals results in the cessation of bile flow,
although only slight morphological disturbances to the liver can
be seen by light microscopy (Heikel et al.,1960).  Other compounds
closely related to icterogenin, e.g. 22β-angeloyloxyoleanolic acid
and are even more active cholestatic agents, and a precise stereochemical relationship has been demonstrated between cholestatic
activity and molecular structure in the substances (Brown et al.,
1963).  The structure of these agents are shown in Figure 8.

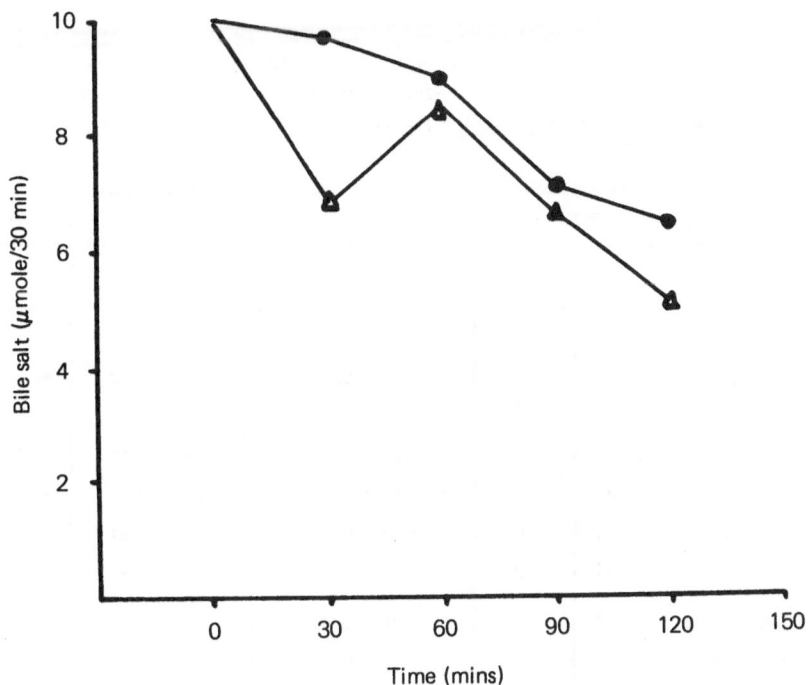

LEGEND FOR FIGURE 6

Effect of fructose (40 mmoles/kg body wt.) on bile salt excretion
in the rat.  The points shown are the means of 4 animals in each
group.  Symbols: ●, saline control; Δ, fructose treated.

 

 

      These agents are virtually insoluble in aqueous media and in
other biologically innocuous solvents.  The use of the isolated
perfused rat liver preparation allowed the addition of these compounds dissolved in a small amount of ethanol and the study of their
direct action on the liver of a known amount.  All three agents
gave a rapid cholestasis (Bullock et. al.,1974).  When bile flow
had ceased the livers were perfused <u>in situ</u> with fixative after
the perfusate had been washed out.  The morphology of these livers
was then studied by electron microscopy.

      Sporidesmin produced a major morphological disturbance in the
structure of the canalicular membranes, with the loss of the microvilli from large areas of the canaliculus.  The microvilli appeared
to be thickened and more closely packed into the canalicular lumen
in icterogenin poisoned livers, while very little alteration in
canalicular morphology was observed after 22β-angeloyloxyoleanic
acid administration (Eakins et al.,1973; Bullock et al.,1974).

TABLE 1

Effects of 2,4 dinitrophenol (DNP) plus sodium salicylate,
sodium salicylate, sodium chloride and fructose on the concentration
of ATP in rat liver and on the percentage of ATP in the supernatant
fraction S.

The number of rats used are in parentheses. Mean values
are given ± S.E.M.

| Treatment | Time (min) | ATP in whole liver μmols/g wet wt. | ATP in fraction μmols/g wet wt. | S % |
|---|---|---|---|---|
| Untreated  (4) | – | 1.95 ± 0.37 | 1.15 ± 0.22 | 59 ± 1 |
| DNP + sodium salicylate (5) | 30 | 1.41 ± 0.05 | 0.87 ± 0.17 | 62 ± 6 |
| Sodium salicylate      (4) | 30 | 2.07 ± 0.14 | 1.40 ± 0.20 | 67 ± 5 |
| Sodium chloride        (4) | 30 | 2.03 ± 0.18 | 1.21 ± 0.21 | 60 ± 6 |
| Fructose               (4) | 30 | 1.29 ± 0.12 | 0.48 ± 0.06 | 38 ± 6 |
| DNP + sodium salicylate (5) | 120 | 1.16 ± 0.05 | | |
| Sodium salicylate      (4) | 120 | 2.00 ± 0.20 | | |
| Sodium chloride        (4) | 120 | 2.26 ± 0.18 | | |

From the results of these experiments together with the lack
of correlation between the fall in bile flow and in the hepatic
cell sap ATP level, it was suggested that the triterpene acids may
act by inhibition of the enzymes resoonsible for bile secretion
especially the canalicular ATPases.  This hypothesis was examined
by preparing rat liver plasma membranes and investigating the
activity of these 3 agents agsinst the canalicular ATPases in vitro
(Table 2).  Both icterogenin and 22β-angeloyloxyoleanic acid proved
to be potent inhibitors of the $Na^+$-$K^+$-ATPase (50% inhibition at
less than 100μM) and to produce a partial inhibition of $Mg^{2+}$-ATPase
at a concentration of 400μM.  Sporidesmin was a weak inhibitor of
$Mg^{2+}$-ATPase at 400μM concentration and did not inhibit the $Na^+$-$K^+$-
ATPase (Eakins et al.,1973).  These results, taken together with
the evidence shown by the electron micrographs of the perfused
livers, indicate that the triterpene acids and sporidesmin act in a
different way upon the canalicular membrane.  Sporidesmin is seen
to disrupt the organisation of the canalicular membrane and this
fact is supported by the evidence of sporidesmin's powerful toxic
action on membranes in general.  When administered to rats, the

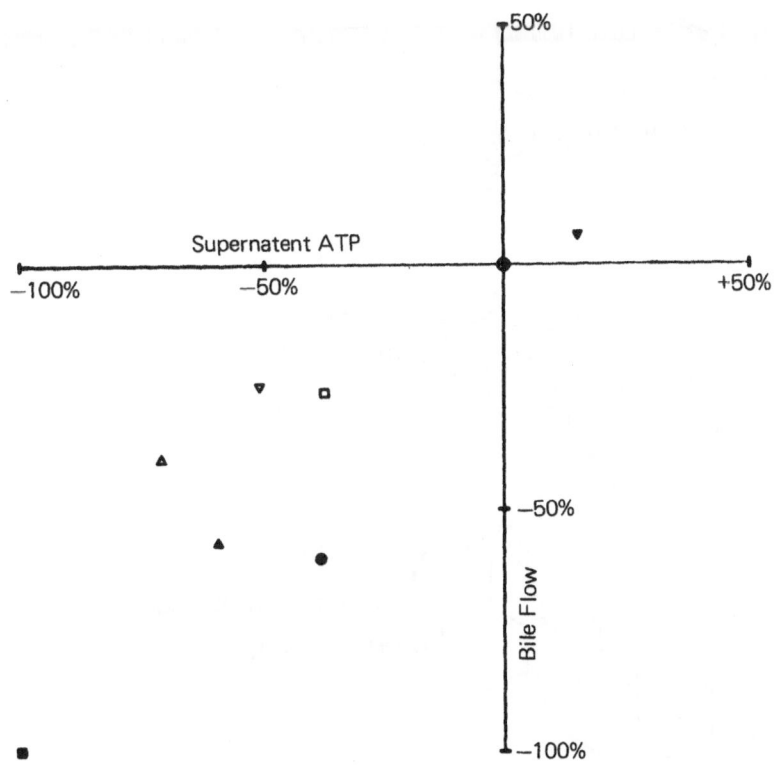

LEGEND FOR FIGURE 7

Effects of various agents on bile flow rate and cell sap ATP in
the rat.    Symbols :    ●, sodium malonate (30 min);
O, CCl₄ (2 h);    ◻ , 2,4-dinitrophenol plus sodium salicylate (30
min);    ▼ , sodium salicylate (30 min);    ▲, fructose (30 min);
▰ , 2,4-dinitrophenol, perfused liver (1 h);    ∇, ethionine
(90 min);    Δ, ethionine (3 h).
The values in parenthesis are the times after dosing.


major response appears to be an inflammation reaction especially in
the form of ascites and pleural effusions (Slater et al.,1964).
Slater (1972) has suggested that this reactivity involves an interaction of the disulphide bridge in sporidesmin with membrane bound
sulphydryl groups.   Icterogenin may act by inhibition of the activity
of a canalicular ATPase which is involved in bile secretion.

     Having discussed briefly the possible reasons why icterogenin
and sporidesmin did not fit the general correlation between bile
rate and cell sap ATP found for other agents, it is necessary to

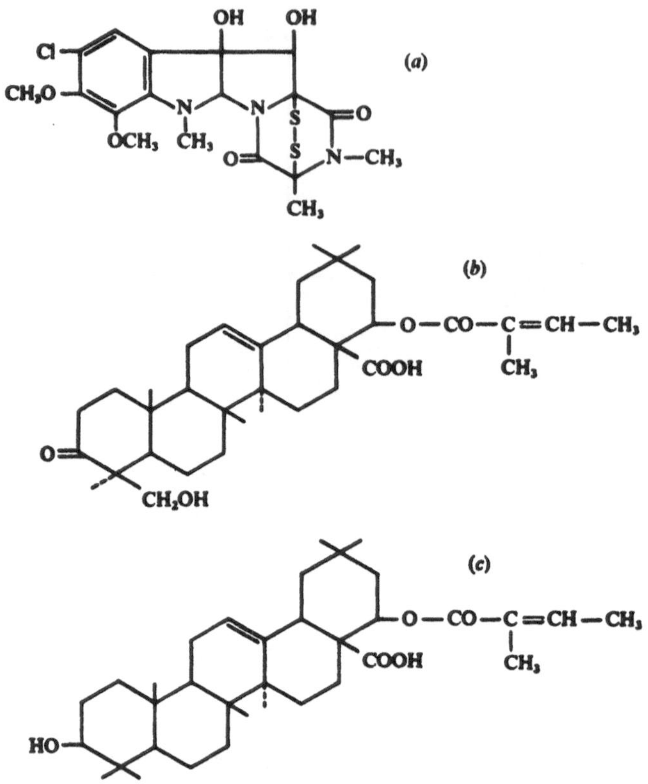

Figure 8.   Structures of (a) sporidesmin, (b)icterogenin, and
    (c) 22β-angeloyloxy-3β-dihydroxyolean-12-en-28-oic acid.

consider now the remaining exception to the correlation i.e.
sodium taurocholate.  The administration i.p. of sodium tauro
cholate (50mg/100g body wt.) produced a large and rapid increase
in bile flow in the rat (Slater and Delaney,1971) whilst producing
a small but significant decrease in cell sap ATP (Slater and
Delaney,1970).

    It has recently been reported that a rapid administration of
sodium taurocholate as a pulse to a rat previously subjected to
biliary drainage for 12 h. did not increase bile flow rate despite
a rapid increase occurring in the taurocholate concentration in
the bile (Klaassen,1974).  A similar observation has been made using
the isolated perfused rat liver preparation to which no taurocholate had been infused for 4 h. to replace the bile salts

TABLE 2

Effects of ethanol, icterogenin, sporidesmin and 22β-angeloyloxy-3β-dihydroxyolean-12-en-28-oic acid on rat liver plasma membrane enzyme activities.

Icterogenin, 22β angeloyloxyoleanolic acid and sporidesmin were dissolved in 50 μl of ethanol and incubated at a concentration of 400 μM.

Values are given as μmoles Pi liberated/mg protein/hour ± S.E.M.

| Additions | $Mg^{2+}$-stimulated ATPase | % of control | $Na^+$-stimulated ATPase | % of control |
|---|---|---|---|---|
| None | 32.8 ± 0.6 (5) | | 6.0 ± 0.3 (5) | |
| Ethanol | 34.5 ± 0.3 (6) | | 6.6 ± 0.1 (6) | |
| Icterogenin | 12.4 ± 0.1 (6) | 38 | 0.6 (0.5–0.7 (3) | 9 |
| Sporidesmin | 31.4 ± 0.3 (5) | 96 | 7.4 (6.9–7.7 (3) | 112 |
| 22β-angeloyloxyoleanolic acid | 18.7 ± 0.4 (4) | 57 | 0 (4) | 0 |

secreted in bile;   after 45 min under such conditions there is only a small content of bile salts present in the bile secretion.  After 4 h. a large pulse of sodium taurocholate was added to the perfusate and this produced only a very small increase in bile flow rate yet was associated with a much elevated bile salt concentration in the bile (Eakins,1972).

Klaassen (1974) applied his procedure outlined above to the dog and rabbit as well as the rat.  In the rabbit and dog the taurocholate pulse was associated with a large increase in bile flow rate so that the rat may be unusual in this respect.  Even so, these observations suggest the possibility that the effect of bile salts on bile flow may be more complex than suggested by Sperber (1959):   some feed-back interaction between bile salt dependent and bile salt independent flow seems to operate and this phenomenon requires close investigation.

The occurrence of a bile salt independent fraction has been demonstrated by the use of inhibitors of $Na^+$-$K^+$-ATPase.  In the rabbit, for example, ouabain ethacrynic acid and amiloride suppressed or at least decreased this fraction (Erlinger et al., 1970) as did scillarin in the isolated perfused rat liver (Boyer,

TABLE 3

Effect of Caerulein (0.1–20 $\mu$g) on $Mg^{2+}$ – ATPase and $(Na^+ – K^+)$–
ATPase of plasma membranes.   The values are expressed as means
$\pm$ S.E.M; the number of experiments are given in parentheses.

| Caerulein $\mu$g | $\mu$moles Pi per mg protein per h | |
| | $Mg^{2+}$ – ATPase | $(Na^+ – K^+)$–ATPase |
| --- | --- | --- |
| 0 | $32.8 \pm 0.6$  (5) | $6.0 \pm 0.3$  (5) |
| 0.1 | $28.8 \pm 0.6$  (3) | $6.3 \pm 0.3$  (5) |
| 1 | $29.0 \pm 0.6$  (5) | $6.4 \pm 0.3$  (6) |
| 10 | † $42.5 \pm 0.4$  (5) | $6.5$  (2) |
| 20 | † $46.6 \pm 0.6$  (8) | $7.0$  (2) |

† $p < 0.01$

1971).  Ouabain, however, has little effect on bile flow rate in
the rat (Slater, T.F. and Delaney, V.B. unpublished data).
Caerulin an octapeptide of similar composition to cholecystokinin
stimulates the $Mg^{2+}$ -ATPase and to a lesser extent the $Na^+$-$K^+$-ATPase
of rat liver plasma membranes in vitro (Table 3).  Caerulin
stimulates bile flow rate and bile salt output;  it is especially
active in the chicken (Angelucci and Linan,1971) and has similar
effects on the rat.

     In summary, it appears from the data outlined previously that
one determinant of bile flow is the concentration of ATP in the
cell sap;  another parameter is the level of activity of ATPase
enzymes in the canalicular membrane.  Changes in cell sap ATP or
in ATPase may thus be associated with changes in bile flow rate.
A third possibility suggested from the work with sporidesmin is
the structural organisation of the canalicular membrane.  Recent
studies with other membranes have shown the importance of membrane
fluidity to biological function (for example, see Stier and
Sackmann,1973) and we feel that comparable studies on canalicular
membrane fluidity in the presence of endogenous materials such as
bile salts would give data of considerable interest and importance.

REFERENCES

Angelucci, L., Baldier, M. and Linari, G. (1970) Eur.J.Pharmacol., 11, 217.

Anton, A.H. (1960) J.Pharmacol.Exp.Therap., 129, 282.

Berthelot, P., Erlinger, S. and Dhumeaux, D. (1970) Amer.J. Physiol., 219, 809.

Bizard, G. (1965) in 'The Biliary System' NATO Symposium, ed. W. Taylor, p.315.

Boyer, J.L. (1971) Amer.J.Physiol., 221, 1156.

Boyer, J.L. and Klatskin, G. (1970) Gastroenterology, 59, 853.

Boyer, J.L. and Bloomer, J.R. (1974) J.Clin.Invest., 54, 773.

Brauer, R.W., Leong, G.F. and Holloway, R.J. (1954) Amer.J. Physiol., 177, 103.

Brown, J.M.M., Rimington, C., and Sawyer, B.C. (1963) Proc.Roy. Soc., B, 157, 473.

Bullock, G., Eakins, M.N., Sawyer, B.C. and Slater, T.F. (1974) Proc.Roy.Soc., B, 186, 333.

Burch, H.B., Max, P., Chyn, K. and Lowry, O.H. (1969) Biochem. Biophys.Res.Commun., 34, 619.

Christensen, L.K., Hansen, J.M. and Kristensen, M. (1963) Lancet, II, 1298.

Delaney, V.B. and Slater, T.F. (1970) Biochem.J., 116, 299.

Eakins, M.N. (1972) Ph.D. thesis, University of London.

Eakins, M.N., Slater, T.F. and Delaney, B.V. (1969) Biochem.J., 115, 62P

Eakins, M.N., Slater, T.F., Sawyer, B.C. and Bullock, G. (1973) Biochem.Soc.Trans., 1, 170

Eiseman, J.L., Gehring, P.J. and Gibson, J.E. (1972) Toxicol. Appl. Pharmacol., 21, 275.

Erlinger, S., Dhumeaux, D. Berthelot, P. and Dumont, M. (1970) Amer.J.Physiol., 219, 416.

Essner, E., Novikoff, A.B. and Musek, B. (1958) J.Biophys. Biochem.Cytol., 4, 711.

Faupel, R.P., Seitz, H.J., Tarnowski, W., Thiemann, V., and Weiss, C.H. (1972) Arch.Biochem.Biophys., 148, 509.

Heikel, T., Knight, B.C., Rimington, C., Richie, H.D. and Williams, E.J., (1960) Proc.Roy.Soc.,B, 153, 43.

Judah, J.D. (1951) Biochem.J., 49, 271.

Klaassen, C.D. (1974) Canard.J.Physiol., 52, 334.

Mäenpää, P.H., Raivio, K.O. and Kekomaki, M.P. (1968) Science, 161, 1253.

Malloy, H.T. and Evelyn, K.A. (1937) J.Biol.Chem., 119., 481.

Mortimer, P.H. (1963) Res.Vet.Sci., 4, 166.

Novikoff, A.B. and Essner, E. (1960) Amer.J.Med., 29, 102.

Paumgartner, G., Herz, R., Sauter, K. and Schwarz, H.P. (1974) Naunym-Schmiederberg's Arch.Pharmakol., 165, 285.

Platt, D.S. and Thorp, J.M. (1966) Biochem.Pharmacol., 15, 915.

Preisig, R. Cooper, H.L. and Sheeler, H.O. (1962) J.Clin. Invest., 41, 1152.

Pugh, P.M. and Stone, S.L. (1968) J.Physiol., 198, 39.

Schersten, T., Nilsson, S., Cahlin, E., Filipson, M., Brodina-
          Persson, G. (1971) Eur.J.Clin.Invest., 1, 242.

Schimassek, H. (1968) in "Stoffwechsel der isoliert perfundierten
          Leber" p.116, Eds. W.Staib and R.Scholz, Springer-Verlag.

Slater, T.F. (1972) in "Free Radical Mechanisms in Tissue Injury"
          Pion Ltd., London.

Slater, T.F. and Griffiths, D.B. (1963) Biochem.J.88, 60P.

Slater, T.F., Strauli, U.D. and Sawyer, B.C., (1964) Res.Vet.Sci.,
          5, 450.

Slater, T.F. and Delaney, V.B. (1970) Biochem.J., 116, 303.

Slater, T.F. and Delaney, V.B. (1971) Toxicol.Appl.Therapeut,
          20, 157.

Spencer, H.C., Rowe, V.K., Adams, E.M. and Irish, D.D. (1948)
          J.Industr.Hyg.Toxicol., 30, 10.

Sperber, I. (1959) Pharmac.Rev., 11, 109.

Sperber, I. (1965) in 'The Biliary System', p.457, NATO Symposium,
          ed. W. Taylor.

Stier, A. and Sackman, E. (1973) Biochim.biophys.Acta, 311, 400.

Stone, S.L. (1965) in 'The Biliary System', p.277 NATO Symposium,
          Ed., W. Taylor.

Thorp, J.M. (1963) J.Atherscler.Res., 3, 351.

Vanlerenbergh, J. (1965) in 'The Biliary System', p.265, NATO
          Symposium, Ed., W. Taylor

Vanlerenbergh, J., Bel, C., Trupin, N. and Guislain, R (1970)
          Arch.int.Physiol.Biochem., 78, 935.

Vogel, A.I. (1970) in 'A textbook of practical organic chemistry'
          p.678, 3rd ed. Longman Group Ltd., London.

Weinbach, E.C., Garbus, J., and Claggett, C.E. (1966) J.Biol.Chem.,
          241, 3708.

Woods, H.F., Eggleston, L.V. and Krebs, H.A. (1970) Biochem.J.
          119, 501.

DISCUSSION OF COMMENTARY BY T.F. SLATER

Popper:    I have two questions.   Do any of these compounds, such
as the icterogenins, produce cholestatic jaundice?   Secondly, you
showed a photomicrograph of the sporidesmin lesion.   As with
lithocholate treatment and other conditions, the microvilli and
tight junctions are perfectly preserved.   These observations may
have important physiological significance;   have you any ideas
about this?

Slater:    Icterogenin and the hydroxyoleanolic acids certainly do
cause jaundice.    In South Africa where the sheep may eat foods
containing these types of compounds, they develop oedema in the
face and look jaundiced, so that the condition is called 'yellow
big head'.   This was described in the 1930's.    Then in the 1950's
it was found that icterogenin produces a conjugated type of
jaundice at a low dose level.    If the dose is increased there
are effects on the conjugating system in the endoplasmic reticulum.
So the type of hyperbilirubinaemia is dose-dependent.    As for
your second question;   it is true that one sees relatively normal
structures, for example nuclei and mitochondria, distant from the
canaliculus.    But stripping of the microvilli can be seen, whereas
at the same time the tight junctions are intact.    We have seen
microfilaments spreading out from the microvilli.    However, I have
no explanation for this action of sporidesmin.

Boyer:    We have also done work on the role of ATPases, particularly
the Na/K-ATPase, in bile secretion.    We use a canalicular membrane-
enriched fraction (CMF) from rat liver.    This preparation has
enrichment of such enzymes as 5'-nucleotidase, Mg-ATPase and Na/K-
ATPase when compared with the whole liver homogenate.    Other cell
fractionation marker enzymes are low.    We have been particularly
interested in the role of the Na/K-ATPase in bile formation, and
in comparing the CMF with the isolated perfused rat liver.    The
latter is quite resistant to ouabain, and with the CMF we need very
high concentrations, up to $10^{-3}$ molar, to inhibit the Na/K-ATPase.
This concentration is very similar to that required to inhibit bile
secretion in the perfused liver.    In contrast, scillarin, a more
potent cardiac glycoside, begins to be effective as an inhibitor
of the Na/K-ATPase in vitro at much lower concentrations.    This
corresponds to the effect on bile flow in the perfused liver.

We have investigated the effect of temperature on both Mg-ATPase and Na/K-ATPase to try to relate these to the classic work on the effect of temperature on bile production in the perfused liver;  here we are dealing with the bile salt independent bile flow.  In our system there is good correlation between the Na/K-ATPase, but less with Mg-ATPase, and bile flow.  The temperature optimum for bile secretion by the perfused liver and the activity of Na/K-ATPase in the CMF is about $42^{\circ}C$, whereas this optimum for the activity of the Mg-ATPase is about $30-35^{\circ}C$.

Since it has been suggested that one of the major thermogenic effects of thyroid hormone is by regulation of Na/K-ATPase, we turned our attention to the effects of thyroid hormone in our systems.  We used erythritol clearance as a marker of canalicular bile flow and compared this with bile acid excretion.  In livers from control rats the bile salt independent bile flow was about 1.8 microlitres per minute per gram of liver.  This flow was significantly increased in hyperthyroid animals and significantly decreased in those with hypothyroidism.  We then compared these results with the activity of Na/K-ATPase in the CMF prepared from similarly treated rats.  It was found that Na/K-ATPase activity is less than normal in tissue from hypothyroid animals, but in tissue from hyperthyroid animals it is almost double that of the control animals.  On the other hand, the Mg-ATPase activity is somewhat low in tissue from hypothyroid animals, but there is no significant difference between the values for the activity of this enzyme in tissue from normal and hyperthyroid animals.  If hypothyroid animals are treated with L-thyroxin, bile salt independent bile flow is restored to normal within 24 hours. The Na/K-ATPase activity in the CMF of animals treated in the same way is increased, but there are no effects on other plasma membrane enzymes.

So our studies support those of Professor Slater in that Na/K-ATPase is one mechanism we must consider in bile salt independent bile secretion.

Slater:  Of course, I am very pleased to hear that your results are so similar to ours.  I was particularly interested in your thyroid work because it throws some light on work we did some years ago but could not explain at that time.  We had found that the drug Atromid (I.C.I.), which is known to displace thyroxin into the liver caused a small but definite increase in bile flow.  Your work obviously provides the probable explanation for what was a mysterious effect to us.

ON THE STRUCTURE AND FUNCTION OF LIGANDIN AND Z PROTEIN

I.M. Arias, G. Fleischner, I. Listowsky, K. Kamisaka,
S. Mishkin and Z. Gatmaitan
The Liver Research Center
Albert Einstein College of Medicine
1300 Morris Park Avenue, New York, N.Y. 10461

A large number of organic neutral and anionic compounds are
noncovalently bound to two proteins in the 100,000 x g supernatant
fraction of homogenates of liver from various animals and man
(Table I).  Binding occurs when the various ligands are either
added in vitro and/or injected in vivo prior to homogenization of
liver.  This report will consider the following with respect to the
binding proteins: (i) their structure, composition and several
forms; (ii) quantitation, tissue and cell distribution, and biological regulation; (iii) site and mechanism of ligand binding; (iv)
enzymatic activity and its relationship to binding of ligands; (v)
transfer of ligands from serum albumin, and (vi) biological function.

In 1967, we began to study the mechanisms responsible for
rapid transfer of bilirubin from plasma into the liver. For at
least four decades it has been known that following injection of
"physiologic" amounts of bilirubin and other organic anions, a
large proportion of the injected dose is recovered within the
liver within a few minutes.  The mechanism responsible for this
rapid and seemingly selective transfer from plasma remains unknown; however, several hypothesis have been tested experimentally.

(i) Hypothesis: Bilirubin is noncovalently bound to serum
albumin and enters the liver cell by pinocytosis as a pigment: albumin complex. This hypothesis is unlikely because when $^{131}I$ albumin and $^{14}C$ bilirubin are injected simultaneously into a rat, the
bile pigment enters the liver at a rate many times faster than
does albumin.  (ii) Hypothesis: An active transport system exists
in the plasma membrane of the parenchymal liver cell. This is unlikely because hepatic uptake takes place despite inhibitors of

TABLE I. Compounds bound to Ligandin in vitro and/or in vivo (1-7)

  I. Covalently bound

    azodye carcinogen

    methylcholanthrene metabolite

  II. Noncovalently bound

    azodye GSH conjugate

    estrogens, cortisol and their metabolites, gastrin
    benzprene, methyl cholanthrene

    bilirubin, bilirubin glucuronide

    BSP, ICG, Rose Bengal, DBSP, T-1824, vasoflavine

    glutathione (GSH), BSP glutathione

    hematin, heme, hematoporphyrin, phylloerythrin

    cholecystographic and renographic agents

    tri- and tetra-iodothyronine

    various fatty acids

    probenecid, p-aminohippurate

    penicillin, chloromycetin, cephalothin, cephlex, tetra-
    cyclines, nitrofurantin, various sulfonamides

    ethacrynic acid, furosemide metabolites

energy metabolism, and 'throughput' studies by Goresky and others
reveal bidirectional bilirubin fluxes consistent with a passive
process. (iii) <u>Hypothesis</u>: <u>Hepatic bilirubin uptake is determined
by hepatic blood flow and a high extraction ratio</u>. Although hepatic
blood flow must influence perfusion of hepatic lobules; definitive
studies of this parameter have not been performed with respect to
bilirubin. Up to 25% increase or decrease in hepatic arterial flow

does not alter net hepatic uptake of bilirubin per unit time. (iv)
Hypothesis: "Unbound" bilirubin in plasma is transferred across the
plasma membrane of the liver cell by simple or facilitated diffusion. Net flux may be determined by intracellular binding of bilirubin, subsequent metabolism or excretion, and/or a plasma membrane
carrier system. Kinetic studies by Goresky, Paumgartner and others
indicate that the uptake process is saturable which precludes
simple passive diffusion. These studies do not reveal the nature
or site of the carrier mediated mechanism. In theory, facilitated diffusion can result from specific membrane molecules or pores,
and/or cytoplasmic proteins having high affinity for bilirubin
which enters the plasma membrane by virtue of its lipid solubility.

Our studies have resulted in purification and partial characterization of ligandin (Y protein) and Z, two organic anion
binding proteins in liver, as well as studies regarding their
function. Our hypothesis is that these proteins, particularly
ligandin, influence the net uptake of organic anions into the liver
specifically by regulating efflux from the cell into the plasma.
It seems obvious that there is no way in which a substance in
plasma can know what is in the liver and, therefore, influx must
be independent of cytoplasmic binding proteins.

In 1968, we determined that approximately 80% of intrahepatic
bilirubin is associated with the 100,000 x g supernatant fraction
of liver after radioactive bilirubin was injected into a rat (8).
Fractionation by gel filtration revealed that radiobilirubin was
found in two nonalbumin containing peaks called Y and Z. In subsequent years, a specific Y and a specific Z protein were purified
and accounted for approximately 85% of the bilirubin binding in
their respective fraction (1,7,9,10).

Ligandin. Ligandin (Y protein, azo carcinogen binding protein
(Ketterer) (11), cortisol metabolite binding protein II (Litwack)
(12), GSH Transferase B (Jakoby) (10)) was purified from rat liver
and kidney by TEAE ion exchange chromatography, Sephadex G-100 gel
filtration and QAE-A-50 chromatography (7,13). Purity was established by isoelectric focusing in ampholyte and gels; electrophoresis on acrylamide with and without added SDS, repeated amino
acid analysis and the ability to produce monospecific precipitating antibody. Identity between Y protein and the Ketterer, Litwack
and Jakoby proteins was established by immunoelectrophoresis,
-diffusion and precipitation as well as comparison of physical-
chemical features (3). Ligandin is a basic protein, pI 9.0 of
46,000 daltons consisting of two apparently identical monomeric
subunits. Circular dichroism studies reveal an ordered structure
with a high degree of $\alpha$ helix conformation (6). The protein from
rat kidney gives identical structural and cross-immunologic responses (7). Physical-chemical properties of ligandin isolated
from rat and human liver and kidney are presented in Table II.

TABLE II.  Physical-chemical properties of ligandin purified from
           rat and human liver

|                                    | Rat     | Human   |
|------------------------------------|---------|---------|
| Molecular Weight                   |         |         |
|    Monomer          | 23,000  | 22,000  |
|    Dimer            | 46,000  | 44,000  |
| Sedimentation Constant ($S^{\circ}W$) | 3.5S | 3.5S    |
| Diffusion Coefficient ($D^{\circ}_{20}W$) | 7.5 | 7.4   |
| Isoelectric Point                  | 9.1     | 8.9     |
| N-Terminal amino acid              | Proline | Proline |

Homogenous preparations of rat and human ligandin were used
to prepare monospecific precipitating antibodies (14,15).  Antibodies were prepared in domestic American goats, 4-6 months of age,
by immunization of 50-75 $\mu$gm of protein in complete Freund's adjuvant administered intracutaneously.  Weekly bleedings were taken
and a second immunization was performed 3 weeks later employing
100-125 $\mu$gm protein in incomplete Freund's adjuvant.  The majority
of animals had a maximal response (titre 1:500) within 7-10 days
following the second immunization; serum was harvested at weekly
intervals, and IgG globulin was prepared. Monospecificity of antisera was verified by immunodiffusion, immunoelectrophoresis, and
quantitative precipitin reactions.  Serologically identical antigens to hepatic ligandin were found in renal and small intestinal
supernatants but were not detected with any tissue, blood, urine
or bile (14,15).  Antibody to purified rat renal ligandin demonstrated immunologic identity with hepatic and small intestinal
supernatants and gave equivalent quantitative ligandin precipitation in these tissues (7).  Direct specific-immunofluorescent studies were performed with a rhodamine conjugate of the gamma globulin
fraction of monospecific antisera to determine the localization of
rat ligandin.  Fluorescent staining was diffusely observed in
hepatocytes throughout the liver lobule with absent membrane and
nuclear staining.  Kupffer cells, vascular structures and portal
triads lacked fluorescence.  Renal fluorescence was localized to
proximal tubular cells in the cortical area with absence of stain
in glomeruli or vascular structures.  Small intestinal villus
cells showed fluorescence with predominance in the tip and weak
staining in the crypts.  The proximal small bowel showed more in-
tense fluorescence than did the distal ileum.  Other rat tissues
failed to demonstrate specific fluorescence.  Additional fluores-

cent studies were performed with hamster tissue where the antibody against rat ligandin demonstrated partial immunologic identity and gave similar results to that observed in rats. We have been unable to identify ligandin in liver cell plasma membranes and other organelles using immunologic techniques.

Anti-rat ligandin prepared in the goat showed no cross-reactivity by immunodiffusion against liver supernatants from several strains of guinea pig and mice, Rhesus monkey, Shetland ponies, chickens, rabbits, fish, amphibia or reptiles (14). Structural and immunologic comparison of rat ligandin with an aminoazodye carcinogen-binding protein isolated by Ketterer and corticosteroid binder IB isolated by Litwack showed all three proteins to be identical and resulted in the term "ligandin" being proposed for the protein (3). Following purification of four glutathione S-transferases (A,B,C,E) from rat liver (16), comparison of each of these proteins with anti-ligandin revealed selective antigenic identity to glutathione S-transferase B. Additional supports for their identity are common physicochemical properties, catalytic activity,and inducibility following phenobarbital treatment in rats (10). The possibility that ligandin has GSH transferase activity was initially suggested by Kaplowitz et al (23).

Quantitation of ligandin (glutathione S-transferase B) content of hepatic, renal and small intestinal supernatants was performed by radial immunodiffusion in normal rats and animals treated with a variety of xenobiotics which induce drug metabolism (Table III) (15,16). In control rats, ligandin accounts for 5% of hepatic supernatant protein, and 2% of supernatant proteins in homogenates of kidney and small intestinal mucosa. By virtue of the fact that the proximal tubular contains about 40% of total kidney cells, the concentration of ligandin in proximal tubular cells approximates that found in rat liver cells. Treatment of rats with phenobarbital, DDT, dieldrin or pregnane-16$\alpha$-carbonitrile caused a 2-2.5 fold increase in hepatic ligandin concentration but did not effect the ligandin content in kidney or small intestinal mucosa. TCDD (tetrachlorodibenzo-p-dioxan) 1 $\mu$g/100g body weight given as a single dose seven days previously doubled the concentration of hepatic and renal ligandin (7).

Five basic GSH transferases ($\alpha$-$\xi$) have been purified from human liver (17) and kidney (18). In contrast with the 4 distinct basic GSH transferases in rat liver, the human proteins have identical amino acid analysis, substrate specificity, ability to bind bilirubin and other ligands (19), and response after administration of TCDD in monkeys.

Monospecific antisera were prepared in goats to a preparation of ligandin from human liver and to each of five homogenous GSH transferases ($\alpha$-$\xi$) isolated from human liver (16). Irrespective

TABLE III.   Ligandin concentration in rat tissues

| Tissue | Control µg/mg ± S.E.M. | Phenobarbital (8mgm/100G per day for 7 days) treated µg/mg ± S.E.M. |
|--------|--------|--------|
| liver | 44.7 ± 2.1 | 124.0 ± 8.9 |
| kidney | 22.4 ± 2.7 | 18.7 ± 3.7 |
| small intestinal mucosa | 17.2 ± 1.9 | 16.7 ± 2.9 |

of the antigen used, all antisera showed identity by immunodiffusion against human ligandin or the five human glutathione transferases, whether comparing antigens or antisera.  Immunoelectrophoresis of each antiserum in agarose (1%) in two systems using barbital buffer pH 8.6 and pH 6.8, and homogenous protein and supernatants of human liver and kidney revealed a single precipitin arc with zero mobility.  Immunofluorescent studies using a direct rhodamine conjugate demonstrated hepatic and renal fluorescence similar to that seen in rats; other human tissues have not been sufficiently studied.  Antisera against each of the human proteins revealed identity with Rhesus monkey hepatic supernatant.  No cross-species reaction was observed with rat ligandin.

Recent studies of acute proximal tubular necrosis produced in rats by mercuric chloride revealed ligandinuria as detected immunologically and enzymatically 10-12 hours after treatment and prior to the onset of oliguria.  "Ligandinuria" appears to be a specific marker of proximal tubular necrosis and may be useful in studies of renal tubular pathology (20).

Table IV gives the results of immunoquantitation of human hepatic ligandin from radial immunodiffusion studies (16).  The concentration of ligandin in human liver is approximately 40% of that found in rat liver.  In the mid-trimester fetus, levels were undetectable ($<$ 5µg/mgm).  By the third trimester, ligandin was detectable and constituted a third of adult values.  Hepatic samples obtained from 10-21 day old infants undergoing surgical procedures for which hepatic biopsy was indicated, showed ligandin content approaching adult levels.  These results in the human fetus and newborn are similar to those reported for Rhesus monkey and guinea pig.  In five adults treated with phenobarbital, hepatic ligandin content showed a 2-3 fold increase demonstrating that hepatic ligandin is inducible in human liver.  Ligandin was not detected in normal human serum, bile and urine and does not appear in serum during acute liver injury.

TABLE IV.  Ligandin concentration in human liver

| Source of liver | No. | Hepatic content $\mu$g/mgm ± S.E.M. |
|---|---|---|
| normal adult | 13 | 17.9 ± 3.6 |
| fetus | | |
|     early | 4 | "too low" |
|     late | 6 | 6.8 ± 2.2 |
| newborn,10-21 days old | 6 | 13.2 ± 2.9 |
| phenobarbital-treated adults | 5 | 40.6 ± 4.7 |

Using $I^{125}$ radio labelled ligandin and antisera prepared
against ligandin, the ability to displace label was studied using
the 5 glutathione S-transferase ($\alpha$-$\varepsilon$) at equivalent concentrations
to unlabelled ligandin (2-0.025$\mu$gm) (16).  All five proteins produced displacement curves with similar slopes which were shifted
to the right except for epsilon which was essentially identical to
ligandin.  The five human glutathione S-transferases have a common
antigenic site.  The varied ability to displace radiolabelled
human ligandin from antibody suggests that differences are present
when sensitive techniques are employed.  Each of the isolated
human glutathione S-transferases has similar amino acid content,
substrate specificities, and ability to bind ligands which are not
substrates, such as bilirubin.  The observed charge differences
probably result from intracellular degradation of a primary gene
as illustrated by the various post translational degradative forms
of tyrosine amino transferase and cytochrome C in rat liver, and
rabbit muscle aldolase.

The control of the protein in rat liver has been partially
characterized (4,13,14,21,22).  Following pulse-labeling with $C^{14}$-
guanidino-arginine and immuno-precipitation, the half life for
ligandin is 2.3 days (Fig. 1).  Dose response studies indicate
that a new steady-state of approximately 220% of basal concentrations is reached following administration of phenobarbital, DDT,
dieldrin, 16 $\alpha$-pregnenecarbonitrile, tetrachlorodibenzodioxan
(TCDD), methyl cholanthrene and benzpyrene.  Phenobarbital administration did not change the half-life of degradation of ligandin
as determined after pulse-labeling with $^{14}$C-guanidino-arginine.
These results indicate that phenobarbital increases synthesis of
ligandin in rat liver.  In mice and rats deprived of pituitary or
thyroid glands, hepatic ligandin concentration is increased by an
average of 30% over basal levels.  In many hormonal replacement
studies, only thyroxine in physiological doses restores hepatic

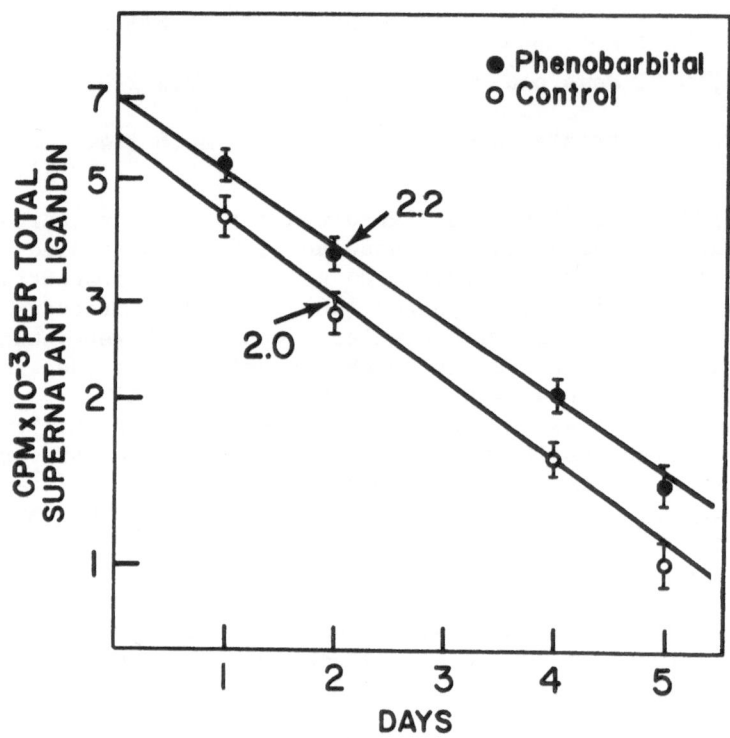

<u>Figure 1.</u>  Degradation of pulse-labeled ligandin isolated by immunoprecipitation from livers of rats treated with saline or phenobarbital.

ligandin concentration to normal.

Ligandin is responsible for at least 80% of the organic anion binding by Y fraction from rat kidney or liver, or human liver. This was proven by quantitation of bilirubin or BSP binding to Y fraction before and after addition of monospecific anti-ligandin IgG with nonspecific IgG serving as control.

The mechanisms responsible for increased ligandin concentration in liver in relationship to drug administration and thyroid hormone insufficiency were also studied using the double isotope method of Arias, Doyle and Schimke (21) an immunoprecipitation. Groups of 5 normal, hypophysectomized and thyroidectomized rats received, for 5 days, daily intraperitoneal injections of isotonic saline, phenobarbital (8mgm/100G) or l-thyroxine (5μg/100G). On the sixth day, each rat received an intraperitoneal injection of 50 μCi leucine $-^{14}C$, was permitted to eat ad libitum and received daily administration of phenobarbital, thyroxine or saline as before. Seventy-two hours later, each rat received an intraperitoneal injection of 250 μCi leucine $H^3$. Four hours later, rats were killed by ether anesthesia. The livers were quickly removed and ligandin was measured immunologically in 100,000 x g supernatants.

Immunoprecipitation was performed by adding 0.5 ml of 100,000 x g liver supernatant to 4 ml of non-specific anti-ligandin IgG. The mixture was kept at room temperature for 1 hour and thereafter at 4°C for 72 hours. Following centrifugation at 18,000 x g for 30 minutes at 4°C, the supernatant was removed and discarded. The precipitate was rinsed three times with 0.001 phosphate buffer, pH 7.4, dissolved by boiling for 1 minute in SDS-dithioerythritol and subsequently electrophoresed on a 10% SDS acrylamide gel. The distribution of $^{14}C$ and $^3H$ in the gel was determined by counting sequential 1 mm slices. Radioactivity was localized to a single region corresponding to the band obtained when pure rat or human ligandin was simultaneously electrophoresed in the same system. The results were expressed as $^3H/^{14}C$ ratio in ligandin as well as a Turnover Index (22).

To determine if $^3H$ and $^{14}C$ were incorporated only as leucine into ligandin, approximately 1 mg of ligandin was purified from liver in each test group and hydrolyzed in 6N HCl for 12 hours at 110% under nitrogen. An aliquot of the hydrolysate was chromatographed by high voltage paper electrophoresis (3000 volts x 4 hours) in a solvent system of water-acetic acid-pyridine, pH 3.5. Chromatograms were cut into 0.5 x 0.5 cm sections. Radioactivity in each section was determined by scintillation spectrometry. Only the area where standards of leucine and isoleucine migrated contained radioactivity.

As shown in Table V, thyroidectomy or hypophysectomy increased

the concentration of ligandin in the liver by approximately 30%
over basal levels, reduced the $^3H/^{14}C$ ratio in ligandin but did
not change the Turnover Index. Thyroxine administration to control
rats did not alter the concentration of ligandin or its Turnover
Index. Thyroxine administration to previously thyroidectomized or
hypophysectomized rats reduced the concentration of ligandin to
normal as well as the ratio of $^3H/^{14}C$ in ligandin. Phenobarbital
administration to control rats increased the concentration of
ligandin by 196% over control values but did not alter the $^3H/^{14}C$
ratio in ligandin or the Turnover Index. Phenobarbital administration to thyroidectomized or hypophysectomized rats increased the
concentration of ligandin by 144 and 184% respectively over control
values and reduced the Turnover Index to normal. In thyroidectomized or hypophysectomized rats treated with phenobarbital, ligandin
constitutes up to 18% of liver supernatant protein presumably reflecting enhancement of synthesis as well as stabilization. The
results indicate that phenobarbital increases synthesis (ie.induct-
ion) of ligandin in control, thyroidectomized or hypophysectomized
rats, whereas, thyroidectomy or hypophysectomy partially stabilize
ligandin. Thyroid hormone reverses this process and stabilizes
ligandin.

There is a relationship between the binding of various ligands
by ligandin and its catalytic activity. Bilirubin, p-aminohippurate,
probenecid and various dyes, renographic and cholecystographic
agents bind to a common site on ligandin and also inhibit ligandin's
catalytic activity. An example using Telepaque is shown in Figure 2; the cholecystographic agent noncompetitively inhibits the
GSH transferase activity of rat ligandin using dichloronitro
benzene as the substrate. None of these ligands form GSH adducts
in vivo or in vitro. Other ligands serve as catalytic substrates.
For example, ethacrynic acid and BSP form GSH adducts in vivo and
in vitro in liver and proximal tubular cells.

TABLE V. Studies of the effect of thyroidectomy, hypophysectomy and administration of tetraiodothyronine ($T^4$) and phenobarbital on immunologic quantitation of ligandin in rat liver; $^3H/^{14}C$ ratio in ligandin and proportional to $^3H/^{14}C$ ratio in total liver protein (Turnover Index), liver weight and liver/body weight ratio.

| | No. Rats | Ligandin (μg/mgm prot.) | Ligandin ($^3H/^{14}C$) | Turnover Index | Liver Weight (GM) | % Body Weight |
|---|---|---|---|---|---|---|
| 1. CONTROL | 5 | 59.3 ± 13.3 | 4.99 ± .39 | 0.60 ± .02 | 9.51 ± .75 | 4.21 ± .19 |
| + T4 | 5 | 67.6 ± 11.5 | 5.73 ± .84 | 0.58 ± .03 | 9.85 ± .35 | 5.03 ± .32* |
| + pheno-barbital | 5 | 116.2 ± 19.2* | 4.57 ± .37 | 0.62 ± .03 | 9.94 ± .75 | 4.76 ± .23* |
| 2. THYROIDECTOMY | 5 | 85.8 ± 13.1* | 3.35 ± .49* | 0.69 ± .08 | 5.98 ± .21* | 3.20 ± .25* |
| + T4 | 4 | 62.6 ± 12.8 | 5.01 ± .37 | 0.81 ± .12* | 7.80 ± .88* | 3.75 ± .21 |
| + pheno-barbital | 5 | 140.7 ± 23.2* | 3.69 ± .36 | 0.58 ± .14 | 7.80 ± .90* | 3.75 ± .23 |
| 3. HYPOPHYSECTOMY | 5 | 89.9 ± 17.0* | 3.27 ± .46* | 0.64 ± .07 | 4.00 ± .41* | 2.88 ± .42* |
| + T4 | 4 | 63.4 ± 14.1 | 5.23 ± .51 | 0.72 ± .14* | 4.46 ± .15* | 3.40 ± .22* |
| + pheno-barbital | 5 | 164.6 ± 19.8* | 4.15 ± .16 | 0.59 ± .09 | 5.83 ± .44* | 3.93 ± .22 |

*p $< .05 > .01$

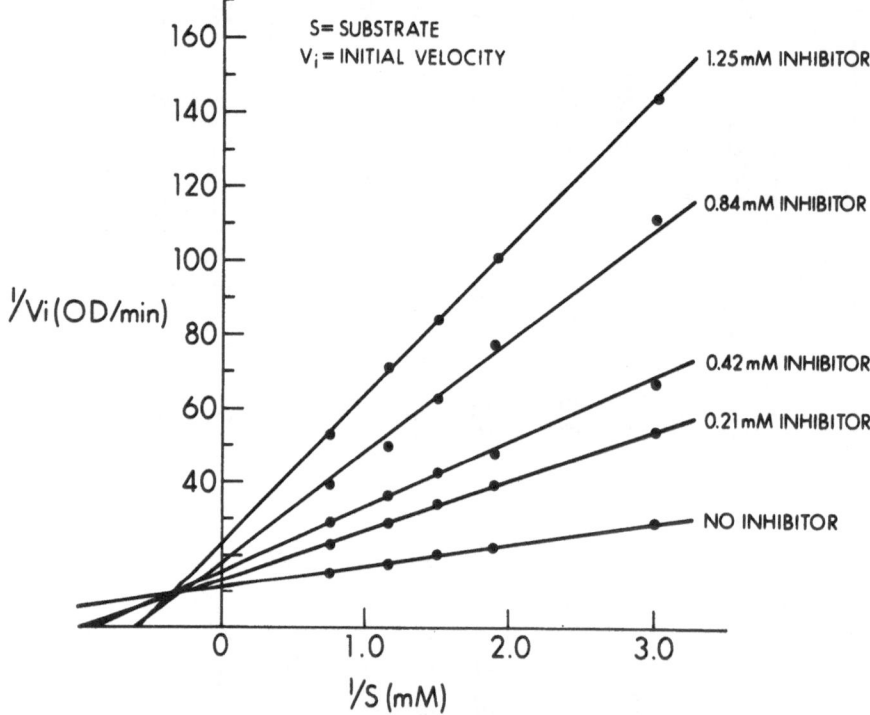

<u>Figure 2</u>.  Lineweaver-Burk Plot for Inhibition by Telepaque of
the Reaction of CDNB + GSH + "Y"

The following studies support the hypothesis that ligandin influences the net organic anion flux specifically by reducing efflux from liver into the plasma.

1. Phyllogenetic study revealed absence of Ligandin by gel filtration of liver supernatants in the presence of added BSP or bilirubin in teleosts, elasmobranchs and several species of amphibia prior to metamorphosis.  These species also have markedly delayed plasma disappearance of injected BSP and/or bilirubin with reduced hepatic uptake.  By contrast, post-metamorphosis amphibia, reptiles, reptiles, birds and mammals have abundant ligandin in their livers and manifest selective hepatic uptake of BSP and/or bilirubin _in vivo_ (23).

2. Ontogenetic studies in newborn guinea pig, rat, monkey and man reveal impaired plasma disappearance and/or reduced hepatic content of BSP and/or bilirubin and other organic anions.  This process matures during the first ten days of life.  Immunoquantitation of ligandin in these species reveals virtual absence of the protein in fetal liver, appearance shortly before or after birth, and maturation to adult concentrations within the first week of life in correlation with maturation of hepatic uptake (24-26) (Table III).

3. Induction of hepatic ligandin following administration of phenobarbital or DDT is associated with increased plasma disappearance of organic anions (bilirubin, BSP, indocyanine green) and increased hepatic content of these organic anions 5 minutes after their intravenous injection.  From 65-80% of intrahepatic exogenous organic anions were in the 100,000 x g supernatant fraction bound to the ligandin peak after gel filtration.  In addition, kinetic studies of relative storage capacity and biliary Tm for BSP in rats treated with phenobarbital for 3 days revealed a significant increase in the former without change in the latter (21, 22).

4. Measurement of the influx and efflux constants, $K_1$ and $K_2$, was performed in dogs with and without phenobarbital administration using a multiple indicator technique and analysis with bilirubin as the test ligand.  Phenobarbital administration for 6 days did not alter $K_1$ but significantly reduced $K_2$.  This finding is consistent with observed induction of ligandin in the liver and reduced efflux of bilirubin from liver into the plasma (unpublished data).

5. Association constants derived from circular dichroism studies of  various organic anions and rat liver ligandin were used to design experiments testing whether or not competition occurs for net transfer of these organic anions from plasma into the liver. For example, tri-iodothyronine binds to ligandin with an association constant of $10^6 M^{-1}$.  Bilirubin in the liver bound to ligandin in UDP glucuronyl transferase deficient (Gunn) rats...or after intravenous administration of unconjugated bilirubin to normal rats...reduced the transfer of $I^{131}$-triiodothyronine from plasma into the liver (2).

6. Induction of renal ligandin in the rat following administration

of TCDD results in increased rate of removal of $^{14}C$-penicillin
from plasma and increased renal content and excretion of the antibiotic. Similar observations were made with respect to Tm p-
aminohippurate in the rat. In addition, BSP and probenecid bind
to ligandin with greater affinity than does penicillin and their
administration reduces renal uptake, excretion and ligandin-bind-
ing of $^{14}C$-penicillin (7,27).

Because ligandin binds various ligands and also has catalytic
activity, it has been proposed that this abundant protein may
function both enzymatically and in influencing net organic anion
flux across the plasma membrane of liver cells. Kinetic studies
reveal that ligandin serves as well as albumin with respect to
various biotransformation reactions found in microsomal membranes
in vitro. The protein may function as a form of "intracellular
albumin". Ketterer et al have suggested that ligandin may facilitate the transfer of heme from mitochondria to apocytochrome
P-450 in the endoplasmic reticulum (28).

Ligandin may also protect cellular elements against 'toxic'
injury. For example, bilirubin uncouples oxidative phosphorylation
in isolated rat liver mitochondria. Such affects are not seen in
liver in vivo even after administration of large amounts of bilirubin; however, uncoupling is observed in brain tissue. The central nervous system lacks ligandin as measured immunologically.
Kinetic studies reveal that ligandin is equally as effective as
serum albumin in protecting isolated liver mitochondria from uncoupling effects of bilirubin (29).

These studies qualitatively support a function for ligandin
in hepatic uptake of various ligands for binding (ex: bilirubin)
or substrates for the catalytic activity (ex: BSP, ethacrynic acid).
Quantitative evaluation of binding sites, affinities and kinetics
is required for further evaluation of our hypothesis as well as
organic anion interaction with albumin, ligandin and Z protein.

Characterization of ligand:protein interactions by dialysis,
ultrafiltration and gel filtration involve physical separation of
the small free ligand molecules from the larger particles of protein and ligand-protein complexes and are often limited by ligand
binding to the supporting gel or membrane, inability to estimate
rapid rates of ligand-unbinding, and difficulties in determining
whether ligands compete at the same or different sites on the protein. Ultraviolet, visible absorption and fluorescence spectros-
copy, optical rotatory dispersion and circular dichroism (CD), and
nuclear magnetic and electron spin resonance have the advantage of
measuring bound and free ligand as well as providing information
on the nature of the ligand-protein interaction. The number of
sites, relative affinities and competition between various ligands
can be rapidly investigated without artificial membranes or gels,

and specific groups on the ligand and protein can be studied in
terms of three dimensional structure.  These considerations are
important in studying the interaction between bilirubin and other
ligands with respect to serum albumin, ligandin and Z protein
from various species including man.

We have studied the three dimensional structure of these
proteins and their ligand complexes primarily using CD (6,30-33).
This method permits rapid and economical study of the site and
affinity of bilirubin binding, specificity of interaction with
competing organic anions, competitive binding of organic anions,
as well as the transfer of bilirubin between albumin and ligandin.

Blauer and King have published CD studies of bilirubin binding to bovine serum albumin (BSA) and human serum albumin (HSA).
We have obtained similar results and, in addition, have studied
the competition between various organic anions for binding of bilirubin by albumin preparations.  Using CD, we analyzed competitive
binding studies to determine the extent and manner in which various
organic anions interact with BSA and HSA.  Because the primary
bilirubin binding sites are of very high affinity and relatively
high protein concentrations ($10^{-5}$ - $10^{-6}$M) were required for the
spectropolarimetric experiments, bilirubin association constants
were too large to be estimated directly from the CD studies.  We
utilized published $K_B$ values for the primary bilirubin binding
site of HSA to calculate relative affinity constants of competitive organic anions according to the following relationship:

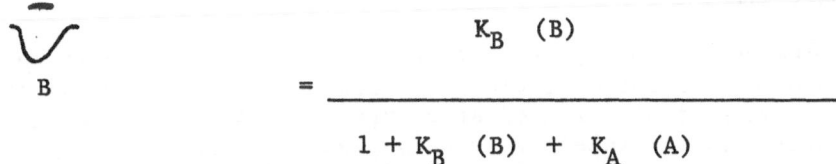

$$\overline{V}_B = \frac{K_B \ (B)}{1 + K_B \ (B) \ + \ K_A \ (A)}$$

Where $\overline{V}_B$ is the average number of moles bilirubin bound, $K_A$ is
the association constant for the competing anion, and $K_B$ = 1.4 x $10^8$
for the HSA bilirubin complex.  (A) is the molar concentration of
free organic anion assuming that the amount of bilirubin displaced
reflects the amount competing organic anion bound to the protein,
and (B) is the concentration of bilirubin displaced by the organic
anion A.  Certain speculations are inherent in this approach, including the assumption that competitive binding occurs at the
bilirubin site exclusively, and that neither complex binding nor
cooperative effects occur.

The ellipticity pattern of the HSA-bilirubin complex was distinct from that of the BSA complex and was characterized by a
positive peak at 460nm, a negative band of 405nm, and a crossover

point at 438nm. An almost linear increase in ellipticity magnitude of both bands was observed after addition of bilirubin up to a molar ratio of 2:1. Between a molar ratio of 2 and 3:1, the slope of ellipticity increase became much shallower and above a molar ratio of 3:1, no further increase in optical activity resulted. Addition of up to 6 moles of BSP or 9 moles of Rose Bengal per mole of a 1:1 HSA-bilirubin complex had little effect on optical activity generated by the complex. Several ligands studied decreased ellipticity magnitudes of HSA-bilirubin CD bands. In bilirubin-HSA 1:1 system, vasoflavine was the most effective competitor on a molar basis. Affinity constants (K) were estimated based on the effectiveness of the organic anions in displacing bilirubin from the primary binding site on HSA. The K values obtained were estimated as $2.5 \times 10^7 M^{-1}$ for vasoflavine, $2.3 \times 10^7 M^{-1}$ for ICG and iodipamide, $7.5 \times 10^6 M^{-1}$ bilirubin glucuronide, $6 \times 10^5 M^{-1}$ for flavaspidic acid, $2 \times 10^5 M^{-1}$ for phenol red, and $5 \times 10^5 M^{-1}$ for Rose Bengal. Under these conditions, the competing anions had no effect on the overall conformation of the proteins as determined from peptide ellipticity bands at 222nm and 208nm. These apparent affinity constants are first approximations because some of the competing anions may displace bilirubin from the primary binding site and the released bilirubin may form a complex at the second binding site. Since the ellipticity values associated with the second site are of the same sign and indistinguishable by CD from those of the first site, the resultant ellipticities after addition of the competing anions reflect both displacement of bilirubin and shifts to a second site. If this occurs, the anion would appear less effective in displacing bilirubin from the primary site.

The CD spectrum of rat liver ligandin reveals a pattern in the peptide absorption region (190-250nm) which is typical for a protein with highly ordered structure and helical content (6,31,33). Computer analysis relative to poly-peptides of known secondary structure reveals that this CD spectrum and 35% random coil. In the 250-300nm region, six bands are evident; and there is no ellipticity above 300nm. On addition of bilirubin, a large increase in ellipticity near 255nm is observed and three new ellipticity extrema appear in the region of bilirubin absorption. These bands are centered at 405, 455 and 515nm. If one plots ellipticity magnirute as a function of amount of bilirubin added, the 405nm band reaches maximum magnitude after addition of 1 mole of bilirubin, and the 455nm band attains about 80% of saturation values after addition of 1 mole. Thus, a 1:1 stoichiometry is reflected in the 405 and 455nm bands. Observations in the 515 and 255nm regions indicate that an additional site(s) is involved after bilirubin is bound to ligandin in excess of 1:1 molar ratio; however, binding to this site(s) generates optically active bands distinct from that associated with the primary site.

Because up to a 1:1 molar ratio, no detectable unbound bilirubin is evident at protein concentrations of $10^{-5}$M, the affinity of bilirubin for ligandin has an association constant of greater than $10^6$M$^{-1}$ associated with the primary binding site.

ICG, BSP, iodipamide, and flavaspidic acid compete with bilirubin for hepatic uptake _in vivo_ and exhibit competitive effects for a bilirubin binding site on ligandin. No Cotton effects are generated when these anions are bound to ligandin. The relative effectiveness of the competing anions and preferential binding to ligandin were monitored by their individual effects on the three observed bilirubin ellipticity bands. Based on the 455nm band, BSP and ICG have similar inhibitory effects, flavaspidic acid has an intermediary effect and iodipamide has a small effect. Association constants are shown in Table VI.

TABLE VI. Binding Affinities of Various Ligands to Ligandin

| Substance | Association Constant (K)M$^{-1}$ |
|---|---|
| Bilirubin | $5 \times 10^7$ |
| Indocyanine green, T-1824, oleic acid, hematoporphyrin, sulfobromophthalein | $10^6$ |
| Cortisol, hemin, benzpyrene, 1-triiodothyronine | $10^5$ |
| Thyroxine, chloromycetin | $10^4$ |
| Iodipamide, penicillin, p-aminohippuric acid probenecid | $10^3$ |
| Iophenoxic acid, propanolol, lidocaine, iodobenzene 1, chloro 2,4 dinitrobenzene | $10^2$ |

The CD spectra of bilirubin-RSA complexes have positive ellipticity extrema at 455nm and negative bands at 405nm. This spectrum is virtually the mirror image of the CD spectrum associated with the ligandin-bilirubin complex and permits study of the transfer of bilirubin from ligandin to RSA directly without a need for artificial membranes or supporting gels. The relative affinity of the two proteins for binding bilirubin is readily derived from these CD experiments. If both proteins are present in equimolar amounts, over 90% of the bilirubin is bound to RSA. An isosbestic point is also observed in the CD spectra indicating

that the process is probably a 2 stage system involving transfer
of bilirubin directly from ligandin to RSA. These results indicate
that the association constant of RSA for bilirubin is approximately
one order of magnitude greater than that of ligandin.

Despite the difference in association constants between albumin and ligandin, the latter may participate in hepatic organic
anion uptake in vivo because (i) the plasma membrane of the hepatocyte separates albumin and ligandin in vivo; (ii) there is an
abundance of ligandin within the cell which facilitates the concentration gradient for a specific ligand; and (iii) binding to
ligandin enhances the availability of most organic anions for subsequent biotransformation or excretion in the bile. Both mechanisms constitute "pump"-like mechanisms.

Ketterer, Meuwissen and colleagues (28) reported higher affinity constants for bilirubin and heme binding to ligandin in native
liver supernatant than with purified protein. Purification of
ligandin appears to reduce its affinity substantially. The K values
were $10^9$ and $10^{10}$ respectively in cytosol and $10^6$ and $10^7$ respectively with purified ligandin. If these observations are correct,
transfer of ligands from plasma into liver can proceed on the basis
of facilitated diffusion with ligandin being a major factor in
regulating this process.

GSH, which is a substrate for the glutathione transferase
activity of ligandin, did not decrease the magnitude of ellipticity
but induced spectral shifts and changes in character of the bilirubin-ligandin CD spectrum (6). A major new ellipticity band at
490nm(+) was observed and additional bands at 450nm(-) and 500nm
($\overset{\bullet}{-}$) appeared if GSH was added to ligandin-bilirubin complexes (6).
These results are inconsistent with competitive displacement of
bilirubin, but indicate specific interactions of GSH with ligandin-
bilirubin complexes. GSH induced effects were not observed with
bilirubin-albumin complexes. Concentrations of GSH at 100 fold
excess, as compared to the ligandin-bilirubin complex, did not
change the spectrum.

The mechanism of interaction of GSH with bilirubin-ligandin
complexes is unknown. The CD data are compatible with several
interpretations. (i) Ternary complexes with GSH bound at a site
adjacent or in close proximity to the bilirubin site, could modify
the spatial orientation of the bilirubin-ligandin complex. (ii)
GSH may interact directly with bilirubin bound to the protein
(perhaps with attendant formation of conjugates). GSH-conjugated
sulfobromophthalein induces different shifts in the bilirubin-
ligandin CD spectrum, and its binding apparently involves interaction with, rather than displacement of, bilirubin. The effects
of GSH on organic anion binding to ligandin are unique and worthy
of further attention.

Z Protein. Z protein is an acidic cytoplasmic protein of 14,000 daltons present in the small intestinal mucosa, liver,heart, kidney, skeletal muscle and fat cells (1,9,34,35). It has an unusual binding affinity for long chain fatty acids and their CoA derivatives in vitro. A role for Z in long-chain fatty acid transport has been suggested; however, complete inhibition of hepatic oleate binding in vivo by competition with flavaspidic acid did not reduce plasma t 1/2, hepatic uptake or rate of esterification of oleate (35). Z also has high affinity for cholecystographic but not renographic agents. Other organic anions bind to Z with high affinity in vitro (ie: flavaspidic acid, bunamiodyl) and inhibit hepatic uptake of other less tightly bound organic anions (ie: bilirubin, BSP, etc.) in vivo. Z develops phyllogenetically in parallel with ligandin. Ontogenetic development in guinea pigs, monkeys, and man is rapid in fetal lige and adult concentrations are present in the liver at birth. Drugs and chemicals which induce ligandin have no apparent effect on Z. Clofibrate and Nafenopen, which are hypolipidemic drugs, increase the concentration of Z protein in the liver (36). Z protein has no known enzymatic activity and its functional interrelationship with ligandin has not been fully explored.

# References

1.  Levi, A.J., Gatmaitan, Z., and Arias, I.M.: The Role of Two
    Hepatic Cytoplasmic Proteins (Y and Z) in the Transfer of
    Sulfobromophthalein (BSP) and Bilirubin from Plasma into the
    Liver.  J. Clin. Invest. 48: 2156, 1969.

2.  Lichter, M., Fleischner, G., Kirsch, R., Levi, A.J.,
    Kamisaka, K., and Arias, I.M.: The Role of Ligandin and Z
    Protein in the Transfer of Thyroid Hormones from Plasma into
    the Liver.  Amer. J. Physiol.  (in press).

3.  Litwack, G., Ketterer, B., and Arias, I.M.: Ligandin: An
    Abundant Liver Protein Which Binds Steroids, Bilirubin,
    Carcinogens and a Number of Exogenous Anions.  Nature
    234: 466, 1971.

4.  Arias, I.M.: Transfer of Bilirubin from Blood to Bile.
    Seminars in Hematology 9: 55, 1972.

5.  Goldstein, E., and Arias, I.M.: Ligandin: Interaction with
    Radiographic Contrast Media. Radiology (submitted).

6.  Kamisaka, K., Listowsky, I., Gatmaitan, Z., and Arias, I.M.:
    Interactions of Bilirubin and Other Ligands with Ligandin.
    Biochem. 14: 2175, 1975.

7.  Kirsch, R., Kamisaka, K., Fleischner, G., and Arias, I.M.:
    Structural and Functional Studies of Ligandin, A Major Renal
    Organic Anion Binding Protein.  J. Clin. Invest. 55: 1009,1975.

8.  Bernstein, L.H., Ben-Ezzer, J., Gartner, L.M. and Arias,I.M.:
    Hepatic Intracellular Distribution of Tritium Labeled Un-
    conjugated and Conjugated Bilirubin in Normal and Gunn Rats.
    J. Clin. Invest. 45: 1194, 1966.

9.  Mishkin, S., Stein, L., Gatmaitan, Z., and Arias, I.M.: The
    Binding of Fatty Acids to Cytoplasmic Proteins: Binding to
    Z Protein in Liver and Other Tissues of the Rat.  Biochem.
    Biophys. Res. Comm. 47: 997, 1972.

10. Habig, W., Pabst, M., Fleischner, G., Gatmaitan, Z., Arias,
    I.M. and Jakoby, W.:  The Identity of Glutathione Transferase
    B with Ligandin, A Major Binding Protein of Liver.  Proc.
    Nat'l. Acad. Sci. 71: 3879, 1974.

11. Ketterer, B., Ross-Mansell, P., and Whitehead, J.K.: The
    Isolation of carcinogen-binding protein from livers of rats
    given 4-dimethylaminoazobenzene. Biochem. J. 103:316,1967.

12. Morey, K.S., and Litwack, G.: Isolation and Properties of
    Cortisol Metabolite Binding Proteins of Rat Liver Cytosol.
    Biochem. 8: 4813, 1969.

13. Arias, I.M. and Fleischner, G.: Regulation of Ligandin.
    in GSH-Chemistry and Function. ed. I.M. Arias and W. Jakoby
    Raven Press, New York (in press).

14. Fleischner, G., Robbins, J., and Arias, I.M.: Immunological
    Studies of Y Protein: A Major Cytoplasmic Organic Anion
    Binding Protein in Rat Liver. J. Clin. Invest. 51: 677, 1972.

15. Fleischner, G., Kamisaka, K., Jakoby, W., and Arias, I.M.:
    Immunoanalysis of Rat and Human Ligandins. in GSH-Chemistry
    and Function. ed. I.M. Arias, and W. Jakoby. Raven Press,
    New York (in press).

16. Pabst, M.J., Habig, W.H. and Jakoby, W.B.: Mercapturic Acid
    Formation: the Several Glutathione Transferases of rat Liver.
    Biochem. Biophys. Res. Commun. 52: 1123, 1973.

17. Kamisaka, K., Habig, W.H., Ketley, J.N., Arias, I.M. and
    Jakoby, W.B.: Multiple Forms of Human GSH Transferase and
    their Affinity for Bilirubin. Biochem. (submitted).

18. Kamisaka, K., Gatmaitan, Z., and Arias, I.M.: In preparation.

19. Jakoby, W.B., Ketley, W. and Habig, W.H.: Rat GSH Transferases:
    Binding and Physical Properties.in GSH-Chemistry and Function.
    ed. I.M. Arias and W. Jakoby. Raven Press, New York (in press)

20. Kirsch, R., Fleischner, G., Feinfeld, D., Goldstein, E.,
    Kamisaka, K., and Arias, I.M.: Renal Ligandin: Structure,
    Function and Role in Diagnosis.

21. Arias, I.M., Doyle, D. and Schimke, R.T.: Studies on the
    Synthesis and Degradation of Proteins of the Endoplasmic
    Reticulum of Rat Liver. J. Biol. Chem. 24: 3303, 1969.

22. Dehlinger, P.J. and Schimke, R. T.: Size Distribution of
    Membrane Proteins of Rat Liver and Their Relative Rates of
    of Degradation. J. Biol. Chem. 246: 2574, 1971.

23.  Kaplowitz, N., Percy-Robb, I.W., and Javitt, N.B.: Role
     of Hepatic Anion-Binding Protein in Bromsulphthalein Con-
     jugation.  J. Exp. Med. 138: 483, 1973.

24.  Levine, R.J., Reyes, H., Levi, A.J., Gatmaitan, Z., and
     Arias, I.M.: Phylogenetic Study of Hepatic Organic Anion
     Uptake Mechanisms.  Nature 231: 277, 1971.

25.  Levi, A.J., Gatmaitan, Z., and Arias, I.M.: Deficiency of
     Hepatic Anion Binding Protein Impaired Organic Anion Uptake
     by Liver and "Physiologic" Jaundice in Newborn Monkeys.
     New Eng. J. Med. 283: 1136, 1970.

26.  Arias, I.M.: Pathogenesis of "Physiologic" Jaundice of the
     Newborn: A Re-evaluation.  Birth Defects VI 2: 55,1970.

27.  Arias, I.M., Fleischner, G., Kirsch, R., Goldstein, E.,
     Feinfeld, D., and Gatmaitan, Z.: Quantitation of Liver
     Structure and Function.  ed. R. Preiseg, Plenum Press,
     New York 1975.

28.  Ketterer, B., Tipping, E., Beale, D., and Meuwissen,J.A.T.P.:
     Ligandin, Glutathione Transferase and Carcinogen Binding.
     in GSH-Chemistry and Function.  ed. I.M. Arias, and W. Jakoby
     Raven Press, New York (in press).

29.  Kamisaka, K., Gatmaitan, Z., Moore, C., and Arias, I.M.:
     Ligandin Reverses Bilirubin Inhibition of Liver Mitochon-
     drial Respiration in Vitro.  Ped. Res. (in press).

30.  Kamisaka, K., Listowsky, I., Betheil, J., and Arias, I.M.:
     Competitive Binding of Bilirubin, Sulfobromophthalein,
     Indocyanine Green and Other Organic Anions to Human and
     Bovine Serum Albumin.  Biochem. Biophys. Acta
     365: 169, 1974.

31.  Kamisaka, K., Listowsky, I., Fleischner, G., Gatmaitan, Z.,
     and Arias, I.M.: Studies of the Binding of Bilirubin and
     Other Organic Anions to Serum Albumin and Ligandin (Y Pro-
     tein).  Birth Defects (Original Article Series) National
     Foundation, 1974 (in press).

32.  Kamisaka, K., Listowsky, I., Gatmaitan, Z., and Arias, I.M.:
     Circular Dichroism Analysis of the Secondary Structure of
     Z Protein and Its Complexes with Bilirubin and Other
     Organic Anions.  Biochem. Biophys. Acta 393: 24, 1975.

33. Listowsky, I., Kamisaka, K., and Arias, I.M.: Circular Dichroism Studies of Y Protein (Ligandin), a Major Organic Anion Binding Protein in Liver, Kidney and Small Intestine. Bulletin, N.Y. Acad. Sci. 226: 148, 1973.

34. Ockner, R.K.: Fatty Acid-Binding Protein in Small Intestine. Identification, Isolation, and Evidence for its Role in Cellular Fatty Acid Transport. J. Clin. Invest. 54: 326, 1974.

35. Mishkin, S., Stein, L., Fleischner, G., Gatmaitan, Z., and Arias, I.M.: Studies on the Role of Z Protein and Other Cytoplasmic Proteins in the Hepatic Uptake and Esterification of Long Chain Fatty Acids. Amer. J. Physiol. 1974 (in press).

36. Meijer, D.K.F., Arias, I.M., Levine, W.G., Gatmaitan, Z., Gluck, R., and Fleischner, G.: Effect of the Hypolipidemic drugs nafenopin and clofibrate on ligandin and Z, two hepatic cytoplasmic organic anion-binding proteins. BBRC (submitted)

DISCUSSION OF A LECTURE BY I. ARIAS

Forker:   Would you comment further on your data on the increase in P.A.H. $T_m$ with induction of ligandin in the kidney.

Arias:   In the liver, we think that transfer from blood into the cell appears to have no energy requirement, whereas transfer into bile requires energy.   In the proximal convoluted tubule the evidence indicates that the transfer from the blood into the cell is largely energy-dependent, whereas the transfer into the lumen is by diffusion.   There are diffusion factors which affect both of these, of course.   So it is difficult to see what the benefit is of increasing cytoplasmic protein.   This would tend to reduce, or at least not increase, the P.A.H. $T_m$.   So the nephrologists are as confused as we are about the mechanism of transport.

Brooks:   Have you tried adding your antibody to the perfusate in isolated liver and determining the effect on the net flux of some of the anions you have been studying?

Arias:   Yes, we have done that.   We literally filled the animal and the liver with as much antibody as we could and still have the animal survive.   But the results were very inconclusive, both in the perfused liver and the whole animal.

Bouchier:   Is there more ligandin present in acute liver failure or acute liver necrosis, and is the ligandin released into the plasma?

Arias:   We have done careful immunological studies looking for ligandin in patients and animals with a variety of acute and chronic liver injury, but we do not find any.   But in the early stages of acute tubular necrosis in man, ligandin appears in the urine, whereas normally there is none in urine.

Boyer:   There is very little ligandin in marine species, especially the elasmobranchs, and there is also very little albumin in the plasma of these species.   In the dogfish, shark and skate, the liver of these species can take up B.S.P., taurocholate and dibromosulphothalein and secrete it into the bile of these species over a period of several days.   Would not this

104

kind of observation support your thought that ligandin is acting
more as a sort of intracellular albumin than as a protein which
is critical for the selective uptake and ultimate excretion of
these substances.   Could you comment on that, and on the
evolutionary parallel between albumin and ligandin?

Arias:    Our original hypothesis was one which could be tested:
namely, is this protein within the liver responsible for influencing the net flux from plasma into the liver.   The hypothesis was
put in that way because there was no way of working with the
plasma membrane of the hepatocyte which could throw light on the
kinetic data presented earlier in terms of carrier proteins and
so on.   So the question was put, is this protein the determinant
of the net transfer?   Well it turns out that there are many
situations in which ligandin is not the total determinant.   Some
of these anions are not liphophilic;   indeed they are quite water-
soluble, and they have widely varying properties.   So one has to
admit that ligandin is not the sole determinant of the flux.
However, the evidence we have so far supports the hypothesis that
it is a determinant of net flux.   I suspect that until we can
design experiments to measure the anion transport on both sides
of the membrane we will have difficulty in coming to any definite
conclusions.   Now if it turns out that the purification processes
alter the binding properties of the protein, that would substantially depress our ability to produce models of how it might
function.   But the proof of its function remains a very difficult
problem.

Dianzani:    In my presentation I stated that the flux of non-
esterified fatty acids into the liver cells needs more attention
particularly with regard to the pathogenesis of fatty liver.   I
would like to know if it is possible to calculate how much influx
of fatty acids is due to protein Y and to protein Z.   There is a
type of fatty liver produced by phenobarbital in which there is
no decrease in biliary lipoprotein secretion, oxidation in mitochondria nor levels of non-esterified fatty acids in plasma.
However, you stated that there is 100 per cent increase in protein
Y, and therefore one might suppose that this type of fatty liver
is caused by an increased synthesis of non-esterified fatty acids,
and therefore an increase in supply of these acids to form more
triglycerides.   And just another small question, do you know
if flavospidic acid is active in vivo?   If it is, we might be
able to modify some types of fatty liver.

Arias:   Neither of these is a small question.   Let me try to
answer your second question first.   Flavospidic acid both in
vivo and in vitro, and without prior metabolism, binds with very
high affinity to protein Z.   When this binding occurs it
completely blocks free fatty acid binding both in vitro and in

vivo, but it has no effect on the hepatic uptake, esterification and utilisation of free fatty acids.

As for your first question about whether we can calculate what the role of either of these proteins could be in the control of free fatty acids. The answer is no. No more than we can calculate what the role is with respect to other substances, for the reasons which I mentioned. We can make associations, study binding characteristics and we can change variables and show net changes in movement, but I know of no way to make the calculation you are asking about. Z protein avidly binds long chain fatty acids, particularly the unsaturated types, but there is no evidence at the moment that this protein is specifically concerned with esterification, uptake or utilisation of fatty acids.

Preisig: You alluded to the fact that there is no animal model lacking ligandin. Yet several groups, including our own, have described patients who appear to lack the ability to store B.S.P. Have you had the opportunity to study such patients, and are they possibly ligandin-lacking models?

Arias: Yes, we have looked at such patients, including one of your own. They are possible models, as you suggest, but I would like to have some more solid facts before I make any comments about this. There are several situations in which people have described what would appear to be very low storage phenomena for organic anions, and we should certainly investigate this important area more fully.

Paumgartner: You mentioned that in previous studies, using a non-purified ligandin, it was not possible to show binding of bile acids to ligandin. It is interesting to learn now that if you use the purified preparation and circular dichroism, binding can be demonstrated. I would like to know if it is possible to calculate primary binding constants for these binding phenomena, and whether you can say anything about the specificity of this binding for bile acids?

Arias: All the substances shown in the circular dichroism experiments showed very low affinities. We have not done a complete study on bile acid binding to these proteins. We did some work with tracer amounts of labelled bile acids, but these did not bind at all to either protein. It is not surprising that with a purified protein a ligand could bind, whereas it might not do so in a more complex system in which the ligand could interact with other constituents such as lipids or other proteins and so on. But there is none of the specificity which prevails with bile salts that prevails with the dyes, bilirubin and some of the other ligands.

<u>Popper</u>:    I want to refer to the distribution of ligandin within the liver, and its possible relation to liver necrosis.    Since we do not know what initiates liver necrosis do you know if ligandin begins to disappear before liver injury, or only after necrosis has become established?

<u>Arias</u>:    We have done immunofluorescent studies with hamsters in which acetominophin and phenacetin over different times were used to induce liver injury, and just by examination of immunofluorescent pictures, it seems that there is no intermediate stage.    Necrotic cells do not seem to show any immunofluorescent reaction, whereas intact, and presumably normal, cells do.    There is nothing to suggest a zonal loss or reduction with any of the toxins we have looked at.

# EXCRETION OF XENOBIOTIC COMPOUNDS IN BILE

PETER MILLBURN

DEPARTMENT OF BIOCHEMISTRY

ST. MARY'S HOSPITAL MEDICAL SCHOOL, LONDON W2 UK

Most foreign compounds (xenobiotics) are metabolised in vivo
producing conjugates (e. g. glucuronides, sulphates, amino acid
conjugates), which are fairly strong organic acids and are readily excreted in either the urine or bile (see Williams and Millburn, 1975).
Compounds excreted in the bile may eventually be eliminated in the
faeces but prior to this they can undergo an enterohepatic circulation or
be metabolised in the intestine by the enzymes of the gut microflora.  The
latter can carry out a considerable number of reactions on xenobiotics,
particularly hydrolytic and reductive reactions, and in certain instances
this can lead to the production of toxic metabolites (see Williams 1972).
If the excretion of a compound in the bile leads to an enterohepatic
circulation this will prolong the presence of the compound or its
metabolites in the body.   This increases the chances of toxic reactions
occurring and may prolong the pharmacological effects of some
substances.   It is, therefore, important to know the types of xenobiotic
compounds excreted in bile and whether this excretory pattern varies
with species.

Before about 1950 the bile was relatively poorly investigated as a
route of excretion for xenobiotics; most work was concerned with the
identification of urinary metabolites of foreign compounds (see Williams,
1947).   In the past 25 years it has become increasingly apparent that
the bile is an important excretory channel for certain compounds and that
the extent of biliary excretion is related to molecular size.   Thus,
Brauer (1959) pointed out that substances which are highly concentrated
in bile are usually organic carboxylic acids with molecular weights of

the order of 300 or greater.  Sperber (1963) stated that ''the majority of the compounds efficiently secreted by the renal tubules have a relatively low molecular weight (200-400), whereas the substances excreted efficiently into bile usually have larger molecules (molecular weight above 400). ''

Since the early 1960's the factors that influence the extent of biliary excretion of xenobiotics have been studied in this laboratory.  Both physicochemical factors such as molecular weight, polarity, lipid solubility and molecular structure, and biological factors, namely species, metabolic transformations and, in rats, sex determine the extent to which organic compounds are excreted in bile.

## ORGANIC ANIONS

For organic anions the dominant factors governing the extent of their biliary elimination are molecular weight, polarity and species.  Thus, a relatively high molecular weight and the presence of a polar anionic group in the molecule are needed for extensive biliary excretion to occur. Many compounds acquire the necessary molecular weight and polarity by metabolism, particularly on conjugation with agents such as glucuronic acid.   The following two examples illustrate these points.

Phenol, a weak acid possessing an OH group, conjugates with glucuronic acid to form phenylglucuronide (mol. wt. 270).   The latter is a fairly strong acid (pKa 3. 4) which is almost completely ionized at physiological pH values and is readily excreted by the kidney, e. g. in the rat, guinea pig and rabbit some 50–95% of a dose of phenol is excreted in the  urine in 24 hours (Capel et al, 1972).   The biliary excretion of phenol is, however, low being only about 5% of the dose in the rat (Abou-El-Makarem et al. , 1967 a).  Phenolphthalein, like phenol, is conjugated with glucuronic acid in vivo.   But, in contrast to phenyl-glucuronide, phenolphthalein glucuronide (mol. wt. 495) is extensively excreted in the bile.   Thus, in the rat 85% of the dose of phenolphthalein is found in the bile as the glucuronide, and in the guinea pig and rabbit 20-30% (Abou-El-Makarem, 1967).

Therefore, both phenol and phenolphthalein are metabolized to water soluble conjugates, which are readily excreted.  However, relatively low molecular weight (below about 300) compounds such as phenylglucuronide are eliminated in the urine, irrespective of species (Abou-El-Makarem et al. 1967 a,b) whereas higher molecular weight compounds (above 300) are excreted in the bile, to an extent which varies with species (Abou-El-Makarem et al 1967 b).

There is a minimum (or threshold) molecular weight at which the elimination of compounds in the bile becomes appreciable (i. e. defined as 10% or more of the dose by Millburn et al. , 1967). For organic anions this threshold varies with species being about 325 ± 50 for the rat, 400 ±50 for the guinea pig and 475 ± 50 for the rabbit (Hirom et al. , 1972 a). Relatively little data is available for man, but the molecular weight threshold in our species is probably in the region of 500 (see Millburn, 1970). Organic anions with molecular weights above 500 appear to be extensively excreted in the bile by most species, including man. These thresholds are illustrated in Table 1, which shows the biliary and urinary excretion of six organic anions in four species, one of which is man.

The first two compounds in Table 1, namely benzoic acid (No. I) and 4-aminohippuric acid (No. II), are metabolised _in vivo_ to low molecular weight conjugates. In most species the major metabolite of benzoic acid is its glycine conjugate ; hippuric acid (mol. wt. 179 ; Bridges et al, 1970). 4-Aminohippuric acid (mol. wt. 194) is excreted both unchanged and as its acetylated product ; 4-acetamidohippuric acid (mol. wt. 236). The Table shows that these conjugates are eliminated almost entirely in the urine in the rat, guinea pig, rabbit and man, with less than 10% of the dose in the bile. Benzoic and 4-aminohippuric acids have a similar low biliary excretion in other species such as the dog, cat and hen (Abou-El-Makarem et al. , 1967 b).

The next compound, succinylsulphathiazole (No. III), in Table 1 has a molecular weight of 355 and is extensively (nearly 40% of the dose) excreted unchanged in the bile in the rat, but not in the guinea pig or rabbit. The biliary excretion of succinylsulphathiazole differs between the rat and rabbit in several respects (Abou-El-Makarem et al. , 1967 c). Thus, not only is the excretion in the bile much higher in the rat than in the rabbit, but in the rat succinylsulphathiazole readily enters the liver and biliary excretion occurs against a concentration gradient from liver to bile. Furthermore, in the rat the excretory process can be saturated and can be depressed by the simultaneous administration of phenol-phthalein glucuronide or bile salts. In the rabbbit this sulphonamide does not readily enter the liver from the blood, there is no transfer of the drug from the hepatic cells into the bile against a concentration gradient, and no saturation or depression of the biliary excretion of succinylsulphathiazole is found. Thus, the rat appears to have an hepatic mechanism for the concentrative transfer of succinylsulphathiazole from blood into bile, whereas the rabbit does not appear to possess such a mechanism for this compound.

Table 1      The relationship of the molecular weight of organic anions to their biliary and urinary excretion

The compounds were injected into bile-duct-cannulated animals or patients with biliary T-tube drainage. The % of dose excreted in bile and urine are given. B = Bile ; U = Urine

| Compound No.* (Mol. wt.) | RAT | | GUINEA PIG | | RABBIT | | MAN | |
|---|---|---|---|---|---|---|---|---|
| | B | U | B | U | B | U | B | U |
| I (179) | 1 | 90 | 2 | 90 | 1 | 90 | – | 99 |
| II (194) | 1 | – | 7 | – | 3 | – | 2 | 64 |
| III (355) | 36 | 58 | 6 | 29 | 1 | 80 | – | – |
| IV (461) | 49 | 23 | 48 | 30 | 8 | 58 | 2 | 84 |
| V (505) | 90 | 2 | 75 | 12 | 85 | 8 | – | – |
| VI (752) | 82 | 0 | 97 | 0 | 94 | 0 | 66 | 0 |

* The compounds are identified by their numbers in the text.

Following succinylsulphathiazole is morphine (No. IV in Table 1), which is metabolized to morphine-3-glucuronide (mol. wt. 461). This glucuronide has a high biliary excretion (nearly half the dose of the administered morphine) in the rat and guinea pig but not in the rabbit or man.

The last two compounds in Table 1, namely Lissamine Fast Yellow (No. V) and Indocyanine Green (No. VI), are both organic anions with molecular weights above 500 and are excreted unchanged predominantly in the bile of all species so far investigated.

Table 1 also illustrates the inter-relationship of the urine and bile as excretory routes for xenobiotic compounds. Thus, urine and bile are complementary pathways ; the extent of urinary excretion is greatest for organic anions of low molecular weight and tends to decrease as molecular weight increases and biliary excretion becomes more extensive. The inter-relation between the excretory roles of the liver and kidney is further illustrated in Table 2, which shows the urinary and biliary excretion of three organic anions in the rat and the effect of preventing either urine or bile formation on the pattern of elimination of these compounds. The compounds are benzoic acid (No. 1), glutarylsulphathiazole (No. VII) and Indocyanine Green (No. VI). Glutarylsulphathiazole is structurely-related to succinylsulphathizole discussed above, and like-wise is excreted unchanged (Hirom et al. , 1972 b).

Benzoic acid is excreted mainly as its glycine conjugate in the urine of rats. Hippuric acid has molecular weight (179) below the threshold value for appreciable biliary excretion in the rat and even when urinary excretion is prevented, by ligating the renal pedicles, only 5% of the dose of benzoic acid (No. I) is excreted in the bile (Table 2). In contrast, glutarylsulphathiazole (No. VII) has a molecular weight (369) within the threshold region and between 40 and 50% of the dose is found in the bile and a similar amount in the urine. When renal excretion is prevented over 80% of the dose of this compound is found in the bile, and on obstructing the bile duct a similar percentage is excreted in the urine. Glutarylsulphathiazole, therefore, is excreted in large amounts by both the liver and kidneys and when one of these two excretory routes is blocked the amount excreted by the other increases markedly. Indocycanine Green (No. VI ; mol. wt. 752 ; above the biliary threshold value) is predominantly eliminated in the bile of rats and none is found in the urine even on obstructing the bile duct.

Table 2        The inter-relationship of urinary and biliary excretion for three
xenobiotics in the rat

The compounds were injected intravenously into either (a) bile-duct-cannulated rats, (b) bile-duct-cannulated rats with their renal pedicles ligated to prevent urine formation or (c) rats with their bile ducts ligated to prevent bile formation.

| Compound Administered * | Hepatic Excretion | Renal Excretion | % of dose excreted in 3 h | |
|---|---|---|---|---|
| | | | Bile | Urine |
| (mol. wt.) | | | | |
| I (179) | intact | intact | 1 | 90 |
| | intact | prevented | 5 | – |
| VII (369) | intact | intact | 42 | 47 |
| | intact | prevented | 85 | – |
| | prevented | intact | – | 83 |
| VI (752) | intact | intact | 82 | 0 |
| | prevented | intact | – | 0 |

* The compounds (all organic anions) are identified by their numbers in the text.

In general, in the rat and probably in other species too, compounds with molecular weights below the threshold value for appreciable biliary excretion are poorly excreted in the bile even when urinary excretion is prevented.   Compounds within the threshold molecular weight range can be excreted in both urine and bile in appreciable amounts and the extent to which they are eliminated by one route can be markedly increased if the other route is blocked.  Xenobiotics with molecular weights above the threshold value appear to have a high affinity for hepatic clearance and only small amounts appear in urine even on biliary obstruction.

The above criteria of molecular weight and polarity appear to apply not only to the biliary excretion of xenobiotic compounds, but to certain endogenous substances as well.   Thus, natural organic components of bile such as the bile acid conjugates, glycocholic acid (mol. wt. 466) and taurocholic acid (mol. wt. 516), and bilirubin diglucuronide (mol. wt. 937) have relatively high molecular weights and are strongly polar. Other endogenous metabolites like the glucuronides and sulphates of steroids, which have molecular weights in the region of 350-500, are eliminated from the body via the bile in considerable amounts (see Millburn, 1970 ; Taylor, 1971 and Smith, 1974).

## ORGANIC CATIONS

The extent to which organic cations, that is quaternary ammonium cations, are eliminated in the bile is also determined by molecular weight.  Quaternary ammonium compounds are very strong bases and their salts are completely ionized at physiological pH values.  Such compounds are used as drugs, detergents and antiseptics.  Hughes et al., (1973 a,b) have made a systematic study of the biliary excretion of both mono- and di-quaternary compounds.   They found that the threshold molecular weight for appreciable biliary excretion of monoquaternary cations is different from that for anions being about 200 ± 50 and in contrast to the anions shows no significant inter-species variations between rats, guinea pigs and rabbits.  It has been suggested by Schanker and Solomon (1963) that the liver has an active secretary process for the transport of quaternary ammonium ions from blood to bile and that this process is different from that for organic anions.   It is, therefore, not surprising that the molecular weight thresholds for organic cations and anions are different.

The relationship of molecular weight to the biliary excretion of monoquaternary cations is illustrated in Table 3, which shows the extent of biliary and urinary excretion of six monoquaternary ammonium cations in the rat, guinea pig and rabbit.

Table 3        Molecular weight and the biliary excretion of monoquaternary cations
in different species

The compounds were injected intraperitoneally into bile-duct-cannulated animals.   The % of dose excreted in
bile and urine are given.    B = Bile ; U = Urine

| Cation Administered* (Mol. wt.) | RAT | | GUINEA PIG | | RABBIT | |
|---|---|---|---|---|---|---|
| | B | U | B | U | B | U |
| VIII (130) | 0.4 | 72 | 0.5 | 75 | 2 | 43 |
| IX (136) | 0.5 | 70 | 0.1 | 17 | 0.4 | 32 |
| X (164) | 6 | 59 | 1 | 33 | 6 | 41 |
| XI (192) | 12 | 65 | 27 | 19 | 13 | 36 |
| XII (226) | 27 | 21 | 41 | 5 | 29 | 20 |
| XIII (302) | 39 | 16 | 38 | 2 | 41 | 10 |

*These cations were administered as either the bromide or iodine salts, and are identified by their numbers
in the text.   Data from Hughes, et al., (1973 a).

These strongly polar compounds are excreted largely unchanged. Tetraethylammonium (No. VIII in Table 3) and trimethylphenylammonium (No. IX) with molecular weights below 150 are very poorly excreted in the bile in all three species ; the urine is the main channel of elimination for these two monocations. The next three compounds in Table 3, namely diethylmethylphenylammonium (No. X), methylphenyldipropylammonium (No. XI) and dibenzyldimethylammonium (No. XII) have molecular weights within the threshold region of 150-250 and the biliary excretion of No. X is below 10% of the dose, but that of the other two cations is greater than this. The last cation in Table 3, namely tribenzylmethylammonium (No. XIII) has a molecular weight (302) above the threshold value for appreciable biliary excretion and about 40% of the dose is found in the bile of all three species. There does not appear to be any very significant inter-species variation in the pattern of biliary and urinary elimination of these six monoquaternary cations. There may be some species difference within the threshold region since the guinea pig differs from the rat and rabbit in the extent of biliary excretion of cations Nos. X, XI and XII. However, this difference is not consistent, since the biliary excretion of cation No. X is lower in the guinea pig than in the rat and rabbit whereas for cations Nos. XI and XII the reverse is true.

The biliary excretion of diquaternary organic cations has been less extensively studied than is the case for monocations and anions. However, the information available is sufficient to make the tentative suggestion that the minimum molecular weight for the appreciable biliary excretion of dications is different from that for monoquaternary compounds and anions and is probably in the region of at least 500-600 (see Hughes et al. , 1973 b). Thus, dications such as paraquat (mol. wt. 186) and decamethonium (mol. wt. 258) are excreted in the bile of rats, guinea pigs and rabbits to the extent of only 1-2% of the dose ; they are eliminated mainly in the urine. In general dications with molecular weights below 500 are excreted in the bile to an extent of less than 10% of the dose. The biliary excretion of only a few dications with molecular weights greater than 500 has been studied. However, the muscle relaxant hexafluorenium (mol. wt. 503), d-tubocurarine (mol. wt. 611) and dimethyltubocurarine (mol. wt. 653) all have a biliary excretion of between about 20 and 40% of the dose in rats (see Hughes et al, 1973 b). At present there is insufficient information to decide whether the molecular weight threshold for more than 10% biliary excretion of these dications varies significantly between species, but it appears to be unlikely.

## GLYCOSIDES

Certain organic compounds that are neither anions nor cations are
excreted in bile.   One important class of compounds which fall into
this category of uncharged organic molecules are glycosides.   Detoxication of foreign compounds by conjugation with glucose, which is of
major importance in insects , is a rare metabolic reaction in
mammals (see Williams & Millburn, 1975).   However, for some classes
of xenobiotic substances conjugation with glucose by mammals may
turn out to be more significant than hitherto thought.   Thus, 3-(4-
pyrimidinyl)-5-(4-pyridyl)-1,2,4-triazole, a potent competitive inhibitor
or xanthine oxidase, is extensively (more than 60% of the dose)
eliminated in the bile of dogs as an N-glucose conjugate (mol. wt. 386 ;
Duggan et al. , 1974).   Important glycosides that are widely used in
medicine are the cardioactive glycosides, which are found in certain
plants.   A number of cardioactive glycosides have been shown to be
excreted in the bile following their administration to experimental
animals (see Millburn, 1970 ; Smith, 1973), although their biliary
excretion has not been systematically studied as is the case for organic
anions and cations.   Such compounds have relatively high molecular
weights and because of their sugar residues are polar, two properties
which they share with organic anions and cations that are eliminated in
bile in considerable amounts.

## MOLECULAR WEIGHT, LIPID SOLUBILITY AND BILIARY EXCRETION

The above studies indicate that a xenobiotic molecule requires both
a polar, water soluble group (either anionic, cationic or possibly a
sugar residue) in its structure and a minimum molecular weight for its
biliary excretion to be appreciable.   That the molecular weight of a
compound influences its biliary excretion is an empirical finding.
Naturally, molecular weight in itself does not determine the extent to
which a molecule is excreted by the liver into the bile.   Preliminary
studies with both organic anions and cations indicate that their molecular
weights are closely related to their lipid solubilities (Hirom et al. , 1974).
Thus, although polar conjugates of xenobiotics are usually thought of as
water soluble excretory products, certain conjugates (e. g. phenolphthalein
glucuronide) have some lipophilic character.   This is estimated by
measuring the partition ratios of compounds between octan-1-ol and
0.1$\underline{M}$-phosphate buffer, pH 7.4, a model system for both biological
lipid and aqueous phases.   In general, the high molecular weight organic
anions and cations, which are excreted in bile, appear to be relatively
more lipophilic than the low molecular weight polar compounds , which

are eliminated in urine.   Furthermore, the extent to which penicillins are excreted in the bile in the rat appears to be related to the balance between non-polar and polar groups within their molecular structures (Ryrfeldt, 1971).   One can, therefore,  tentatively suggest that the threshold molecular weight values given above reflect the underlying physicochemical property of a minimum lipid solubility of these polar organic molecules.   This may imply that a certain balance between hydro-phobic and hydrophilic properties (amphiphilicity) is required before a compound can cross liver cell membranes and be excreted in the bile.

## STRUCTURAL FACTORS IN BILIARY EXCRETION

Provided the above requirements of molecular weight and polarity are satisfied, the extent of biliary excretion can be influenced by several facets of molecular structure (Hirom et al. , 1972 b).   Thus, the glucuronic acid conjugate of 4, 4'-dihydroxybiphenyl (mol. wt. 362) has a much higher biliary excretion (about 90% of the dose) in the rat than 4-hydroxybiphenylglucuronide (mo. wt. 346 ; 60% of dose in bile) and yet these two molecules differ in structure by only a single -OH group (Millburn, et al. , 1967).

Excretion in the bile can also be influenced by the shape of the mole-cule.   This structural factor is shown by the three compounds, phthalyl-, 1, 2, 3, 6-tetrahydrophthalyl - and hexahydrophthalyl-sulphathiazole, in Table 4.   These three sulphonamides all have molecular weights of about 400 and yet, in the rat and guinea pig, the extent of biliary elimination of the last two is considerably higher than that of the first (e. g. the biliary excretion of hexahydrophthalylsulphathiazole is about 3-4 times that of phthalylsulphathiazole).   This increase may be related to the fact that phthalylsulphathiazole contains a flat benzene ring whereas the tetra- and hexa-hydro compounds are different in shape having puckered six mem-bered rings in their structures.   In the rabbit, this structural factor is relatively unimportant for these compounds.   Thus, although the extent of biliary excretion of hexahydrophthalylsulphathiazole is higher than that of phthalylsulphathiazole, it is still not appreciable (ie. 10% of more of the dose), since the molecular weights of   both   compounds are below the threshold value for the rabbit (475 $\pm$ 50).   This illustrates that the primary requirement for the appreciable biliary excretion of a polar molecule is that it satisfies the molecular weight thresholds given above.

The position of polar groups in a molecule's structure may also influence biliary excretion.   Thus, Iga and coworkers (1970 ; 1971) on studying the elimination of some dyes in the bile of rats, found that the shift of a single $SO_3^-$ group from one position to another within the

Table 4          Structural factors in biliary excretion

The compounds were injected intravenously (100 μmol/kg) into bile-duct-cannulated animals.

| COMPOUND | MOL. WT | % DOSE IN BILE | | |
| --- | --- | --- | --- | --- |
| | | RAT | GUINEA PIG | RABBIT |
| Phthalylsulphathiazole | 403 | 22 | 16 | 2.5 |
| 1,2,3,6-Tetrahydrophthalyl-sulphathiazole | 407 | 45 | 25 | – |
| Hexahydrophthalyl-sulphathiazole | 409 | 80 | 44 | 8.1 |

Data from Hirom, et al., (1972 a).

molecule caused a 4-8 fold change in the extent of biliary excretion.

## SEX DIFFERENCES IN BILARY
## EXCRETION

There is a marked sex difference in the biliary excretion in the rat of food dye Tartrazine, but not of the structurely-related compound Lissamine Fast Yellow.    This sex difference is not found in the guinea pig or rabbit.    Thus, female Wistar albino rats excrete about 30% of the dose of Tartrazine in the bile, whereas the biliary excretion of this organic anion in male rats is only about half this value (Gregson et al. , 1972).    Treatment of male rats with oestradiol increases the biliary excretion of Tartrazine to that found in normal females, and , conversely, treatment of female rats with testosterone decreases the biliary excretion of Tartrazine to that found in normal males (Bertagni et al. , 1972). In contrast to Tartrazine, the extent of biliary elimination of Lissamine Fast Yellow is about 80-90% of the dose in rats, guinea pigs or rabbits of either sex.    There are a few other reports on sex differences in the extent of biliary excretion of xenobiotic compounds in the rat (Gregson et al. , 1972).

## MECHANISM OF EXCRETION OF
## XENOBIOTICS IN THE BILE

It has been shown above that the liver selectively excretes relatively high molecular weight polar compounds into bile.  The biochemical basis for this preference and the nature of the mechanism involved in the hepatic transfer of xenobiotic compounds from blood into bile are not known.   The overall process of biliary excretion can be considered to take place in three stages ; (a) uptake of compounds into the liver from the blood, (b) events occuring within hepatic cells, and (c) passage of compounds from the liver cells into the bile.

As regards hepatic uptake, two proteins "Y" and "Z" have been separated from liver cytoplasm by gel filtration (Levi et al. , 1969).   These proteins bind bilirubin, sulphobromophthalein and other anionic substances such as Indocyanine Green.  Arias and his co-workers have proposed that these proteins are  involved in the selective transfer of organic anions from blood into the liver (see Fleischner et al. , 1972).   Y protein appears to be identical to a carcinogen-binding hepatic protein and also to another protein binding certain steroids and their metabolites, & has been called ligandin. (Litwack et al. , 1971). Recently the roles of the Y and Z binding proteins in the hepato-biliary transport of organic anions has been investigated by

Takada, et al. , (1974).   Of five organic anions studied, all were bound
to Y protein (ligandin), but only those for which the liver/plasma concentration ratios were greater than one were bound to Z protein.   It is
interesting that these workers found that Bromophenol Blue (mol. wt. 670),
which has a high biliary excretion, was much more extensively bound to
a rat liver cytoplasmic protein fraction than 4-acetamidohippuric acid
(mol. wt. 236), which has a low biliary excretion.

One clearly important biochemical event occurring within the liver
cells is the metabolic transformation of xenobiotics into water soluble
conjugates.   This introduction of a polar grouping into the molecule is a
crucial step in the formation of a substance with the requisite parameters
of molecular size and polarity for appreciable biliary excretion.   Although experimentally one tends to use polar compounds which are not
metabolised to study biliary excretion - this avoids any complications
due to metabolism ; for example differences in rates of metabolism
between species - the majority of foreign compounds encountered by the
body are metabolised prior to excretion.

The importance of metabolism for the biliary excretion of xenobiotic
compounds is shown by the following experiments (Levine et al. , 1970).
The metabolic transformations of xenobiotics occur mainly in the hepatic
endoplasmic reticulum and the enzymes carrying out this metabolism
can be induced by phenobarbitone and inhibited by agents such as SKF
525 -A.   Pretreatment of rats with phenobarbitone for several days
almost doubles the extent of biliary excretion of biphenyl, which has to
be hydroxylated and then conjugated with glucuronic acid before appearing
in bile.   Phenobarbitone treatment also enchances the biliary excretion
of phenolphthalein and stilboestrol by rats.    Both compounds are
conjugated w ith glucuronic acid before their elimination in bile.   However,
phenobarbitone treatment does not stimulate the hepatic transport into bile
of administered phenolphthalein glucuronide and stilboestrol glucuronide,
which are excreted without prior metabolism.   This  suggests that the
increased rate of excretion of phenolphthalein and stilboestrol is due to
their accelerated rate of glucuronide formation following phenobarbitone
treatment.   Conversely, SKF 525 - A, which inhibits glucuronide synthesis,
reduces the biliary excretion of phenolphthalein and stilboestrol by the rat.

Probably the commonest conjugates of xenobiotics found in bile are
glucuronides.   The enzyme catalysing the glucuronidation of xenobiotics
is UDP-glucuronyltransferase (E. C. 2. 4. 1. 17), which is located in the
endoplasmic reticulum of liver cells. The activity of this enzyme is
dependent on the integrity of the endoplasmic reticulum structure and a

number of biochemical investigations have suggested that UDP-glucuronyltransferase is located in the deep layers of the microsomal membrane.
Thus,  treatment of hepatic microsomes with agents which tend to
remove the outer layers of the membrane such as surfactants (Vainio
and Hanninen, 1972) and chaotropic agents (e. g. $SCN^-$, $I^-$, $NO_3^-$ and
urea ; Vainio, 1973 a) result in an increase of measurable UDP-
glucuronyltransferase activity, but inhibit hydroxylation reactions.  The
oxidising enzymes are, therefore, thought to be more superficially
located in the endoplasmic reticulum membranes than is the glucuron-
idating enzyme.  Vainio (1973 b) has speculated that there may be a
multienzyme complex (consisting of the xenobiotic oxidising enzymes
together with UDP- glucuronyltransferase) which functions vectorially
in transporting metabolic products (ie. glucuronides) into the reticular
lumen before excretion from the liver.

Following  hepatic metabolism conjugates of xenobiotics such as
phenolphthalein glucuronide and stilboestrol glucuronide are thought
to cross liver cell membranes into the bile canaliculae.  One major
problem that has yet to be overcome technically is that of obtaining
primary bile ; canalicular bile.  Our understanding of the mechanisms
involved in renal excretion (ie. tubular reabsorption and secretion)
depended largely on experiments in which samples of the glomerular filtrate
were obtained from the various regions of the kidney tubules.  At present
we do not know the composition of primary bile, but it has been suggested
by several authors that as the bile passes down the biliary tract its
composition may be altered by the reabsorption of water and solutes(see
Clark et al. , 1971 for references).  In particular, recent work by
Peterson and Fujimoto (1973) suggests that, in the rat, bile is concentrated
by the extensive reabsorption of water from the biliary tree.

Preliminary studies in this laboratory (Hirom, 1970 ; Clark et al. ,
1971) suggest that low molecular weight organic anions, which on intravenous or intraperitoneal administration are poorly excreted in the bile,
are readily absorbed from the biliary tree of the rat.  In contrast,
relatively high molecular weight organic anions, which are extensively
excreted in bile, appear to be relatively poorly absorbed from the biliary
tract (see Table 5).   The first three conjugates in Table 5, namely
hippuric acid, 3-aminophenylsulphate and 2-aminophenylglucuronide, have
molecular weights below 300 and on intravenous administration are poorly
(less than 10% of dose) excreted in the bile.  When these compounds are
infused into the biliary tree less than 15% of the dose is recovered in the
bile within 30 min.  These three low molecular weight conjugates, there -
fore, appear to be rapidly absorbed from the biliary system, and following

Table 5    Absorption of some conjugates from the biliary tree compared with their biliary excretion in the rat

The conjugates were administered to bile-duct-cannulated rats either (A) intravenously or (B) by retrograde intrabiliary infusion into the biliary tree.

| Conjugate (mol. wt.) | (A) % dose excreted in bile in 3 h. | (B) % dose recovered in bile at | | |
|---|---|---|---|---|
| | | 5 min. | 15 min. | 30 min. |
| Hippuric acid (179) | 5 | 12 | 14 | 14 |
| 3-Aminophenylsulphate (189) | 1 | 6 | 7 | 7 |
| 2-Aminophenylglucuronide (285) | 4 | 12 | 13 | 14 |
| Stilboestrol glucuronide (445) | 92 | 43 | 68 | 78 |
| Phenolphthalein disulphate (479) | 76 | 31 | 47 | 65 |
| Phenolphthalein glucuronide (495) | 96 | 29 | 41 | 65 |

Date from Clark, et al., (1971)

the intrabiliary administration of hippuric acid nearly 50% of the amount infused is recovered in the urine in 30 min., and 70% in 1 hour.  The last three conjugates in Table 5, namely stilboestrol glucuronide, phenolphthalein disulphate and phenolphthalein glucuronide have molecular weights in the region of 450-500, and by comparison with the above low molecular weight conjugates, appear to be more slowly absorbed from the biliary tract, since following their retrograde intrabiliary infusion, relatively large amounts (30-40% of the amount infused) are recovered in the bile 5 min. after stopping the infusion.  However, some absorption of these higher molecular weight xenobiotics from the biliary tree, followed by excretion into the bile, probably occurs.   Thus, after their retrograde biliary infusion, the amounts recovered in bile at 30 min are higher than at 5 min., whereas for the low molecular weight conjugates the amounts recovered at 5 and 30 min are about the same (see Table 5). Phenolphthalein glucuronide has been detected in the systemic blood following its retrograde biliary administration to rats (Gustafson and Benet 1974), confirming that some absorption of this glucuronide from the biliary tract does take place.

The absorption of succinylsulphathiazole  from the biliary tract has been compared in two species, namely the rat and rabbit (Hirom, 1970). Succinylsulphathiazole shows a marked species difference in the extent of its biliary excretion (compound No. III in Table 1) ; about 40% of the dose appearing in the bile in the rat, but only 1% in the rabbit.   This xenobiotic shows a more extensive absorption from the biliary system of the rabbit than of the rat.   Thus, following the infusion of succinylsulphathiazole into the biliary tree of the rabbit, less than 1% of the amount infused is recovered in the bile in 30 min. , compared with nearly 30% in the rat. This observation raises the question as to whether intra-species variations in the extent of biliary excretion of xenobiotics are related to species differences in the extent to which such compounds are reabsorbed from the biliary system.

Xenobiotics, therefore, appear to be absorbed at differing rates from the biliary system of the rat.  This may at least partly explain the empirical finding that high molecular weight compounds are more extensively excreted in the bile than low molecular weight substances. Thus, organic anions of relatively low molecular weight appear to be readily absorbed from the biliary tract, whereas higher molecular weight compounds are relatively poorly absorbed. This hypothesis should be tested with a wide variety of foreign compounds and the absorption of xenobiotics from the biliary system needs to be compared in different species.

REFERENCES

Abou-El-Makarem, M. M. (1967). Studies on the Biliary Excretion of Some Foreign Organic Compounds in Different Species. Ph. D. Thesis. University of London.

Abou-El-Makarem, M. M., Millburn, P., Smith, R. L. and Williams, R. T. (1967 a). Biliary Excretion of Foreign Compounds ; Benzene and its Derivatives in the Rat, Biochem. J. 105, 1269-1274.

Abou-El-Makarem, M. M., Millburn, P., Smith R. L. and Williams R. T. (1967 b). Biliary Excretion of Foreign Compounds ; Species Differences in Biliary Excretion, Biochem. J. 105, 1289-1293.

Abou-El-Makarem, M. M., Millburn, P., and Smith R. L. (1967 c) Biliary Excretion of [$^{14}$C]Succinylsulphathiazole in the Rat and Rabbit, Biochem. J. 105, 1295-1299.

Bertagni, P., Hirom, P. C., Millburn, P., Osiyemi, F. O., Smith, R. L., Turbert, H. B. and Williams, R. T. (1972) Sex and Species Differences in the Biliary Excretion of Tartrazine and Lissamine Fast Yellow in the Rat, Guinea Pig and Rabbit. The influence of Sex Hormones on Tartrazine Excretion in the Rat, J. Pharm. Pharmacol. 24, 620-624.

Brauer, R. W. (1959) Mechanisms of Bile Secretion, J. Amer. Med. Ass., 169, 1462-1466.

Bridges, J. W., French, M. R., Smith, R. L. and Williams, R. T. (1970) The Fate of Benzoic Acid in Various Species, Biochem. J. 118, 47-51.

Capel, I. D., French, M. R., Millburn, P., Smith, R. L. and Williams R. T. (1972). The Fate of [$^{14}$C] Phenol in Various Species, Xenobiotica 2, 25-34.

Duggan, D. E., Baldwin, J. J., Arison, B. H. and Rhodes, R. E. (1974) N-Glucoside Formation as a Detoxification Mechanism in Mammals, J. Pharmacol. Exp. Ther. 190, 563-569.

Fleischner, G., Robbins, J., and Arias, I. M. (1972) Immunological Studies of Y Protein. A Major Cytoplasmic Organic Anion-Binding Protein in Rat Liver, J. Clin. Invest. 51, 677-684.

Gregson, R. H. S. , Hirom, P. C. , Millburn, P. , Smith ,R. L., Turbert, H. B. and Williams, R. T. (1972) The Biliary Excretion of Tartrazine. Sex Differences in the Rat and Species Differences in the Rat, Guinea Pig and Rabbit, J. Pharm . Pharmacol 24, 20-24.

Gustafson, J. H. , and Benet, L. Z. (1974) Biliary Excretion Kinetics of Phenolphthalein glucuronide after intravenous and retrograde biliary administration, J. Pharm. Pharmacol. 26, 937-944.

Hirom, P. C. (1970) Factors Influencing the Biliary Excretion of Organic Compounds, Ph. D. Thesis, University of London.

Hirom, P. C. , Millburn, P. , Smith, R. L. , and Williams, R. T. (1972 a). Species Variations in the Threshold Molecular-Weight Factor for the Biliary Excretion of Organic Anions, Biochem. J. 129, 1071-1077.

Hirom, P. C. , Millburn, P. , Smith, R. L. and Williams, R. T. (1972 b). Molecular Weight and Chemical Structure as Factors  in the Biliary Excretion of Sulphonamides in the Rat. Xenobiotica, 2, 205-214.

Hirom, P. C. , Hughes, R. D. and Millburn, P. (1974) The Physicochem- ical Factor Required for the Biliary Excretion of Organic Cations and Anions. , Biochem. Soc. Trans. 2, 327-330.

Hughes, R. D. , Millburn, P. , and Williams, R. T. (1973 a). Molecular Weight as a Factor in the Excretion of Monoquaternary Ammonium Cations in the Bile of the Rat, Rabbit and Guinea Pig, Biochem. J. 136, 967-978.

Hughes, R. D. , Millburn, P. , and Williams, R. T. (1973 b) Biliary Excretion of Some Diquaternary Ammonium Cations in the Rat, Guinea Pig and Rabbit  Biochem. J. 136, 979-984.

Iga, T. , Awazu, S. , Hanano, M and Nogami, H. , (1970) Pharmacokinetic Studies of Biliary Excretion I. Comparison of the Excretion Behaviour In Azo Dyes and Indigo Carmine, Chem. Pharm. Bull. Tokyo, 18, 2431-2440.

Iga, T. , Awazu, S. , and Nogami, H. (1971) Pharmacokinetic Study of Biliary Excretion II.  Comparison of Excretion Behaviour in Triphenylmethane Dyes, Chem. Pharm. Bull. , Tokyo, 19, 273-281.

Levi, A. J., Gatmaitan, Z. and Arias, I. M. (1969) Two Hepatic
Cytoplasmic Protein Fractions, Y and Z, and their Possible Role in
the Hepatic Uptake of Bilirubin,Sulfobromophthalein, and other Anions.
J. Clin. Invest. 48, 2156-2167.

Levine, W. G., Millburn, P., Smith, R. L. and Williams, R. T. (1970)
The Role of the Hepatic Endoplasmic Reticulum in the Biliary Excretion of Foreign compounds by the Rat. The Effect of Phenobarbitone
and SKF 525-A (Diethylaminoethyl Diphenylpropylacetate), Biochem.
Pharmacol. 19, 235-244.

Litwack, G., Ketterer, B., and Arias, I. M. (1971) Ligandin : A Hepatic
Protein which binds Steroids, Bilirubin, Carcinogens and a Number of
Exogenous Organic Anions, Nature, Lond., 234, 466-467.

Millburn, P. (1970) Factors in the Biliary Excretion of Organic Compounds
In Metabolic Conjugation and  Metabolic Hydrolysis (Fishman,W. H.,
ed.) Vol. 2. pp. 1-74, Academic Press, London.

Millburn, P., Smith, R. L. and Williams, R. T. (1967) Biliary Excretion
of Foreign Compounds ; Biphenyl, Stilboestrol and Phenolphthalein
in the Rat : Molecular Weight, Polarity and Metabolism as Factors in
Biliary Excretion. Biochem. J. 105, 1275-1281.

Peterson, R. E. and Fujimoto, J. M. (1973) Retrograde Intrabiliary Injection : Absorption of Water and Other Compounds from the Rat
Biliary Tree, J. Pharmacol. Exp. Ther. 185, 150-162.

Schanker, L. S. and Solomon, H. M. (1963). Active Transport of
Quaternary Ammonium Compounds into Bile. Amer. J. Physiol.
204, 829-832.

Smith, R. L. (1974) Biliary Excretion and Hepatotoxicity of Contraceptive
Steroids. Acta Endocr., Copenh. 75, Suppl. 185, pp. 149-168.

Ryrfeldt, A. (1971) Biliary Excretion of Penicillins in the Rat, J. Pharm.
Pharmacol., 23, 463-464.

Smith, R. L. (1973) The Excretory Function of Bile. Chapman and Hall,
London.

Sperber, I., (1963) Biliary Excretion and Choleresis. In Proceedings
of the First International Pharmacological Meeting, August 22-25,
1961, Vol. 4, Drugs and Membranes. (Hogben, C. A. M., ed) pp.
137-143, Pergamon Press Ltd., London.

Takada, K., Ueda, M., Ohno, M. and Muranishi, S. (1974) Biopharm-
aceutical Study of the Hepato-Biliary Transport of Drugs II.   Roles
of the Liver Cytoplasmic Y and Z Binding Proteins and T Binder on
the Hepato-Biliary Transport of Organic Anionic Compounds.
Chem. Pharm. Bull., Tokyo, 22, 1477-1486.

Taylor, W.   (1971) The Excretion of Steroid Hormone Metabolites in
Bile and Faeces, Vitam. Horm. (New York) 29,  201-285.

Vainio, H. (1973 a)  Action of Chaotropic Agents on Drug-Metabolizing
Enzymes in Hepatic Microsomes, Biochim. Biophys. Acta, 307, 152-
161.

Vainio, H. (1973 b) On the Topology and Synthesis of Drug-Metabolizing
Enzymes inHepatic Endoplasmic Reticulum, M. D. Thesis, University
of Turku, Finland.

Vainio, H. and Hanninen, O. (1972) Effect of Surfactants on Drug
Metabolism in Hepatic Microsomes, Suomen Kemistilehti (Finn. Chem.
J.) B 45, 56-61.

Williams, R. T. (1947) Detoxication Mechanisms, Chapman and Hall,
London

Williams, R. T. (1972) Toxicologic Implications of Biotransformation by
Intestinal Microflora. Toxicol. Appl. Pharmacol. 23,  769-781.

Williams, R. T. and Millburn, P. (1975) Detoxication Mechanisms ;
The Biochemistry of  Foreign Compounds, in MTP International
Review of Science, Biochemistry Series One, Vol. 12. Physiological
and Pharmacological Biochemistry. (Blaschko, H. K. F., ed) pp. 211-
266, Butterworths, London.

DISCUSSION OF LECTURE BY P. MILLBURN

Bradley:   I would like to make a comment as a renal physiologist.
I am sure the same problem has occurred to many other people here.
In renal physiology we have been plagued for years with the
problem of how to evaluate disappearance curves.   Some 50 years
ago now the clearance concept was introduced primarily as a means
of dealing with this problem because disappearance curves coupled
with recovery of a dose in urine is extremely difficult to
interpret in terms of mechanisms of transport and renal excretion
owing to the multifactorial systems that are involved.   One must
cope with the problem of protein binding, of transfer maxima which
are extremely important in evaluating disappearance curves and in
particular recovery in the urine, the changing blood level and
the character of the change in terms of bolus injections versus
infusions.

Now when one couples this with comparisons of hepatic
removal, one gets into considerable difficulty.   We have been
interested in this for a long time in renal physiology from the
standpoint of evaluating bromosulphothalein disappearance.   I
would suggest that an appropriate comparison could only be made
in terms of clearance determinations and comparisons with constant
blood levels, at levels definitely below the transfer maximum to
make it possible to determine the true differences between the
kidney and liver in terms of excreting these materials.

I should say too, that there are large differences between
species in different phylla.   Fish for example secrete B.S.P.
much more effectively via the hepatic route than the renal route.
Again, one wonders about probable protein binding, and of the
problem of delivery.   Delivery to the kidney and liver in man
are approximately the same, but this is not true of every species.
So I would suggest that there may be more complications than your
measurements and conclusions would seem to suggest.

Ostrow:   Dr. Millburn, you have presented us with a mass of data
that has been very useful because this has not been available on
such a wide basis before.

However, I was rather surprised that you did not once

mention protein binding in your entire talk.   A very simple
observation suggested that this may be extremely critical and
probably may be the way in which the lipid solubility relates
to whether a substance goes out in the liver or kidney.   If you
have cholestasis, these compounds and conjugates that you have
been talking about that are highly excreted in the bile, will
back up and go out predominantly in the urine.   In fact, it has
been shown that virtually every conjugate that has been studied
is less well protein-bound than its corresponding unconjugated
more lipid-soluble derivative to both ligandin and serum albumin.
Despite the fact that these compounds when conjugated are greater
in molecular size, they will, by clearance studies, be actually
more readily and more rapidly cleared in the urine than the
unconjugated compounds from which they came.   I would think that
protein binding probably more than any of these other features
might be the thing that would be the real key determinant.

        Evans Blue, which is very tightly protein-bound, is not very
well excreted by the liver at all but it does not go out in the
urine either.

Millburn:   We have done a rather limited comparative study on
protein binding with about 5 or 6 compounds that were excreted
unchanged so there is no complication of species differences in
metabolism.   We looked at the extent to which they were bound
to the plasma proteins of the rat and the rabbit.   These compounds
were extensively excreted in the bile by the rat but not by the
rabbit and yet, in our studies, there was no real difference in
the protein binding in the two species.   We found a difference
in the amount that appeared in bile in the canulated animal, but
when we looked at the binding to plasma proteins by the ultrafiltration method there was really no difference between the rat
and the rabbit.   So for that group of compounds that did not
seem to be a determining factor.   Of course, it would be interesting to compare the binding of some of these compounds with
ligandin in some of these various species.   Maybe Dr. Arias will
have something to say on that.

Coleman:   This is probably a very naive question but the
structure of these molecules is essentially a big hydrophobic part
and a carboxyl which looks very much like say glycocholic acid.
Does glycocholic acid compete with these compounds for excretion,
or do they compete with it?

Millburn:   I showed you excretion of phenobarbital and succinylsulphathiazole.   There was a big difference between the rat and
the rabbit.   The succinylsulphathiazole was excreted against the
concentration gradient in the rat and not in the rabbit.   In the
rat we found that both taurocholate and glycocholate did compete

with the foreign compound for excretion.

We have done a few compounds but we have not obviously done 20, 30 or 40.

Coleman:   Could I ask then, does this mean that there might be a normal mechanism rather than a special mechanism?

Millburn:   It could be.   I do not think any of us knows what we mean by the term mechanism, in the sense that it depends on where you start.   If you start in the plasma you can say there is a mechanism for uptake and a mechanism for metabolism and a mechanism for excretion.   But if we confine ourselves to excretion, certainly looking at the structures of a lot of endogenous compounds such as the bile acid conjugates, say thyroxine glucuronide or thyroxine sulphate and many steroids conjugates, they would fit in with the molecular weight hypothesis.   We do not know whether they all go by the same mechanism or by more than one mechanism for different groups of anions.

Bergan:   I have some problem in understanding how your retrograde injection could in any way tell anything about normal readsorption, because you have to use an increased hydrostatic pressure of about 30 centimetres of water.   That makes conditions more like the acute phases of cholestasis and you have the problem of regurgitation rather than reabsorption.   If you had some way of intravenous injection to keep the hydrostatic pressure at the normal or physiological level, then you could say something about normal reabsorption.

Millburn:   I think the reabsorption experiments are obviously difficult to interpret.   The one point about them is that there is a comparison using the same technique between two different groups of compounds, but in the last two or three years there have been a number of papers in the literature concerning the technique of reabsorption itself, and the technique of retrograde biliary infusion.   I think the current estimate of the volume of the biliary tree of the rat is 50 microlitres.   One group of investigators say that you should not exceed this and distend the biliary tree by retrograde injection.   Otherwise, this would influence the results.   Yet another group say that in their opinion it was a very good thing to distend the biliary tree. Perhaps this is a matter of opinion, but I think that the sort of experiments that I described at the very end are very tentative experiments and I just suggested them as a discussion point.   One needs, as you said, to do more rigorous experiments to see whether that concept holds up or not.

Bergan:   Did you sample for more than 30 minutes?

<u>Millburn</u>:  Yes, we sampled in some cases up to about an hour.
It seemed as though we were getting a good total recovery if you
include both bile and urine after about 30 minutes.  Many of these
conjugates are cleared very quickly.

<u>Bergan</u>:  Yes, because you have to expect some delay because of
thoracic duct regurgitation.

<u>Millburn</u>:  I think that could be a complicating factor.  The
reason we found it interesting was because we were aware of it
when we did the work.  We were struck by the marked difference
between the two compounds.  One group seemed to be very extensively reabsorbed, and another group that was reabsorbed to some
but much lower extent.  Maybe this means something or may be it
does not.  We really must do another set of experiments to
evaluate this further.

<u>Dowling</u>:  What was the dose of substances which you gave, and is
the per cent of the given dose related to the total excretion of
the dose?

   Secondly, following on Dr. Coleman's question, are all of
these substances choleretics, and if so, is this in proportion to
the molecular weight of the substance?  Do they in fact have
mutually inhibitory or stimulatory effects on, say, bile lipids
as well as bile acids?  A few years ago it was found that with
some of these substances, such as B.S.P. and the cholangiographic
agents, there was a marked change in the pattern of the biliary
lipid secretion during the infusion of these substances.  I
wondered if you had had a chance to look at this.

<u>Millburn</u>:  We have not looked at any of the biliary lipids in
any of our experiments.

   With regard to the dose of the organic anions, we try to
have a dose of either 50 to 100 micromoles per kilogram as a sort
of standard molar dose between the various species.  With cations
it is lower because they are more toxic.  For some compounds we
have done this at a variety of doses and obviously for some
compounds you can saturate the mechanism by increasing the dose.
However, in our experiments, there does seem to be a wide range
of doses where you get essentially the same amounts in bile at
whichever dose you use.

<u>Dowling</u>:  Yes, it was a little bit difficult to tell from your
slides because I think for the most part you showed us mean values
and that very much relates to Dr. Bradley's question and comments
about saturating the plasma mechanism or the transfer mechanism;
that is, whether or not you are operating at optimal conditions.

Millburn:    Yes, in all the data I only showed mean values
otherwise there would have been too many figures on the slides,
but all the data that I showed was at a dose level that would be
below saturation.

GENERAL DISCUSSION OF SESSION I

<u>Taylor</u>:   Dr. Millburn and I have known each other for many years
and have had discussions and indeed confrontations about his
molecular weight hypothesis.

First of all I would question the criterion that 10 per cent
amounts to a "substantial excretion".

The discussions that we have had previously have centred
around the excretion of steroid hormone metabolites in bile and
urine.   These have a molecular weight of about 600 as glucuronides.

I think a lot of this work, and in fact a lot of this work on
the biliary system in general, has been bedevilled by the use of
the rat as the standard laboratory animal.   I have selected for
purposes of my own argument some of the results of Dr. Millburn's
group.   If we look at the biliary excretion of succinyl-sulphathiazole in the rat with the renal pedicules ligated or not ligated
we see that in fact what Dr. Millburn says is quite right, namely
that with the renal pedicules ligated more goes out in the bile.

In the rabbit with ligated renal pedicules, you cannot force
succinyl-sulphathiazole out into bile.   There is something which
seems to be obstructing the biliary excretion of the succinylsulphathiazole in the rabbit but not in the rat.

If we look at the species differences in the excretion of a
number of steroid hormone metabolites, we find that the rat is a
good excretor of steroid hormone metabolites in bile.   Taking
cortisone as the example, the molecular weight of the major
metabolites is about 600 plus.   The highest figure that has been
obtained for biliary secretion is about 5 per cent.   The oestrogens
are rather different, but there are these very peculiar species
differences when we come to steroids.   Certainly in man, the major
route of excretion of the polar corticoids with high molecular
weights is via urine and not via the bile.

If we consider some of Dr. Millburn's results there are many
anomalies.   There are about 5 compounds which have a fairly high,
or by his criterion, substantial excretion, and yet they can vary

in molecular weight from 120 up to 300.

What I have suggested elsewhere is that what we should be
looking at in these compounds is not only their molecular weight,
their polarity or the other properties he mentioned, but in fact
we should look at the molecular models to see what their shape is.
I have suggested that what in fact determines whether or not
something goes out in the bile is the nature of the proteins in
the bile canaliculus and these structural differences between the
compounds and the acceptance or the recognition by the canalicular
protein in the membrane will determine what goes out in bile.    It
is not molecular weight or polarity;  it is the structure of the
compounds, and the relationship of this structure to binding sites
of canalicular membrane proteins.   What I would like to see is
models made to see how these fit.   There are many anomalies in
their results which are quite fascinating, but the basic hypothesis
that you can draw a line at a molecular weight of 350, 450, 600 is
not what matters because, I imagine, that as you increase the
molecular weight of the compound you increase its molecular shape
and complexity.   Therefore, a particular compound will be more or
less acceptable to canalicular membrane proteins than smaller
molecules.   Also there are the species differences to explain.
I have suggested that the rat has rather "primitive" proteins in
the canalicular membrane which will accept almost anything of a
given molecular weight, whereas in other species the canalicular
proteins have become more selective.   In man, the canalicular
protein simply will not accept certain molecules for excretion in
bile.

Millburn:   We have had lots of interesting discussions over the
years on the molecular weight hypothesis.   I think Dr. Taylor
may have misunderstood what I was saying about our definition of
appreciable biliary excretion.   What I was saying was that we
regarded something that had an excretion of less than 10 per cent
of the dose as relatively insignificant, which is a little different
from the way he put it.   If we look at the molecular weight threshold values, we find that in the rat there is a group of compounds
whose molecular weight is below 300 and less than 10 per cent of
the dose appears in the bile.   We felt that once biliary excretion
became greater than 10 per cent, it became more significant.   So,
as molecular weight increases biliary excretion of the compounds
becomes more substantial.   The same trend is shown by other
species.   Let us consider the complementary roles of biliary and
urinary excretion.   Succinyl-sulphathiazole has a molecular
weight of 350, which is in the threshold region of biliary excretion
for the rat.   Therefore, it is not surprising that biliary excretion of the drug increases when the renal pedicles are ligated.   In
the rabbit, the drug is excreted predominantly in the urine, and for
many other compounds there is very little biliary excretion.   So

I think our results on renal ligation are consistent with the
hypothesis of molecular weight and threshold.   Surprisingly few
anomalies are found.

Obviously molecular weight in itself is not the sole
determining factor in biological systems.   I did stress that
these compounds have polar and non-polar parts which may bind to
the proteins which Dr. Taylor has suggested occur in the canalicular membrane, but, of course, such proteins may not occur.

There are some compounds with molecular weights below 200
which are substantially excreted in bile, but he seems to have
selected the molecular weight of the compound administered, whereas
we are concerned with the molecular weight of the metabolites which
appear in bile.   Important examples are the biphenyl and hydroxy-
biphenyl compounds which are excreted in the bile as glucuronides.

I still think that the molecular weight idea is useful in a
practical way in that you can look at the molecular weight of a
compound and make some prediction about the extent of its biliary
excretion.   But obviously it tells us nothing about binding
within the liver cell or at the canaliculus.

Fevery:   In this comparison of rat and rabbit it so happens that
with bilirubin and oestrogens, the rabbit is a very good glucoside
former, whereas the rat does not produce glucosides of bilirubin.
So you may simply be comparing the ability of the animals to form
glucosides rather than glucuronides, and if one takes this into
account the concept may change.

Haslewood:   I do not accept Dr. Taylor's idea that man has
reached the peak of the evolutionary tree, and that the rat is a
primitive species.   In fact the rat is a very advanced and
successful mammal.

Taylor:   I suggested that the canalicular membrane proteins are
"primitive", which is not the same as saying that the species
itself is primitive.

Popjak:   What is known about species differences in the permeability of the glomerular membrane, and has this any role in the
excretion of substances in bile or urine?

Bradley:   There are species differences in this respect, but
they have not been defined in any systematic way.   For instance,
the male rat has a lot of protein in the urine, but I do not think
that this implies that there is high permeability to protein at
the glomerular level.   In fishes there is an even larger loss of
protein in the urine.   However, the whole problem of glomerular

permeability to protein is a vexed question at this time.
Current ideas based on the micropuncture work in rats, dogs and
rabbits are that there is no appreciable glomerular permeability
to plasma proteins, and that the unbound, or free, fraction which
must be taken into account when considering excretion by glomerular
filtration independent of secretion and absorption.   Now most of
these materials are secreted by the renal tubular cells, and
filtration is not really involved.   Some undergo reabsorption
and this may be augmented by non-ionic diffusion.   Therefore
a lot depends on the acid-base balance of the body and the pH of
the urine, and one should control these factors before talking
about excretion in urine relative to excretion by the liver.   The
confusion in my own mind arises from thinking about this from a
pharmacological rather than a physiological point of view.   In
pharmacology it is important to know about the partitioning,
breakdown and excretion of substances, and this may not be relevant
to physiological problems, and that in turn may not be related to
biochemical processes.   Therefore we may be talking about
processes far removed from fundamental mechanisms.

<u>Popper</u>:   Dr. Millburn, what are your ideas about liver injury,
which is a key question for a lot of us.   In such injury, peculiar
circumstances may arise.   You showed a very nice diagram of the
UDPG-transferase being decreased, yet it is well known that these
transferases are increased in liver injury because the superficial
layer where the cytochrome P450 is may be removed.   So really I
am adding pathological aspects to what Dr. Bradley has already
said.

<u>Millburn</u>:   For the sake of argument let us consider a compound
which is completely excreted in bile and 80 to 90 per cent of it
is unchanged.   In the rat, if you tie off the bile duct, the
substance could not be excreted in the urine.   So, presumably,
in liver injury it would stay around in the body, assuming it
could not be excreted in the bile.   With another type of compound
which has to be conjugated as a glucuronide before excretion, then
the increase in glucuronyl transferase would increase the excretion.
But that is pure speculation on my part.

<u>Hofmann</u>:   I have a question, a comment and a proposed experiment
for Dr. Millburn.   The question is:  when you did your retrograde
injections into the biliary tree, did you include polyethylene
glycol which is an acceptable marker for membrane permeability,
and if so, what kind of recovery did you get?   My comment is
that your group, which does such good experiments, may be doing
yourselves a disservice by using the term "increasing molecular
weight".   In fact, what you are actually doing is adding
additional methyl groups, but if you were to increase the molecular weight, by adding, say, sulphonic acid groups, you would

get a totally different effect.    In other words, some of the
controversy might subside if you were more specific in describing
how you increase the molecular weight.

Millburn:   We have not used polyethylene glycol as you suggested.
I agree that for the organic cations the molecular weight was
usually increased by adding additional methyl groups.    However,
we have studied about a hundred organic anions, and the molecular
weight has been increased in a number of different ways.    I
admit that if you add extra polar groups this would make a
difference.   We do not have enough data yet, but my guess is
that there is a balance between lipid and water solubility.   If
we had enough data we could compare compounds with one or two
negative charges and this would be interesting to do.

Hofmann:   My proposed experiment is concerned with the possibility
of association of these compounds with micelles as they pass down
the biliary tree.    For example, it would be feasible to produce
taurocholate-lecithin micelles in an aqueous phase and determine
the partition coefficient between the aqueous phase and octanol.
If the formation of micelles in the aqueous phase altered the
partition coefficient, this would indicate that there was
association between the micelles and, say, the drug conjugates.
This would provide a clue about the mechanisms involved.    It
seems to me that what the micelle provides is an amphiphilic
surface on which adsorption of drug metabolites can occur.   The
advantage of forming an amphiphilic metabolic product of a drug is
that the partition into octanol is decreased and therefore there
is a decrease in non-ionic diffusion along the biliary tree, or
in effect, an increase in biliary secretion of the metabolite.
So I think that the experiment I propose would give some indication
of micellar associations.

Millburn:   The retrograde infusion experiments I described were
preliminary work, but I think we ought to do experiments of the
kind you have suggested.

Javitt:   Some of us have reservations about Dr. Millburn's concept
because it is too general in its nature to be useful.

        Let us consider the tetrabromo-sulphothalein monosulphate,
B.S.P. which is dibromo-sulphothalein, and the corresponding
tetrasulphonate.    The monosulphate is totally excreted in bile
but the tetrasulphonate is almost completely excreted in urine
even though the tetrasulphonate has a higher molecular weight.
B.S.P. is excreted in bile and urine, irrespective of whether it
is conjugated or not.    I should add that the tetrasulphonate is
not metabolized in any way.    So I think that we must consider
what Professor Ussing said;   that there are some very clever and

specific exchange proteins, possibly myriads of them which we have not yet identified.   After all we know that there are some proteins which require only sodium at one place and glucose at another to cross the membrane.   Therefore I think we are generalising too much about these compounds to come up with a concept which would help us to come to grips with the problem of hepatic excretion.

Taylor:   I would like to endorse these comments of Dr. Javitt. I am sure it is the proteins we should be thinking about.

Coleman:   Professor Lucy mentioned that there is a problem in that the liver is secreting a detergent, and detergents damage membranes.   The answer to this problem may lie either in the nature of the detergents or with the nature of the membrane. So we have looked at the effects of different detergents on membranes.   Our work is done at 37°C, at neutral pH in an iso-tonic medium.   Under these conditions deoxycholate appeared to solubilise the membrane of erythrocyte ghosts.   However cholate solubilised all phospholipids from the membrane, but only produced about 40 per cent solubilisation of membrane protein.   When we looked at the proteins in the residue, we found that it was not a random collection of proteins which had been solubilised.   The proteins in the residue were mainly the intrinsic membrane proteins, such as band III;   and only spectrin-like molecules had been removed.   The residual protein still maintained structural organisation.   The ghosts had lost their lipids and all the spectrin and showed internal vesiculation, but the membrane-like profile remained.   So it seems as though cholate can remove the lipid and yet the membrane is not too badly damaged.

When conjugated bile acids were used we were surprised to find that there was a depression in the ability to solubilise lipids from the membranes although the same amount of protein was solubilised.   So we conclude that the conjugated bile salts are not so damaging as we might think.   Small has suggested that the bile salts penetrate the canalicular membrane and remove some of the lipid and cholesterol.   There are some problems about this concept.   It has not been proved that the lipids are removed from the plasma membrane.   As far as I can tell from the literature, the bile salts within the liver cell appear to be present below the critical micellar concentration, whereas outside the cell there are micelles.   All bile salts tested so far solubilise a range of phospholipids from membranes.   I would suggest that the bile salts being secreted have been engineered by the liver to reduce their membrane-damaging properties.   The bile salts are actively pumped out of the cell and only the plasma membrane is exposed to bile salt micelles, and even though something may be removed from the plasma membrane there is no real damage to the

liver cell.   We have shown that bile contains a number of plasma
membrane enzymes.   It might be possible to remove lipid from
membranes without lysis to the cells.   Using intact red cells and
measuring haemoglobin and phospholipid release, we have found that
with glycocholate, and to some extent taurocholate, up to 20 per
cent of phospholipid can be removed before lysis occurs.   We do
not know exactly where this phospholipid comes from as yet.

Lucy:   With respect to what Dr. Coleman has said, others have
shown that by using a combination of enzymes which can degrade
phospholipids it is possible to release up to 60 per cent of the
phospholipid of red cells without causing lysis.   So it is
possible that phospholipids are removed from the liver cell
membrane during bile secretion, and this is very interesting.

Fisher:   We have also been studying plasma membranes and bile
secretion, and we fell that our canalicular enriched membrane
fraction is enzymatically, chemically, ultrastructurally and
biosynthetically quite distinct from the other parts of the
liver plasma membrane.   The incorporation of labelled glycerol
into total canalicular membrane phospholipids is biphasic, quite
unlike that found with other cell fragments.   We have studied
the solubilisation of the canalicular membrane and other organelles by various bile acids.

     Chenodeoxycholate and deoxycholate have similar effects.
Microsomes are solubilised linearly with respect to increasing
bile acid concentration, and are completely dissolved when the
bile acid:phospholipid ratio is 20:1.   The non-canalicular
plasma membrane is no less resistant, and again, solubilisation
is dependent on bile acid concentration in a linear way.   However,
solubilisation of phospholipid from the canalicular membrane is
clearly biphasic with a marked change in the slope at a bile
acid:phospholipid ratio of about 30:1.   At a bile acid:phospho-
lipid ratio of 20:1 the dihydroxy bile acids solubilise approximately 40-50 per cent of the canalicular membrane phospholipids.
About half of this is phosphatidyl choline and 40 per cent
phosphatidyl ethanolamine.   At a bile acid:phospholipid ratio
of 100:1 all of the canalicular membrane phospholipid is
solubilised.   About 50 per cent of this is phosphatidyl serine,
inositol, sphingomyelin and lysolecithin.   At a ratio of 20:1,
the phospholipids taken out of the canalicular membrane are quite
different from those left in, but which are solubilised when the
ratio is increased to 100.   Those phospholipids solubilised at
the lower ratio are remarkably similar to those found in bile.
The dienes are the predominant molecular species in the phospholipids found in bile.   At a ratio of 20:1 the fatty acid
composition of solubilised phospholipid dienes is quite different
from what is left in but is very similar to that found in bile.

So we conclude that there can be selective solubilisation of phospholipids from the canalicular membrane, but we do not know if this occurs <u>in vivo</u>.   Our results are compatible with the hypothesis that the phospholipids in bile originate from the canalicular membrane itself.

<u>Boyer</u>:   I want to add a cautionary word to those using canalicular enriched fractions.   They certainly are enriched, but they are not pure.

<u>Fisher</u>:   I certainly agree that we must be careful in the use of these canalicular fractions.

<u>Sjövall</u>:   I have real difficulty in believing in this hypothesis of the origin of biliary phospholipids.   How can the hypothesis explain species differences?   There are wide differences in the types of bile acids excreted by different animals and also differences in concentration of phospholipids in bile.   For instance, the guinea pig produces hardly any phospholipids, and the major bile acids are chenodeoxycholate and 7-ketolithocholate. Also, the fatty acid compositions of rat and human biliary lecithin is quite similar, yet the bile acids excreted are markedly different. Yet you have been describing different degrees of solubilisation by different bile acids.   How can one reconcile these conflicting data?

<u>Fisher</u>:   We certainly cannot explain this;  we are simply reporting data from the rat, and find it difficult enough to explain our findings in this one animal species.

<u>Boyer</u>:   What may be critical in this is the concentration of bile acid in the canaliculus, and might this not vary considerably from species to species irrespective of the type of bile acid.

<u>Sjövall</u>:   I agree that this could be the explanation.   I was talking about the type and concentration of bile acids obtained from a bile fistula.   But it is possible that the situation could be quite different higher up the biliary tree.

# Structure and Function in the Hepatobiliary System

# THE FINE STRUCTURE OF LIVER CELLS

Francesco Orlandi and Maurizio M. Koch

Digestive Disease Unit, University of Ancona
and
Division of Gastroenterology, General Hospital of Ancona

The first electron micrographs of liver cells were published 25
years ago by Dalton, and the first comprehensive report of the
fine structure of the rat liver cell was published by Fawcett in
1955. Since then, there have been several review articles or
monographs about the qualitative patterns and morphological features
of normal liver cells both in animals and in man (Brown et al.,
1957; Hampton, 1960; Novikoff and Essner, 1960; Jezequel, 1962;
Rouiller and Jezequel, 1963; Cossel, 1964; David, 1964; Bruni and
Porter, 1965; Oudea et al., 1967; Tanikawa, 1968; Elias and
Sherrick, 1969; Ma and Biempica, 1971; Jezequel and Orlandi, 1972;
Schaffner and Popper, 1972; Ma et al., 1972; Trump et al., 1973).
The methods of tissue processing for electron microscopy have
become gradually standardized and some differences in interpreta
tion of ultrastructural findings have been resolved. Moreover the
observation of liver cell changes in numerous experimental situa
tions has increased the basic "pool" of information and has
permitted to establish a pattern of normal fine structure of liver
cells, largely free from misinterpretations or acritical evaluations.
In the last years both the adequacy of techniques and the back
ground of knowledge have allowed the application of morphome
tric methods to the study of the normal liver cell in rat (Loud, 1968;
Wiener et al., 1968; Weibel et al., 1969; Hope, 1970; Rohr et al.,
1971; Riede et al., 1972; Sturgess and De La Iglesia, 1972;
Dobbins et al., 1972; Oudea et al., 1973; Herzfeld et al., 1973),
in dog (Hess et al., 1973a, 1973b, 1973c), in the lactating cow

(Reid, 1973) and in man (Jezequel et al., 1974, 1975a, 1975b;
Slabodsky-Brousse et al., 1974; Jezequel et al., in press; Rohr
et al., unpubl. obs.).

According to the present feeling of most electron microscopists,
ultrastructural morphometry has not been applied to the study of
liver diseases. Electron microscopy of the liver tissue has provi
ded few, if any, diagnostic criteria useful in the management of
patients (Schaffner and Popper, 1972). The early, sometimes rough
trend to apply to the electron microscopic studies the conventional
approach of diagnostic light microscopy has been a transitory, in
some way unavoidable, but often uninformative step in liver resea
rch. The risk of subjectivity and of anedoctal descriptions has
been emphasized by competent hepatologists (Steiner et al., 1964;
Chalmers, 1969). A major attention is now paid to the morphological
responses of the liver cell to stimuli and to their correlations
with biochemical changes of liver tissue or cellular fractions. The
verbal descriptions inherited from the conventional histo-pathologi
cal practice become often inadequate. They restrict morphological
information to semiquantitative evaluation sometimes based on
subjective judgement alone, and a proper correlation of biochemical
data is impossible (Weibel et al., 1969).

The following considerations will concern the fine structure of the
normal liver cells as a dimensional problem. The emphasis will be
placed on some methodological aspects connected with this type of
investigation.


THE MEANING OF NORMAL LIVER CELL


Perhaps the greatest defect in current expressions about normality
of the fine structure of liver cells is the lack of information
about the reference population. While it has been well established
that the general pattern of organelle morphology is common to the
liver cell of various species, a proper approach needs a separate
evaluation and a better delineation of different types of normal
liver cells related, first of all, to the species and strains.
Certain misinterpretations of ultrastructural findings have occurred
taking the pattern of a species as a reference for the evaluation
of another (Jezequel and Orlandi, 1972). Monoparticulate glycogen
present in endothelial cells of human liver, but not in the rat,
has been mistaken by some for virus particles. Normal patterns of
the smooth endoplasmic reticulum in man have been evaluated as

"hypertrophic" with respect to the normal rat liver cell. Beside
species and strain, the reference population includes sex, age,
diet, environmental factors in all the individuals considered, intra
personal variations and other bias.

The idea of an abstract normal liver cell as a static and ideal re
ference, such as we could perhaps consider the liver cell of a
germ-free animal, is therefore replaced by the present feeling of
normality as a multivariate problem and as an area of the "continuum"
from health to disease.

Delineation of normality is largely dependent on the methodological
approach. Both in histopathological work and in research the hepa
tologist makes judgement (statement) of "normal morphology" by
reviewing his own information incorporated from specimens previously
examined, usually integrated with clinical or biological data. He
delineates his own zone of normality according to negative criteria
referring to some innocuous or ideal morphological situations.

At the borderline of this area, the observation of minimal changes
such as rare fat droplets or isolated abnormalities of organelles
are often interpreted in the light of the protocol of the inve
stigation. Such ambiguous limits of normality are well known also
in light microscopy. Infiltration of portal tracts, f.e., can be
disregarded or else make the diagnosis of chronic persistent hepa
titis according to the clinical data (Soloway et al., 1971; Orlandi
et al., unpubl. obs.). Evidence of cytolysomes can be related to
the normal organelle turnover or to an organelle injury, according
to their "frequency" on micrographs. Mitochondrial filamentous
inclusions and giant mitochondria can be described as a pathological
finding (Jezequel, 1959) or as an occasional feature of normal
liver cells (Rouiller and Jezequel, 1963; Mugnaini, 1964; Wills,
1965; Ma and Biempica, 1971). Intranuclear glycogen can be related
to diabetes (Dominici and Orlandi, 1961) or evaluated as an occa
sional finding in normal liver (Ma and Biempica, 1971). Many
ultrastructural features of the liver cell can be considered or not
in the zone of normality according to their frequency rather than
to their qualitative aspect (Steiner et al., 1965). The non-dimen
sional characteristics of conventional morphology is therefore its
major methodological drawbeck in studies integrated with functional
observations. These handicaps become even more evident when various
types of data are to be involved in the morphological statement: the
process of histopathological diagnosis making is sometimes regarded
as an art-like, occasionally mystical, often intuitive procedure.

Such a morphology sometimes allows, just as certain clinical habits
(Feinstein, 1967), a rationale that need not to be overtly rational,
and reasons that need not to be particularly reasonable.

On the other hand quantification of fine morphology is regarded by
some hepatologists as a rough approach to the problem carrying a
risk of negligence of soft data, with a loss of important informa
tions and with a dangerous simplification in research. This opinion
is entirely shared by biostatisticians. The belief that mathematical
analysis alone will serve to make dinstiction between normal or
abnormal findings is erroneous and to come under the spell of calcu
lations is a great risk for the investigator (Feinstein, 1970 and
1974; Elveback, 1972 and 1973).

There is a general agreement between morphologists that the qualita
tive examination of the tissue remains the primary approach to the
evaluation of the ultrastructural findings. Quantitative techniques
nevertheless complement descriptive morphology in an increasing part
of research. They are particulary needed for a proper evaluation
of the normal base-line data of the liver cell.


THE SELECTION CRITERIA

Quantification of ultrastructural findings implies checking the whole
profile of the investigation, passing from the conventional protocols
focused on qualitative and elegant findings to an objective and con
trolled evaluation. The selection procedure concerns first of all
a random choice of the individuals examined.

Criteria for the selection of normal animals are relatively simple.
It is nevertheless necessary to emphasize here that the meaning of the
quantitative final data depends on many "details" of the protocol.
Some diurnal variations of the liver cell ultrastructure have been
observed (Rohr et al., 1970) and the hour of sacrifice should be
always mentioned.

Different rat strains and procedures and different protocols have
been used in quantitation of the normal fine structure of liver cells.
Loud (1968) choosed 5-month-old female Columbia-Sherman rats, given
laboratory chow ad  libitum until sacrificed between 10:00 and 11:00
a.m. Weibel and coworkers (Weibel et al., 1969; Staubli et al.,
1969) used male albino rats, Wistar-derived, 8-9 weeks old and
weighing 176-227 g., fed ad libitum with standardized laboratory chow

and fasted for 24 hours before sacrifice to deplete glycogen. Oudea and coworkers (1973) used 5 normal male Charles River rats weighing from 160 to 170 g. and given solid food plus water. Dobbins and coworkers (1972) used male Sprague-Dowley rats weighing 150 to 200 g. and caged individually, fed Purina chow and water; the animals were killed between 8:00 and 10:00 a.m. after 1-3 hours of starvation. Riede and coworkers (1972) compared morphometric findings in male Wistar rats (average weight 252 g.) with those of Desert rats. Herzfeld and coworkers used Kx rats 90-100 days old. Sturgess and De La Iglesia (1972) sacrificed male Wistar rats after overnight fasting. In some studies rats were sacrificed after anesthesia with ether (Weibel et al., 1969; Hope, 1970; Sturgess and De La Iglesia, 1972).

Base-line morphometric data on Freiesian-Ayrshire dairy cows were collected in animals in lactation (Reid, 1973). Liver tissue was obtained by the biopsy method of Hibbit and Baird (1967). Hess and coworkers (1973a, 1973b) used dog liver in view of the fact that dog is increasingly used for pharmacological studies. The study of liver function can be better achieved in dog than in small animals such as the rat and experimental observations can be followed on the same animal by serial needle biopsies. Mongrels and beagle dogs fed standard diet were submitted to needle biopsies and, under deep anesthesia with pentobarbital, to surgical biopsies.

Selection of normal individuals is obviously more difficult in man. The ethical handicaps can be overcome by selecting eligible specimens in the course of a large diagnostic or clinicopharmacologic activity. Moreover the risk of heterogeneity is higher in man than in laboratory animals, due to the genetic background, conditions of living, nutrition habits and a difficulty to evaluate exposure to environmental agents. As elsewhere, broad criteria of admission give results representative of a larger reference population. However a low threshold in selection can increase the heterogeneity of admitted individuals, the size of the sample needed and the complexity of the protocol. The random sampling of clinical populations is a debated problem of biostatistics (Feinstein, 1970b). Jezequel and coworkers (1974) selected needle liver biopsies obtained from four in-patients fed a standard normocaloric and no-ethanol diet. Biopsies were performed at 10:00 a.m. after overnight starvation. The four selected patients were 21, 24, 27, 48 years old and two of them were male. False diagnosis of hepatomegaly or false suspicion of granulomatous diseases possibly involving liver

tissue motivated biopsies. Only Xylocain to obtain local anesthesia
was given before the biopsy. The selection procedure considered the
clinical evaluation and the routine functional tests, such as BSP
retention, serum aminotransferases, bilirubin and alkaline phospha
tase, HBsAg and HBsAc, etc. Special attention was paid to the
drug-taking history including self-medication. Three "drug-free"
weeks, abstinence from smoking and an ethanol consumption of less
than 50 g. per day were requested for eligibility. The selection
also took into account the light microscopy findings on a routinely
processed portion of the specimen. Evidence of mild steatosis or
other slight changes excluded 6 out 10 candidate specimens.
Slabodsky-Brousse and coworkers (1974) examined needle or surgical
liver biopsies from 10 patients with gastric ulcer or uncomplicated
gallstone disease. Rohr and coworkers (unpubl. obs.) have examined
liver specimens from four healthy volunteers fed normocaloric diet
and abstinent from smoking, ethanol and drugs during two weeks prior
to biopsy; normal clinical, biochemical and histologic evaluations
including HBsAg in blood and liver tissue were requested for
admission.


                              THE SAMPLE


The results of a study on the normal liver cell are obviously impro
ved increasing the number of individuals examined. In general, the
number needed depends on the experimental conditions and on the goal
of the study. The hepatologist should first estimate the difference
to be considered as morphologically important between normal group(s)
and experimental group(s), the variability of the morphological
values and the level of false positive and false negative errors. These
preliminary estimations influence the sample size needed and should
never be delegated to the statistician, who has not usually a specific
experience in hepatology. If deputed, he is forced to introduce
foreign evaluations in the profile of the investigation.

Moreover, biostatisticians remind us that the size of the sample
should be always kept in mind considering both the intermediary and
the final results. A statistical test of significance is sometimes
thought to be an automatic rule for making a decision either to
"accept" or "reject" a null hypothesis. This attitude should be
avoided. The hepatologist should add to the evidence of calculations
the knowledge accumulated from his own past work and from the work

of others. With a small sample, the test is likely to produce a
significant result only if the null hypothesis is very badly wrong.
With a large sample, on the other hand, small departures from the
null hypothesis can be detected as statistically significant.
However the difference can be estimated too small to be of practi
cal importance (Snedecor and Cochran, 1968).

It is not yet established how the individual sample size which is
representative for the morphometric findings of a liver must be
defined and determined (Hess et al., 1973a). The stepwise procedure
defined and detailed by Weibel (Weibel, 1966; Weibel et al., 1969)
ensures a compromise between the size of the area of tissue
investigated,which must be large enough to include the entire
distribution of structures, and high magnifications required for
a proper measurement of organelles. The micrographs are examined
on a viewing screen fitted with different types of grids for
measurement of liver cell components, i.e. a quadratic lattice
screen at 1000 x primary magnification for volume and number of
nuclei, a double-lattice grid at 2500 x for volumes of extrahepato
cytic space, of liver cell cytoplasm, of nucleus and mitochondria;
a multipurpose grid with 18 lines at 10.000 x for volume and
surface densities of endoplasmic reticulum and mitochondria. This
stepwise procedure has given reproducible results in the experience
of other investigators. The sampling area is about 14.000 square
microns and contains profiles of some 180 hepatocytes (Hess et al.,
1973a).

Needle biopsy in local anesthesia is obviously the most preferable
procedure both in big animals and in man (Menghini and Orlandi,
1957). Surgical biopsies show morphological changes especially if
they are not performed at the beginning of intervention
(Zamcheck et al., 1949; Keller and Smetana, 1950). The disadvanta
ges of the needle biopsy are the small quantity of tissue obtained
(between 8 and 50 mg.), and the frequent ecapsulation of portal
tracts when 1-1.2 mm. sized aspiration needles are used. A morpho
metric comparison between needle and surgical biopsy specimens
in normal dogs supported the view that needle biopsy specimens
offer the possibility of a reliable analysis. It was sometimes
necessary to use blocks derived from two needle biopsies (Hess et
al., 1973b). In man the strikingly small variations of individual
values obtained on single needle biopsies (Jezequel et al., 1974;
Rohr et al., unpubl. obs.) and the significant morphometric changes
observed between the group of controls and the patients given

drugs inducing microsomal enzymes, or in cholestasis (Jezequel et
al., 1974; Capurso et al., 1975) are in favor of the representati
vity of the specimens. Of course, the data from needle biopsy
material  should be compared with base-line data obtained by the
same procedure.

Electron microscopic techniques do not permit the study of the fine
structure of hepatocytes on large portions of the liver. In these
conditions the representativity of the limited samples can be
assured only with a strictly systematic random sampling of the
blocks of embedded tissue of the light microscope fields and the
electron micrographs.


## PROCESSING OF THE TISSUE

In the last 10 years the procedures of liver tissue preparation for
electron microscopy have become less heterogeneous than in the
previous period. Most morphometric studies have been made following
schedules essentially based on fixation with phosphate-buffered
osmium tetroxide, dehydration with acetone or alcohol-propylene
oxide, embedding with Araldite or Epon or a mixture Epon-Araldite.
It is evident however that a persisting variety of protocols among
investigators is another serious handicap to a proper comparison of
the morphometric results.

A strict standardization of high-level techniques in each laboratory
is an elementary need for quantitative studies. Tissue-processing
artifacts are the most important source of systematic errors. They
can be eliminated almost entirely if the fixative and processing
media are isotonic (Loud et al., 1965; Weibel et al., 1966).

Morphometric evaluation of histochemical findings of the liver
cells are still lacking in electron microscopy. Unfortunately most
histochemical methods give a different pattern at the center and at
the periphery of the blocks, an aspect in contrast  with the prere
quisites of quantitative studies.


## MORPHOMETRIC TECHNIQUES

The stereological methods introduced for the quantification of liver
cell structures (Loud, 1968; Weibel et al., 1969) derive from
techniques developed by geologists and metallurgists (Delesse,

1947; Glagoleff, 1933; Chayes, 1956) applied to biomorphological pro
blems (Weibel, 1963,1966 and 1969; Weibel and Elias,1967). Detailed
modalities of analytic procedures are reported elsewhere (Weibel
et al., 1966; Loud, 1968; Weibel et al., 1969).

These techniques can be applied to the liver cell studies assuming
that (a) hepatocytes and their organelles are present in large num
bers; (b) the cells are homogeneously distributed throughout the lobu
le and the liver and the organelles throughout the cells; (c) hepato
cytes are isotropic enough, i.e. they do not show preferential orien
tation with respect to shape and internal organization (Weibel,1973).

Morphometric data are relative measurements. Volume, surface, area,
and number of components are expressed in relation to a "countaining
space": body weight, liver weight, liver tissue, hepatocytes, liver
investigators according to the morpho-functional relationship
wanted or to other elements of the experience.

Some investigators have examined the liver cells disregarding sublobu
lar variations and considering "average" cells, as they are essential
ly studied in liver homogenates (Weibel et al.,1969; Oudea et al.,
1973; Hess et al., 1973a; Slabodsky-Brousse et al.,1974; Jezequel et
al.,1974). Loud showed that centrolobular liver cells, especially
the two or three layers surrounding the central veins, are morphome
trically different from the remaining 80 per cent of hepatocytes. So
he gave some separate data on peripheral, midzonal and centrolobular
liver cells (Loud,1968; Wiener et al.,1968). Other authors discard
blocks or part of blocks in whom a centrolobular vein is evident
(Hope, 1970; Dobbins et al.,1972). The choice of the "average" or of
the "sublobular" base-line data can be made in function of the expe
rience planned. The "average" models may be suitable for the study
of relationships with functional data disregarding sublobular findings,
while an expected sublobular difference of the liver cell response,
such as in cholestasis, can justify a separate evaluation of
different sublobular areas also in the normal group.

Morphometric techniques are affected by some intrinsic sources of
systematic errors. The ratio of the section thickness to the mean
diameter of particles is limiting factor. The loss of some profiles,
due to tangential sections of particles, gives an underestimation of
the number of mitochondria or microbodies. The most important aspect
is related to a loss of endoplasmic reticulum membranes and of mito
chondrial cristae of about 30 per cent. Appropriate corrections
can be introduced (Weibel et al., 1969).

VARIABILITY OF MORPHOMETRIC DATA

Observer errors can be an important systematic bias in morphometric
evaluation. Blind examination of micrographs eliminates the potential
trend of the observer to alter the standardized criteria of counting
by selecting the data expected. This procedure implies the indepen
dence of the observers from the investigator who takes the films
at the electron microscope (Jezequel et al., 1974; Capurso et al.,
1975; Jezequel et al., in press).

The variability in data counting can be evaluated by the determination
of the inter-observer and intra-observer errors. These aspects are
estimated by recycling periodically 10 per cent of the micrographs
for a second observation. Table 1 concerns the variability of inter
section-counting of cytoplasmic membranes in one of the samples used
for inter-observer controls. The three observers had attained a com
mon good level of interpretation after a two or three-month training
period. The variability was satisfactorily low and negligeable with
respect to the purpose of the study. However some counting differen
ces in single micrographs led to a re-emphasis of the criteria for
allocation of membranes in rough endoplasmic reticulum (RER) and in
non vesicular profiles of smooth reticulum (SER 2).

Recycling a series of micrographs is also useful as a test for candi
date observers, at the beginning of their morphometric experience.
The initial trend of all the observers was a loss of about 15% in
identification of cytoplasmic membranes. Table 2 shows an example of
the under-estimation of the profiles of cytoplasmic membranes, as it
appeared in a first A1 counting made during observer training. The
reference countings A2 and A3 represent two countings of the same
series of micrographs made at a six months interval each by the same
observer. Counting A2 and A3 account also for an intra-observer con
trol.

A maximum variability of 4 per cent for inter-observer errors has
been attained providing that observers are motivated, that the
maximum individual time for counting is 90 minutes per day and
270 minutes per week, recording facilities are available and
periodical meetings are held, discussing both the intermediary
results and the trends to overestimate or underestimate an element.
The definition of the minimal ultrastructural feature necessary to
identify a structure and the definition of "equivocal" findings
are preliminary requisites in order to minimize observer errors.

Table I

| Observers | A | B | C | mean | SD |
|---|---|---|---|---|---|
| Smooth ER type I | 261 | 272 | 271 | 268.0 | 6.8 |
| Smooth ER type 2 | 62 | 50 | 66 | 59.3 | 8.3 |
| Smooth ER total | 323 | 322 | 337 | 327.3 | 8.4 |
| Golgi | 120 | 118 | 119 | 119.0 | 1.0 |
| Equivocal (SER or RER?) | 18 | 31 | 29 | 26.0 | 7.0 |
| Rough ER | 315 | 311 | 272 | 299.3 | 23.7 |
| ER total | 776 | 782 | 757 | 771.6 | 13.0 |

Inter-observer variations,intersection counting of same micrographs (surface of the liver cell endoplasmic reticulum). Recycling sample No.CFL2.74. Primary magnification of 9,100.

Table 2

| Observer | A3 | A2 | mean | SD | A1 |
|---|---|---|---|---|---|
| Smooth ER type 1 | 140 | 136 | 138.0 | 2.83 | 99 |
| Smooth ER type 2 | 18 | 20 | 19.0 | 1.41 | 19 |
| Smooth ER total | 158 | 156 | 157.0 | 1.41 | 118 |
| Golgi | 131 | 128 | 129.5 | 2.12 | 120 |
| Equivocal (SER or RER?) | 1 | 5 | 3.0 | 2.83 | 3 |
| Rough ER | 142 | 146 | 144.0 | 2.83 | 125 |
| ER total | 432 | 435 | 433.5 | 2.12 | 366 |

Intra-observer variations,intersection counting of the same micrographs(surface of the liver cell endoplasmic reticulum).A3 and A2 are data obtained after a large counting experience. A1 are data collected by the observer during training. Recycling sample K1.K2.K3.7374. Primary magnification of 9,100.

A systematic error can be related to the variability of magnifica
tion power of the electron microscope. The use of carbon grating
replica and a calibration of the microscope within 2 per cent of
the nominal magnification have been recommended (Weibel et al.,
1969; Hope, 1970).


## THE CELL

Although relatively few dimensional studies are still performed,
a quantitative pattern of the fine structure of the normal liver
cell is forming.

The geometrical shape of the liver cell varies according to its
localization in the liver cell plate (Elias and Sherrick, 1969)
and the estimation of the mean liver cell volume must therefore
be interpreted as indicating an order of magnitude (Hess et al.,
1973a). The values based on a cuboidal model are higher than
those assuming a dodecahedral or octahedral shape. Data from adult
rats, dogs and lactating cows are between 4768 and 5540 cubic
microns (Loud, 1968; Weibel et al., 1969; Hess et al., 1973a; Reid,
1973). An increase of these values was evident in the rat perinatal
period (Rohr et al., 1971). In lactating cows the mean cell volume
increases from 4768 to 5424 cubic microns after 5 days of starva
tion; the change is mainly associated with the increase of liposo
mes and lipid droplets (Reid, 1973).

In rats, the average diameter of liver cells was found to be
17.7+0.8 microns (Weibel et al., 1969), and no differences were
evident in sublobular areas (Loud, 1968).

The values of the volume of liver cells vary  from 79.3 to 88.0
per cent of the liver tissue. Data derived from electron micro
graphs are more reliable and higher (84.4 versus 70.6 per cent in
dog) than those obtained by light microscopic examination. The
difference seems related to shrinkage of tissue in paraffin section
(Hess et al., 1973a).

The average surface area of a liver cell was estimated to 1680
square microns in rats (Weibel et al., 1969) and 1870 in dogs
(Hess et al., 1973a). The volume to surface ratio was 2.95+0.05
cubic microns per square micron (Hess et al., 1973a).

The liver cell membrane is in contact with the space of Disse, the
biliary canaliculi and the neighboring hepatocytes. The inter-cellu

lar surface can be considered as potentially in contact with the
perisinusoidal space (Matter et al., 1969). Both functional and
kinetics studies (Wheeler et al., 1960; Segre, 1972; Molino and
Milanese, 1975) furnish a compartmental funnel-shaped model of the
liver cell, with a large exchange area at the sinusoidal pole and
a relatively narrow exchange area at the level of the canaliculi.
Morphometric values confirm this model. In Albino rats it has been
estimated that about 2000 square microns of a liver cell membrane
is in contact with the Disse space and 700 square microns with the
biliary canaliculi, with a ratio 3:1 (Weibel et al., 1969). In dogs
the space of Disse and intercellular surfaces have been evaluated
to 900 square cm. and the canalicular surface was found to be 170
square cm per cubic cm of tissue, with ratio 5:1 (Hess et al.,
1973a). In man, the surface densities of canalicular membrane and
of the Disse plus intercellular membrane have been respectively
estimated at 0.05 and 0.30 square microns per cubic micron of
cytoplasm, i.e. a ratio 6:1. The values increase significantly in
cholestatic patients (Capurso et al., 1975; Jezequel et al., in
press).


THE NUCLEUS


Scarse attention has been paid to electron microscopic patterns of
the liver cell nucleus. Both in qualitative and mensurational
morphology, it has been often considered by investigators as an
undifferentiate sphere.

The size distribution of nuclei, derived according to the Wicksell
transformation, vary between 5 and 11 microns. The average diameter
was found to be between 7.6 and 8.3 microns in different strains
of rats (Loud, 1968; Weibel et al., 1969; Dobbins et al., 1972;
Hope, 1970).

The phrase "mean volume of the nucleus" means the mean liver cell
portion related to one nucleus (Weibel et al., 1969). The values
in the literature varie from 277 to 312 cubic microns in different
strains and species (Weibel et al., 1969; Loud, 1968; Hope, 1970;
Hess et al., 1973). In newborn Wistar rats the mean value was 382
(Rohr et al., 1971).

The nuclear volume varies from 5.2 to 6.0 per cent in rats and dogs
and from 7.3 to 8.0 per cent of the liver cell volume in man
(Loud, 1968; Weibel et al., 1969; Oudea et al., 1973; Hess et al.,

1973a; Slabodsky-Brousse et al., 1974; Jezequel et al., in press).
During lactation the waves of mitosis and the increase of binuclear
liver cells yield an increase of the mean nuclear volume in rat
(Hope, 1970). An increase from 268 to 350 cubic microns was also
evident in lactating cows after starvation (Reid, 1973).


## THE CYTOPLASM

The density volume of the liver cell cytoplasm has been estimated
in rats to 0.771 cubic cm. per 1 ml of hepatic tissue (Weibel et
al., 1969). The values for (mononuclear) hepatocytes vary from
4640 to 5337 cubic microns (Loud, 1968; Weibel et al., 1969; Hope,
1970; Sturgess and De La Iglesia, 1972). An increase is evident
in rat gestation and early lactation (Hope, 1970).

The cytoplasmic ground substance varies from 60.4 to 68.1 per cent
of the cytoplasmic volume and from 54.9 to 62.6 per cent of the
liver cell volume in different species (Weibel et al., 1969; Hess
et al., 1973a; Jezequel et al., 1974). The different procedures
of tissue preparation probably influence these results more than
other ultrastructural findings. Centrolobular cells show a higher
percentage rate of ground substance than other hepatocytes (Loud,
1968).

Data about glycogen are lacking in most morphometrical studies, and
some of these were performed after starvation to obtain a glycogen
depletion. In non starved rats the glycogen rosettes occupy about
the same volume as the mitochondria, that is around 20 per cent
(Loud, 1968; Wiener et al., 1968; Dobbins et al., 1972). Loud (1968)
found great variations among rat liver cells: in centrolobular cells
the values are lower and a scattered distribution of particles is
prevalent while larger aggregates were frequently seen in pheriphe
ral cells. The distribution of glycogen within the liver lobule,
as estimated biochemically, supports only in part morphometric intra
lobular findings (Welsch, 1972).


## THE ENDOPLASMIC RETICULUM

The volume of the endoplasmic reticulum has been evaluated from
14.0 to 20.7 per cent of the cytoplasm in different species
(Weibel et al., 1969; Hess et al., 1973a; Jezequel et al., 1974;

Rohr et al., unpubl. obs.). Variations among individuals are surpi
singly low both in animals and in clinical groups. In lactating
cows the values are around 30 per cent (Reid, 1973).

The surface density of the reticulum has been found between 6.2 and
4.0 square microns per cubic microns of cytoplasm in different species
(Oudea et al., 1973; Hess et al., 1973; Jezequel et al., 1974;
Rohr et al., unpubl. obs.). The values obtained by Weibel were higher
(Weibel et al., 1969). The surface density of granular profiles of
the reticulum shows higher values in peripheral cells while smooth
membranes decrease in the periportal areas of the rat liver lobule
(Loud, 1968; Wiener et al., 1968). In the developing rat liver the
surface area of the smooth reticulum accounts for 30 per cent of
adult values (Herzfeld et al., 1973). An increase of the volume
density of the rough  reticulum is evident during gestation (Hope,
1970) and in the perinatal rat liver at the first day post partum
(Rohr et al., 1971). A decrease of the rough profiles is evident in
lactating cows during starvation (Reid, 1973). The two lowest
mean values of surface density of rough membranes have been obser
ved in man: 0.9+0.22 (Jezequel et al., 1974) and 1.2 (Rohr et al.,
unpubl. obs.) versus 2.4 to 3.4 square microns per cubic micron of
cytoplasm in animals (Loud, 1968; Wiener et al., 1968; Hope, 1970;
Hess et al., 1973a).

Species differences become more evident comparing the smooth-to-rough
reticulum ratios. The surface ratio was found to be between 0.74
and 1.15 in rats (Loud, 1968; Wiener et al., 1968; Weibel et al.,
1969; Oudea, 1973), 1.50 in dogs (Hess et al., 1973) and between
2.50 and 3.24 in man (Jezequel  et al., 1974; Rohr et al., unpubl.
obs.). Values in lactating cows are close to the human data (Reid,
1973), suggesting a basic predominance of smooth endoplasmic reti
culum in out-bred species.

The reticulum profiles show marked differences in distribution
among species. The stacks of narrow cisternae studded with riboso
mes are a prominent arrangement in rat liver cell, while in man
the rough endoplasmic reticulum is usually distributed along the
nucleus, along the sinusoidal border and around mitochondria. The
rest of the cytoplasm is occupied by smooth membranes, usually
arranged as round and relatively small vesicles (Jezequel and
Orlandi, 1972; Jezequel et al., 1974).

Moreover, two different arrangements of the smooth endoplasmic
reticulum are evident in man. Treatment with therapeutic agents

inducing microsomal enzymes such as Phenobarbital or Hydantoine
gives an extensive increase (up to 5.0 square microns per cubic
micron of cytoplasm) of cytoplasmic areas occupied by densely
packed smooth membranes. In these areas the profiles are arranged
in an intricated network where cisternal lumina are not clearly
recognizable, and a finely tubular appearance is often evident. Such
a dense packing, indicated as "type 2 smooth profiles" (Jezequel
et al., 1974, 1975a, 1975b), is evident also in limited cytoplasmic
areas of the control group. Its surface density in normal humans is
0.68 square microns per cubic micron of cytoplasm, with a ratio
type 1(smooth vesicular) to type 2 profiles of 3:1. The drug-induced
focal proliferation together with other findings suggest that in man
the type 2 configuration represents the newly formed smooth membranes
(Jezequel et al., 1974, 1975a, 1975b; Koch et al., 1974, 1975).

Golgi areas have been evaluated together with smooth endoplasmic
reticulum by most investigators. In developing liver of rats from
3 to 7 weeks old, the Golgi membranes show at 5 weeks a transient
increase to 4.5 per cent of cytoplasmic volume, which represents
25 per cent of the volume of the endoplasmic reticulum. The propor
tion of rough membranes was highest at 3 weeks, whereas the smooth
membranes reached maximum values at 7 weeks or later (Sturgess
and De La Iglesia, 1972). Some values of Rohr and coworkers (1971)
are consistent with these observations. In man, the Golgi membranes
account for 1.0 per cent of the cytoplasmic volume (Jezequel et
al., 1975a, 1975b; Koch et al., 1974, 1975).


THE MITOCHONDRIA


The volume density of liver cell mitochondria shows a relatively
stable range of mean values among different samples, strains and
species. It varies between 19 and 26.2 per cent of the cytoplasm
volume in rats (Loud, 1968; Wiener et al., 1968; Weibel et al.,
1969; Hope, 1970; Riede et al., 1972; Dobbins et al., 1972; Oudea
et al., 1973; Berger, 1973). In dog the mean value is 24 per cent
(Hess et al., 1973a), in lactating cows 23.5 per cent (Reid, 1973).
In man it has been evaluated at 14.2 (Jezequel et al., unpubl. obs.),
17.0 (Slabodsky-Brousse et al., 1974) and 19 per cent (Rohr et
al., unpubl. obs.). The scattering of individual measurements is
usually small, as expressed in standard errors of only 2 per cent
of the mean in rats (Weibel et al., 1969).

The chondrioma seems to have a high capacity to compensate the ada ptive changes of the organelles by preserving its relative dimensio ns in the liver cell. Comparative observations of Riede and cowor kers (1973) showed that in Wistar rat mitochondria have a mean volu me about half that of desert rats, while the number is about twice.

The liver cells surrounding the central veins show a chondrioma significantly less developed than in other liver cells, with a decrease of the volume density from 19.1 to 12.9 per cent of the cytoplasm, a decrease of the mean volume from 0.95 to 0.41 cubic microns, and of the mean diameter from 0.56 to 0.32. On the contra ry the number of mitochondria per 100 cubic microns of the cytopla sm is increased from 20 to 31 and the ratio surface-to-volume from 13.8 to 23.0 (Loud, 1968).

Moreover, three-dimensional reconstruction techniques show that the variety of mitochondrial profiles is largely due to the presence of rod-shaped and V-shaped mitochondria, distributed in a two-to-one ratio (Berger, 1973). A combined morphometric and biochemical study has shown that in gestational and postnatal periods the mitochon dria are larger than in adult rat liver (Herzfeld et al., 1973). Both the mean volume density and the surface density increase transiently at birth (Rohr et al., 1971).

The surface area of mitochondria varies from 1.0 to 1.7 square mi crons per cubic micron of cytoplasm (Hess et al., 1973; Slabodsky- -Brousse et al.,1974; Jezequel et al.,unpubl. obs.; Rohr et al., unpubl. obs.). The surface of the inner membrane with cristae has been found 4 times larger than the external membrane surface of the organelle (Weibel et al., 1969). In man the ratio between the surface density of the cristae considered alone and the mem brane has been found to be 0.6. The values of the cristae increa se significantly in cholestatic patients (Capurso et al., 1975; Jezequel et al., in press). In a size distribution study of mito chondria in man a maximum diameter of 4.5 microns was found in the control group, while in Gilbert's syndrome part of the mitochondria exibited a larger size (Slabodsky-Brousse et al., 1974).


THE PEROXISOMES

Extensive studies on microbodies have been conducted in various species (Hruban and Rechigl, 1964). A cristalline nucleoid is evident in most microbodies of rat liver cell and contains the enzyme urate oxidase. A core is occasionally evident also in normal human liver (Ma and Biempica, 1971), while the enzyme is absent in our species.

The volume density of microbodies has been evaluated between 1.1 to 1.9 per cent of the cytoplasmic volume in different strains of rats (Loud, 1968; Wiener et al., 1968; Weibel et al., 1969; Hope, 1970; Dobbins et al., 1972; Oudea et al., 1973; Wedel and Berger, 1975). It has been found that one rat liver cell contains about 370 microbodies. During gestation there is a transient early increa se of the volume of the organelles (Hope, 1970) and in the newborn rat is evident an increase  at birth (Rohr et al., 1971). In man the volume density is similar to that of the rat: 0.97 per cent (Jezequel et al., in press) and 1.3 per cent (Rohr et al., unpubl. obs.). Higher values of 3.19 per cent for dog (Hess et al., 1973) and 3.9 per cent in lactating cow (Reid et al., 1973) have been found. In dogs, the number of peroxisomes per unit of cytoplasmic volume is manifold higher than in rats, a species characteristic (Hess et al., 1973a).

## THE LYSOSOMES AND OTHER PARTICLES

The ambiguous limits for allocation of a particle to the lysosomal class are a handicap for mensuration criteria. Primary and secon dary lysosomes, lipid bodies, liposomes, dense bodies and lipofuc sins are still a group of particles variably evaluated. The dense bodies show a high volume density in human liver where they account for 1.33 (Jezequel et al., in press) and 2 per cent (Rohr et al., unpubl. obs.) of the cytoplasmic volume. In dog the value  is 0.77 per cent (Hess et al., 1973a) and 0.18 per cent in the rat (Oudea et al., 1973).

The volume density of fat droplets varies in different series of observations. It was found to be 0.33 per cent in rats (Oudea et al., 1973), 0.14 in dogs (Hess et al., 1973a), 0.18 in lactating cow (Reid et al., 1973), 0.24 (Jezequel et al., in press) and 0.43 (Rohr et al., unpubl. obs.) per cent in man. These differences may be related to species differences, to nutritional factors or may represent the habitual morphology in the populations considered.

DATA FROM NEEDLE BIOPSY IN MAN

In hepatology most experimental studies are performed in connection
with clinical problmes, and morphometric data obtained from needle
liver biopsies deserve a special attention. Most results from our
group (Jezequel et al., 1974, 1975; Capurso et al., 1975; Koch et
al., 1975) and from other investigators (Slabodsky-Brousse et al.,
1974; Rohr et al., unpubl. obs.) have been reported in the precee
ding paragraphs. We would like to emphasize here some additional
aspects concerning the variability of base-line data in our series
of observations.

Variations among the values obtained from different blocks of the
same subject were low. Expressed as the standard deviation of the
means, they never exceeded 10 per cent. This is in agreement with
the substantial homogeneity of the normal liver cell, as defined
by Loud (1968) and assumed by other investigators. In cholestasis
the data obtained in centrolobular areas differed greatly from those
in other areas of the tissue (Capurso et al., 1975).

The morphometric data obtained in each subject, their mean and the
standard deviations are shown in Table 3. The values of cell volume,
cytoplasmic ground substance volume, total endoplasmic reticulum
and mitochondrial volume and surface densities show standard devia
tions between subjects from 1.8 to 10 per cent of the mean. Standard
deviation between 10.1 and 20.0 per cent of the mean are found for
the volumetric density of the extra-hepatocytic space, nuclei,
smooth endoplasmic reticulum type 1 and rough endoplasmic reticulum,
and for both the volume and surface density of the total smooth
endoplasmic reticulum. The surface densities of the cell membrane
of its sinusoidal and canalicular fronts and of mitochondrial cristae show standard deviations between 20.1 and 30.0 per cent of the
mean. The values of smooth membranes type 2, peroxisomes and
dense bodies show a high variability.

The number of the individuals considered here is too small to
permit extrapolations. We can note however that differences in
inter-individual variability among organelles systems were and
seem predictable, in view of the different role of the organelles
in the liver cell metabolism and their different involvement in the
response to various stimuli. The chondrioma and the total endopla
smic reticulum seem to have relatively stable intracellular dimen
sions. On the contrary, the smooth membranes type 2, the most
responsive ultrastructural component to microsomal enzyme inducing

Table 3

Inter-individual variations of ultrastructural findings in needle liver biopsies from 4 healthy humans

| Component | sex and age(years) | | | | | |
| --- | --- | --- | --- | --- | --- | --- |
| | F21 | F24 | M27 | M48 | mean | SD |
| °Extrahepatocytic sp,vol | 13.76 | 12.99 | 10.89 | 10.32 | 11.99 | 1.65 |
| °Liver cell,vol | 86.24 | 87.01 | 89.11 | 89.68 | 88.01 | 1.65 |
| °Nuclei,vol | 6.84 | 7.64 | 5.52 | 8.16 | 7.04 | 1.15 |
| Cell membrane,surf | 0.43 | 0.26 | 0.41 | 0.32 | 0.36 | 0.079 |
|   sinusoidal,surf | 0.39 | 0.20 | 0.34 | 0.27 | 0.30 | 0.083 |
|   canalicular,surf | 0.036 | 0.060 | 0.066 | 0.050 | 0.053 | 0.013 |
| °Ground cytop.subst,vol | 54.05 | 52.29 | 56.71 | 57.06 | 55.14 | 2.26 |
| Endopl.reticulum,surf | 3.77 | 4.43 | 4.08 | 3.95 | 4.06 | 0.28 |
|               vol | 0.143 | 0.172 | 0.150 | 0.152 | 0.154 | 0.012 |
| Rough ER,surf | 0.86 | 0.86 | 0.68 | 1.20 | 0.90 | 0.22 |
|         vol | 0.0447 | 0.0475 | 0.0337 | 0.0525 | 0.0446 | 0.008 |
| Smooth ER,surf | 2.54 | 3.56 | 3.09 | 2.49 | 2.92 | 0.51 |
|         vol | 0.0828 | 0.1210 | 0.1011 | 0.0898 | 0.0987 | 0.017 |
| Smooth ER,type 1,surf | 2.04 | 2.96 | 1.89 | 2.06 | 2.23 | 0.49 |
|               vol | 0.0815 | 0.1130 | 0.0946 | 0.0886 | 0.0944 | 0.013 |
| Smooth ER type 2,surf | 0.50 | 0.60 | 1.20 | 0.43 | 0.68 | 0.35 |
|               vol | 0.0012 | 0.0082 | 0.0068 | 0.0012 | 0.0044 | 0.004 |
| Golgi,surf | 0.37 | 0.13 | 0.30 | 0.26 | 0.26 | 0.10 |
|     vol | 0.0157 | 0.0037 | 0.0150 | 0.0096 | 0.0110 | 0.005 |
| Equivocal,surf | | | | | 0.001 | |
|     vol | | | | | 0.009 | |
| Mitochondria,surf | 1.03 | 0.99 | 1.07 | 0.90 | 1.00 | 0.073 |
|           vol | 0.149 | 0.150 | 0.140 | 0.130 | 0.142 | 0.009 |
|   cristae,surf | 0.68 | 0.63 | 0.72 | 0.40 | 0.61 | 0.14 |
| Peroxisomes,surf | 0.0719 | 0.0590 | 0.0471 | 0.1101 | 0.0720 | 0.027 |
|         vol | 0.0103 | 0.0074 | 0.0061 | 0.0150 | 0.0097 | 0.004 |
| Dense bodies,vol | 0.0126 | 0.0110 | 0.0254 | 0.0044 | 0.0133 | 0.009 |
| Fat droplets,vol | 0.0041 | 0.0053 | 0.0004 | 0.0000 | 0.0024 | 0.003 |

°per cent of the liver tissue. Other components are related to the cy toplasm. Volume densities are expressed as cubic microns per cubic micron, surface densities are expressed as square microns per cubic micron.

agents demonstrate an elevated variability in untreated subjects.

Inter-individual variations of the same order of magnitude have been observed in inbred dogs (Hess et al., 1973b).


## CONCLUSIONS

Both the morphometric approach to the fine structure of the liver cells and the related methodology emphasize the need to compare any experimental change with the variability of baseline findings. Although biostatisticians remind us to be aware of the difficulties in the delineation of a "normal range" (Feinstein, 1974), morphometric data on diurnal fluctuations in the rat liver cell (Rohr et al., 1970) and on the inter-individual variability in dog and human liver cells represent a first mensurational approach to such a fundamental problem.

The fine structure of the liver cell is obviously richer in details than the relatively few available morphometric data. Dr. Phillips will give in this meeting an example of fascinating aspects related to the recent identification in situ of a network of actin-like microfilaments attached to the cell membrane, a contractile system perhaps providing the motive force for endocytosis, transport of vesicles and biliary flow (Wagner et al., 1971;and 1973; Jahn, 1973; Stein et al., 1974; Redman et al., 1975; French and Davies, 1975).

If we agree that the activity of the liver cell depends on an interrelationship between structural and functional components, fine morphology should be evaluated in coordinated analytic models such as those proposed by Bolender (1974), where biochemical data from cellular fractions and sterological data from intact cells are considered together with morphometric values obtained from cellular fractions, another relatively recent application of the stereological techniques (Baudhuin et al., 1967; Baudhuin and Berthet, 1967; Wibo et al., 1971; Loud, 1973).

Dimensional morphology is a time-consuming work (Weibel et al., 1969; Loud, 1968). Its usefulness and necessity in liver research are related to the type of ultrastructural information required. Statistical and stereological techniques have received major attention. It is to be noted however that together with the technical machinery, stereological contributions have emphasized some fundamental aspects of the research planning in liver morphology, such as the need of randomized protocols.

*This work has been supported by grants N. 72.00003.04 and 73.00691.04 of the Consiglio Nazionale delle Ricerche, Roma.*

REFERENCES

Baudhuin  P, Evrard P, Berthet J (1967). Electron microscopic exa mination of subcellular fractions. I. The preparation of represen tative samples from suspensions of particles. J. Cell. Biol. 32, 181-191.
Baudhuin P, Berthet J (1967). Electron microscopic examination of subcellular tractions. II. Quantitative analysis of the mitochondrial population isolated from rat liver. J. Cell. Biol., 35, 631-648.
Berger ER (1973). Two morphologically different mitochondrial populations in the rat hepatocyte as determined by quantitative three-dimensional electron microscopy. J. Ultrastruct. Res., 45, 303-327.

Brown DB, Delor CJ, Greider H, Frajda WJ (1957). The electron microscopy of human liver. Gastroenterology, 32, 103-118.

Bruni C, Porter KR (1965). The fine structure of the parenchymal cell of the normal rat liver. I. General observations. Am. J. Pathol., 46, 691-755.

Capurso L, Freddara U, Jezequel AM, Orlandi F (1975). Organelle changers of liver cell during cholestasis in man. A morphometric study. Rendiconti Gastroent., in press.

Capurso L, Koch MM, Freddara U, Lorenzini I, Jezequel AM, Orlandi F. Contribution of morphometry to the study of cholestasis in man. Proc. 10th Meeting Europ. Assoc. Study Liver, Barcelona, 1975. Digestion, in press.

Chalmers TC (1969). A challenge to clinical investigators. The presidential address. Gastroenterology, 57, 631-635.

Chayes F (1956). Petrographic modal analysis. Wiley and Sons Publ., New York.

Cossel L (1964). Die manschliche Leber im Elektronenmikroskop. G. Fisher Publ., Jena.

Dalton AJ, Kahler H, Striebich MJ, Lloyd B (1950). Finer structure of hepatic, intestinal and renal cells of the mouse as revealed by the electron microscope. J. Nat. Cancer Inst., 11, 439-461.

David H (1974). Submicroscopic ortho- and patho-morphology of the liver. Mac Milla Publ., New York.

Delesse MA (1847). Procédé mécanique pour déterminer la composition des roches. C.R. Acad. Sci. (Paris), 25, 544-545.

Dobbins WO, Rollins EL, Brooks SG, Fallon HJ (1972). A quantitative morphological analysis of ethano effect upon rat liver. Gastroenterology, 62, 1020-1033.

Dominici G, Orlandi F (1961). Ultrastructural and micro-analytical observations on human hepatic tissue removed by puncture biopsy in diabetic subjects. Proceed. Internat. Congr. Gastroenterol., 125-128. Excerpta Med. publ., Amsterdam.

Drochmans P, Wanson JC, Mosselmans R (1975). Isolation and subfractionation on Ficol gradiens of adult rat hepatocytes. J. Cell Biol., 66, 1-22.

Dunnill MS (1968). Quantitative methods in histology. In Rec. Adv. Clin. Pathol., Series V. S.C. Dyke eds, pp. 401-416. Churchill, London.

Elias H, Henning A, Schwartz DE (1971). Stereology: applications to biomedical research. Physiol. Rev., 51, 158-200.

Elias H, Sherrick JC (1969). Morphology of the liver. Academic Press, New York.

Elveback LR (1972). How high is high? A proposed alternative to the normal range. Mayo Clin. Proc., 47, 93-97.

Elveback LR (1973). The population of healthy persons as a source of reference information. Human Pathol., 4, 9-16.

Fawcett DW (1955). Observations on the cytology and electron microscopy of hepatic cells. J. Nat. Cancer Inst., 15, 1475-1503.

Feinstein AV (1967). Clinical Judgment. Williams and Wilkins Publ., Baltimore.

Feinstein AV (1970a). Clinical biostatistics. I. A new name and some order changers of the guard. Clin. Pharmacol. Ther., 11, 135-148.

Feinstein AV (1970b). Clinical biostatistics. II. Statistics versus science in the design of experiments. Clin. Pharmacol. Ther., 11, 282-292.

Feinstein AV (1974). Clinical biostatistics. XXVII. The derangements of the "range of normal". Clin. Pharmacol. Ther., 15, 528-540.

French SW, Davies PL (1975). Ultrastructural localization of actin-like philaments in rat hepatocytes. Gastroenterology, 68, 765-774.

Glagoleff AA (1933). On the geometrical methods of quantitative mineralogic analysis of rocks. Trans. Inst. Econ. Mineral. (Moscow), 59.

Hampton JC (1960). A re-evaluation of the submicroscopic structure of the liver. Texas Rep. Biol. Med., 18, 602-624.

Herzfeld AM, Federman M, Greengard O (1973). Subcellular morphometric and biochemical analyses of developing rat hepatocytes. J. Cell Biol., 57, 475-483.

Hess FA, Weibel ER, Preisig R (1973a). Morphometry of dog liver: normal base-line data. Virchows Arch. Abt. B Zellpath., 12,303-317.

Hess FA, Gnägi HR, Weibel ER, Preisig R (1973b). Morphometry of dog liver: comparison of wedge and needle biopsies. Europ. J. Clin. Invest., 3,451-458.

Hess FA, Preisig R, Weibel ER (1973c). The validity of needle biopsies for liver cytomorphometry, 58-61, In "The liver. Quantitative aspects of structure and function". G. Paumgartner and R. Preisig eds. S. Karger Publ., Basel.

Hibbitt KG, Baird GD (1967). An induced ketosis and its role in the study of primary spontaneous ketosis in the bovine. Vet. Rec., 81, 511-517.

Hope J (1970). Stereological analysis of the ultrastructure of liver parenchymal cells during pregnancy and lactation. J.

Ultrastruct. Res., 33, 292-305.

Howard RR, Lee JC, Pooch LA (1973). The fine structure, potassium content and respiratory activity of isolated rat liver parenchymal cells prepared by improved enzymathic techniques. J. Cell Biol., 57, 642-658.

Hruban Z, Recheigl NJ (1969). Microbodies and related particles. Academic Press, New York.

Jahn W (1973). Similarity between the effect of experimental congestion of the isolated perfused rat liver and the action of cytochalasin B. Naunyn Schmiedebergs Arch. Pharmacol., 278, 431-434.

Jezequel AM (1959). Degenerescence myelinique des mitochondries de foie humaine dans un epithelioma du cholédoque et un inctère viral. J. Ultrastruct. Res., 3, 210-215.

Jezequel AM (1962). Microscopie électronique du foie normal. Pathol. Biol. Semaine Hôp., 10, 501-525.

Jezequel AM, Koch MM, Capurso L, Lorenzini I, Freddara U, Orlandi F. Fine structure of the liver cells (in press).

Jezequel AM, Koch MM, Orlandi F (1974). A morphometric study of the endoplasmic reticulum in human hepatocytes. Gut, 15, 737-747.

Jezequel AM, Koch MM, Orlandi F (1975a). Liver response to drugs in man. A correlated morphometric and functional study. In Diseases of the Liver and biliary tract. Karger Publ., Basel.

Jezequel AM, Koch MM, Galeazzi R, Capurso L, Lorenzini I, Freddara U, Quattrini A, Orlandi F (1975b). Changes induced by Diphenylhydantoin and Phenobarbital in human liver. Correlated morphometric and functional data. J. Microsc. Biol. Cell, 22, 94.

Jezequel AM, Orlandi F (1972). Fine morphology of the human liver as a tool in clinical pharmacology, 145-192, in "Liver and Drugs", F. Orlandi and A.M. Jezequel eds., Academic Press Publ., New York.

Keller TC, Smetana HF (1950). Artefacts in liver biopsies. Amer. J. Clin. Pathol., 20, 738-747.

Koch MM, Galeazzi R, Lorenzini I, Jezequel AM, Orlandi F (1975). Changes of the liver cell endoplasmic reticulum in patients treated with Diphenylhydantoine and Phenobarbital. Morphometric and functional data. Rendiconti Gastroent., in press.

Koch MM, Jezequel AM, Orlandi F (1974). Endoplasmic reticulum of the human liver cell: morphometric evaluation in normal subjects and changes induced by drugs. Rendiconti Gastroent., 6, 213.

Loud AV (1962). Method for the quantitative estimation of cytopla smic structure. J. Cell Biol., 15, 481-487.

Loud AV (1967). Ultrastructure equilibria in liver cell cytoplasm. In Proc. 2nd Internat. Congr. Stereology, 72, H. Elias Ed., Springer- -Verlag, New York.

Loud AV (1968). A quantitative stereological description of the ultrastructure of normal rat liver parenchymal cells. J. Cell Biol., 37, 27-46.

Loud AV (1973). A quantitative electron microscopic view of liver cell fractions. In The Liver. Quantitative aspects of structure and function, 13-20, G. Paumgartner and R. Preisig eds., S. Karger Publ., Basel.

Loud AV, Barany WC, Pack BA (1965). Quantitative evaluation of cytoplasmic structures in electron micrographs. Lab. Invest., 14, 996-1008.

Ma MH, Biempica L (1971). The normal human liver cell, cytochemi cal and structural studies. Am. J. Pathol., 62, 353-390.

Ma MH, Goldfisher S, Biempica L (1972). Morphology of the normal liver cell, 1, 17, in "Progress in Liver Diseases", H. Popper and F. Schaffner eds., Grune and Stratton Publ., New York.

Matter A, Orci L, Rouiller C (1969). The study on the permeability barriers between Disse's space and the bile canaliculi. J. Ultras structure Res. (suppl.), 11, 1-71.

Menghini G, Orlandi F (1957). La puntura-biopsia epatica, Strumenti, Metodi, Pratica Clinica. Il Pensiero Scientifico Publ., Roma.

Molino G, Milanese M (1975). Structural analysis of compartmental models for the hepatic kinetics of drugs. J. Lab. Clin. Med., 55, 865-878.

Mugnaini E (1964). Filamentous inclusions in the matrix of mitochondria in human liver. J. Ultrastruct. Res., 11, 525-544.

Novikoff AB, Essner E (1960). The liver cell, some new approaches to its study. Am. J. Med., 29, 102-131.

Orlandi F. An AISF seminar on liver needle biopsies and laparo photographs in chronic hepatitis and cirrhosis. 2.3.1974, in press.

Oudea MC, Collette M, Oudea P (1973). Morphometric study of ultra structural changes induced in rat liver by chronic alcohol intake. Amer. J. Digest. Dis., 18, 398-402.

Oudea P, Domart-Oudea MC (1967). L'ultrastructure hépatique. I. Le foie normal. Rev. Franc. Etude. Clin. Biol., 12, 527-543.

Paumgartner G, Preisig R eds. (1973). The Liver. Quantitative aspects of structure and function. S. Karger Publ., Basel.
Redman CM, Banerjee D, Howell K, Palade GE (1975). Colchicine inhibition of plasma protein release from rat hepatocytes. J. Cell Biol., 66, 42-59.
Reid IM (1973). An ultrastructural and morphometric study of the liver of the lactating cow in starvation ketosis. Exper. Molec. Path., 18, 316-330.
Riede UN, Kuepfer A, Rasser Y, Rupp S, Rohr HP (1972). Vergleichende Ultrastrukturell-morphometrische untersuchung der Leberparenchym zellen der Wistarratten und der Wuestenratten. Z. Zellforsch, 123, 240-250.
Rohr HP, Bianchi L, Hundstad AC, Eckert H (1970). Morphometrisch--ultrastrukturelle untersuchungen ueber die durch die tageszeit induzierten veranderungen der rattenleberparenchymzellen. Acta Anat., 76, 102-113.
Rohr HP, Luthy J, Gudat F, Oberholzer M, Gysin C, Stalder G, Bianchi L (1975). Stereology: a new complement to the study of human liver biopsy specimens. Proc. 2nd Internat. Gstaad Symp., in press.
Rouiller CH, Jezequel AM (1963). Electron microscopy of the liver, in "The liver", Vol. I, 195-264, C.H. Rouiller ed. Academic Press Publ., New York.
Schaffner F, Popper H (1972). Electron microscopy of the liver, 50-83, in "Diseases of the liver", L. Schiff ed. Lippincott Publ., Philadelphia.
Segre G (1972). Kinetics of drugs in the hepatobiliary system. In "Liver and Drugs", F. Orlandi and A.M. Jezequel eds. Academic Press Publ., New York.
Slabodsky-Brousse N, Feldmann G, Brousse J, Dreyfus P (1974). Etude stéréologique de la fréquence des mitochondries géantes hépatiques dans la maladie de Gilbert. Comparaison avec le sujet normal. Biol. Gastroenterol. (Paris), 7, 179-186.
Snedecor GW, Cochran WG (1968). Statistical methods. Iowa Univ. Press Publ., Ames.
Soloway RD, Baggenstoss AH, Schoenfield LJ, Summerskill WHI (1971). Observer error and sampling variability tested in evaluation of hepatitis and cirrhosis by liver biopsy. Amer. J. Digest. Dis., 16, 1082-1086.
Staubli WS, Hess R, Weibel ER (1969). Correlated morphometric and biochemical studies on the liver cell. II. Effect of Phenobar bital on rat hepatocytes. J. Cell Biol., 42, 92-112.

Stein O, Sanger L, Stein Y (1974). Colchicine-induced inhibition
of lipoprotein and protein secretion into the serum and lack of
interference with secretion of biliary phospholipids and choleste
rol by rat liver in vivo. J. Cell Biol., 62, 90-103.
Steiner JW, Phillips MJ, Miyai K K (1964). Ultrastructural and
subcellular pathology of the liver. In Internat. Rev. Exper.
Pathol., Vol. 3, 65-167, G.W. Richter  and Epstein M.A. eds.
Academic Press Publ., New York.
Sturgess JM, De La Iglesia FA (1972). Morphometry of the Golgi
apparatus in developing liver. J. Cell Biol., 55, 524-530.
Tanikawa K (1968). Ultrastructural aspects of the liver and its
disorders. Springer-Verlag Publ., New York.
Trump BF, Dees JH, Shelburne JD (1973). The ultrastructure of
the human liver cell and its common patterns of reaction to injury,
80-120, in "The Liver", E.A. Gall and F. K. Mostofi eds. Williams
and Wilkins Publ., Baltimore.
Wagner RC, Rosenberg MD (1973). Endocytosis in Chang liver cells:
the role of microtubules in vacuole orientation and movement.
Cytobiologie, 7, 20-27.
Wagner RC, Rosenberg MD, Estensen R (1971). Endocytosis in Chang
liver cells. Quantitation by sucrose-3H uptake and inhibition by
cytochalasin B. J. Cell Biol., 50, 804-817.
Weibel ER (1963). Morphometry of the human lung. Academic Press
Publ., New York.
Weibel ER (1969). Stereological principles for morphometry in
electron microscopic cytology. Internat. Rev. Cytol., 26, 235-302.
Weibel ER (1973). Stereological methods for the qualification of
hepatic structures, 2-12, in "The Liver. Quantitative aspects of
structure and function", G. Paumgartner and R. Preisig eds.
S. Karger Publ., Basel.
Weibel ER, Elias H (1967). Quantitative methods in morphology.
Springer-Verlag Publ., Berlin.
Weibel ER, Kistler GS, Scherle WF (1966). Practical stereological
methods for morphometric cytology. J. Cell Biol., 30, 23-38.
Weibel ER, Staubli W, Gnägi HR, Hess FA (1969). Correlated morpho
metric and biochemical studies on the liver cell. I. Morphometric
model stereologic methods, and normal morphometric data for rat
liver. J. Cell Biol., 42, 68-91.
Welsch FA (1972). Distribution of glycogen within the liver lobule.
J. Histochem. Cytochem. Cytochem., 20, 112-115.
Wheeler HO, Meltzer JI, Bradley SE (1960). Biliary transport and
hepatic storage of sulfobromophtalein   sodium in the unanesthethi

zed dog, in normal man, and in patients with hepatic disease. J. Clin. Invest., 39, 1131-1144.

Wibo M, Amar-Cortesec A, Berthet J, Beaufay H (1971). Electron microscopic examination of subcellular fraction. III. Quantitative analysis of the microsomal fraction isolated from rat liver. J. Cell Biol., 51, 52-71.

Wiener J, Loud AV, Kimberg DV, Spiro D (1968). A quantitative description of cortisone-induced alterations in the ultrastructure of rat liver parenchymal cells. J. Cell Biol., 37, 47-61.

Wills EI (1965). Crystalline structures in the mitochondria of normal human liver parenchymal cells. J. Cell Biol., 24, 511-514.

Zamcheck N. Chalmers TC, Davidson CS (1949). Pathologic and functional changes in the liver following upper abdominal operations. Amer. J. Med., 7, 409-420.

DISCUSSION OF LECTURE BY F. ORLANDI

Altmann:    There is a big difference between the ultrastructure
of liver cells from the central and peripheral regions of the
lobule.    Also you know that there are different regional
reactions to drugs and such toxins as carbon tetrachloride.    So,
if you are comparing a first and second liver biopsy from the same
animal, whether it be man or dog, how can you be sure that you are
looking at changes from the same type of liver cell?

Orlandi:    Eighty per cent of liver cells are ultrastructurally
homogeneous, and about 20 per cent exhibit a different ultrastructural picture, as you have said.    You can choose an "average"
liver cell, or sublobular type of cell according to our protocol.
There are some values which lie outside the normal range.    For
example, if you wish to compare cells from normal and cholestatic
conditions you must have baseline data from centrolobular, midzonal and peripheral cells to make such a comparison possible.

Bradley:    Your work seems to me to be very important from the
standpoint of cell physiology.    But I do have reservations about
the contribution this type of work can make to an understanding
of the liver as an organ.    Have you given any thought to the
hepatic vasculature, because the liver is of great importance in
the cardiovascular system?    The liver is ordinarily distended
under different kinds of pressures in different parts of the
cardiovascular system.    So intrahepatic pressures must have
some effect on the configuration of structures.    Therefore I
think it is very important that work be carried out to see how
the ultrastructure of hepatocytes is related to changing
conditions in the hepatic vasculature.    Have you any data which
might relate to my remarks?

Orlandi:    No, we have not.

Coleman:    Have you ever observed any structures which we could
call vesicles which might be carrying material to the canaliculus
for secretion across the canaliculus?

Orlandi:    We have counted vesicles, but made no observations
about what they might be doing.

<u>Coleman</u>:   Have you ever seen any of these vesicles fusing with the canalicular area?

<u>Orlandi</u>:   This is an easy question.   The answer is, no, we have never seen what you describe.

<u>Popper</u>:   This is important and interesting work, but we should all remind ourselves that we are looking at artefacts in electron microscope preparations.   We should be fully aware that we have not reached the ultimate in the recognition and definition of the entire organelle system.   There is no doubt that there is an intercellular system of "cavities", but for simple optical reasons we cannot demonstrate this.   We have come a long way in the past 25 years, but we still have no idea of what kind of intracellular transport really takes place.   As a further example of our ignorance I would mention that we have knowledge of intercellular contractile proteins which can be defined in biochemical or biophysical ways, but we cannot see these with the electron microscopes available today.

To comment on Dr. Bradley's valid statements:  by electron microscopy it is quite impossible to answer the questions he raised because of the fixation and other processes needed to present the artefact we see under the microscope.   So I think that, at the present time, we should take full advantage of the morphometric technique, but bearing in mind this problem of artefact formation and the important points raised by Dr. Altmann and Dr. Bradley.   We electron microscopists look at the kind of cell we like best, and then prove from the cell we know best what we want to prove.   The kind of work Professor Orlandi is doing is moving us away from that terrible habit.

<u>Phillips</u>:   I think it should be pointed out that it is only when you have done some morphometry do you begin to realise what an enormous amount of work is involved.   When you examine, say, a human liver, there is an enormous range of variation of normal to be seen, even in the same piece of liver.   So I would like to see ranges of normal values given for morphometry, just as we have ranges of normal values for clinical biochemical values.

<u>Orlandi</u>:   But what is a <u>normal</u> liver?

<u>Phillips</u>:   Of course, that is <u>the</u> problem.

<u>Hofmann</u>:   For those of us with no experience of this kind of work, it seems to me that it should be possible to define such things as precision, accuracy and so on, because these measurements are very similar to those which exist for the usual clinical testing.   There we are concerned with reproducibility within one

laboratory, differences between laboratories and then what the
clinical chemists call "long term drift" or systematic changes
with time.   So large serum banks and standards have been set up,
and samples for analysis can be sent out to different laboratories
from time to time to assess the reliability of assays.   Would
such an arrangement be possible in morphometric studies, and if it
would be, what efforts are pathologists making to set up a system
of quality control?

Orlandi:   Such arrangements may be somewhat ambiguous, even in
routine clinical chemistry testing.   For example, if you use in-
patients as your normal standard values, you may get one set of
results, and other types of normal subjects may give different
values.   The situation in pathology is particularly difficult
and, as far as I know, no such pathological standards are being
set up.

Case:   You said that about 20 per cent of the liver cell consists
of mitochondria.   Do you have any information from serial sections
about the way in which mitochondria are organised in the liver?
Do they exist as numerous individual bodies, or is there some
form of organisation into coiled tubes for example?

Orlandi:   There appear to be two types of mitochondria in
hepatocytes:   some are rods and some are crescent-shaped.   I
think that mitochondria exist in the cell as discrete bodies,
since I have no evidence that their distribution is organised in
any way.

Ostrow:   I have been wondering about how the different alcoholic
drinking habits of different countries might affect what we may
consider normal.   Do you think alcohol intake may affect your
results?

Orlandi:   One can only assume that the alcohol consumption of
your normal population is fairly constant.

Steiner:   I would like to make an iconclastic statement.   I
admire Professor Orlandi's patience and all the work he has done.
But as a pathologist and morphologist myself I am really not
convinced that morphometry contributes anything to the pathologist.
My reason for saying this is because as long as biochemists,
physiologists and pharmacologists will believe that pathologists
really can, by morphometry, assess changes we will be living in
a "never-never" land.   I think it is important for everyone to
understand that morphology is really a form of witchcraft;   mostly
guesswork based on experience.   The accuracy which is implied in
morphometry really contributes very little in either diagnosis or
the assessment of both what is normal and what pathological.

<u>Bouchier</u>:   With respect to Dr. Ostrow's question, there seems to me to be no particular reason for picking on alcohol, because, as we know, our environment and diet contain so many compounds which might affect the fine structure of liver cells.   So it is almost impossible to decide what a normal environment is.

<u>Erlinger</u>:   You mentioned that the intercellular spaces were potentially in connection with the space of Disse.   This is an important point in relation to biliary secretion.   Do you mean to imply that under certain conditions this connection does not exist?

<u>Orlandi</u>:   I do not know, because it has not been established.

<u>Erlinger</u>:   Your main topic was on normal liver cells.   Have you been able to look at animal models such as Gunn rats or mutant Corriedale sheep that have the Dubin-Johnson syndrome?

<u>Orlandi</u>:   It has not been done as far as I know.

<u>Fisher</u>:   Do you have any idea how your estimate of canalicular surface might be altered by considering the microvilli?

<u>Orlandi</u>:   There are two levels of estimation.   In one you can estimate values on the basis of a smooth membrane, and also by considering the microvilli.   When comparing these the ratio of canalicular membrane varies from one to three or one to four.

ULTRASTRUCTURAL CHANGES INDUCED BY DRUGS

IN THE LIVER

A.M. Jezequel

Cell Pharmacology
University of Ancona
Ancona, Italy

Drugs represent useful tools in the study of various cellular metabolic pathways and it is of interest to analyze the early stages of drug-induced response of the liver to chemical injury. Too often in the past the ultrastructural studies have led to an accumulation of data, often purely anecdotal, and to a dispersion of the information. Only in the past decade, the application of stereological methods has permitted to obtain quantitative morphological data in normal conditions and in various pathological situations, and also to study some correlations with biochemical data. Until now most of these studies have been conducted on animal material, only a few in man.

Alterations induced by drugs involve changes in the configuration or in the amount of organelles, and also overload of the cell by substances not usually present or present in small amount in the cytoplasm such as biliary material, fat, iron, etc. The structural modifications often appear prominent at the level of one system of organelles(nucleus, mitochondria, peroxisomes, endoplasmic reticulum) but they are rarely isolated, rather part of a complex response involving other components as well. These associated modifications may escape purely qualitative observation. Conversely, focal changes may affect groups of hepatocytes, and by concentrating the attention of the observer on a limited area, they lead to false conclusions as to the organ as a whole, an error which may be avoided by a statistical analysis of randomized pictures. This review is too brief to cover all the changes induced by drugs in hepatocytes. It is rather an illustration of some of the most characteristic alterations of the liver cell ultrastructure. Organelle changes in drug-induced cholestasis are not considered here since they are being dealt with in another chapter.

## THE NUCLEUS

Nuclear changes are produced following the administration of
inhibitors of DNA or RNA synthesis, some antibiotics and antimeta
bolites, carcinogens and other unrelated substances (Bernhard and
Monneron, 1971; Monneron, 1971). More characteristic is the nucleo
lar segregation which leads to a sorting out and rearrangement of
nucleolar constituents in three distinct areas : the granules, the
fibrils and the protein matrix (Fig.1). Actinomycin D is the most
well  known of the agents capable of producing this alteration
(Stenram, 1965; Bernhard, 1971) and acts as an inhibitor of DNA
dependent RNA polymerase. But other drugs, acting at different le
vels can induce the same configurational changes such as acute in
toxication with mithramycin (Kume et al.,1967), anthramycin (Harris
et al., 1968a), 4-Nitroquinoline N-oxide (Reynolds et al.,1963),
senecio alkaloids (Svoboda and Soga, 1966), dimethylnitrosamine(DMN)
and methylazoxymethanol (MAM) (Ganote and Rosenthal, 1968), tannic
acid (Racela et al.,1967), aflatoxin (Bernhard et al.,1965; Svoboda
et al.,1966). It is interesting that with DMN or MAM, nucleolar
changes seem to be more prominent in centrolobular areas (Ganote
and Rosenthal, 1968). Accompanying cytoplasmic alterations involve
loss of ribosomes with an increase of smooth endoplasmic reticulum
(SER) and formation of whorled membranes. In contrast with acute
intoxication, chronic administration of aflatoxin leads to the for
mation of hepatomas without notable changes in nuclear or cytoplas
mic morphology (Svoboda et al.,1966). Also in the latter experiments,
strain  differences have been observed, with a marked periportal ne
crosis in rats and ducklings and predominance of focal cell necro
sis in monkey giving a picture somewhat similar to viral hepatitis
in man. The formation of nuclear "spheres", the retraction of chro
matin from the nuclear membrane, the clumping of interchromatin gra
nules are less characteristic events than the nucleolar segregation
and may be associated or not with it (Bernhard, 1971). It has been
suggested that the formation of "spheres" represent condensation of
ribonucleoproteins (Monneron, 1971). The giant nucleolar hypertro
phy produced by thioacetamide is rather unique and is accompanied
by increased rates of synthesis of high molecular weight RNA (Steele
et al.,1965). Giant nucleoli are almost exclusively composed of gra
nules with very few fibrils (Suter and Salomon, 1966) and they exhi
bit a sensitivity to the action of Actinomycin D or aflatoxin as
shown by the segregation of the various components after a brief
exposure to the drugs (Suter and Salomon, 1966). On the contrary,
thioacetamide is able to prevent the nucleolar cahnges induced by
Actinomycin (Kume and Chiga, 1967).

Inhibition of RNA synthesis follows the administration of
ethionine as well as Actinomycin D and other agents inducing nucleo
lar segregation but the nuclear alterations produced by these drugs
are not identical. After ethionine the disorganization and fragmen
tation of the nucleoli in small masses dispersed in the nucleoplasm

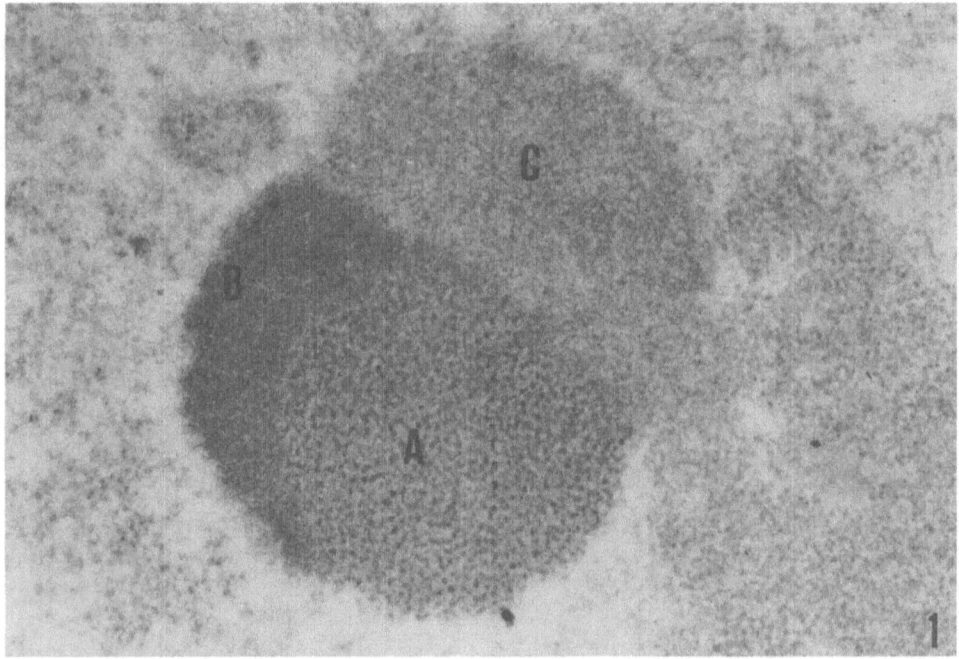

Fig.1. Segregation of nucleolar components induced by Actinomycin D.
A :granular component, B: fibrillar component, C: matrix
56000 X

is associated with aggregates of interchromatin granules and conden
sation of chromatin (Miyai and Steiner, 1967; Shinozuka et al.,1968).
The changes are likely to be related to the ATP deficiency induced
by ethionine and they are prevented or reversed by adenine or methio
ne (Shinozuka et al.,1968). The associated cytoplasmic changes,
disorganization of the rough endoplasmic reticulum, increase of the
smooth endoplasmic reticulum with formation of lamellar bodies,
seem to depend on mechanisms different from nuclear changes, maybe
related to intracellular differences in ATP metabolism, since the
spontaneous or the glucose-induced restitution of nucleolar integri
ty takes place notwithstanding persistent cytoplasmic alterations
(Shinozuka et al.,1970; Miyai et al.,1970). Low doses of D-galacto
samine which do not produce cell necrosis, allow the development
of nuclear alterations with fragmentation of nucleoli and formation
of fibrillar bodies somewhat similar to the changes occuring after
ethionine. These changes are prevented or reversed by uridine and
are probably related to the inhibition of RNA synthesis (Shinozuka
et al.,1973). A break-up of nucleoli with separation of granules

from fibrils also follows the administration of α-amanitin, an in
hibitor of RNA polymerase II (Marinozzi and Fiume, 1971). Rats seem
to recover better than mice after a single injection of the drug.

Most of the nuclear alterations we have described follow acute expe
riments performed in laboratory animals and, except perhaps for
α-amanitin, have no counterpart in human pathology. Clumping of
chromatin which is frequently observed in necrotic cells usually
precedes karyolysis. On the contrary, a variety of changes induced
at the cytoplasmic level can be observed in experimental animals as
well as in man.

## THE CYTOPLASM

### Smooth Endoplasmic Reticulum (SER)

Changes in the configuration of the SER are among the more pro
minent cytoplasmic alterations induced by drugs and they have arou
sed much interest since the SER is the site of a number of drug-meta
bolizing enzymes, and configurational changes of the membranes are
often related with changes in enzymatic activity. Phenobarbital (PB)
is the prototype of compounds capable of inducing both an increase
of microsomal membranes and an increase of drug-metabolizing enzy
mes (Remmer and Merker, 1963a; 1963b). The increase of the smooth
membranes appears early (2 to 4 days) in the rat or hamster treated
with PB and is accompanied by a depletion of liver glycogen (Jones
and Fawcett, 1966) (Fig.2), and the appearance of dense bodies dis
placing cristae in mitochondria (Burger and Herdson, 1966). Changes
of other cell components are not appreciable with qualitative obser
vations. However morphometric studies show that there is an early
rise in the surface density of both SER and rough endoplasmic reti
culum (RER) during the first 16 hours after administration of PB to
rats; thereafter the SER continues to increase whereas the RER de
creases progressively to return to control values by the fifth day
of treatment. The SER increase is positively correlated with the in
crease of microsomal drug-metabolizing enzymes such as Cytochrome
P-450, NADPH cytochrome c reductase and N-demethylase (Staubli et
al.,1969). In addition, there is an increase in the volume and num
ber of nuclei, whereas the increase in the specific number of mito
chondria and peroxisomes is accompanied by a decrease in their mean
volume (Staubli et al.,1969). Some discussion remains about the lo
bular distribution of changes induced by PB. The SER increase has
been said to occur first in peripheral hepatocytes (Remmer and Mer
ker, 1963a; 1963b), in centrolobular areas (Burger and Herdson, 1966)
or to vary from cell to cell (Orrenius and Ericsson, 1966). Recent
studies, based on density gradient centrifugation allow to distin
guish between two types of hepatocytes in the rat : "light" hepato
cytes, rich in SER would correspond to centrolobular cells and
"heavy" hepatocytes rich in glycogen would correspond to perilobular
cells. In PB-treated rats, the increase of the SER seems predominant
in the "light" cells (Wanson et al.,1975). However the localization

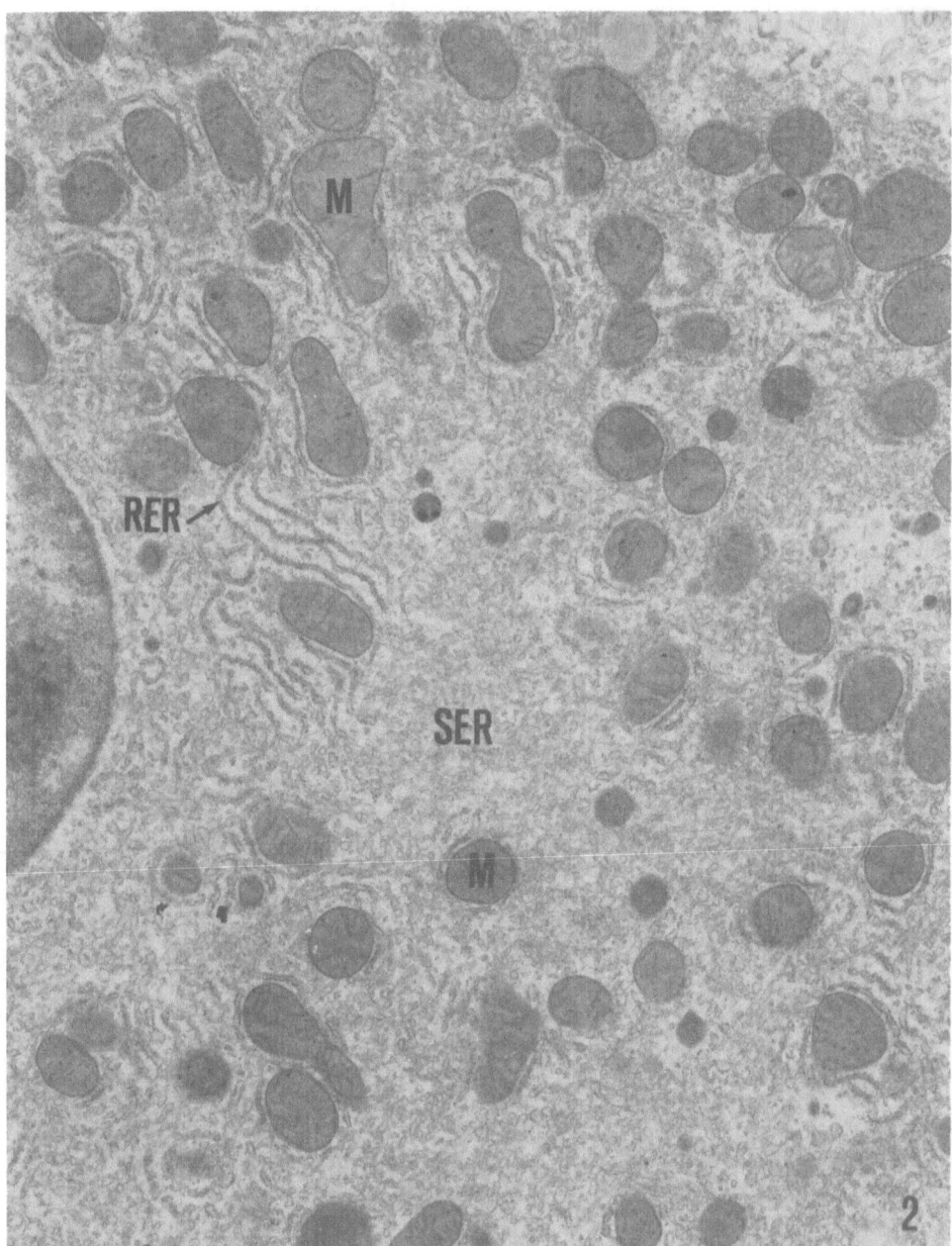

Fig.2. Part of a hepatocyte of rat given Phenobarbital(80 mg/kg/day) for 4 days. Small SER vesicles are numerous and diffuse throughout the cytoplasm. Flat cisternae of RER are located next to mitochondria (M). No glycogen particles are seen in this field. Compare with Fig.3, same magnification.                    11250 X

of "light" cells in the lobule is in contradiction with previous results (Castagna and Chauveau, 1969) and remains speculative in the absence of a specific marker for the cells of the various zones of the lobule. Suspenzion of PB administration leads to a progressi ve disappearance of excess smooth membranes. The return to a normal morphology is obtained in 5 days and is associated with an increase in number and volume of autophagic vacuoles containing ER membranes, showing the existence of a specific cellular mechanism in the turno ver of cytoplasmic membranes (Bolender and Weibel, 1973).

The increase of smooth membranes is not specifically correlated with enzymatic induction. A number of substances act on the model of PB such as Chlordane (Fouts and Rogers, 1965), DDT (Ortega, 1966), Thiohydantoin (Herdson et al.,1964), butylated hydroxytoluene (Con ning and Mc Elligott, 1970), progesterone (Emans and Jones, 1968). However polycyclic aromatic hydrocarbons such as 3-methylcholanthre ne and 3,4 benzpyrene, although inducers of microsomal enzymes, sti mulate a more limited number of metabolic pathways and give an in crease of a variant of cytochrome P-450 (P-448) but no change in NADPH-cytochrome c reductase (Hernandez et al.,1967) and no signifi cant changes in the amount of smooth membranes (Fouts and Rogers, 1965). Spironolactone produced an increase of smooth membranes (Kovacs et al.,1970) but no change or even a decrease of Cytochrome P-450 together with an increase in NADPH-cytochrome c reductase (Stripp et al;,1971). A normoactive hypertrophic SER has been obser ved in D-galactosamine induced hepatitis (Koff et al.,1973). The SER increase which follows chronic administration of pyrazole is accompanied by a depression of a number of microsomal enzymes (Lie ber et al.,1970). Dieldrin has a biphasic effect characterized by an early increase followed by a decrease of microsomal enzymes toge ther with a persistence of increased smooth membranes (Hutterer et al.,1968). On the other handn when PB is associated with aminotria zole, an inhibitor of heme synthesis, the increase of smooth membra nes occurs without changes of cytochrome P-450 (Raisfeld et al.,1970). Thus enzymatic induction is a complex phenomenon and variations of drug metabolism are mediated through several mechanisms which cannot be related to a single specific enzymatic component. In the same way, alterations in the distribution or amount of smooth membranes cannot be specifically related to modifications of a single metabo lic pathway, for instance to an increase of Cytochrome P-450, or another component of the group of microsomal enzymes. Indeed, even in the presence of inhibitors of Cytochrome P-450 such as carbon tetrachloride ($CCl_4$) there is an early increase of smooth membranes associated with a degranulation of rough membranes. This might repre sent denaturation rather than proliferation of SER (Reynolds and Ree, 1971). The conspicuous increase in smooth membranes produced in the rat by a diazafluoranthen derivative ( AC-3579) is not due to an increased synthesis of membranous components but to a decrea sed breakdown of phospholipids. This is accompanied by the presence of numerous lamellated lysosomes, probably related to the impairment of the normal breakdown of SER membranes by the lysosomal enzymes (Thys et al.,1973; Hildebrand et al,,1973). These alterations recall those occuring after triparanol (Hruban et al.,1965c) or chloroqui ne (Abraham et al.,1968). Such a mechanism may be responsible for the alterations ("phospholipidosis") induced in human liver by a coronary dilating agent (Itoh and Tsukada, 1973; dela Iglesia et al. 1974). It could also account, at least in part, for the early in crease of smooth membranes following halothane (Bombeck et al., 1969; Ross and Cardell, 1972) in relation with the binding of a me tabolite of halothane to microsomal phospholipids (Van Dyke and Wood, 1975).

Formation of whorls or "fingerprints" also follows the adminis tration of inducing agents (Herdson et al.,1964) and a variety of other substances (Stenger, 1970). These lamellar formations have been variably interpreted as evidence of degeneration or regenera tion phenomena (Stneger, 1970). In rats given cyclizine or chlorcy clizine, the accumulation of smooth cisternae occurs around lipid droplets (perilipidic smooth cisternae) and the smooth membranes occasionally show transition with rough cisternae. These membranous components have been thought to be involved in lipid metabolism (Hruban et al.,1974).

The study of changes of the endoplasmic reticulum following ethanol administration are still controversial. A proliferation of the SER has been described in rat and in man together with an in crease of various drug-metabolizing enzymes (Rubin et al.,1968; Lieber, 1973) but the increase of SER membranes does not appear as a constant feature (Koff et al.,1970). Quantitative studies suggest that the increase of smooth membranes might be partly due to a de granulation of the RER (Oudea et al.,1973) while others have found a true decrease of the SER (Dobbins et al.,19727. Differences in the experimental procedure or in the diet may account for these dis crepancies.

Structural changes of the SER occur not only in experimental conditions in animals given high dosage of a drug, but also in hu mans given therapeutic doses. A few observers have reported an in crease of SER in man after administration of alcohol (Rubin et al., 1968), PB (Crigler and Gold, 1969; Whelton et al.,1968), Rifampicin (Jezequel et al.,1971), Triacetyloleandomycin (Jezequel and Orlandi, 1972), oral contraceptives (Perez et al.,1972), benzodiazepin (Jeze quel et al.,1974 ; Orlandi et al.,1975), hydantoin alone or associa ted with other anticonvulsant agents (Jezequel et al., 1975a, 1975b). However studies in man are often hampered by the lack of base-line data and ethical problems make it difficult to dispose of biopsies of normal untreated patients for comparison purposes. This together with the subjectivity of the observer makes quantitation of data especially useful in the study of drug-induced changes in human li ver. In fact, morphometric studies have shown that contrary to the rat, the SER is more abundant than the RER in normal untreated pa

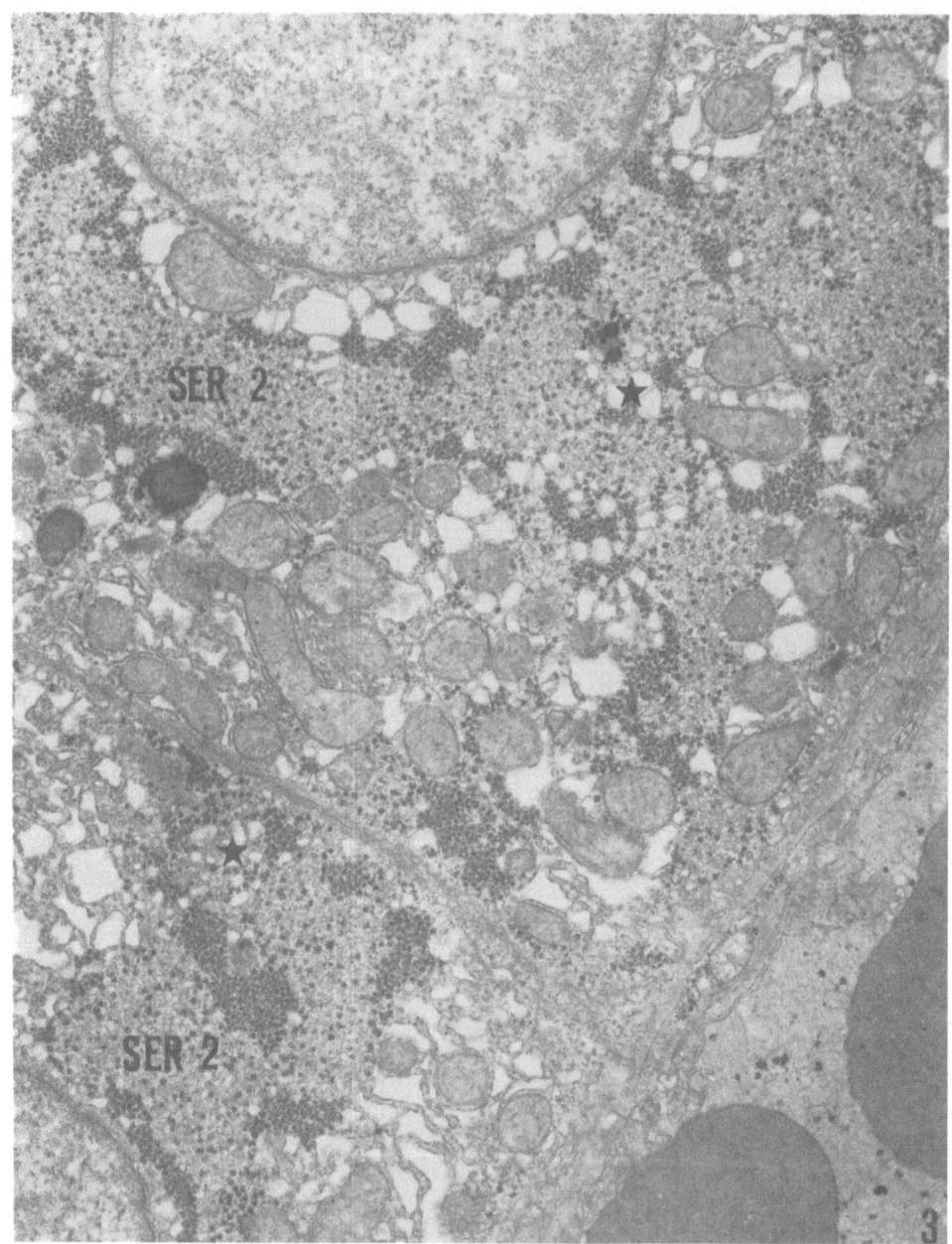

Fig.3. Liver biopsy in a patient under combined anticonvulsant thera
py for 9 years. Two hepatocytes in the field contain vast areas of
densely packed smooth membranes(SER 2). Some smooth surfaced vesci
cles are also present(stars). Compare with Fig.2, same magnification
for the different pattern of membrane proliferation.      11250 X

tients and it may be divided in two components, the SER type 1 or
vesicular and the SER type 2 compact or non vesicular (Jezequel et
al.,1974). Under treatment with benzodiazepin, the amount of SER
almost doubled after 2 to 4 days treatment (Jezequel et al.,1974;
Orlandi et al.,1975). Changes appeared only after 14 days treatment
and despite an early fall in serum bilirubin, in a patient with
Gilbert's syndrome treated with PB while in one patient with Cri
gler-Najjar syndrome treated with hydantoin, the increase in smooth
membranes was evident only after one of treatment (Jezequel et al.,
1975 a, 1975b). In all these cases, the increase affected mainly
the SER 2 component. On the other hand, changes following anticon
vulsant therapy were evident after 3 weeks of treatment and persis
ted in patients treated up to 15 years : the SER 1 was increased up
to threefold and the SER 2 increased up to eightfold. The overload
of hepatocytes by smooth membranes led to a profound modification
of the liver cell architecture (Jezequel et al.,1975b)(Fig. 3) and
this was observed in all cells in the lobule, except for a row of
hepatocytes next to the protal areas corresponding to the limiting
plate.

     In man as in animals, an increase of smooth membranes is not
indicative per se of an induction of microsomal enzymes and of a
stimulation of drug metabolism. However this finding provides a va
luable information in the study of the properties of a substance or
in the screening of new drugs. Besides the kinetics of drugs, addi
tional information useful in the interpretation of morphological
data in humans can be gained by the evaluation of some drug-metabo
lizing enzymes in liver biopsy material. Rifampicin for instance
increases the Cytochrome P-450 (Schoene et al.,1972a) and hydantoin
therapy increases the level of NADPH cytochrome c reductase (Jeze
quel et al.,unpublished results). Besides these two enzymatic sys
tems, other microsomal enzymes can be measured on biopsy material
(Schoene et al.,1972b; Gang et al.,1972). The data concerning drug
metabolism in vitro and the estimation of some functional parameters
such as the urinary excretion of D-glucaric acid (Hunter et al.,
1972, 1973) allow the study of correlations with the morphological
quantitative data as already made in rat (Staubli et al.,1969) or
in the guinea-pig (Hunter et al.,1973). It is of interest that in
man the increase in surface density of the SER 2 was positively cor
related with the hepatic cholesterol synthesis in benzodiazepin-trea
ted patients (Orlandi et al.,1975) and it was correlated with the
urinary D-glucaric output in PB or DPH-treated subjects (Jezequel et
al.,1975b). No correlation was found with the values of gamma gluta
myl transpeptidase.

     The intense cytoplasmic acidophilia observed with the light
microscope in man after administration of methandrostenolone -an ana
bolic steroid- is due to a diffuse increase of smooth membranes in
the hepatocyte with a localization of mitochondria and RER around
the nucleus and along the cell membrane (Jezequel and Orlandi, 1962;

Orlandi and Jezequel, 1966). An increase of the SER also follows
the administration of oral contraceptives (Larsson-Cohn and Stenram,
1965; 1967; Perez et al.,1969). Steroids are naturally occuring sub
strateds for drug-metabolizing enzymes (Kuntzman, 1969) and an inter
ference of these compounds with normal microsomal metabolism may
explain some of their adverse effects on the liver function, maybe
on a genetical basis (Aldercreutz and Tehunen, 1970; Metreau et al.,
1972).

The induction of microsomal enzymes in the fetal liver is still
a controversial subject. Glucagon accelerates the structural diffe
rentiation and the development of SER in fetal hepatocytes (Chu and
Phillips, 1970). On the other hand, there is some evidence that the
administration of inducing agents like pregnelonone 16 $\alpha$-carbonitri
le to pregnant rats have little or no effect on fetal liver (Tuchwe
ber et al.,1972). However these experimental findings cannot be ex
trapolated to man since notable species differences exist in the pat
tern of development of microsomal enzymes in the fetal liver (Gillet
te and Stripp, 1975).

### Rough Endoplasmic Reticulum (RER)

Disorganization of the RER is a common reaction to injury and
follows the administration of a number of substances such as ethio
nine and puromycin (Villa-Trevino et al.,1964; Wood, 1965), azaseri
ne (Hruban et al.,1965b), phenylalanine analogues (Hruban et al.,
1963, 1965a), taurolithocholate (Schaffner et al.,1966), CC14
(Smuckler et al.,1962; Ganote et al.,1968) ethanol (Thorpe and Sho
rey, 1966; Oudea et al.,1970) 3'methyl-4-dimethylaminobenzene (Por
ter and Bruni, 1959; Ketterer et al.,1967; Arcasoy et al.,1968),
cycloheximide (Harris et al., 1968b; Verbin et al.,1969) and various
other compounds (Stenger, 1970) including extensive damage produced
by chenodeoxycholic acid on isolated perfused rat liver (Miyai et
al.,1971). The disorganization of the RER is often accompanied by a
fragmentation and a dilatation of the cisternae but these alterati
ons are highly unspecific and may be observed in non related condi
tions such as ischemia (Bassi and Bernelli-Zazzera, 1964), shock
(Boler and Bibighaus, 1967; Blair et al.,1968) and also in autolysis
(Trump et al.,1965). In man alterations of the RER have also been
seen after ethanol (Rubin and Lieber, 1967), treatment with 6-mer
captopurine (Orlandi and Jezequel, 1971) and a variety of conditions
(Feinman et al.,1972). It is generally believed that swelling of the
RER is due to cellular uptake of water and this may also occur as a
passive phenomenon during technical preparation of the samples for
electron microscopy, introducing artefacts in the specimen. Thus al
terations described as "swelling" of the endoplasmic reticulum should
always be interpreted with great caution.

On the contrary, changes in the distribution and number of ribo
somes, degradation of polysomes,accompanied by biochemical changes,
mainly impaired protein synthesis and decreased aminoacid incorpo

ration have been well documented for instance after intoxication
with actinomycin D (Smuckler and Benditt, 1964), CC14 (Smuckler et
al.,1962; Smuckler, 1963, 1966; Recknagel et al.,1973), ethionine
(Farber et al.,1964; Steiner et al.,1964; Meldolesi et al.,1967),
phosphorus and thioacetamide (Barker et al.,1963) and dimethylnitro
samine (Hultin et al.,1960; Emmelot and Benedetti, 1960; Ganote and
Rosenthal, 1968). Still more specific is the formation of "helical
polysomes" which follow  the injection of lasiocarpin or aflatoxin
and which have been considered as a special type of polysomes, due
to a change in the nature of the messenger RNA (Monneron, 1969).
A special mention must be made about the Mallory bodies (alcoholic
hyalin) which are often observed in man in alcoholic hepatitis.
Originally supposed to originate from altered RER membranes (Biava,
1964), they appear to result from an accumulation of actin-like pro
teins identified by immunofluorescence in the liver cell cytoplasm
(Nenci, 1975) and probably represent ethanol-induced alterations of
the network of actin-like filaments recently described (French and
Davis, 1975) in hepatocytes.

## Mitochondria

Mitochondrial alterations are one of the most noticeable-al
though non specific- alterations following alcohol administration in
man or in rats and include the presence of megamitochondria with fi
lamentous inclusions, enlarged mitochondria with dense bodies, stacks
of cristae (Svoboda and Manning, 1964; Rubin and Lieber, 1967; 1970;
Oudea et al.,1970). These are probably related to various alterations
in the enzymatic equipment of mitochondria such as a diminished abi
lity to oxidize various substrates together with an increase of
$\delta$ -amino levulinic acid (ALA) synthetase (Rubin et al.,1970; Fein
man et al.,1972). Morphometric measurements show that the increase
in volume density of mitochondria occurs without a change in the
number of these organelles which suggest that the increase in volu
me results from an adaptive change (Oudea et al.,1973). A similar
adaptive phenomenon might occur in animals given thyroxine (Harman
and Sheldon, 1971), cuprizone (Suzuki, 1969) or cortisone (Wiener
et al.,1968) which develop greatly enlarged mitochondria. With cor
tisone, the mean volume of mitochondria shows up to a fourfold in
crease together with  a decrease in the number of mitochondria per
cell so that the total mitochondrial volume per cell remains unchan
ged (Wiener et al.,1968). Similar observations have been made in rats
given triiodothyronine (Reith, 1973). Thus, apparent "swelling" of
mitochondria, or "bizarre" shapes, should not necessarily be conside
red as a degenerative change of these organelles. On the contrary,
electron opaque masses made up of aggregates of electron-dense granu
les or of needle-like structures present in the mitochondria of
CC14-intoxicated rats result from cell injury and have been shown to
contain calcium bound to glycoproteins (Reynolds, 1965; Bonucci et
al.,1973). The filamentous inclusions observed in mitochondria du
ring steroid-induced cholestasis (Perez et al.,1969) are non-speci

fic since they are observed with a variable frequency in the liver
of normal subjects (Rouiller and Jezequel, 1963; Wills, 1965, Mugnai
ni, 1965; Ma and Biempica, 1971). They seem to be often associated
with steatosis. Optical diffraction studies show that in normal or
in pathologic human liver, these inclusions are actually crystals
with a periodical structure. They are not made up of simple phospho
lipids, but rather of phospholipid micelles or of relatively large
protein molecules. Although suggested, their relationship with mito
chondrial cristae has not been demonstrated (Sternlieb and Berger,
1969). In steroid-induced cholestasis, as in other forms of chole
stasis, "curled" cristae are often present in mitochondria. Morpho
metric studies show that this is associated with an increase of the
ratio mitochondrial cristae/external mitochondrial membrane, i.e. a
true increase of the surface density of mitochondrial cristae (Ca
purso et al.,1975).

## Peroxisomes

Drug-induced increase in the number of peroxisomes has been
first reported after administration of ethyl chlorophenoxyisobutyra
te (CPIB) (Hess et al.,1965; Svoboda and Azarnoff, 1966) and is also
part of the response to other hypolipidemic agents such as nafenopin
(Su-13437) (Hess and Bencze, 1968; Reddy et al.,1974) or unrelated
compounds such as salicylates, some antihistaminics and aminogluthe
timide (Hruban et al., 1974a; 1974b). Numerical changes are associa
ted with the appearance of fibrillar material in the matrix, a de
crease in the number of cores, an increase of the SER and an increa
se of the catalase, a peroxisomal enzyme, thus representing another
type of enzymatic induction. Study of the interrelationships between
these various elements and also of the relationship with cholesterol
metabolism may help to understand better the role of peroxisomes in
cell metabolism. Only male rats and mice seem to respond to the  ac
tion of CPIB whereas no sex difference is appreciable  in nafenopin-
treated animals (Reddy et al.,1974). A proliferation of peroxisomes
has also been observed in man under treatment with 6-Mercaptopurine
(Orlandi and Jezequel, 1971) (Fig.4). It is likely that many of the
organelles described as "mitochondria-like bodies" in patients recei
ving contraceptive steroids (Larsson-Cohn and Stenram, 1965; 1967)
are in fact peroxisomes increased in size and number. On the contra
ry a decrease in the number of peroxisomes occurs in rats receiving
cortisone (Wiener et al.,1968) and it is of interest that this is
associated with a decrease of the SER, perhaps indicating a rela
tionship between the two phenomena.

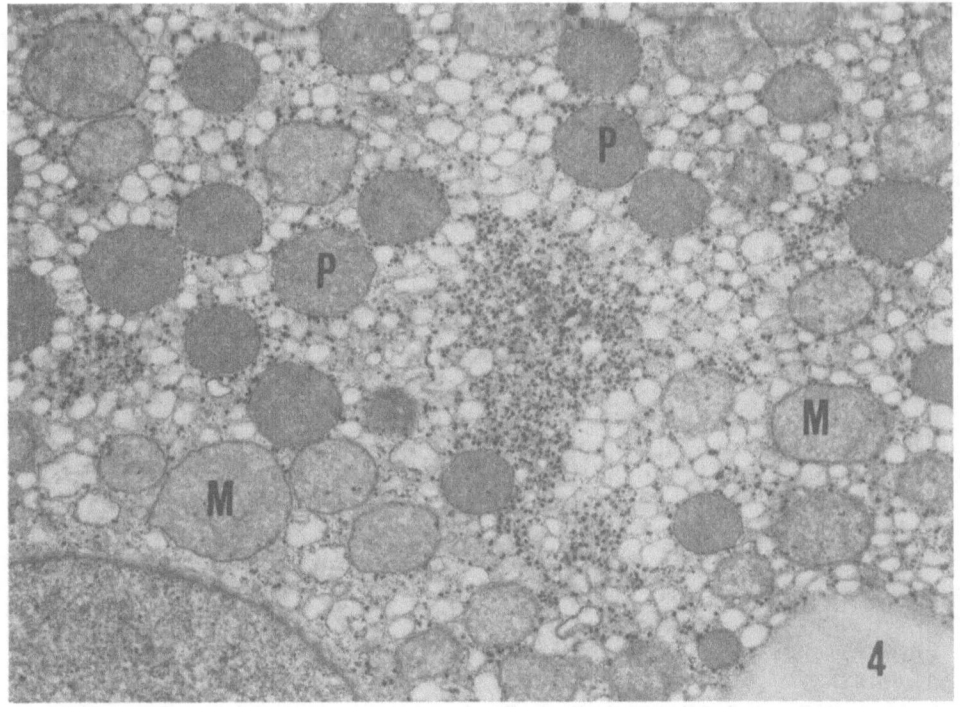

Fig. 4. Increase of the number of peroxisomes (P) in a patient under treatment with 6-Mercaptopurine (Purinethol). The ratio peroxisomes/ mitochondria (M) is close to 1 to 1.     15000X

## Golgi Apparatus

Alterations in the conformation of the Golgi apparatus often appear as part of an unspecific response to a great variety of agents. However the alterations induced by colchicine recently described (Redman et al., 1975) have indicated this drug as a useful tool in the study of the movement of secretory proteins : in vivo as in vitro colchicine causes an accumulation of secretory products inside the hepatocytes especially at the level of the Golgi complex and Golgi-derived vacuoles. Although an interaction of colchicine with micro tubules has been postulated, there was no morphological evidence for such a mechanism (Redman et al.,1975). The involvement of the Golgi apparatus and of some smooth-surfaced vesicles in the transport of lipoproteins to the space of Disse also results from radioauto graphic studies of the liver in ethanol-treated rats (Stein and Stein, 1967).

## CONCLUDING REMARKS

1. There is a general feeling that the morphological types of response of the liver cell to pharmacological stimuli are few and aspecific. This short review shows however that experimental models allow the study of a variety of changes at the level of the nucleus or of the cytoplasm.

2. These changes do not necessarily have a predictive value for humans, since the experimental models are often distant from the real life situations.

3. The range of use of electron microscopy in pharmacology is situated between the normal base-line data and the development of fine structural changes of the organelles. Necrosis and gross morphological alterations are beyond this range. In this field of study, various types of information can be obtained.
a) a morphology still normal, but with dimensional variations of the components. This can be obtained also with the study of cell fractions.
b) alterations of the architecture and arrangement of structures, for instance the smooth endoplasmic reticulum. This can be analysed only in situ.
c) alterations in the topographical relationship between the cell components, for instance the "polarization" of the organelles. This also can be seen only in situ.

4. The quantitative analysis of the cellular components does not replace the qualitative observation, but it represents an additional and valuable source of information in this field of study.

## REFERENCES

ABRAHAM R, HENDY R and GRASSO P. Formation of myeloid bodies in rat liver lysosomes after chloroquine administration. Exp.Mol. Path. 1968,9,212
ALDERCREUTZ H and TENHUNEN R. Some aspects of the interaction between natural and synthetic female sex hormones and the liver. Am.J.Med. 1967,42,341.
ARCASOY M, SMUCKLER EA and BENDITT EP. Acute effects of 3'Methyl-4-Dimethylaminobenzene intoxication on rat liver. Am.J.Path.1968, 52,841.
BARKER EA, SMUCKLER EA and BENDITT EP. Effects of thioacetamide and yellow phosphorus poisoning on protein synthesis in vivo. Lab.Inv.1963,12,955.
BASSI M and BERNELLI-ZAZZERA A. Ultrastructural cytoplasmic changes of liver cells after reversible and irreversible ischemia. Exp.Mol.Path. 1964,3,332.

BERNHARD W. Drug-induced changes in the interphase nucleus. In "Advances in Cytopharmacoloty", Vol.1, F.Clementi and B.Ceccarelli eds. Raven Press, N.Y. 1971, p.49.

BERNHARD W, FRAYSSINET Ch., LAFARGE Ch. and LE BRETON E. Lesions nucleolaires précoces provoquées par l'aflatoxine dans les cellules hépatiques du rat. Comptes Rendus Acad.Sci.Paris, 1965,261,1785

BIAVA C. Mallory alcoholic hyalin : a heretofore unique lesion of hepatocellular ergastoplasm. Lab. Inv. 1964,13,301

BLAIR OM, STENGER RJ, HOOKINS RW and SIMEONE FA. Hepatocellular ultrastructure in dogs with hypovolemic shock. Lab.Inv. 1968,18,172

BOLENDER RP and WEIBEL ER. A morphometric study of the removal of phenobarbital-induced membranes from hepatocytes after cessation of treatment. J.Cell Biol. 1973,56,746

BOLER RK and BIBIGHAUS AJ. Ultrastructural alterations of dog livers during endotoxin shock. Lab.Inv. 1967,17,537

BOMBECK CT, AOKI T, SMUCKLER EA and NYHUS LM. Effects of halothane, ether and chloroform on the isolated perfused bovine liver. Am.J. Surg. 1968,117,91

BONUCCI E, DERENZINI M and MARINOZZI V. The organic-inorganic relationship in calcified mitochondria. J.Cell Biol. 1973,59,185

BURGER PC and HERDSON PB. Phenobarbital-induced fine structural changes in rat liver. Am.J.Path. 1966,48,793

CAPURSO L, KOCH MM, FREDDARA U, LORENZINI I, JEZEQUEL AM and ORLANDI F. Contribution of morphometry to the study of cholestasis in man. Proc. 10th Meeting Europ. Assoc. Study Liver, Barcelona 1975 Digestion (in press)

CASTAGNA M and CHAUVEAU J. Separation des hepatocytes isoles de rat en fractions cellulaires distinctes. Exp.Cell Res. 1969,57,211

CHIU HF and PHILLIPS MJ. Glucagon induces premature structural differentiation of fetal hepatocytes. Lab.Inv. 1974,30,305

CONNING DM and McELLIGOTT TF. Quantitation of the proliferative response of smooth endoplasmic reticulum to dietary butylated hydroxytoluene and its toxicological significance. Proc.Eur.Soc. Study Drug Tox. 1970,11,203

CRIGLER JF Jr. and GOLD NI. Effect of sodium phenobarbital on bilirubin metabolism in an infant with congenital non hemolytic, unconjugated hyperbilirubinemia and kernicterus. J.Clin.Invest.1969.48,42

DE LA IGLESIA F, FEUER G, TAKADA A and MATSUDA Y. Morphologic studies on secondary phospholipidosis in human liver. Lab.Inv.1974,30,539

DOBBINS WO III, ROLLINS EL, BROOKS SG and FALLON MJ. A quantitative morphological analysis of ethanol effect upon rat liver. Gastroenterology 1972,62,1020

EMANS JB and JONES AL. Hypertrophy of liver cell smooth surfaced reticulum following progesterone administration. J.Histochem. Cytochem. 1968,16,561

EMMELOT P and BENEDETTI EL. Changes in the fine structure of rat liver cells brought about by dimethylnitrosamine. J.Biophys.Biochem. Cytol. 1960,7,393

FEINMAN L, RUBIN E and LIEBER CS. Adaptation of the liver to drugs.

In "Liver and Drugs", F.Orlandi and AM Jezequel eds. Acad.Press, London, 1972, p.41

FOUTS JR and ROGERS LA. Morphological changes in the liver accompanying stimulation of microsomal drug metabolizing enzyme activity by Phenobarbital, Chlordane, Benzpyrene or methylcholanthrene in rats. J.Pharmacol.Exp.Therap. 1965,147,112

GANG H, LIEBER CS and RUBIN E. Aniline hydroxylase microassay suitable for needle biopsy specimens : effects of phosphate and pyrophosphate on aniline hydroxylation. J.Pharmacol.Exp.Therap.1972,183, 218

GANOTE C and ROSENTHAL AS. Characteristic lesions of methylazoxymethanol-induced liver damage. Lab.Inv. 1968,19,383

HARMAN J and SHELDON H. On the increase in size of mitochondria and appearance of new intramitochondrial enzyme following treatment with L-thyroxine. Lab.Inv. 1971,24,433

HARRIS C, GRADY H and SVOBODA D. Segregation of the nucleolus produced by anthramycin. Canc.Res. 1968a,28,81

HARRIS C, GRADY H and SVOBODA D. Alteration in pancreatic and hepatic ultrastructure following acute cycloheximide intoxication. J. Ultrastr.Res. 1968b,22,240

HERDSON PB, GARVIN PJ and JENNINGS RB. Reversible biological and fine structural changes produced in rat liver by a thiohydantoin compound. Lab.Inv.1964,13,1014

HERNANDEZ PH, MAZEL P and GILLETTE JR. Studies on the mechanism of action of mammalian hepatic azoreductase. Biochem.Pharmacol.1967, 16,1877

HESS R and BENCZE WL. Hypolipidemic properties of a new tetralin derivative (CIBA 13,437-Su) Experientia, Basel, 1968,24,418

HESS R, STAUBLI W and REISS W. Nature of the hepatomegalic effect produced by ethyl chlorophenoxy-isobutyrate in the rat. Nature, 1965,208,856

HILDEBRAND J, THYS O and GERIN Y. Alterations of rat liver lysosomes and smooth endoplasmic reticulum induced by the Diazafluoranthen derivative AC-3579. II.Effects of the drug on phospholipid metabolism. Lab.Inv. 1973,28,83

HRUBAN Z, GOTOH M, SLESERS A and CHOU S. Structure of hepatic microbodies in rats treated with acetylsalicylic acid, clofibrate and dimethrin. Lab.Inv. 1974a,30,64

HRUBAN Z, MOCHIZUKI Y, GOTOH M, SLESERS A and CHOU S. Effect of some hypocholesterolemic agents on hepatic ultrastructure and microbody enzymes. Lab.Inv. 1974b,30,474

HRUBAN Z, SWIFT H, DUNN FW and LEWIS DE. Effect of $\beta$-3 Furylalanine on the ultrastructure of the hepatocytes and pancreatic acinar cells. Lab.Inv. 1965a,14,70

HRUBAN Z, SWIFT H and SLESERS A. Effect of azaserine on the fine structure of the liver and pancreatic acinar cell. Canc.Res.1965b, 25,708

HRUBAN Z, SWIFT H and SLESERS A. Effect of triparanol and diethanolamine on the fine structure of hepatocytes and pancreatic acinar cells. Lab.Inv. 1965c,14,1652

HRUBAN Z, SWIFT H and WISSLER RW. Alterations in the fine structure of hepatocytes produced by β-3-thienylalanine. J.Ultrastr.Res. 1963,8,236

HULTIN T, ARRHENIUS E, LOW H and MAGEE PN. Toxic liver injury: inhibition by dimethylnitrosamine of incorporation of labelled aminoacids into proteins of rat liver preparation in vitro. Biochem.J. 1960,76,109

HUNTER J, MAXWELL JD, CARELLA M, STEWARD DA and WILLIAMS R.Urinary D-glucaric excretion as a test for hepatic enzyme induction in man. Lancet, 1971,1,572

HUNTER J, MAXWELL JD, STEWART DA and WILLIAMS R. Urinary D-glucaric acid excretion and total liver content of cytochrome P-450 in guinea-pigs. Biochem.Pharmacol. 1973,22,743

HUTTERER F, SCHAFFNER F, KLION F and POPPER H. Hypertrophic hypo-active smooth endoplasmic reticulum; a sensitive indicator of hepatotoxicity exemplified by dieldrin. Science, 1968,161,1017

ITOH S and TSUKADA Y. Clinico-pathological and electron micro-scopical studies on a coronary dilating agent: 4-4'-diethylamino-ethoxyexestrol-induced liver injuries. Acta Hepato-Gastroent. 1973,20,204

JEZEQUEL AM, KOCH MM, GALEAZZI R, CAPURSO L, LORENZINI et al. Changes induced by Diphenylhydantoin and/or Phenobarbital in human liver. J.Microsc.Biol.Cell. 1975,22,94

JEZEQUEL AM, KOCH MM, GALEAZZI R, LORENZINI I and ORLANDI F. Liver response to drugs in man. A correlated morphometric and functional study. In "Diseases of the liver and biliary tract". S.Karger (Basel) 1975b.(in press)

JEZEQUEL AM, KOCH MM and ORLANDI F. A morphometric study of the endoplasmic reticulum in human hepatocytes. Correlation between morphological and biochemical data under treatment with some drugs. Gut, 1974,15,737

JEZEQUEL AM and ORLANDI F. Electron microscopy of the human liver after methandrostenolone adminstration. In "Aktuelle Probleme der Hepatologie", GA Martini ed., G.Thieme Verlag, Stuttgart,1962,p.41

JEZEQUEL AM and ORLANDI F. Fine morphology of the human liver as a tool in clinical pharmacology. In "Liver and Drugs", F. Orlandi and AM Jezequel eds. Acad.Press, London 1972, p.145

JEZEQUEL AM, ORLANDI F and TENCONI LT. Changes of the smooth endo-plasmic reticulum induced by rifampicin in human and guinea-pig hepatocytes. Gut, 1971,12,984

JONES AL and FAWCETT DW. Hypertrophy of the agranular endoplasmic reticulum in hamster liver induced by phenobarbital. J.Histochem. Cytochem. 1966,14,215

KETTERER B, HOLT SJ and ROSS-MANSELL P. The effect of a single dose of the hepatocarcinogen 4-dimethylaminobenzene on the rough surfaced endoplasmic reticulum of the liver of the rat. Biochem.J. 1967, 103,692

KOFF RS, CARTER EA, LUI S and ISSELBACHER KJ. Prevention of the

ethanol-induced fatty liver in the rat by phenobarbital. Gastroenterology, 1970,59,50

KOFF RS, DAVIDSON LJ, GORDON G and SABESIN S. D-galactosamine
hepatotoxicity. III.Normoactive smooth endoplasmic reticulum and
modification by phenobarbital. Exp.Mol.Path. 1973,19,168

KOVACKS K, BLASCHECK JA and GARDELL C. Spironolactone-induced
proliferation of smooth-surfaced endoplasmic reticulum in the
liver of rats. Zeitsch.ges.Exp.Med. 1970,152,104

KUME F and CHIGA M. Inhibition of the actinomycin-induced
nucleolar change by thioacetamide in mouse hepatic parenchymal
cells. Lab.Inv.1967,17,767

KUME F, MARUYAMA S, d'AGOSTINA AN and CLUGA M. Nucleolar change
produced by mithramycin in rat hepatic cells. Exp.Mol.Path.1967,
6,254

KUNTZMAN R. Drugs and enzyme induction. Ann.Rev.Pharmacol.1969,9,21

LARSSON-COHN U and STENRAM U. Jaundice during treatment with oral
contraceptives. J.A.M.A. 1965,193,422

LARSSON-COHN U and STENRAM U. Liver ultrastructure and function in
icteric and non-icteric women using oral contraceptive agents.
Acta Med.Scand. 1967,181,257

LIEBER CS. Hepatic and metabolic effects of alcohol. Gastroenterology, 1973,65,821

LIEBER CS, RUBIN E, DE CARLI M, MISRA P and GANG H. Effects of
pyrazole on hepatic function and structure. Lab.Inv.1970,22,615

MA M and BIEMPICA L. The normal human liver cell. Cytochemical and
ultrastructural studies. Am.J.Path. 1971,62,353

MARINOZZI V and FIUME L. Effect of $\alpha$-amanitin on mouse and rat
liver cell nuclei. Exp.Cell Res. 1971,67,311

MELDOLESI J, CLEMENTI F, CHIESARA E, CONTI F and FANTI A. Cytoplasmic changes in rat liver after prolonged treatment with low
doses of ethionine and adenine. Lab.Inv. 1967,17,265

METREAU JM, DHUMEAUX D and BERTHELOT P. Oral contraceptives and
the liver. Digestion, 1972,7,318

MIYAI K, PRICE VM and FISHER MM. Bile acid metabolism in mammals.
Ultrastructural studies on the intrahepatic cholestasis induced by
lithocholic and chenodeoxycholic in the rat. Lab.Inv. 1971,24,292

MIYAI D, RAICK A and RITCHIE AC. Effect of glucose on the subcellular structure of the rat liver cells in acute ethionine
intoxication. Lab.Inv. 1970,23,268

MIYAI K and STEINER JW. Fine structure of interphase liver cell
nuclei in acute ethionine intoxication. Lab.Inv. 1967,16,677

MONNERON A. Experimental induction of helical polysomes in adult
rat liver. Lab.Inv. 1969,20,178

MONNERON A. Action of some drugs on liver nuclei and polysomes. In
"Advances in Cytopharmacology", Vol.1, F.Clementi and B. Ceccarelli
eds. Raven Press, N.Y. 1971, p.131

MUGNAIGNI E. Filamentous inclusions in the matrix of mitochondria
from human livers. J.Ultrastr. Res. 1965,11,525

NENCI I. Identification of actin-like proteins in alcoholic hyalin
by immunofluorescence. Lab.Inv. 1975,32,257

ORLANDI F, BAMONTI F, DINI M, KOCH M and JEZEQUEL AM. Hepatic
cholesterol synthesis in man. Effect of Diazepam and other drugs.
Europ.J.Clin.Invest. 1975,5,139

ORLANDI F and JEZEQUEL AM. On the pathogenesis of the cholestasis
induced by 17-alkyled steroids. Rev.Int.Hepatol. 1966,16,331

ORLANDI F and JEZEQUEL AM. A comparative study of liver response to
6-Mercaptopurine in patients with normal liver or with chronic
aggressive hepatitis. Digestion, 1971,4,169

ORRENIUS S and ERICSSON JLE. Enzyme-membrane relationship in phenobarbital induction of synthesis of drug-metabolizing enzyme system
and proliferation of endoplasmic membranes. J.Cell Biol,1966,28,181

ORTEGA P. Light and electron microscopy of Dichlorodiphenyl-trichlor-
ethane(DDT) poisoning in the rat liver. Lab.Inv. 1966,15,657

OUDEA MC, COLLETTE M and OUDEA P. Morphometric study of ultrastructural changes induced in rat liver by chronic alcohol intake.
Am.J.Dig.Dis. 1973,18,398

OUDEA MC, LAUNAY AN, QUENHERVE S and OUDEA P. The hepatic lesions
produced in the rat by chronic alcoholic intoxication. Histological,
ultrastructural and biochemical observations. Rev.Europ.Et.Clin.
Biol. 1970,15,748

PORTER K and BRUNI C. An electron microscope study of the early
effect of 3'MeeDAB on rat liver cells. Canc.Res. 1959,19,997

PEREZ V, GORODISCH S, DEMARTIRE J, NICHOLSON R and DI PAOLA G.
Oral contraceptives: Long-term use produces fine structural changes
in liver mitochondria. Science,1969,165,805

RACELA A, GRADY H and SVOBODA D. Ultrastructural nuclear changes
due to tannic acid. Canc. Res. 1967,27,1658

RAISFELD IH, BACCIN R, HUTTERER F and SCHAFFNER F. The effect of
amino 1,2,4 triazole on the phenobarbital-induced formation of
hepatic microsomal membranes. Mol.Pharmacol. 1970,6,231

RECKNAGEL RO, UGAZIO G, KOCH RR and GLENDE EA JR. New Perspectives
in the study of experimental carbon tetrachloride liver injury. In
"The Liver", EA Gall and FK Mostofi eds. Williams and Wilkins Co.
Baltimore, 1973, p.L50

REDDY JK, AZARNOFF DL, SVOBODA DH and PRASAD JD. Nafenopin-induced
hepatic microbody (peroxisome) proliferation and catalase synthesis
in rats and mice. Absence of sex difference in response. J.Cell
Biol. 1974,61,344

REDMAN CM, BANERJEE D, HOWELL K and PALADE GE. Colchicine inhibition
of plasma protein release from rat hepatocytes. J.Cell Biol. 1975,
66,42

REITH A. The influence of triiodothyronine and riboflavine
deficiency on the rat liver with reference to mitochondria. Lab.Inv.
1973,29,216

REMMER H and MERKER HJ. Drug-induced changes in the liver endoplasmic reticulum : association with drug-metabolizing enzymes.
Science, 1963a,142,1657

REMMER H and MERKER HJ. Enzyminduktion und Vermehrung von endoplas-
matichem Reticulum in der Leberzelle während der Behandlung mit

Phenobarbital (Luminal). Klin.Wochschr. 1963b,41,276
REYNOLDS ES. Liver parenchymal cell injury. III. The nature of
calcium-associated electron-opaque passes in rat liver mitochondria
after poisoning with carbon tetrachloride. J.Cell Biol. 1965,25,53
REYNOLDS RC, MONTGOMERY PO and KARNEY D. Nucleolar "caps", a morpho-
logical entity produced by the carcinogen 4-Nitro-quinoline-N-oxide.
Cancer Res. 1963,23,525
REYNOLDS ES and REE HJ. Liver parenchymal cell injury. VII. Membrane
denaturation following carbon tetrachloride. Lab.Inv. 1971,25,269
ROSS WT and CARDELL RR Jr. Effects of halothane on the ultrastructure of rat liver cells. Am.J.Anat. 1972,135,5
ROUILLER Ch. and JEZEQUEL AM. Electron microscopy of the liver. In
"The Liver" Ch. Rouiller ed., Vol.1, Acad.Press, N.Y. 1963, p.195
RUBIN E, BEATTIE DS and LIEBER CS. Effects of ethanol on the bio-
genesis of mitochondrial membranes and associated mitochondrial
functions. Lab.Inv. 1970,23,620
RUBIN E, HUTTERER F and LIEBER CS. Ethanol increases hepatic smooth
endoplasmic reticulum and drug-metabolizing enzymes. Science,
1968,159,1469
RUBIN E and LIEBER CS. Early fine structural changes in the human
liver induced by alcohol. Gastroenterology, 1967,53,1
SCHAFFNER F and JAVITT NB. Morphologic changes in hamster liver
during intrahepatic cholestasis induced by taurolithocholate.
Lab.Inv. 1966,15,1783
SCHOENE B, FLEISCHMANN, RA and REMMER H. The cytochrome P-450 and
the activities of various microsomal enzymes in human liver.
Proc. Europ. Soc. Study Drug Tox. 1972a,13,249
SCHOENE B, FLEISCHMANN RA, REMMER H and Von OLDERSHAUSEN HF.
Determination of drug-metabolizing enzymes in needle biopsies of
human liver. Europ.J.Clin.Pharmacol. 1972b,4,65
SHINOZUKA H, GOLDBLATT PJ and FARBER E. The disorganization of
hepatic cell nucleoli induced by ethionine and its reversal by
adenine; J.Cell Biol. 1968,36,313
SHINOZUKA H, MARTIN JT and FARBER JL. The induction of fibrillar
nucleoli in rat liver cells by D-galactosamine and their subsequent
reformation into normal nucleoli. J.Ultrastr.Res. 1973,44,279
SHINOZUKA H, REID IM, SHULL KH, LIANG H and FARBER E. Dynamics of
liver cell injury and repair. Lab. Inv. 1970,23,253
SMUCKLER EA. Studies on carbon tetrachloride intoxication. IV.
Effect of carbon tetrachloride on liver slices and isolated
organelles in vitro. Lab.Inv. 1966,15,157
SMUCKLER EA and BENDITT EP. Carbon tetrachloride poisoning in rats.
Alterations in ribosomes of the liver. Science, 1963,140,308
SMUCKLER EA and BENDITT EP. The early effects of actinomycin on rat
liver. Changes in ribosomes and polysomes. Lab.Inv. 1964,14,1699
SMUCKLER EA, ISERI OA and BENDITT EP. An intracellular defect in
protein synthesis induced by carbon tetrachloride. J.Exp.Med.
1962,116,55
STAUBLI W, HESS R and WEIBEL ER. Correlated morphometric and

biochemical studies on the liver cell. II.Effect of phenobarbital on rat hepatocytes. J.Cell Biol. 1969,42,92

STEELE WJ, OKAMURA and BUSCH H. Effects of thioacetamide on the composition and biosynthesis of nucleolar and nuclear ribonucleic acid in rat liver. J.Biol.Chem. 1965,240,1742

STEIN O and STEIN Y. Lipid synthesis, intracellular transport, storage and secretion. J.Cell Biol. 1967,33,319

STEINER JW, MIYAI K and PHILLIPS MJ. Electron microscopy of membrane-particles arrays in liver cells of ethionine-intoxicated rats. Am.J. Path. 1964,44,164

STENGER RJ. Organelle pathology of the liver. The endoplasmic reticulum. Gastroenterology, 1970,58,554

STENRAM U. Electron microscopic study on liver cells of rats treated with actinomycin D. Z.Zellforsch. 1965,65,211

STERNLIEB I and BERGER JE. Optical diffraction studies of crystalline structures in electron micrograph. II. Crystalline inclusions in mitochondria of human hepatocytes. J.Cell Biol. 1969,43,448

STRIPP B., HAMRICK M, ZAMPAGLIONE NG and GILLETTE JR. The effect of spironolactone on drug metabolism by hepatic microsomes. J. Pharmacol.Exp.Therap. 1971,176,766

SUTER E and SALOMON JC. Effet de l'actinomycine D sur la structure fine du nucleole des hépatocytes de rat intoxiques par la thioacétamide. Exp.Cell Res. 1966,43,248

SUZUKI K. Giant hepatic mitochondria : production in mice fed with cuprizone. Science, 1969,163,81

SVOBODA DJ and AZARNOFF DL. Response of hepatic microbodies to a hypolipidemic agent, ethylchlorophenoxyisobutyrate (CPIB). J.Cell Biol. 1966,30,442

SVOBODA DJ, GRADY H and HIGGINSON J. Aflatoxin B$_1$ injury in rat and monkey liver. Am.J.Path. 1966,49,1023

SVOBODA DJ and MANNING RT. Chronic alcoholism with fatty metamorphosis of the liver. Am.J.Path. 1964,44,645

SVOBODA DJ and SOGA J. Early effects of pyrrolizidine alkaloids on the fine structure of rat liver cells. Am.J.Path. 1966,48,347

THORPE MEC and SHOREY CD. Long term alcohol administration. Its effects on the ultrastructure and lipid content of the rat liver cell. Am.J.Path. 1966,48,557

THYS O, HILDEBRAND J, GERIN Y and JACQUES PJ. Alterations of rat liver lysosomes and smooth endoplasmic reticulum induced by the Diazafluoranthen derivative AC-3579. I. Morphological and biochemical lesions. Lab.Inv. 1973,28,70

TRUMP BF, GOLDBLATT PJ and STOWELL RE. Studies of necrosis in vitro of mouse hepatic parenchymal cells. Ultrastructural alterations in endoplasmic reticulum, Golgi apparatus, plasma membrane and lipid droplets. Lab.Inv. 1965,14,2000

TUCHWEBER B, SOLYMOSS G, KHANDEKAR JD, KOVACKS K, GARG BD et al. Effect of pregnenolone 16$\alpha$-carbonitrile on the hepatic ultrastructure, glucogen content and ethylmorphine N-demethylase activity in pregnant, fetal and newborn rat. Exp.Mol.Path. 1972, 17,281

VAN DYKE RA and WOOD CL. In vitro studies on irreversible binding
of halothane metabolite to microsomes.  Drug Metab.Dispos. 1975,
3,51
VERBIN RS, GOLDBLATT PJ and FARBER E. The biochemical pathology of
inhibition of protein synthesis in vivo. The effects of cycloheximide on hepatic parenchymal cell ultrastructure. Lab.Inv. 1969,
20,529
VILLA-TREVINO S, FARBER E, STAHELIN T, WETTSTEIN O and NOLL H.
Breakdown and reassembly of rat liver ergosomes after administration of ethionine or puromycin.  J.Biol.Chem. 1964,239,3826
WANSON JC, DROCHMANS P, MAY C, PENASSE W and POPOWSKI A. Isolation
of centrolobular and perilobular hepatocytes after phenobarbital
treatment. J.Cell Biol. 1975,66,23
WEINER J, LOUD AV, KIMBERG DV and SPIRO D. A quantitative
description of cortisone-induced alterations in the ultrastructure
of rat liver parenchymal cells. J.Cell Biol. 1968,37,47
WOOD RL. The fine structure of hepatic cells in chronic ethionine
poisoning and during recovery. Am.J.Path. 1965,46,307
WHELTON MJ, KRUSTEV LP and BILLING BH. Reduction in serum bilirubin
by phenobarbital in adult unconjugated lyperbilirubinemia.  Am.J.
Med. 1968,45,160

DISCUSSION OF COMMENTARY OF ANNE-MARIE JEZEQUEL

Low-Beer:  When the enterohepatic circulation of bile salts is interrupted there is an increase in bile salt synthesis.  Have you looked at any morphological counterparts to this situation? That is, when patients have a bile-salt losing state, do you see any changes in the endoplasmic reticulum?

Jezequel:  We have not studied this.

Low-Beer:  Are there any sex differences in man, particularly with respect to the time in the menstrual cycle at which samples are taken.

Jezequel:  We have studied only two normal men and two normal women, and that is not enough for any sort of statistical evaluation.

Low-Beer:  How did you mention cholesterol synthesis?

Jezequel:  This was done on liver biopsy specimens _in vitro_ by scaling down macromethods for measuring incorporation of $^{14}C$-acetate into cholesterol.

Heirwegh:  In connection with your work on Gilbert's disease and Crigler-Najjar patients, you measured development of smooth endoplasmic reticulum and also demonstrated changes in bilirubin levels.  It seems that the bilirubin glucuronyl transferase, at least in the rat, is more abundant in the rough endoplasmic reticulum, whereas for some substrates such as phenolphthalein the transferase is in the smooth endoplasmic reticulum.  Did you also see and quantitate any changes in rough endoplasmic reticulum accompanying various treatments?

Jezequel:  There were no morphological changes that we could observe.

Heirwegh:  In the normal, or near-normal metabolic state the bilirubin-transporting system in the cytosol ligandin is an essential component and may be a rate-limiting step in bilirubin transport.  Phenobarbitone induces ligandin more rapidly than the transferase enzyme, so the rapid decrease in bilirubin you observed could be due to enhancement of the bilirubin transfer system.    In our studies in rats we have found that the content of the binding of bilirubin-binding cytosol proteins increases markedly within 24 hours when fasting rats are given food.

Jezequel:    What you say is probably correct.    It seems that the transferase enzymes are quite low and ligandin increases much earlier.

Danielsson:    I have a comment pertinent to Dr. Low-Beer's question.    Several groups, including our own, have shown that total cytochrome P450 is completely unchanged in the rat during biliary drainage.    We have also measured NADPH-cytochrome P450 reductase and this is also unchanged.    Hence one would not expect to see an increase in the endoplasmic reticulum.

Arias:    I would like to respond to Dr. Heirwegh's comments. Firstly, we have to take into account the rate at which a protein such as ligandin changes its concentration.    It is determined by its half-life, which is 2-3 days in the rat, but we have no idea what it is in man.    But when we consider the UDP-glucuronyl transferase system, this is not a pure protein and so we cannot study its half-life.    We can measure the half-life of the total enzyme activity, but this may be greatly influenced by changes in other cellular constituents.    So the rate at which the enzyme activity changes compared with that change in a specific protein which we can measure is full of difficulty, especially if we attempt any physiological interpretation as to what is actually rate-limiting.

      Secondly, we have no idea what a particular percentage in reduction of enzyme activity really means.    This is particularly difficult in man, because, as Dr. Jezequel has pointed out, we have great difficulty in getting a sufficient number of specimens to measure turnover rates and so on.    So we can only make tenuous guesses at this stage, and certainly morphological studies do not present any of the answers.

Boyer:    As a biliary physiologist, I have been intrigued by the fact that methyl cholanthrene will stimulate endoplasmic reticulum and microsomal enzyme function, but does not apparently stimulate biliary secretion.    Other drugs, such as phenobarbital stimulate both.    Are there any morphologic counterparts to this situation, which might provide a clue to this apparent anomaly?

Jezequel:    There is no increase in membranes with methyl cholanthrene.

Boyer: We generally consider the Golgi apparatus as an extension of the smooth endoplasmic reticulum. Do you know of any compounds which selectively stimulate the Golgi apparatus without affecting the endoplasmic reticulum?

Jezequel: Colchicene seems to block secretion of proteins at the level of the Golgi apparatus, but does not affect protein synthesis. An effect on the microtubules has been postulated to explain this, but we have no morphological evidence for this, although there is hypertrophy of the Golgi apparatus.

Mitropoulus: Do membranes in general go through a formation, turnover and loss series of changes, or are they changed into another form? For instance, is the smooth endoplasmic reticulum ever converted to rough endoplasmic reticulum?

Jezequel: I think the reverse happens. Smooth endoplasmic reticulum components are formed at the level of rough endoplasmic reticulum. In experiments with phenobarbitol, there is synthesis of phospholipids _in situ_ in the smooth endoplasmic reticulum, but not the rough. But with diazofluoranthane the increase in membranes is due to an inhibition of breakdown of membranes. In other words, it is not a matter of synthesis, but delayed breakdown.

# LIVER DAMAGE AND REGENERATION AFTER POISONING

M.U. Dianzani

Institute of General Pathology
University of Turin
Turin, Italy

The liver is probably the organ most studied under both biochemical and morphological points of view.Its toxic damage represents,
therefore,a good model for the study of the elementary changes in
injured cells. As the substances injuring liver cells are very numerous,one has to select poisons having some essential features:I)
they must provoke reproducible damage in short time;2)they must be
active in low doses;3)the difference between the injurying dose and
the lethal dose must be reasonable. For different reasons,haloalkanes,
white phosphorous,ethanol and several inhibitors of protein synthesis have been preferred as models for liver toxicity.
In general terms,it can be stated that liver cells respond in a rather uniform way to toxic damage.Electron microscopy shows that in
most cases the structure primarily affected is the endoplasmic ret-
iculum.Mitochondria become affected usually later and lysosomal involvement,when present,is a late event.Only in some cases(for instance in amanitine poisoning) nuclear damages may be seen  before
any cytoplasmic involvement.Most liver poisons produce rather early
fatty infiltration;other types of degeneration(glycogenosis,after
chronic dinitrophenol;vacuolar degeneration after phalloidin in rats;
cloudy swelling after dyphteria toxin in guinea pigs or after Sal-
monella typhi murium toxin in rats)are less common. The series of
derangements produced by poisons,that may be somehow different in
their sequence according to their different nature,may lead the cells
to die.Cell death is followed by regeneration,provided the animal
survives.In some instances,and especially after chronic poisoning,
repeated episodes of cell death and regeneration may be followed by

cirrhosis and/or cancerization. In the present review,the problems
of the most frequent elementary changes following acute poisonings,
i.e. fatty degeneration,cell death and regeneration,will be shortly
discussed.So,cirrhosis and cancerization will remain out of this
survey.
Fatty liver is a very common event.Its frequency is caused by the
peculiar position this organ occupies in lipid metabolism.The net
amount of triglycerides(TG)present within the liver at any given
time is the result of the balance between the input and the output
of these substances from the local pool.The output is mostly concerned with secretion of lipoproteins(LP)from liver cells into the blood.
Much less importance has the hydrolysis by liver lipase.An acid lipase located within lysosomes may be concerned with TG degradation
during focal autolysis.Its congenital deficiency is responsible for
the Wolman's disease,the only type of intralysosomal fatty infiltration. The input of TG into the liver pool is dependent upon their synthesis from fatty acids and glycerol.The net result of this reaction
depends both from the activity of triglyceride synthetase and from
the availability of the substrates.The intrahepatic concentration
of fatty acids is influenced by several factors.It is increased by
their increased arrival from the blood,where they circulate either
in the form of chylomicrons,or as not-esterified fatty acids bound
to albumin,mostly released from depôt fat.Increase of fatty acids
may result also from increased synthesis,or from decreased oxidation in mitochondria.On the contrary,decreased arrival from the blood,
decreased local synthesis or increased oxidation may provoke decreased
supply of fatty acids to TG synthesis.
All the substances producing fatty liver act sometimes preferentially on some point in this scheme,but very rarely they affect an unique
site.in Most cases,several sites may be affected,depending upon the
phase of intoxication.For instance,$CCl_4$ mostly affects secretion
of LP(Recknagel et al.,1960),this impairment occurring early and in
good cohincidence with fat accumulation(Lombardi and Ugazio,1965).
In later stages,however,severe mitochondrial changes,characterized
by swelling,dissociation of oxidative phosphorylation and decreased
oxidation of fatty acids,contribute to fat accumulation(reviews by
Dianzani,1974 and 1975;Recknagel,1967;Slater,1972).Moreover,$CCl_4$-
treatment provokes an early increase in fat mobilization,that is
permissive for development of fatty liver.Very similar phenomena
have been observed with white phosphorus(Dianzani,1973)and with e-
thionine(Hutterer,1963).  In acute ethanol poisoning,several types
of derangements have been observed,but also denied:increased supply
of fatty acids by the blood,increased local synthesis from acetyl-

-CoA,favoured by the increase in the ratio of reduced to oxidized
pyridine nucleotides,decreased oxidation of fatty acids due to early mitochondrial damage(reviews by Lieber,1971,1975).
In order to fully understand the mechanisms for the development of
fatty livers produced by different substances,therefore,one has to
consider chronologically all the possibly involved variables.
Fatty liver and necrosis are separate events,but they are the consequence of the same primary causes.A good model for the study of the
relationships between fatty liver and necrosis is $CCl_4$-poisoning.
$CCl_4$ is known as a liver poison since a number of years.Outside the
liver,it damages especially the kidney(swelling od endoplasmic reticulum and of mitochondria,uncoupling of oxidative phosphorylation,
cloudy swelling),the lungs(edema),the adrenals and eventually the
platelets. Independently of the administration way(oral,inhalatory,
parentheral),$CCl_4$ accumulates rapidly in the liver,the amount being
present in other organs being negligible.The intrahepatic concentration remains high for a few hours and then decreases,becoming very
low after 24  hours. The toxicity of $CCl_4$ is depending upon its metabolization in the smooth endoplasmic reticulum(SER)by the local
oxidative chain,usually called as drug metabolizing system(DMS).
This produces the homolytic cleavage of the haloalkane,that leads
to the formation of the free radicals $CCl_3^{\cdot}$ and $Cl^{\cdot}$ .These are very
reactive and subtract hydrogen to all the possible donors they contact,so forming respectively $CHCl_3$ and HCl,whereas the donors become
activated and transformed into other  free radicals.So,a chain reaction is initiated. As SER is very rich in unsaturated lipids,that are
rather prone to activation,these substances become easily involved
in the chain reaction,leading to lipid peroxidation.Initially,free
radicals of the fatty acids are produced;they are,however,unstable
and undergo to a series of transformations,including the shifting
of double bonds to give diene configuration.The appearing absorption
band at 235 nm is very suitable for chemical estimations.In the presence of oxygen,fatty acids free radicals are transformed into lipid
peroxides.These are also very reactive and can start other reactions,
involving lipids,proteins and other cell constituents.Such interactions may lead to the formation of lipofuscins,rapidly segregated
within secondary lysosomes,or to protein polymerization,as well as
to the production of membrane damages(Roubal and Tappel,1966 a,b;
Recknagel,1967;Reynolds and Ree,1971).Furthermore,lipid peroxides
(Roubal and Tappel,1967)and possibly free radicals are able to damage nucleotides:this may represent an impact for mutation and event-
ual cancerization.  The free radicals from $CCl_4$,on the other hand,
can also act directly with other substances or cell constituents,

causing the production of new compounds containing covalently bond
$CCl_4$-metabolites.This may be another cause for inactivation of enzymes or for destruction of functions. In addition,also the substances derived from the lipoperoxidative disintegration of fatty acids
(for instance,aldehydes;malonaldehyde decreases the template activity
of DNA,according to Klamerth and Levinsky,1969)may contribute to
damage. Oxidation,covalent binding,lipid peroxidation and interaction
with substances coming from lipid disintegration may represent the
most important mechanisms of damage.
Several other haloalkanes are metabolized by DMS,but at different
rates.It is noteworthy that the both rate of metabolization and toxicity depend upon the values of the bond dissociation energy.$CBrCl_3$,
that has a bond dissociation energy lower than $CCl_4$,is cleaved more
rapidly and is therefore more toxic than $CCl_4$(Ugazio et al.,1973;
Burdino et al.,1975).$CHCl_3$,having a much higher bond dissociation
energy,is less easily cleaved and therefore less toxic.
Causes affecting the functional state of DMS modify haloalkane toxic-
ity.Several haloalkanes being normally little or non-toxic,become
much more toxic when the rate of their metabolism is increased by
inducing the DMS.This is,for instance,the case of halothane(Ugazio
et al.,1973;Reynolds and Moslen,1974)and also of trieline(Ugazio et
al.,1973),that become toxic after pretreatment with phenobarbital.
Pretreatment with phenobarbital strongly increases the toxicity also
of $CCl_4$(Garner and McLean,1969)and of $CBrCl_3$(Torrielli et al.,1974).
On the contrary,pretreatment with methylcholanthrene,that is a minor
inducer producing increase of a special type of cytochrome P,character-
ized by an absorption band at 448 nm(whereas phenobarbital induction
increases cytochrome $P_{450}$)doesn't increase $CCl_4$-toxicity(Pani et al.,
1973). Decreased rates of metabolism,either due to insufficient development of DMS(for instance,in newborn rats:Dawkins,1963),or to its
pathological involvement,afford,on the contrary,protection towards
haloalkanes. So,hypoproteic diets are protecting(McLean and McLean,
1966);also protecting is the treatment with SKF 525-A,that damages
the DMS(Smuckler and Hultin,1966;Recknagel,1973).The last substance,
however,is not effective when $CCl_4$is given by inhalation,suggesting
also a mechanism of protection based also on a decrease of the intestinal absorption of $CCl_4$(Burdino et al.,1975).Pretreatment with
low doses of $CCl_4$,damaging the DMS,is also protective(Ugazio et al.,
1972).Surgical hepatectomy,followed by regeneration,also protects,
possibly due to the incomplete development of DMS in the young cells
(Ugazio et al.,1973b;Burdino et al.,1975). Another type of protection is afforded by substances metabolized by the same DMS chain cleaving $CCl_4$,when given immediately before this poison.For instance,pheno-

barbital,that increases the toxicity of $CCl_4$ when used as an inducer,
protects when given in an unique dose immediately prior $CCl_4$. Also
some substances used as antioxidants,like propylgallate(Torrielli and
Slater,1971;Ugazio and Torrielli,1969)and DPPD(Torrielli et al.,1974;
Gabriel et al.,1974),act at least partially in this way.
Possibly the same are the mechanisms of the interactions between ethanol and $CCl_4$.Repeated pretreatments with ethanol enhance $CCl_4$-toxic-
ity,probably by increasing the efficiency of DMS,that metabolizes
also ethanol(Lieber,1971,1975).When ethanol is given,however,immediat-
ely prior $CCl_4$,a decrease in toxicity of this substance is seen.
Reversely,$CCl_4$-pretreatment enhances ethanol toxicity,probably due
to the destruction of the microsomal system metabolizing ethanol.
It has not been concluded as yet at which site of the DMS chain
the cleavage of $CCl_4$ occurs.According to Slater(1972),only two sites
in this chain may be involved:the flavoprotein and the $cytP_{450}$ sites,
both having a lipid environment.According to McLean(1967),$CCl_4$ would
interact with $cyt.P_{450}$ producing a difference spectrum ressembling
that seen with other drugs.$Cyt.P_{450}$ level decreases strongly after
$CCl_4$-poisoning(Recknagel et al.,1973;Castro et al.,1972),the destruction of the cofactor being effected either by lipoperoxides(Recknagel
et al.,1975)or by free radicals(De Toranzo et al.,1975).According to
Slater,however,the primarily affected site would be flavoprotein.In
fact,$CHCl_3$ and $CFCl_3$,which are not very active on lipid peroxidation
and very slightly metabolized,interact with $cyt.P_{450}$ with the same
intensity as $CCl_4$. In addition,the incubation with a partial atmosphere of CO,which binds to reduced $P_{450}$,increases the malonyldialdehyde
production normally seen with $CCl_4$.The same happens by using SKF 525-A,
that binds strongly with $P_{450}$,or p-chloromercuribenzoate,that blocks
the electron transport chain between flavoprotein and $P_{450}$.The last
facts strongly suggest that the interaction of $CCl_4$ with the chain
is in the neighbouring of flavoprotein.
We described above that damage to cell structures may be provoked
through different mechanisms,i.e.by the free radical themselves,or
by lipid peroxides,or also by their degradation products,as aldehydes. Free radicals are so reactive,that it is difficult to conceive
that they may act on cell structures not placed in the immediate
neighbouring of the site where they are produced.So,one may accept
the idea that free radicals are directly responsible for inactivation of $P_{450}$(De Toranzo et al.,1975),notwithstanding the different
opinion of Recknagel et al.(1975),who think that this damage is done
by lipoperoxides.Other early types of damage,occurring at certain
distances from the SER,seem,however,less easily attributable to free
radicals.Reynolds(1967)reported several years ago that metabolism of

$CCl_4$ is followed by covalent binding to lipids or proteins amounting
to about 40% of the injected poison in 2 hours.Recknagel et al.(1975)
has quite recently reported data showing the practically total metabolization of $CCl_4$ in 90 minutes in an in vitro anaerobiotic system,
35% of the substance being converted into $CHCl_3$ and the remainder
becoming covalently bound to microsomal lipids and proteins.So,the
production of free radicals is so big,that the possibility that they
may diffuse and act at certain distances from the production sites
cannot be disregarded.
Among the early damages produced by $CCl_4$,the loss in glucose-6-phos-
phatase and the impairment in protein synthesis have been particularly
studied.Glucose-6-phosphatase is sited in the SER membranes.So,it
becomes affected quite early by $CCl_4$(Comporti et al.,1965b;Recknagel,
1967;Cignoli and Castro,1971).It is rapidly destroyed also when microsomes or homogenates are incubated in vitro in conditions favouring
lipid peroxidation,in the absence of $CCl_4$,whereas the prevention of
this fenomenon by EDTA protects towards the loss of the enzymatic act-
tivity(Comporti et al.,1965a). So,there is good evidence that the impairment in the enzymatic activity can be due to lipoperoxidation
itself,even if the hypothesis that $CCl_4$-free radicals may be also
active cannot be ruled out.
As far as it regards protein synthesis,it has been firstly shown by
Smuckler and Benditt(1965) that $CCl_4$-treatment produces decreased
incorporation of aminoacids into proteins,as well as dissociation
of polyribosomal profiles.As the last event is prevented by prior
administration of substances blocking chain elongation(cycloheximide,
Gravela and Dianzani,1970;Farber et al.,1971 ;tenuazoic acid:Farber
et al.,1971;emetine:Dianzani and Gravela,1974 ),there is reason to
think that $CCl_4$ is a poison of recycling,acting on some step of the
initiation reaction. As the damage is prevented also by prior administration of glutathione,it seems very probable that an oxidative
reaction is involved.Gravela(1973)has shown a few years ago that ribosomes from $CCl_4$-treated livers bind preferentially to the newly synthesized mRNA instead of the 'old' mRNA,so indicating that a decrease
in the life-span of preexisting mRNA may be involved.Of course,this
experiment doesn't rule out the hypothesis that initiation reaction
is damaged also by other mechanisms,for instance at the level of ribosomes or of the initiation factors.
As far as it regards the nature of the inhibiting substances,we were
able to show recently that the initiation reaction is blocked also
by aldehydes,that are known to block -SH groups(Dianzani and Gravela,1974;Dianzani et al.,1975). In vitro,these substances are active
at concentrations ranging from 0.1 to 2.5 mM,that are rather high,

but might be not necessarily requested in vivo.In fact,the possibility exists that lower amounts,produced in the neighbouring of key sites,might be sufficient to block protein synthesis.In experiments done with $CBrCl_3$ added in vitro,it was seen,however,that anaerobiosis,preventing the formation of both lipoperoxides and aldehydes,but not the metabolism of the haloalkane,doesn't prevent the impairment in protein synthesis. Moreover,conditions favouring in vitro lipid peroxidation don't increase the inhibition as provoked by $CBrCl_3$. So,it is clear that in vitro,in anaerobiotic conditions,$CBrCl_3$--derived free radicals are able to block protein synthesis by themselves.Of course,this doesn't rule out the hypothesis that in vivo, where aerobiotic conditions are encountered and where the diffusion of free radicals from the production sites is probably less effective, aldehydes may act or contribute on the inhibition.

White phosphorus poisoning is another interesting model.As red phosphorus is non-toxic,we have here an example of an element whose toxicity is only a matter of its physical state.White phospshorus,like $CCl_4$,provokes mitochondrial swelling,loss of oxidative phosphorylation and of fatty acids oxidation,changes in lysosomes and derangement in the endoplasmic reticulum(review in Dianzani,1973).Also in this case there is an early impairment in protein synthesis. With high dosage,dissociation of polyribosomal profiles,also in this case prevented by cycloheximide and glutathione,occurs at I-2 hours after poisoning.So,it seems evident that also white phosphorus behaves as a poison of recycling and that its type of damage is oxidative in nature.Some difference from $CCl_4$ does,however,exist.For instance, there is  no preferential binding of the ribosomes to the 'new'mRNA. In addition,notwithstanding contrary reports by Ghoshal et al.(I969), we were unable to detect in this case any diene conjugation band in microsomal lipids,and there was no increased production of malonyldialdehyde in vitro. So,the mechanism of action of this substance is not lipid peroxidation.The fact that SKF 525-A protects also towards this type of poisoning(Torrielli et al.,I973),might allow the conclusion that in any case phosphorus-toxicity is mediated through something happening in the DMS.There is,however,the possibility that also in this case SKF 525-A may modify the intestinal absorption of the poison. The studies on white phosphorus are complicated by the fact that it is impossible to follow the intracellular destiny of the poison.In fact,[32]P is non-toxic and we cannot draw any conclusion from the knowledge that,after its administration to rats,it is found especially in the soluble part of the homogenate and,in little amounts, also in microsomes(Ghoshal et al.,I97I).

Severe liver damages are produced also by several other inhibitors

of protein synthesis.The comparative study of such substances gives
interesting information on the mechanisms of fatty liver and of cell
death. It is noteworthy,first of all,that not all the inhibitors of
protein synthesis in the liver produce such types of damages.Actino-
mycin D,for instance,is very poorly steatogenic;ethionine is steatogenic,but not necrogenic,when given in a single dose.Cycloheximide,
that is poorly steatogenic,is able to decrease the extent of fatty
infiltration as provoked by $CCl_4$(Gravela and Poli,I974),as well as
that of cell death(Farber et al.,I97I;Flaks and Nicoll,I974;Gravela
and Poli,I974).Whereas the partial protection towards fatty liver is
probably a problem of TG balance(cycloheximide decreases the supply
of free fatty acids from the blood to the liver)the protection against
necrosis seems much more interesting.The same type of protection is
elicited also towards D-galactosamine-induced necrosis(Keppler,I975),
as well as towards that induced by 2-acetylaminofluorene,3'-methyl-
4-dimethylamino-azobenzene and diethylnitrosamine(Flaks and Nicoll,
I974).The hypothesis has been put forward that cell death is mediated through the synthesis od some 'killer' proteins.This is a very
important tool for future experiments.
If we compare the onset times for fatty infiltration after treatment
with different inhibitors of protein synthesis,we can observe that
most substances produce fatty infiltration as early as 5-6 hours
after poisoning or sometimes later,the only exceptions in our experience being $CCl_4$,$CBrCl_3$ and emetine.The two haloalkanes are effective as early as I hour after poisoning,emetine at 3 hours.As the
block in the aminoacids incorporation into proteins begins a few
minutes after treatment in most cases,the question arises how this
chronological discrepancy can be explained. Among the possible reasons,
one has to consider that it is known that the same apolipoprotein
molecules can work several times in extracting TG from the liver and
in vehiculating them throughout the blood. So,a poison of protein
synthesis is expected to produce fatty infiltration only when a sufficient amount of preexisting apolipoprotein molecules have been exhaust-
ed. The differences in chronology among the two haloalkanes and the
other poisons might be explained either by supposing that the last
substances increase the life-span of preexisting apolipoprotein molecules,as a difference from haloalkanes,or by thinking that the early
fat infiltration caused by the two haloalkanes is dependent upon
reasons other than the block in protein synthesis. Some experiments
in vitro(Dianzani and Ugazio,1973)suggest the possibility of a denaturation of preexisting apolipoprotein molecules by $CCl_4$-metabolites.
However,there is no evidence that these results can be adapted to
what happens in vivo. Other possibilities might also be represented

by a damage to the cell sites(endoplasmic reticulum or Golgi apparatus)where the different components of lipoproteins are mounted up.
During the last months,we begun to consider another possibility,
that of a damage to intracellular transport of lipoprotein micelles.
The knowledge on the mechanism of lipoprotein secretion is still
rather obscure.The fact that lipoproteins become enriched with plas-
mamembrane components (Scanu,1973)suggests that secretion involves
some type of membrane fusion,like in the case of the extrusion from
the cell of lysosomal enzymes(Poole,1973).This consideration,as well
as the demonstration(Le Marchand et al.,1973;Stein and Stein,1974)
that colchicine,that blocks the intracellular movements,decreases
lipoprotein secretion by the liver,led us to test if a block in the
intracellular traffic due to impairment of the contractile system
(microtubules or microfilaments)may be involved. It is generally
thought that the contraction of intracellular contractile proteins
depends upon the local concentration of cAMP.When cAMP,or cAMP/cGMP
ratio,is high,contraction doesn't take place and the movements are
blocked;on the contrary,low values favour intracellular movements.
In our $CCl_4$-treated rats,we found  40% increase in cAMP at 2 hours
after poisoning,and about 100% increase at 6 hours.With progress of
time,cAMP concentration decreased again.cAMP/cGMP ratios were very
high during the first hours after treatment.So,the hypothesis of a
a block in the intracellular traffic of lipoproteins has its background.
The second important point in the study of liver damage is that of
the mechanism of cell death. Our knowledge on this point is much less
complete than that we have in the case of steatosis. There is no necessary parallelism between the steatogenic and the necrogenic effi-
ciencies of single poisons.This becomes clear after having considered
that steatosis is a problem of TG balance,that may be affected in
several ways,not necessarily leading to cell death. What is really
intriguing,however,is to understand why an injured cell dies.Different
lesions to different important organelles or functions have been
claimed to be of key importance for cell death:damage to the endoplasmic reticulum or to the nucleus leading to block in protein synthesis,damage to mitochondria provoking energetic unbalancement,
damage to lysosomes provoking autolysis .
The substances blocking protein synthesis may be necrogenic,but very
often big chronological discrepancies exist between the time of inhibition of protein synthesis and that of necrosis.For instance,am-
anitin blocks in few minutes RNA polymerase II in the nucleus,but
cell death is a matter of several hours.With actinomycin D (Chiga
et al.,1966)and with cycloheximide(Verbin et al.,1969,1971)the seq-

uence is very similar. With $CCl_4$,however,cell death occurs much earlier,notwithstanding the fact the block in protein synthesis is not
stronger.In addition,pretreatment with cycloheximide affords protection towards necrosis induced by $CCl_4$ or by other poisons.So,there
is no reason to think that cell death is primarily due to the block
in protein synthesis.
Uncoupling of oxidative phosphorylation in mitochondria occurs rather
early(2 hours in my hands with high $CCl_4$ dosage)and leads to big
ATP depletion.In this case,ATP depletion and cell death seem to be
sufficiently fitting.Experiments by the Farber's group,however,have
shown that in ethionine poisoning ATP depletion is even higher,never-
theless no necrosis is present(Farber,1973).Also in kidney ischemia
cell death seems rather independent from low ATP values.So,in absolute,we cannot accept the idea that mitochondrial damage is the unique
responsible for cell death.
The importance of lysosomal damage for cell death has been emphasized for long time.The conclusion was,however,that the solubilization
of lysosomal enzymes is not an early event in liver damage(Dianzani,
1963;Slater et al.,1963).The release of the enzymes from latency,
i.e. the appearance of a 'free' activity still sedimentable with
the particles,occurs earlier.There are now reasons to think that
this type of change is not due to gradual damage of lysosomal membranes,but to the reabsorption of enzyme molecules previously solub-
ilized(Dianzani,1972;Baccino and Zuretti,in press).So,the thesis
that lysosomal enzymes may act in early times is put forward again.
Some conditions exist,however,in which both 'free' and 'soluble'
activities are increased in the absence of necrosis.This happens,
for instance,in ethionine-poisoning(Zuretti and Baccino,1975),or
during blast transformation of lymphocytes(Hirschhorn et al.,1968).
So,one may conclude that lysosomes changes may perhaps cooperate
in leading damaged cells to the non-return point,but they are hardly
conceivable as the primary agents of cell death in the majority of
cases. The key point for cell death is probably to define the reasons
for irreversibility of damages;this is at present impossible.Tenta-
tively,one may suppose that cell death is a problem of energetic
unbalancement.This may be influenced by several factors,included
those described above;irreversibility might take place when the unbalancement has been prolonged for a certain extent of time,so producing the loss of integrated functions.
The problem of cell regeneration is only a facet of that of the regulation of cell multiplication and of organ development.The basical
point is to understand why differentiated cells having practically
lost their multiplicative properties,recover them after damage.

Table I

Effect of $CCl_4$ (2.5 ml/kg Body Wt) on ATP and cAMP
Levels in Rat Liver

| TREATMENT | ATP | | | cAMP | | |
|---|---|---|---|---|---|---|
| | NUMBER OF RATS | µMOLES/G LIVER (MEANS ± SD) | PERCENT | NUMBER OF RATS | NMOLES/G LIVER (MEANS ± SD) | PERCENT |
| CONTROLS | 8 | 1.07 ± 0.09 | (100) | 6 | 15.24 ± 2.15 | (100) |
| $CCL_4$ 1 H | 6 | 0.99 ± 0.11 | 93 | 6 | 14.12 ± 1.95 | 93 |
| $CCL_4$ 2 H | 8 | 0.75 ± 0.09 | 70 | 6 | 21.20 ± 1.76 | 139 |
| $CCL_4$ 6 H | 8 | 0.62 ± 0.10 | 58 | 6 | 31.67 ± 2.35 | 208 |
| $CCL_4$ 12 H | 4 | 0.63 ± 0.22 | 55 | 4 | 29.73 ± 1.13 | 195 |
| $CCL_4$ 24 H | 4 | 0.84 ± 0.08 | 78 | 4 | 22.16 ± 2.42 | 145 |

Foetal liver contains cells that multiply frequently,but this ability is progressively lost until the adult situation is reached.Adult
liver has very low multiplication rates.During the last years the
concept of 'contact inhibition' has been developed,especially with
regard to what happens in cancer cells. According to recent views
(Emmelot,1973),contact inhibition would be the result of mutual com-
pression.Peculiar receptors on the cell surface would be able to
transform pressorial stimuli into chemical signals producing activation of membrane-bound adenylcyclase and consequently increased synthesis of cAMP.This would be able to block both intracellular movements and multiplication. Cancer cells might have lost their contact
inhibition due to membrane changes. If we try to insert this scheme
into the problem of cell regeneration,it would become clear that cell
death,accompanied by loss of parenchyme,might lead to decreased mutual compression among the residual cells.So,the onset of regenerat-

ion might be considered as a problem of release from mutual compres-
sion.In our experiments on $CCl_4$,we found that cAMP levels,increased
during the first hours,returned to lower values at 24 hours.This
chronology would fit with the hypothesis said above.In fact,it is
generally thought that the time needed to start regeneration after
hepatectomy is longer than 20 hours;in the case of $CCl_4$ it may be
delayed due to the prolonged presence of $CCl_4$ in the organ after the
administration.
Another facet of the problem of regeneration is that of the possible
participation of lysosomes.Lysosomal involvement has been suggested
in cell multiplication,included that occurring in liver regeneration,by several authors(Allison et al.,1964,1965;Robbins and Gonatas,
1964;Kent et al.,1965;Adams,1963;Verity et al.,1975;Poole,1973;Carr,
1965;Butterworths,1970;Hirschhorn and Hirschhorn,1965).Very clear
experiments by Hirschhorn et al.(1968)have shown that blastic transformation of lymphocytes induced by phytohaemoagglutinin is characterized by an early increase in both free and soluble activities of lysosomal enzymes.As far as it regards $CCl_4$-treatment,we observed several
years ago(Dianzani,1963)that both free and soluble activities of lysosomal enzymes increase at 2-6 hours after poisoning and that the tot-
al(specific)activity increases very much between 24 and 144 hours,
after the onset of regeneration.The explainations for the participation of lysosomes in cell multiplication are very hypothetical.A few
among them have now only historical value.For instance,that suggesting digestion by lysosomes of nuclear or centriolar envelopes,or also the mitotic apparatus after anaphase(Mazia,1961).According to
other authors(Hisrchhorn and Hirsccchorn,1965;Hirschhorn et al.,1968,
1969),lysosomal enzymes might digest repressors of cell multiplication,or possibly cytoplasmic RNA to supply pyrimidine and purine
bases to the synthesis of new nucleic acids.The first idea is supported by the fact that lysosomes from polymorphonuclear leukocytes
(Davies et al.,1971)and probably also from liver cells(Rita,unpubl-
ished results),contain a histonase able to split histones,that are
thought to act as repressor of DNA replication.Nuclei from stimulated lymphocytes contain DNA having template activity(Hirschhorn et
al.,1969);treatment of isolated nuclei from liver cells with a lysosomal extract in vitro is also able to increase the amount of DNA
having template activity(Rita and Baccino,1970).
The new liver cells are more resistant to poisoning than the old
cells,at least in the case of $CCl_4$.This may be due to at least two
reasons:1)the fact that DMS cleaving $CCl_4$ is rather poor in young
cells;2)the fact that young cells contain much higher amounts of
natural antioxidants than the adult ones.This has been shown for

cancer cells(review in Ugazio et al.,1969)and also for regenerating
liver(Zicha et al.,1966).According to Burlakova(1967)a high level
of antioxidants within the cells would facilitate the onset of mit-
osis.This might be,therefore,an additional mechanism of regulation
of mitotic rates in regenerating liver.
It is clear from these short and incomplete comments that also the
problem of liver regeneration is far from resolved.We have now,
however,some interesting ideas to develop.

## REFERENCES

Adams R.L.D.,1963,Periodic activation of lysosomal enzymes during
regeneration of the liver,Biochem.J.,87:532

Allison A. and Mallucci L.,1964,Lysosomes in dividing cells,with
special reference to lymphocytes,Lancet,ii:1371

Allison A. and Paton G.R.,1965,Chromosome Damage in Human Diploid
Cells following Activation of Lysosomes,Nature,207:1170

Burdino E.,Gabriel L.,Dianzani M.U.,Poli G.,Sena L.,Torrielli M.V.
and Ugazio G.,1975,Haloalkane toxicity in different experimental
conditions,in Advances in Biochemical Pathology:Toxic Liver Injury,
1975(in press)

Burlakova E.B.,1967,O vozmozhnoi roli svobodnoradikalnovo mekhanizma
b reguliatzii razmozheniia kletok,Biofizika,12:82

Butterworth S.T.G.,1970,Changes in Liver Lysosomes and Cell Junctions
close to an invasive Tumour,J.Pathol.,101:227
Carr A.J.,1965,The Relation to Invasion of Glycosidases in Mouse
Tumours,J.Path.Bact.,89:239

Castro J.A.,Diaz Gomez M.I.,de Ferreyra E.C.,de Castro C.R.,D'Acosta
N. and de Fenos O.M.,1972,Carbon tetrachloride effect on rat liver
and adrenals related to their mixed-function oxygenase content.Biochem.
Biophys.Res.Comm.,47,315

Chiga M.,Kume F. and Millar R.C.,1966,Nucleolar Alteration produced by
Actinomycin D and the Delayed Onset of Hepatic Regeneration in Rats,
Lab.Inv.,15:1403

Cignoli E.V. and Castro J.A.,1971,Lipid peroxidation,necrosis and the
in vivo depression of liver glucose-6-phosphatase by $CCl_4$,Exp.Mol.Path.
14:43

Comporti M.,Rita G.A. and Della Corte E.,1965a,Azione protettiva
dell'EDTA sulla inattivazione da $CCl_4$ -n vitro della glucoso-6-fosfatas
microsomiale.Boll.Soc.Ital.Biol.Sper.,41:678

Comporti M.,Saccocci C. and Dianzani M.U.,1965b,Effect of $CCl_4$ in vitro and in vivo on lipid peroxidation of rat liver homogenates and subcellular fractions,Enzymologia,29:185

Davies P.,Rita G.A.,Krakauer K. and Weissmann G.,1971,Characterization of a neutral protease from lysosomes of rabbit polymorphonuclear leucocytes,Biochem.J.,122:559

Dawkins M.J.R.,1963,Carbon tetrachloride poisoning in the liver of new born rats,J.Path.Bact.,85:189

De Toranzo E.G.D.,Diaz Gomez M.I. and Castro J.A.,1975,Mechanism of in vivo carbon tetrachloride-induced liver microsomal cytochrome $P_{450}$ destruction,Biochem.Biophys.Res.Comm.,64:823

Dianzani M.U.,1963,Lysosomes changes in liver injury,Ciba Found. Symposium on Lysosomes,A.V.S.DeReuck and M.P.Cameron eds.,Churchill, London,335

Dianzani M.U.,1973,Il concetto di lesione lisosomiale,Quaderni Sclavo di Diagnostica,8:54
Dianzani M.U.,1973,Liver Steatosis induced by White Phosphorus,Morgagni,5:1
Dianzani M.U.,1974,Trattato di Patologia Generale,U.T.E.T.,Torino

Dianzani M.U.,1975,Biochemical Mechanisms of Fatty Liver,in Biochemical Mechanissms of Liver Injury,T.F.Slater ed.,Acad.Press,in press

Dianzani M.U.,Gabriel L.,Gravela E. and Paradisi L.,1975,Interference of $CCl_4$ metabolites with subcellular structures,Recent Advances in Biochemical Pathology:Toxic Liver Injury,Minerva Medica,in press

Dianzani M.U. and Gravela E.,1974,Inhibition of protein synthesis in $CCl_4$-induced liver injury,IV Workshop on Experimental Liver Injury, Freiburg im Breisgau,in press

Dianzani M.U. and Ugazio G.,1973,Lipoperoxidation after $CCl_4$ poisoning in rats previously treated with antioxidants,Chem.-Biol.Inter.6:67

Emmelot P.,1973,Biochemical Properties of Normal and Neoplastic Cell Surfaces;a review.Europ.J.Cancer,9:319

Farber E.,1973,ATP and cell integrity,Fed.Proc.,32:1534

Farber E.,Liang H. and Shinozuka H.,1971,Dissociation of effects on protein synthesis and ribosomes from membrane changes induced by carbon tetrachloride,Amer.J.Path.,64,601

Flaks B. and Nicoll J.W.,1974,Modification of toxic liver injury

in the rat.I.Effect of inhibition of protein synthesis on the action of 2-acetylaminofluorene,carbon tetrachloride,3'-methyl,4-di-
methylaminoazobenzene and diethylnitrosamine.Chem.-Biol.Interactions,
8:135

Gabriel L.,Burdino E.,Torrielli M.V. and Ugazio G.,1974,Interference
of DPPD with hepatic drug metabolizing enzyme system.Pharmacol.Res.
Comm.,6:127

Garner R.C. and McLean A.E.M.,1969,Increased susceptibility to carbon
tetrachloride poisoning in the rat after pretreatment with oral
phenobarbitone.Biochem.Pharmacol.,18:645

Ghoshal A.K.,Porta E.A. and Hartroft W.S.,1969,The role of lipoperoxidation in the pathogenesis of fatty livers induced by phosphorus
poisoning in rats.Amer.J.Pathol.,54:275

Ghoshal A.K.,Porta E.A. and Hartroft W.S.,1971,Isotopic Studies on
the Absorption and Tissue Distribution of White Phosphorus in Rats,
Exp.Mol.Path.,14:212

Ghoshal A.K. and Recknagel R.O.,1965,On the mechanism of carbon tetrachloride hepatotoxicity.Cohincidence of loss of glucose-6-phosphatase
activity with peroxidation of microsomal lipid.Life Sci.,4:2195

Gravela E.,1973,Evidence for a reduced life-span of messenger RNA in
liver of rats poisoned with carbon tetrachloride,Exp.Mol.Path.,19:79

Gravela E. and Dianzani M.U.,1970,Studies on the mechanism of CCl$_4$-
-induced polyribosomal damage,FEBS Letters,9:93

Gravela E. and Poli G.,1974,Modifications of carbon tetrachloride-
-induced liver steatosis and necrosis by cycloheximide and emetine.
IRCS,2:1534

Hirschhorn R.,Brittinger G.,Hirschhorn G. and Weissmann G.,1968,
Studies on Lysosomes.XII.Redistribution of Acid Hydrolases in Human
Lymphocytes Stimulated by Phytohaemoagglutinin.J.Cell Biol.,37:412

Hirschhorn R. and Hirschhorn K.,1965,Role of lysosomes in the lymphocyte response,Lancet,ii:1046

Hirschhorn R.,Troll W.,Brittinger G. and Weissmann G.,1969,Template
Activity of Nuclei from Stimulated Lymphocytes,Nature,222:1247

Hutterer F.,1963,Role of Impaired Transmethylation of Epinephrine in
Ethionine-Induced Hepatic Fat Accumulation,Exp.Mol.Pathol.,2:541

Kent G.,Minick O.T.,Orfei E.,Volini F.I. and Madera-Orsini F.,1965,
The movement of iron-laden lysosomes in rat liver cells during mitosis,Amer.J.Path.,46:803

Keppler D.,1975,RNA Synthesis Inhibition and Cell Necrosis induced
by selective Uridine Triphosphate Deficiency in Liver and Ascites
Hepatoma Cells,Recent Advances on Biochemical Pathology:Toxic Liver
Injury,Minerva Medica,in press

Klamerth O.L. and Levinsky H.,1969,Template activity in liver DNA
from rats fed with malondialdehyde,FEBS Letters,3:205

LeMarchand Y.,Singh A.,Assimacopoulos-Jeannet F.,Orci L.,Rouiller C.
and Jeanrenaud B.,1973,A role for the microtubular system in the
release of ve-y low density lipoproteins by perfused mouse livers ,
J.Biol.Chem.,248:6862

Lieber C.S.,1971,Metabolism of ethanol and its effects upon the liver,
Quaderni Sclavo di Diagnostica,7:861

Lieber C.S.,1975,Alcoholic Fatty Liver,its Pathogenesis and Precursor
Role for Hepatitis,Recent Advances on Biochemical Pathology:Toxic
Liver Injury,Minerva Medica,in press

Lombardi B. and Ugazio G.,1965,Serum lipoproteins in rats with carbon
tetrachloride-induced fatty liver,J.Lipid Res.,6:498

Mazia D.,1961,Mitosis and the Physiology of Cell Division,in The Cell,
ed.by J.Brachet and A.E.Mirsky,Acad.Press,New York,3:77

McLean A.E.M.,1967,Effect of hexane and carbon tetrachloride on microsomal cytochrome P450,Biochem.Pharmacol.,16:2030

McLean A.E.M. and McLean E.K.,1966,Effect of diet and of 1,1,1-tri-
chloro-2,2bis-(p-chlorophenyl)ethane(DDT)on microsomal hydroxylation
enzymes and on sensitivity of rats to carbon tetrachloride poisoning,
Biochem.J.,100:564

Pani P.,Gabriel L.,Torrielli M.V. and Gravela E.,1973,Interference
by 3-Methylcholanthrene and Phenobarbital on the Development of Liver
Damage Caused by Carbon Tetrachloride and White Phosphorus Poisoning,
Biochem.Soc.Trans.,1:976

Poole A.R.,1973,Tumour lysosomal enzymes and massive growth,in Lysosomes in Biology and Pathology,J.T.Dingle ed.,NorthHolland,Amsterdam,
303

Recknagel R.O.,1967,Carbon Tetrachloride Toxicity,Pharm.Rev.,19:145

Recknagel R.O. and Glende E.A.,1973,Carbon tetrachloride hepatotoxicity:an example of lethal cleavage,Critical Reviews in Toxicology,2: 263

Recknagel R.O.,Hruskewycz A. and Glende E.A.,1975,Absolute Dependence of $CCl_4$ -Induced Loss of Glucose-6-Phosphatase and Cytochrome P-450 on Lipid Peroxidation,Recent Advances on Biochemical Pathology:Toxic Liver Injury,Minerva Medica,in press

Recknagel R.O.,Lombardi B. and Schotz M.C.,1960,A new insight into the pathogenesis of carbon tetrachloride fat infiltration,Proc.Soc. Exp.Biol.Med.,104:608

Reynolds E.S.,1967,Liver Parenchymal Cell InjuryIV.Pattern Incorporation of carbon tetrachloride into chemical constituents of liver in vivo.J.Pharmacol.Exp.Ther.,155:117

Reynolds E.S. and Moslen M.T.,1974,Liver injury following halothane anesthesia in phenobarbital-pretreated rats.Biochem.Pharm.,23:189

Reynolds E.S. and Ree H.J.,1971,Liver Parenchymal Cell Injury.VII. Membrane Denaturation following carbon tetrachloride,Lab.Inv.,25,269

Rita G. and Baccino F.M.,1970,Interazione fra lisosomi ed altri costituenti cellulari:effetti litici delle idrolasi lisosomiali su nuclei isolati di fegato di ratti,Boll.Soc.Ital.Biol.Sper.,46:337

Robbins E.and Gonatas N.K.,1964,The ultrastructure of a mammalian cell during the mitotic cycle,J.Cell Biol.,21:429

Roubal W.T. and Tappel A.L.,1966a,Damage to protein,enzymes and aminoacids by peroxidizing lipids,Arch.Biochem.Biophys.,113:5

Roubal W.T. and Tappel A.L.,1966 b,Polymerization of proteins induced by free-radical lipid peroxidation,Arch.Biochem.Biophys.,113150

Roubal W.T. and Tappel A.L.,1967,Damage to ATP by peroxidizing lipids, Biochim.Biophys.Acta,136:402

Scanu A.M.,1972,Structural studies on serum lipoproteins,Biochim. Biophys.Acta,265:471

Slater T.F.,1972,Free Radical Mechanisms in Liver Injury,Pion Ltd., London

Slater T.F.,Greenbaum A.L. and Wang D.Y.,1963,Lysosomal changes during liver injury and mammary involution,in Ciba Found.Symposium on Lysosomes,A.V.D.DeReuck and M.P.Cameron eds.,Churchill,London,311

Smuckler E.A. and Benditt E.P.,1965,Studies on carbon tetrachloride intoxication.III.A subcellular defect in protein synthesis,Biochemistry,$\underline{4}$:671

Smuckler E.A. and Hultin T.,1966,Effects of SKF 525 A and adrenalectomy on the aminoacid incorporation by rat liver microsomes from normal and $CCl_4$-treated rats,Exp.Mol.Path.,$\underline{5}$:504

Stein O.,Sanger L. and Stein Y.,1974,Colchicine-induced inhibition of lipoprotein and protein secretion into the serum and lack of interference with secretion and biliary phospholipids and cholesterol by rat liver in vivo,J.Cell Biol.,$\underline{62}$:90

Torrielli M.V.,Pani P.,Gabriel L. and Gravela E.,1973,The Pathophysiological Significance of Hepatic DMES in the Liver Damage induced by $CCl_4$ and White Phosphorus,Proc.Europ.Soc.Study of Drug Toxicity,$\underline{15}$:294

Torrielli M.V. and Slater T.F.,1971,Inhibition of NADPH-cytochrome c reductase by propylgallate,Biochem.Pharm.,$\underline{20}$:2027

Torrielli M.V.,Torrielli M.V.,Ugazio G.C.,Gabriel L. and Burdino E.,1974a,Time course of protection by $N,N_1$-Diphenyl-p-Phenylendiamine (DPPD)against $CCl_4$-hepatotoxicity,Agents and Actins,$\underline{4}$:383

Torrielli M.V.,Ugazio G.,Gabriel L. and Burdino E.,1974b,Effect of drug pretreatment on $CBrCl_3$-induced liver injury,Toxicology,$\underline{2}$:321

Ugazio G.,Burdino E.,Danni O. and Milillo P.A.,1973,Hepatotoxicity and Lethality of Halogenoalkanes,Biochem.Soc.Trans.,$\underline{1}$:968

Ugazio G.,Burdino E.,Danni O.,Milillo P.A. and Congiu A.M.,1973b, $CCl_4$-toxicity:Protective Action of Surgical Partial Hepatectomy against Lethal Doses of $CCl_4$,Rendiconti di Gastroenterologia,$\underline{5}$:553
Ugazio G.,Gabriel L. and Burdino E.,1969,Perossidazione lipidica e processi proliferativi,Atti Soc.ital.Patol.,$\underline{11}$:325

Ugazio G.,Koch R. and Recknagel R.O.,1972,Mechanisms of protection against $CCl_4$ by prior $CCl_4$-administration,Exp.Mol.Path.,$\underline{16}$:281

Ugazio G.,and Torrielli M.V.,1969,Effect of propylgallate on $CCl_4$--induced fatty liver,Biochem.Pharm.,$\underline{18}$:2271

Verbin R.S.,Goldblatt P.J. and Farber E.,1969,The Biochemical Pathology of Inhibition of Protein Synthesis in vivo.The effects of cycloheximide on Hepatic Parenchymal Cell Ultrastructure,Lab.Inv.,$\underline{20}$:529

Verbin R.S.,Langnecker D.S.,Lian H. and Farber E.,1971,Some observations on the Acute Histopathologic Effects of Cycloheximide in vivo, Am.J.Path.,$\underline{62}$:111

Verity M.A., Travis G. and Cheung M., 1965, Lysosome-vacuolar System Reactivity During Early Cell Regeneration, Exp.Mol.Pathol., 22:73

Zicha B., Benes J., Lejsek K. and Semek J., 1966, quoted by Ugazio et al., 1969, Atti Soc.Ital.Patol., 11:325

DISCUSSION OF COMMENTARY BY M.U. DIANZANI

<u>Javitt</u>:   A few years ago we were working with labelled carbon
tetrachloride, and we had to do the experiments in a fume hood
because most of the radioactivity appears in the expired air.
I was impressed by the fact that the liver takes up only a very
small percentage of the total dose.   In any of your studies, do
you know what fraction of the dose actually got into the liver?
If you take a more toxic compound you may be changing the bond-
energy, but the compound would also be less volatile;   therefore,
the actual amount of the compound getting to the liver would be
greater.   So the protective effects of many of the well-known
drugs could be interpreted in several different ways.   Related to
that question is another;   have you identified the enzymes or
enzyme systems which generate the free radicals, since you suggest
that these are generated enzymatically?   A dehalogenase enzyme
was once postulated;   has this enzyme been identified further?
Further, when one is caring for patients who have been exposed
to carbon tetrachloride, one finds that they have liver damage but
most of them die because they have a complete renal shut-down.
This has a parallel, because a drug such as halothane is occasionally hepatotoxic but does not affect the kidney.   Anaesthetics
such as dimethoxyfluorane can sometimes cause renal shut-down.
In essence, do we know anything about the kidney damage as opposed
to the liver damage?

<u>Dianzani</u>:   In reply to your first point, liver damage occurs if
you give carbon tetrachloride by stomach tube or by several other
routes.   We determine the amount of carbon tetrachloride both by
colorimetry and by using the labelled compound.   We found that,
after a few minutes, most of the carbon tetrachloride is concentrated in the liver.   We have also tried to study the intracellular localisation, but found this to be impossible because
after homogenisation of the liver there is complete redistribution
of the carbon tetrachloride.   Also, because of its volatility,
which you mentioned, a lot of the compound is lost.   Therefore
it is very difficult to say exactly how much of the dose gets
into the liver.   When we give 250 µl of carbon tetrachloride by
stomach tube we found about 2-3 mg in the liver, and the rest
remains in the gut.   If you give 25µl liver damage still occurs.
Therefore, the amount we normally give greatly exceeds the amount

needed to produce hepatotoxicity.

With regard to your second point about the involvement of enzymes, it does seem that drug-metabolizing systems are involved. It has been established that carbon monoxide can block cytochrome P450, and this prevents metabolism of carbon tetrachloride, and metabolism is thought to occur in the neighbourhood of flavo-proteins. But Professor Slater has more information about this than I have.

When I started my work with carbon tetrachloride I also studied the kidney, and I observed effects on oxidative phosphorylation in this organ also, and histological examination revealed cloudy swelling. However, we have not found any evidence for lipid peroxidation, and so it is possible that something passes from the liver to the kidney, and that is what causes the kidney damage.

I think that the reason why carbon tetrachloride causes so much liver damage is because it is metabolized exclusively in the liver. Carbon tetrachloride itself is not hepatotoxic; it is the metabolic products which are toxic.

# TOXIC EFFECTS OF LITHOCHOLATE ON THE LIVER AND BILIARY TREE*

Robert H. Palmer

The Rockefeller University

New York, New York 10021

Lithocholic acid is the major bacterial metabolite of cheno-deoxycholic acid. It is absorbed from the lower intestine and conjugated with taurine or glycine. In man, it is extensively sulphated, but the sulphated lithocholates secreted in bile are not extensively reabsorbed; this results in a small pool of circulating lithocholates with a rapid turnover. The metabolism of lithocholate in healthy man has been carefully studied in Hofmann's laboratory (A.E. Cowen et al, Gastro. 69:59, 67 & 77, 1975).

Lithocholic acid (and certain related bile acids) produces a variety of toxic effects, many if not most of which are presumed to be due to the effect of the bile acid on membrane structure and function. The nature of the interaction is unclear, but apparently it is highly dependent on the molecular configuration of the bile acid. Bile acid haemolysis is the classic example, though the phenomenon can be demonstrated in a number of cells and organelles (A.Kappas and R.H. Palmer, Pharm. Rev. 15:123, 1963).

One of the more subtle effects of lithocholate (as well as its taurine and glycine conjugates, 3-ketocholanate and 3β-hydroxy-5-cholenate) is the production of marked cholestasis when infused in vivo or in isolated liver preparations (A.C. Ivy, JAMA 117:1151, 1941; N.B. Javitt, Nature 210:1262, 1966; J.E. King and L.J. Schoenfield, J.Clin.Invest. 50:2305, 1971; M.M. Fisher, R. Magnusson and K. Miyai, Lab. Invest. 25:88, 1971). The mechanism for

*From the Department of Medicine, University of Chicago Pritzker School of Medicine, the Franklin McLean Memorial Research Institute (operated by the University of Chicago for the Energy Research and Development Administration), and The Rockefeller University.

this cholestasis is not understood.  The cholestasis may be accompanied by biliary precipitates, but they do not appear to be responsible since the ultra-structural morphology differs from that
produced by mechanical obstruction and since sulphated lithocholate
causes cholestasis (though of a lesser degree) without biliary
precipitation (N.B. Javitt, The Liver, p. 355, Karger, Basel,
1973; T.J. Layden, J. Schwarz and J.L. Boyer, Gastro. 69: in press,
1975).  In view of the recent report of Phillips et al (Gastro.
69:48, 1975) on the possible role of microfilament dysfunction in
cholestasis, it would be interesting to see whether lithocholates
might affect microfilament function as they do the structure and
function of so many other organelles.

The ultra-structural changes induced by lithocholate are extremely interesting and unusual.  They consist of focal dilation
of the canaliculi, loss of microvilli, and large evaginations of
pericanalicular ectoplasm (K.Miyai, V.M. Price, and M.M. Fisher.

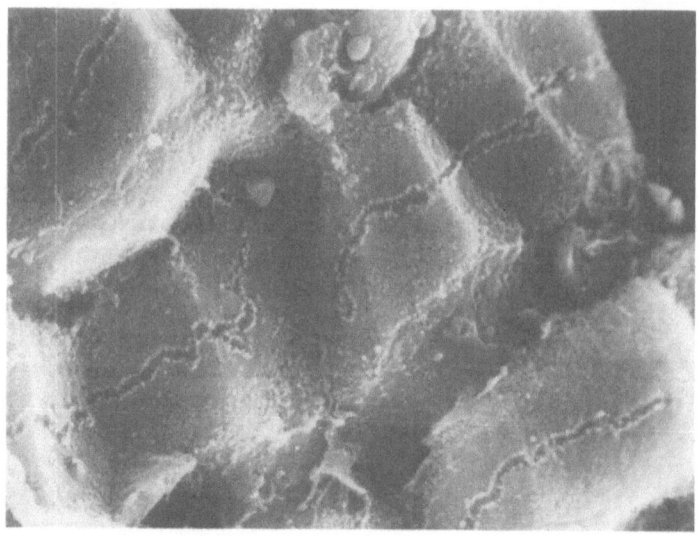

Fig. 1.  Rat Liver.  Normal bile canaliculi showing two end-terminal
portions.  2500x.  Reproduced by permission of Layden, Schwarz, and
Boyer.

Fig. 2.  Top.  Typical end-terminal lesions produced by taurolithocholate infusion (0.6 μmoles/min).  Compare with Fig. 1.  Note
dilation and loss of microvilli.  2500x.  Bottom left.  Normal liver
Sinusoid along left margin, canaliculus along right, inter-cellular
space horizontally.  6200x.  Bottom right.  Lithocholate lesion.
Membranous webs and broad, tongue-like evaginations of pericanalicular ectoplasm (see Fig. 3).  Reproduced by permission of Layden,
Schwarz, and Boyer.

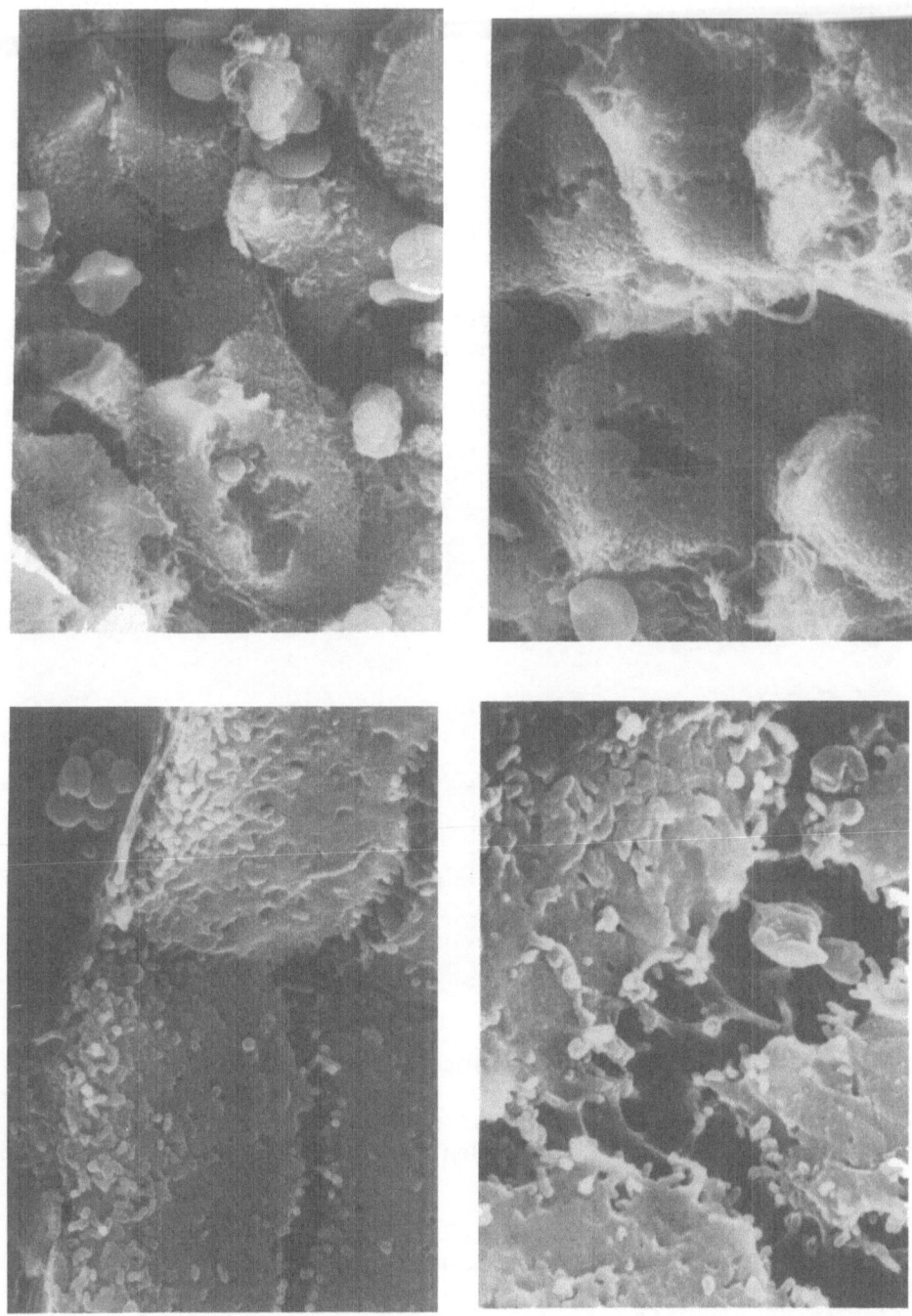

<u>Lab. Invest.</u> 24:292, 1971).  With scanning electron microscopy,
the focal dilation is found to be predominantly limited to blind
or terminal portions of the canaliculi - whether in central or
portal zones of the lobule.  In these areas, membranous evaginations of pericanalicular ectoplasm, corresponding to the lesions
seen in transmission electron microscopy, can be found.  The
changes have been beautifully demonstrated by Layden, Schwarz and
Boyer (see above), and several of their superb illustrations are
reproduced below with their kind permission (figures 1-3).  These
lesions are not observed when sulphated lithocholate is infused
despite the mild cholestasis, so that they must either be associated with changes leading to more severe cholestasis or represent
an independent toxic effect of the bile acid.

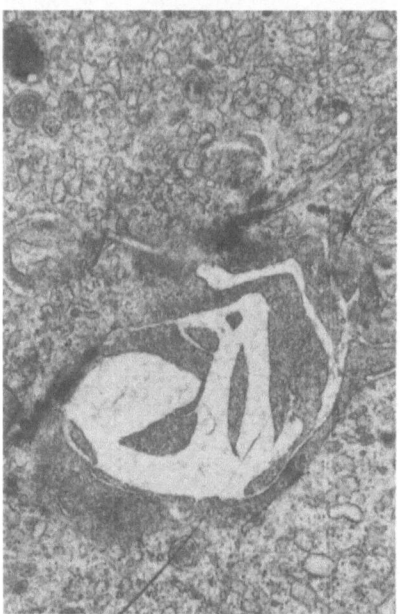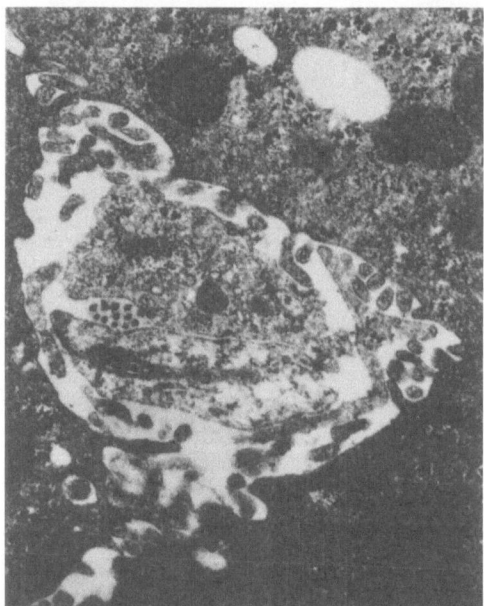

Fig. 3.  Left - Typical end-terminal lithocholate lesion by
transmission electron microscopy.  Right - canaliculus down-stream
showing preservation of microvilli and particulate (cytoplasmic?)
material in the lumen.  From Layden, Schwarz and Boyer.


     The administration of large amounts of lithocholate to intact
animals produces a spectrum of gross pathological changes depending on the species (for review, see R.H. Palmer, <u>Arch. Int. Med.</u>
130:606, 1972).  However the early changes (12-36 hrs) consist of
focal necrotic areas that seem to occur in the middle or outer
portions of the lobule in chickens (H. Eyssen, M. Vandeputte, and

E. Evrard, <u>Arch. Int. Pharmacodyn</u>. 158:292, 1965), or scattered
throughout the lobule with no particular zonal distribution in mice
(S.A. Bagheri, M.G. Bolt, R.H. Palmer and J.L. Boyer, <u>Advances in
Bile Acid Research</u> III Bile Acid Meeting, Freiburg-im-Br., June 13-
15, 1974, in press).  The distribution of the lesions raises the
question of whether they may be related to the end-terminal canalicular lesions demonstrated on scanning electron microscopy - which
are also scattered throughout the lobule.  Typical lesions are
shown in Fig. 4.  There is an interesting similarity between these
lesions and the peliosis hepatis lesions seen in patients following
long term therapy with synthetic anabolic steroids.

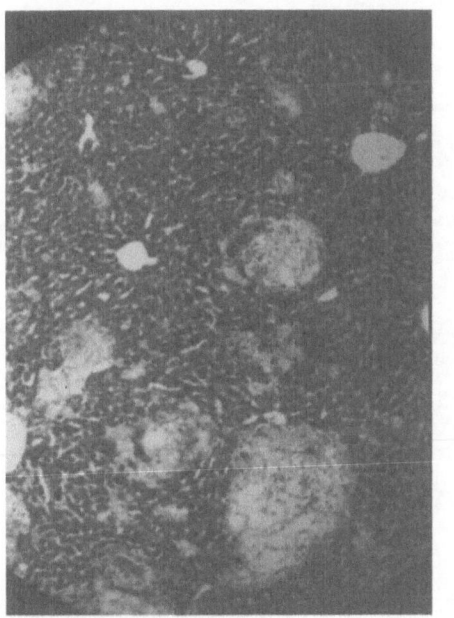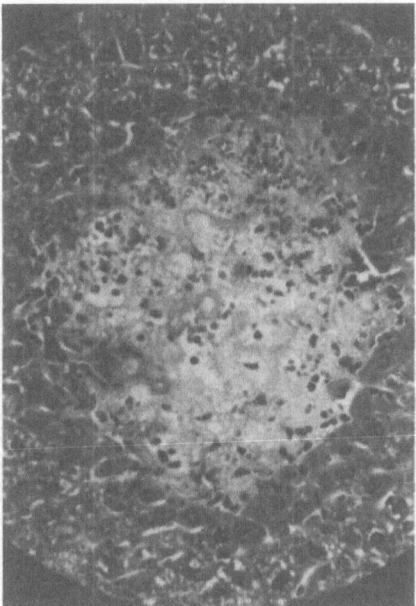

Fig. 4.  Peliosis-like lesions in mouse liver 12 hours following
the oral administration of 25mg lithocholate.  Sinusoids communi-
cating with the necrotic areas result in blood filled spaces a
little later.


    The observations of Bagheri et al (see above) also add more
support to the hypothesis, based on other structure-function relationships, that lithocholate itself, rather than an hydroxylated
metabolite, is involved in the pathogenesis of the lesions.  Administration of the microsomal enzyme inhibitor SK525A increased the
severity of the lesions, while phenobarbital administration pre-

vented the lesions and increased the proportion of the 6βhydroxy
metabolite of lithocholate in bile.  Further, a variety of dihydroxy
bile acids, such as chenic, deoxycholic, hyodeoxycholic and ursodeoxycholic, failed to produce these changes.

    With more prolonged administration of lithocholate, patho-
logical changes of the liver and biliary tract that vary from
species to species can be observed.  Holsti, who first described
the changes in rabbits, noted degenerating liver cells at the
lobular periphery, with connective tissue infiltration around the
lobules leading to a nodular cirrhosis (see Acta Path. Microbiol.
Scand. 54:479, 1962).  In rats, ductular proliferation is particularly striking (Fig. 5).  The changes can be prevented by the
simultaneous administration of cholic acid and cholesterol, but not
be either one alone.

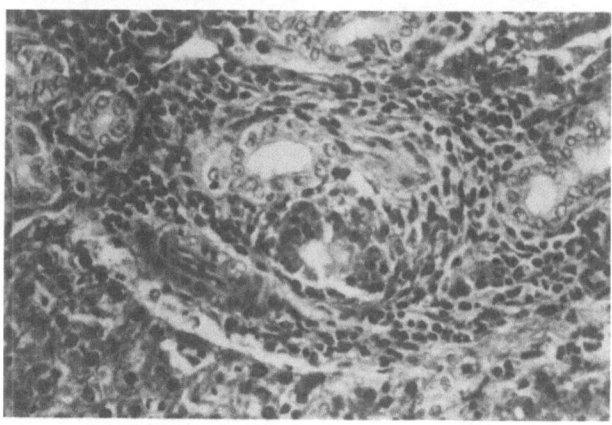

Fig. 5.  Bile duct proliferation in a rat fed lithocholate.

    It is of some interest to consider the amount of lithocholate
necessary for hepatoxicity.  For a mouse, 25mg is a large dose, but
it is not known what fraction of the dose was absorbed and what
proportion of that was then inactivated by 6βhydroxylation.  Bagheri
et al observed that 24 hours after its administration, lithocholate
constituted 18% of the bile acids in the gallbladder bile.  If the
bile acid pool in the mouse is about 5.6mg, it would suggest that
the effective dose may have been only about 1mg.  In any case, 18%
lithocholate in bile corresponds closely with the level of 15% seen
in rabbits that develop typical "litho" lesions while being treated
with chenic acid (E.H. Mosbach, Am. J. Dig. Dis. 19:877, 1974).
Primates, that develop the lesion more slowly, have somewhat lower

levels - around 10% (C.K. McSherry et al, Gastro. 67:815, 1974),
although how much of this is present in the sulphated form is not
well established.  The observations are thus consistent with, though
they provide no direct support for, the hypothesis that the metabolism of chenic to lithocholic acid plays a role in the toxicity
observed in those animal models.  More direct support comes from
recent observation by Salen et al (Lancet 2:1082, 1975) demonstrating that concurrent administration of lincomycin abolishes
lithocholate in bile and prevents lesions otherwise expected in
rhesus monkeys treated with 40mg chenic acid/kg/day.  Thus biliary
concentrations of lithocholate (unsulphated) in excess of 9-10% of
total bile acids should be considered potentially injurious; the
lower limit of potentially toxic concentrations needs to be further
defined in relation to both the sulphated and unsulphated fractions,
since the former can probably be considered to be non-toxic.  Whether
there are species differences in tissue susceptibility, as opposed
to metabolic inactivation (hydroxylation, sulphation) remains to be
established.

In order to study the hyperplasia induced by lithocholate more
carefully, Dr. R.J. Michael Fry, from the Argonne National Laboratory, and I tube fed rats with 18mg lithocholate three times a
day, and then studied proliferative activity in liver cells, bile
ducts, and the common bile duct.  Animals were sacrified in groups
of 3 at 0, 12, 24, 48 and 96 hours.  Mitoses were counted to obtain
a mitotic index, and the incorporation of $^3$H-thymidine (0.5 Ci/gm)
was assessed by autoradiography.  The percent of labeled cells was
determined by scoring at least 1,000 nuclei for the presence of
radioactivity.

The results are shown in Fig. 6.  There was a marked increase
in the number of labeled epithelial cells in the common duct 24
hours after lithocholate was given, and a significant though less
marked increase in the epithelium of the bile ducts in the liver -
still present at 96 hours.  There was also some increase in the
labeling index of hepatocytes at 96 hours.  At 24 hours, there
were a large number of labeled mesenchymal cells, but it was not
considered possible to quantitate this increase.  In general, the
mitotic index paralleled the labeling index.

The rapidity of these changes was confirmed by studies in female
white CFl mice fed a diet containing 0.5% lithocholate (estimated
intake - 25mg/24 hours).  The incorporation of $^3$H-thymidine into
DNA was studied in groups of 6 mice after different time intervals.
Liver specimens were analyzed separately, but gallbladders and
common ducts were arbitrarily combined in groups of two to obtain
sufficient DNA for processing.  The results are shown in Fig. 7.

Peak specific activity in gallbladder tissue was found at 36
hours, although one pair showed evidence of incorporation by 12

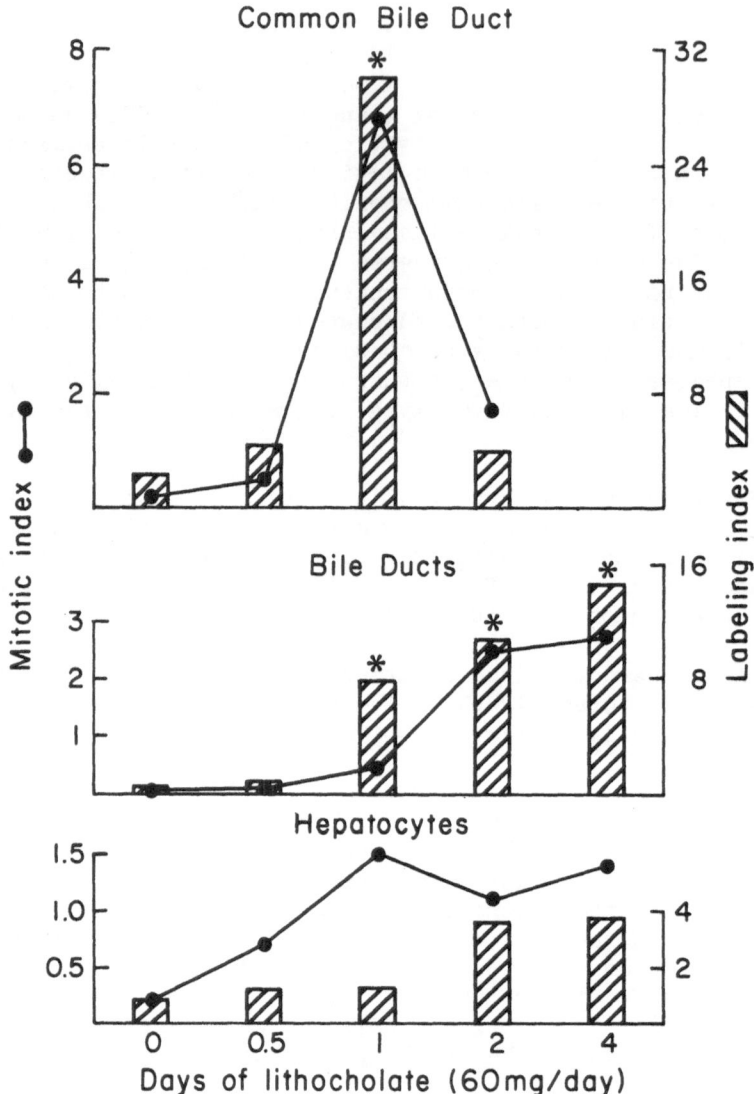

Fig. 6.  Counts of mitoses and labelled cells (determined by autoradiography) in rats fed lithocholate.  Each point is the mean of
three rats.  *Labelling index statistically different from control
(p < .01).

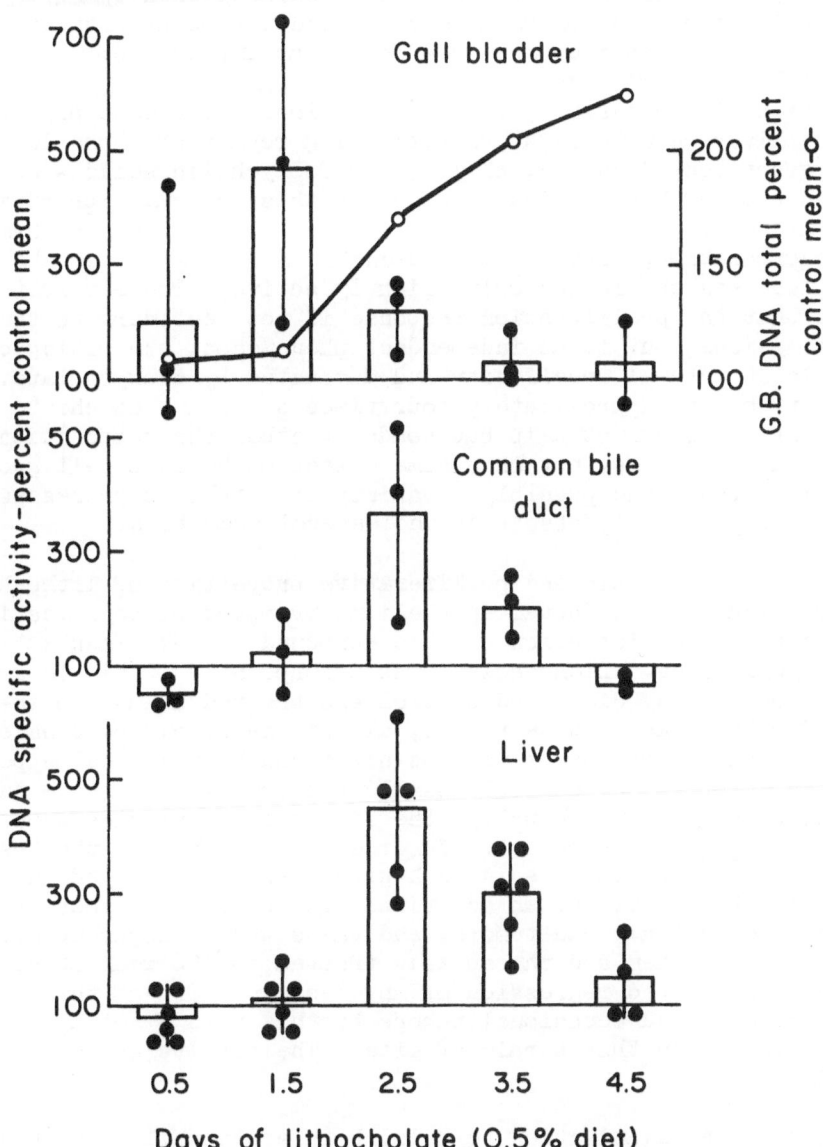

Fig 7.   Incorporation of [3]H-thymidine in mice following lithocholate feeding.   Individual and mean values are shown.   Total DNA
could be measured in gallbladders, which were readily isolated, but
not in other tissues.   Gallbladders and common ducts analyzed in
groups of two.

hours. The subsequent decline in specific activity was accompanied by a reciprocal rise in total DNA. In contrast, peak specific activity in liver and common bile ducts did not occur until 60 hours. However that increase, 3-4 fold, was impressive.

In view of the early histological lesions, it seemed probable that the liver results might be reflecting repair of those lesions. We therefore tested chenic, cholic, and deoxycholic acids - none of which produce histological lesions in this system. Surprisingly, deoxycholic was by far the most active in promoting $^3$H-thymidine incorporation; lithocholic and cholic acids were moderately active, whereas chenic was only slightly active. These results suggest that the proliferation response is not secondary to the hepatic lesions, but is an independent phenomenon, exhibiting considerable structural specificity and dominated by deoxycholate. With deoxycholate approximately four times as active as chenic in this regard, one cannot help but wonder whether the composition of the bile acid pool may not have some effect on hepatic cell growth, hence liver mass, and possibly a variety of metabolic processes such as lipoprotein synthesis or cholesterol secretion.

The important toxic and proliferative properties of lithocholate, particularly on ductal epithelium, prompted us to investigate the long term administration of this compound to C57 black x C3H-F$_1$ hybrid mice. Lithocholate was incorporated (0.5%) in synthetic stock colony diet, and control and treated animals maintained for 50 weeks. At sacrifice, all of the surviving treated mice had hepatic nodules of various sizes and histological appearance. Only four of 27 control animals had abnormal livers - each containing one nodule. Usually, the lithocholate nodules were larger and much more numerous. In order to see whether the lesions would regress, four animals in each group were then placed on laboratory chow diets for an additional 16 weeks. All four of these treated animals had tumors. and there was no apparent difference between them and the animals treated for 50 weeks that might have suggested regression of any lesions. Two of the four control animals had occasional tumors by this time - not an unanticipated finding in this strain of mice. The results are given in Table 1.

Histological examination revealed both eosinophilic and basophilic nodules (see Fig. 8). Cellular pleomorphism was prominent,

Fig. 8. Hepatic nodules induced by long term lithocholate administration in mice. Upper left - Low power view of a nodule with "peliotic lesions" in the adjacent liver. Upper right - Higher power view with nodule above. Lower left - multi-nucleated, pleomorphic cells in a nodule. Lower right - Tumor tissue within a blood vessel.

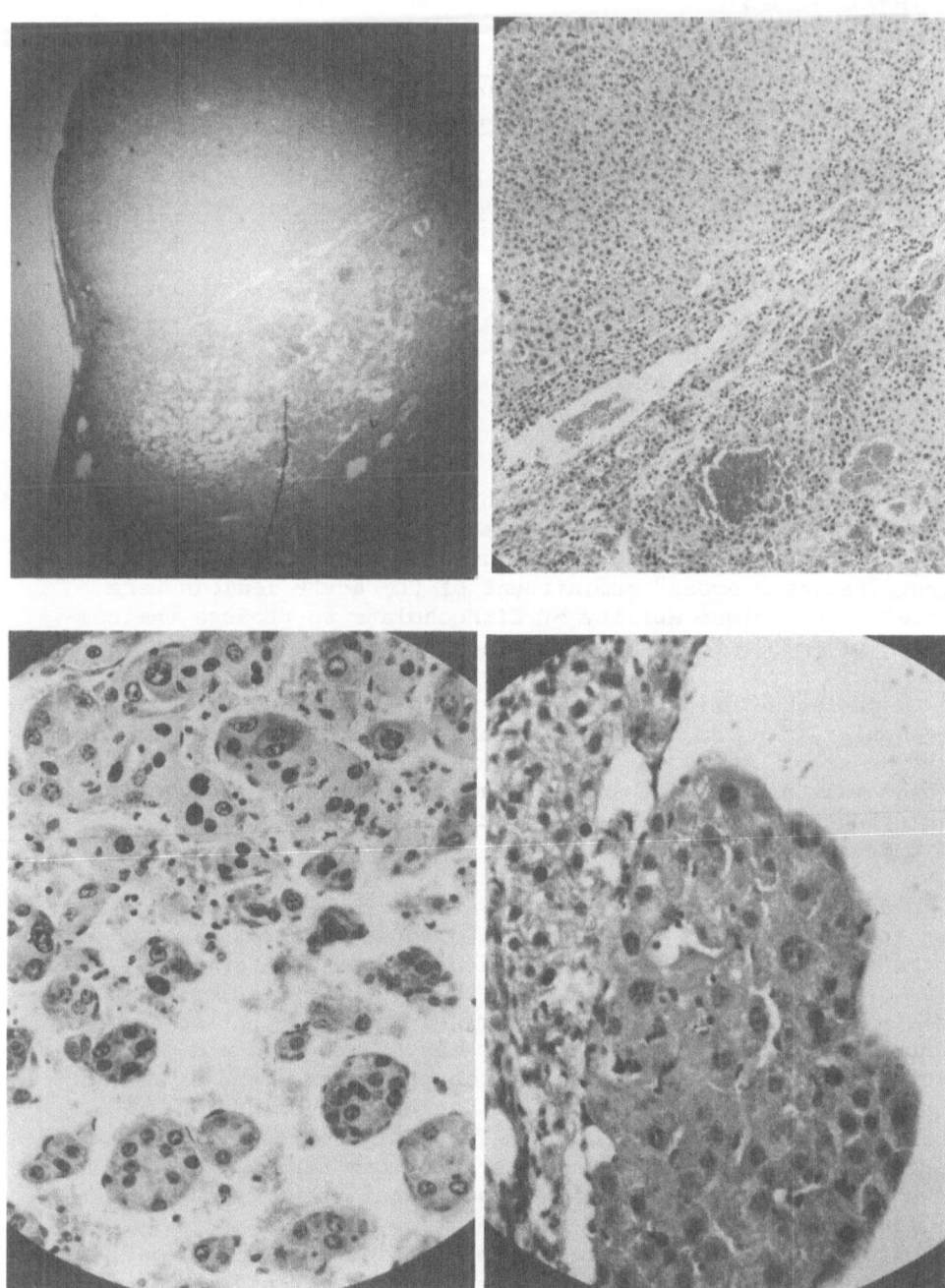

Table 1.  Hepatic Nodules Induced by Lithocholate in Mice

| | A<br>50 weeks<br>study diet | | B<br>A plus 16<br>weeks stock diet | |
| | Control | Litho-<br>cholate | Control | Litho-<br>cholate |
|---|---|---|---|---|
| Died | 0 | 12 | 0 | 1* |
| No nodules | 23 | 0 | 2 | 0 |
| One nodule | 4 | 1 | 1 | 1* |
| Two nodules | 0 | 0 | 1 | 1 |
| Multiple nodules | 0 | 12 | 0 | 2 |
| Total | 27 | 25 | 4 | 4 |

*Same animal

and mitoses frequent.  Despite the histological appearance of
malignancy, no gross metastases were observed; however, in one
section tumor was seen apparently invading a blood vessel.  In most
livers, "peliotic areas" reminiscent of the acute lesions were
observed.  The unique ability of lithocholate to produce the combination of nodule formation and vascular lesions prompts speculation about a possible relation to the peliosis hepatis lesions
seen in patients taking anabolic steroids (mentioned earlier) and
the vascular adenomas seen in patients on contraceptive steroids.
Both classes of compounds contain or are normally metabolized to
steroids that share, with lithocholate, the unusual property of
being pyrogenic - an activity also unique to lithocholate in the
bile acid series.

In summary, lithocholate has several important effects on
liver and bilary tract epithelium.  It causes cholestasis and is
associated with rather specific lesions of the end-terminal canaliculus. It may cause significant areas of hepatocellular necrosis,
possibly in relation to the end-terminal lesions, that go on to
resemble the lesions of peliosis hepatis.  Immediate and long term
effects include hyperplasia of hepatic parenchyma, and of biliary
epithelium in particular, up to and including adenomas and/or
hepatomas in susceptable animals.  The similarities between the
experimental lesions and those seen in humans taking structurally
related synthetic anabolic or progestational steroids suggests a
similar mechanism of action.  The relation of bilary bile acid
composition to hepatic cell mass and function needs further investigation.  The evidence to date suggests that sulphation in man
and hydroxylation in rodents protects against most if not all of
these effects if it can prevent unsulphated lithocholate levels
in bile from rising above certain limits, perhaps 7-8%.

## Bibliography

SA Bagheri, MG Bolt, RH Palmer, and JL Boyer: Lithocholic acid induced peliosis hepatis.  Influence of microsomal enzyme metabolism
on hepatic toxicity.  Advances in Bile Acid Research. III. Bile
Acid Meeting, Freiburg-im-Br., June 13-15, 1974. In press.

AE Cowen, MG Korman, AF Hofmann and OW Cass:  Metabolism of lithocholate in healthy man. I. Biotransformation and biliary excretion
of intravenously administered lithocholate, lithocholylglycine and
their sulfates.  Gastroenterology 69:59-66, 1975.

AE Cowen, MG Korman, AF Hofmann, OW Cass and SB Coffin: Metabolism
of lithocholate in healthy man. II. Enterohepatic circulation.
Gastroenterology 69:67-76, 1975.

AE Cowen, MG Korman, AF Hofmann, and PJ Thomas: Metabolism of
lithocholate in healthy man. III. Plasma disappearance of radioactivity after intravenous injection of labeled lithocholate and
its derivatives.  Gastroenterology 69:77-82, 1975.

H Eyssen, M Vandeputte and E Evrard: Effect of various dietary
bile acids on nutrient absorption and on liver size in chicks.
Arch Int Pharmacodyn 158:292-306, 1965.

CD Fischer, NS Cooper, MA Rothschild and EH Mosbach: Effect of
dietary chenodeoxycholic acid and lithocholic acid in the rabbit.
Am J Digest Dis 19:877-886, 1974.

MM Fisher, R Magnusson, and K Miyai: Bile acid metabolism in
mammals. I. Bile acid-induced intra-hepatic cholestasis. Lab Invest
25:88-91, 1971.

P Holsti: Cirrhosis of the liver induced in rabbits by gastric
instillation of 3-monohydroxycholanic acid.  Nature 186:250, 1960.

P Holsti: Bile acids as a cause of liver injury - cirrhogenic
effect of chenodeoxycholic acid in rabbits. Acta Path Micrbiol
Scand 54:479, 1962.

AC Ivy: The applied physiology of bile secretion and bile salt
therapy. JAMA 117:1151-1154, 1941.

NB Javitt: Cholestasis in rats induced by taurolithocholate.
Nature 210:1262-1263, 1966.

NB Javitt: in The Liver, p.355, Karger, Basel, 1973.

A Kappas and RH Palmer: Selected aspects of steroid pharmacology.
Pharmacol Rev 15:123-167, 1963.

JE King and LJ Schoenfield: Cholestasis induced by sodium taurolithocholate in isolated hamster liver. J Clin Invest 50:2305-
2312, 1971.

TJ Layden, J schwarz and JL Boyer: Scanning electron microscopy of
the rat liver.  Studies on the effect of sodium lithocholate and
other models of cholestasis. Gastroenterology 69: in press, 1975.

CK McSherry, KP Morrissey, RL Swarm and F Glenn: Hepatic function
and morphology in the baboon fed chenodeoxycholic acid for one
year. Gastroenterology 67:815, 1974.

K Miyai, VM Price and MM Fisher: Bile acid metabolism in mammals.
Ultrastructural studies on the intrahepatic cholestasis induced by
lithocholic and chenodeoxycholic acids in the rat. Lab Invest 24:
292-302, 1971.

RH Palmer: Bile acids, liver injury, and liver disease. Arch Int
Med 130:606-617, 1972.

MJ Phillips, M Oda, E Mak, MM Fisher and KN Jeejeebhoy: Microfilament dysfunction as a possible cause of intrahepatic cholestasis. Gastroenterology 69:48-58, 1975.

G Salen, H Dyrszka, T Chen, WH Saltzman and E Mosbach: Prevention
of chenodeoxycholic acid toxicity with lincomycin. Lancet 1:1082,
1975.

DISCUSSION OF COMMENTARY BY R.H. PALMER

Taylor:    You were using lithocholic acid itself in your experiments.    Do you know if lithocholic sulphate or tauro- or glycolithocholate are equally toxic?

Palmer:    I would expect that tauro- and glycolithocholate would
have the same effects.    They have equivalent cytotoxicity in terms
of haemolysis and pyrogenicity.    The sulphate presents a more
difficult problem which I have tried to explore by feeding lithocholate sulphate to see if it produced the same degree of
proliferation, which indeed it did.    But the problem was that
most of the lithocholate was excreted in faeces without the
sulphate moiety, so clearly there was loss of the sulphate during
enterohepatic circulation.    Therefore, it is impossible to say
whether the effects I observed were caused by lithocholate sulphate
or by non-sulphated lithocholate returning to the liver.

Ostrow:    I would be interested in your comment on the hypothesis
that the increase in chenodeoxycholic acid pathway seen in patients
with chronic liver disease might account for some of the liver
damage seen in such patients.

Palmer:    When the amount of chenodeoxycholic acid in the body is
increased by feeding this acid to patients, the lithocholate which
is formed can be reabsorbed and returned to the liver.    It seems
to me that the crucial question about the possibility of this
lithocholate initiating or complicating liver damage in man is
what happens to the sulphating mechanism in such patients.    If
they retain the ability to sulphate lithocholate, I would suppose
that there would be difficulty in sustaining that hypothesis.
On the other hand, if sulphating ability is lost then the hypothesis
would provide a reasonable answer to the problem.

Sjövall:    Is there a sex difference in the effects of lithocholate
in rats?    There is a marked sex difference in the metabolism of
steroids in these animals, such as $6\beta$-hydroxylation, sulphation,
hydrolysis of sulphates and so on.

Palmer:    We have not paid any particular attention to that point,
so I cannot answer your question.

241

Fisher:    There are no sex differences in cholestasis produced
by lithocholate in the isolated, perfused rat liver, but we have
no data on the effects of chronic feeding of lithocholate.   There
are sex differences in the metabolism of cholate and chenodeoxycholate, but none with lithocholate.   Dr. Palmer, would you care
to comment on increased ethionine carcinogenicity in animals fed
lithocholate at the same time?

Palmer:    I am aware of that report, but there are so many possible
interpretations that the conclusions are highly speculative, and I
do not have any real information about this.   Further to Professor
Sjövall's question;  the only thing I know of with regard to sex
differences and lithocholate is related to steroid fever.   As far
as I know, the mechanisms of steroid fever produced by, say,
aetiocholanolone or 11-ketopregnanolone and by lithocholate are
all the same.   It has been definitely shown that females are
relatively more resistant than are males to that type of pyrogenic
activity.

Thaler:    As I understand it, lithocholate does not form micelles
at normal body temperature.   Did you find any evidence for hepatic
secretion and enterohepatic recirculation of lithocholate?

Palmer:    You are correct in thinking that lithocholate does not
form micelles.   It is secreted by the liver and it can be reabsorbed and participate in the enterohepatic circulation, but the
sulphated form is much less readily absorbed than the free form.

Haslewood:    I have doubts about the idea that 6β-hydroxylation is
a defence mechanism against lithocholate.   As far as I know, this
type of hydroxylation is characteristic only of the laboratory rat
and mouse.   It is possible to produce a reasonable evolutionary
theory to explain why this hydroxylation would be an advantage to
the rat and mouse.   I feel that it is just coincidental that this
particular enzyme is there in these animals, and that it has very
little to do with lithocholic acid.   A number of other animals
must be faced by the same problem, but do not have the same
solution available.

Palmer:    You are quite right in taking me to task for using a
teleological explanation for this phenomenon.   The rat is much
more resistant to the effects of lithocholate, but this is not
true for the mouse.

Popper:    These studies on increased thymidine uptake related to
lithocholate and other bile acids have reminded me that the first
studies on increased thymidine uptake by the liver were done in
experimental cholestasis.   Simple ligation of the bile duct
causes increased thymidine uptake in hepatocytes, so it is

reasonable to assume that the increase is due to bile acid retention.

Hofmann: The Rhesus monkey sulphates lithocholate extremely poorly, and this would seem to be the reason for the difference in toxicity of chenodeoxycholate in this monkey and in man. In single-pass studies, we find that the glycine conjugate of litho-cholate is sulphated much more readily than the taurine conjugate. Have you any thoughts why this should be?

Palmer: When we first looked at sulphates, we had the impression that there was more sulphation of the glycine fraction than in the taurine fraction. But our data were not clear enough to establish that point. However, the finding goes along with our general hypothesis that sulphation is a mechanism applied more to less polar compounds. In the bile acid series this hypothesis holds, in that lithocholate is sulphated more than chenodeoxycholate and deoxycholate, and these two are sulphated more than cholate. So it is not surprising that taurolithocholate is not sulphated as much as the glycine conjugate, because the taurine form is a much more polar compound than the glycine form.

# FINE STRUCTURE OF THE BILIARY TREE

M. James Phillips, Masaya Oda, Ellen Mak,
and Jan W. Steiner

Banting Institute, University of Toronto
Toronto, Ontario, Canada

## INTRODUCTION

This paper is divided into three sections. Firstly, there is a review of the normal structure of the biliary passages. The second section deals with the pathology of bile canaliculi with particular emphasis on the fine structural alterations in canaliculi in cholestasis. The final section concerns recent investigations on pericanalicular microfilaments in cholestasis.

## NORMAL BILIARY TREE

The biliary tree includes the bile ducts, ductules, pre-ductules, connecting ducts (canal of Hering, ampulla, intermediate piece or cholangiole) and bile canaliculi. In the past, the usage of some of these terms has not been uniform resulting in unnecessary confusion. The nomenclature pertaining to biliary channels has been reviewed by Steiner et al (75) and is not a current problem. Biliary epithelial cells are much smaller than hepatocytes, have fewer cytoplasmic organelles, and are provided with a basement membrane. Biliary epithelial cells are columnar and are provided with microvilli on their luminal surface. Mitochondria are few in number and much smaller than those in hepatocytes, microfilaments are frequent in the cytoplasm. Bile is formed initially as an intracanalicular secretory product of hepatocytes but there is evidence that bile is modified during its passage through the biliary, ductular system, probably by the secretion of inorganic electrolytes and water and the reabsorption of water(76,82). Recently a method for isolating a liver fraction rich in bile ducts has been described (49) which might facilitate future studies on the role of the bile ducts in biliary excretion.

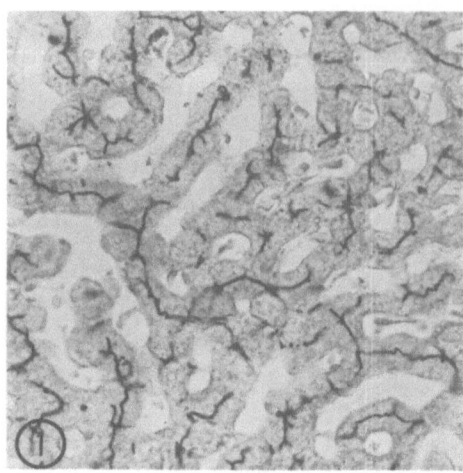 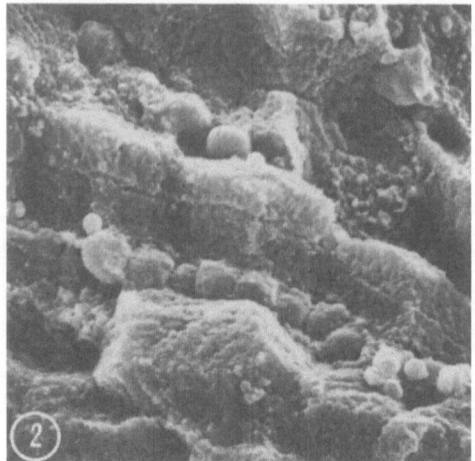

Fig. 1                     Fig. 2

Fig. 1. Hepatic parenchyma showing chicken wire-type network of bile canaliculi. Adenosine triphosphatase "stain". Frozen section X 320.

Fig. 2. Hepatic parenchyma showing freeze-fractured surface. The bile canaliculi are seen en face. Scanning electron micrograph X 2,400

The bile canaliculus is an intercellular space bounded by a specialized region of the plasma membrane of adjacent liver cells. The bile canaliculi are difficult to resolve by routine light microscopy. In histochemical preparations, particularly the adenosine triphosphatase technique described by Wachstein and Meisel (80), bile canaliculi appear as slender channels situated between the hepatocytes. They appear of uniform calibre through-out the liver lobule and have been very adequately described as forming a chicken wire-like network (Fig.1). In the scanning electron microscope, in specimens that have been teased apart after freeze drying, the bile canalicular network is extremely well shown since the hepatocytes separate in this plane exposing the interior of the canaliculi. In such preparations, the anastomosing network of fine biliary channels richly supplied with microvilli are well seen (8) (Fig. 2). In ultrathin sections stained by conventional methods for transmission electron microscopy, the bile canaliculi have been extensively studied (5,12,14,20,29 and others). They appear as focal areas where the cell membranes are separated, are provided with microvilli and are sealed by junctional complexes. Normally, the bile canalicular lumen is small and nearly filled with microvilli. There is a narrow organelle-free zone around the bile canaliculus termed the pericanalicular ectoplasm. In conventional sections, this is a homogeneous granular zone although microfilaments have been described in this zone in both human(5) and calf liver(84). The junctional complexes have strong bonds which serve to form attachments between the cells and separate the lumen of the bile canaliculus from the intercellular and peri-sinusoidal spaces. In uranyl acetate and/or lead stained preparations, the zonula occludens (tight junctions) is always observed but other components of the junctional complex are frequently difficult to identify. With glutaraldehyde perfusion fixation followed by post-fixation in osmium tetroxide, good visualization of the components of the junctional complex is possible. The macula occludens (tight junction), zonula adherens (intermediary junction), desmosome (macula adherens) and nexus, are all well seen (42). A number of studies have been done to assess the permeability of the tight junctions. The tight junctions are generally considered to be impermeable under normal circumstances (5,6,14,19) and in extrahepatic biliary obstruction(61,75). Hampton (25) injected mercuric sulfide or thorotrast into the common bile duct and found no evidence of passage across the tight junctions. Yodaiken (85) injected gum acacia impregnated with lead salts into the portal vein or aorta of rats and suggested passage of the lead across the tight junction. Using the much finer colloidal suspension of lanthanum nitrate(particle size approximately $25°A$ in diameter) of Revel and Karnovsky (58), Schatzki(66) and Matter et al (42) found penetration of the junctional complex in both directions. However the tight junctions were impermeable to horseradish peroxidase (molecular weight 40,000) when injected intravenously or in retrograde manner into the common bile duct(42).

The ruthenium red (RR) technique was used by Cossel et al(13) and by Oda et al (48). Ruthenium red (RR, $Ru_3O_2(NH_3)_{14}Cl_6H_2O$ molecular weight 858.5) is an inorganic dye which probably binds to the acid mucopolysaccharides of tissue glycoproteins. The binding process is thought to involve the formation of ionic complexes between the ammonium groups of RR and the polyanions of acid muco-polysaccharides (39). The high electron density is thought due to the catalytic reduction of osmium tetroxide by an RR-OsO4 coupled reaction after osmification. The RR procedure is excellent for the visualization of the surface coats of cell membranes because these are esaily accessible and composed of glycoprotein but the intracellular distribution of RR-positive material is not defined in intact cells because the RR cannot penetrate the intact plasma membranes (40). In the liver, the distribution of RR positive materials depends upon the penetration of the RR into the liver tissue, much deeper penetration of the tissue is found with perfusion than with immersion techniques. Electron dense deposits, corresponding to RR-positive materials were regularly observed on the external surface of the sinusoidal microvilli, the lateral liver cell membranes, and on the plasma membranes of sinusoidal lining cells, macrophages and blood cells. Bile canaliculi did not usually show the positive RR reaction, but in some instances the RR pepentrated the zonula occludens and was observed on the luminal surface of canalicular microvilli.

Relevant to this discussion is the structure of bile canaliculi in isolated hepatocytes. Liver cells isolated by the technique of Berry and Friend(4) and maintained in Ham's F10 medium enriched with heat inactivated horse serum as described by Jeejeebhoy et al (35) show excellent preservation of fine structure. Most of the cells on isolation are single or paired. In single isolated hepatocytes, the bile canaliculus is invariably near the surface of the cells, but occasionally is deeply intracellular. It is of interest that they are provided with junctional complexes even though deep in the cell cytoplasm. The entire biliary pole of the liver cell remains intact since the close association of the bile canaliculus with lysosomes and Golgi is maintained. In single isolated cells, the entire perimeter of the cell has a RR positive surface coat (52). The isolated cell pairs are of particular interest to this discussion since the contiguous liver cells are joined at their biliary poles and their bile canaliculi appear completely intact. The canalicular lumen is invariably closed. RR penetrates into the canaliculi of liver cells in suspension more easily than into in vivo liver and gives an RR positive reaction in all bile canaliculi observed. The RR positive surface coat measures 200-300 $A^\circ$ thick over the microvilli and is composed of amorphous substance located on the outer(luminal) leaflet of the canalicular membrane (Fig. 3). Small canalicular associated vesicles also stained positively but no other intracytoplasmic structures showed the RR positive reaction since the RR did not cross the undamaged plasma membranes of the isolated cells.

From these various studies, it can be stated conclusively that the bile canalicular membrane is provided with a thick RR-positive surface coat. The question of whether materials can enter the bile canaliculus from the extracellular space and vice versa remains contraversial from electron microscopic studies; for instance, the more easy access of RR into canaliculi of liver cells in suspension might be explained on damage during isolation making the tight junctions more leaky. This question requires further study.

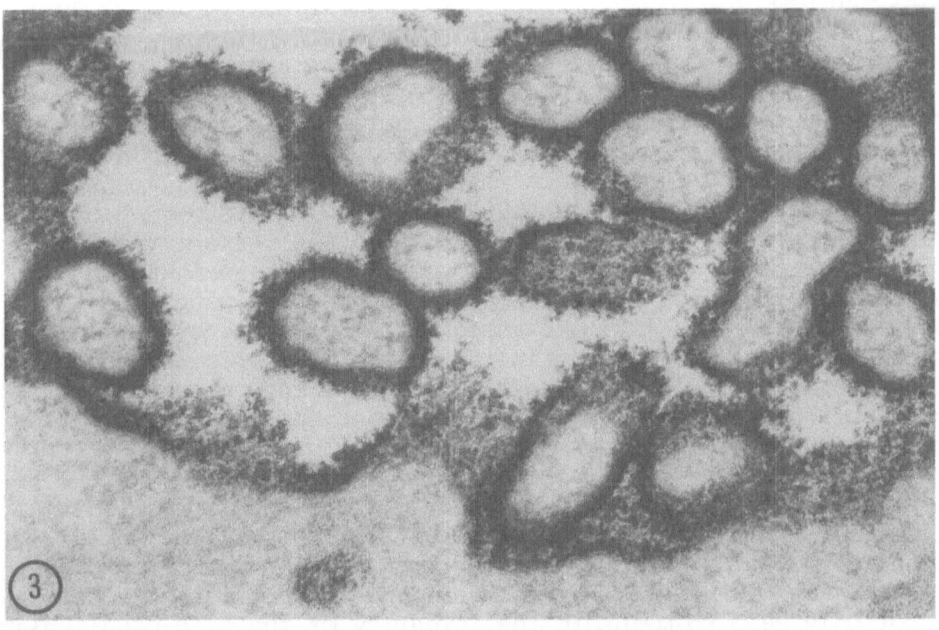

Fig. 3.   Portion of a bile canaliculus from an isolated hepatocyte
preparation showing thick (black) ruthenium red positive surface
coat on canalicular membrane and microvilli.  Note that the canalicular wall is unstained.  Ruthenium red stain  X 125,000

    The examination of in vitro bile canalicular membranes pre-
pared by discontinuous sucrose gradient centrifugation as described
by Song et al (68) and of liver cells which are partly disrupted
during the centrifugation procedure allows excellent visualization
of canalicular and pericanalicular structure.  Isolated bile
canaliculi prepared by this technique are intact with junctional
complexes, a variable length of the lateral cell membranes, microvilli and surface coat all easily identifiable.  In lead stained
preparations, wispy, fuzzy-appearing filamentous material of low
electron density is evident around the canaliculus in the region
corrsponding to the pericanalicular ectoplasm of conventional
transmission electron micrographs.  Filamentous structures in the
pericanalicular ectoplasmic region have been demonstrated previously in in vivo liver(5,6,84), in isolated bile canaliculi(24) and
in association with junctional complexes(19) but in all these
instances they have been poorly visualized.   With the uranyl

acetate-en bloc staining of bile canaliculi in vitro, a rich net-
wotk of microfilaments is shown(48). The microfilaments form a
meshwork around the entire canaliculus and are attached to the
canalicular membrane, they enter the cores of microvilli and insert
into the junctional complex, where they are present in very large
numbers. They are easily divided into two main types, thin and
thick with some intermediary in size. The thin microfilaments are
$50 \overset{o}{A}$ in diameter and the thick $100 \overset{o}{A}$ in uranyl acetate-en bloc
stained preparations, and $70-85 \overset{o}{A}$ and $100-150 \overset{o}{A}$ respectively in RR
stained specimens. Pericanalicular vesicles show an intimate
association with these microfilaments, many appear caught up in
their meshwork. This intimate association with intracytoplasmic
vesicles is even more evident in the partially disrupted hepatocyte preparation. Microfilaments are present throughout the cytoplasm particularly near the plasma membranes and especially in the
pericanalicular region.

There is convincing evidence that microfilaments are important
in cellular motility and contractility(72,81) as well as in the
process of movement of intracellular granules and vacuoles(23,36,
43). We have suggested that the pericanalicular microfilaments
may not only help to maintain the integrity of the bile canalicular
wall but also may regulate the calibre of the canaliculi depending
on the functional state of the liver (48,51).

## THE PATHOLOGY OF THE BILE CANALICULUS

Dilation of bile canaliculi, loss of microvilli and the
deposition of bile pigment in canaliculi and to a lesser extent
within hepatocytes and Kupffer cells are the most characteristic
morphological manifestations of cholestasis (57). The nature and
origin of this pigment is not well understood. It has been
variously considered to be stagnant bile due to impaired bile flow
(16); or abnormally inspissated bile due to reabsorption of water
(7); or abnormally viscous bile resulting from the reabsorption of
water (26), or abnormally viscous bile due to some combination of
dehydration and the addition of proteins from damaged hepatocytes
(56). There is only slight variation in the fine structural
appearance of the canalicular bile pigment in a wide spectrum of
cholestatic disorders(5,6,57,63). The pigment consists of finely
fibrillar material, and less commonly a membranous component.
According to Biava (6) the fibrillar material is derived from precipitated ground substance or pericanalicular ectoplasm, while the
membranous component represents fragmented agranular reticulum and
canalicular cell membranes. Rarely, such as in Byler disease(38),
the biliary material is coarse and particulate and appears to be
derived at least in part from the canalicular membrane and microvilli.

The mechanism of bile secretion is complex and incompletely understood. A widely accepted hypothesis is that bile salts play a major role in regulating biliary secretion(30,69). The mechanism of intrahepatic cholestasis is even less well understood. Early electron microscopic studies of human cholestasis placed the site of initial injury in the bile canaliculus and immediately adjacent structures within the hepatocyte(5,6,59). More recently, it has been postulated that the primary alteration is a disturbance in the secretion of micelles of bile salts mixed with other solids(57). In these studies, emphasis has been placed on bile acid induced alterations in the endoplasmic reticulum to explain the impaired hydroxylation of bile acids and defective micellar formation(15,31, 64). According to these studies, cholestasis is the result of hypoactive hypertrophic smooth endoplasmic reticulum in the hepato-cyte.

Certain bile acids can induce a variety of pathological alterations in hepatic function and morphology. For instance, ductular cell hyperplasia (30,87), fibrosis, cirrhosis(28) and cholelithiasis(87) can be produced by prolonged lithocholic acid administration to experimental animals. A single intravenous injection of sodium taurolithocholate to the hamster induced intra-hepatic cholestasis(34,62). Chenodeoxycholic acid, the taurine and glycine conjugates of chenodeoxycholic acid and lithocholic acid produce cholestasis in the isolated perfused rat liver (22,46). A number of ultrastructural studies on bile acid induced cholestasis on hepatic ultrastructure have been reported(22,46,62,87). The most common changes reported are swelling, shortening or loss of canalicular microvilli, canalicular dilation, thickening of peri-canalicular ectoplasm, prominence of the Golgi apparatus, increased numbers of lysosomes, autophagic vacuole formation, alterations in mitochondrial membranes and disruption of the rough endoplasmic reticulum. These changes are very similar to those described in experimental intrahepatic (65,83) in extrahepatic cholestasis(59, 74) and in human cholestasis(5,6,29,57,86).

In extrahepatic biliary obstruction, scanning electron microscopy of liver prepared by glutaraldehyde perfusion fixation and critical point freezing has shown a progressive dilatation and abnormalities confined to the bile canaliculi(11). The canaliculi instead of being virtually filled with finger-like microvilli, were smoothly flattened. After three days of obstruction, pro-gressive canalicular dilation was followed by sacculations and diverticula formation. The canaliculi became tortuous with dila-tations and angulations following prolonged obstruction but no communications with the space of Disse were observed.

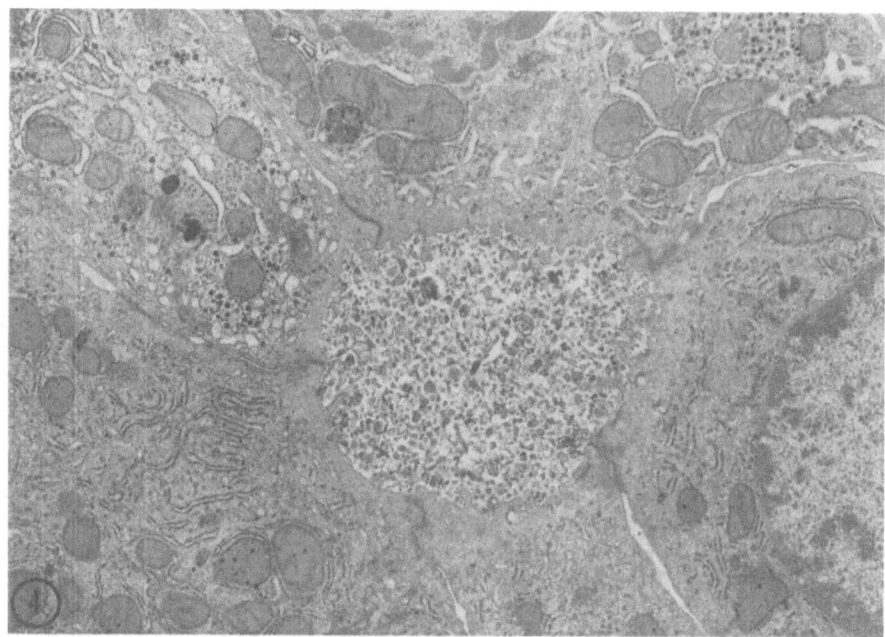

Fig. 4. Human liver from patient with Byler's disease. The bile
canaliculus is dilated, microvilli are reduced, the pericanalicular
ectoplasm is thickened, and the lumen is filled with coarse particulate material. Lead citrate stain  X 12,000

Hence electron microscopic studies have shown that human intrahepatic cholestasis and the cholestasis induced experimentally are
all associated with bile canalicular changes. The problem that has
been difficult to resolve is whether the bile canaliculus itself or
some other structure is the site of primary injury in cholestasis.
It is evident from all the studies cited that there is no single
cause or mechanism of cholestasis.

There are two disorders of particular note in which there is
strong evidence to indicate that the bile canaliculus is the primary
site of injury, namely Byler's disease and lithocholic acid induced
hepatic cell injury; they are worth special mention. Byler's
disease is an inborn error of metabolism characterized by fatal
intrahepatic cholestasis resulting from a defect in transport of

bile salts within hepatocytes (10). Bile acids formed in the liver
are unable to reach the canalicular lumen as shown by elevated
plasma bile acids, reduced intestinal bile salts, increased urinary
loss of bile salts, decreased stool bile salts, increased rate of
bile acid synthesis, delayed plasma disappearance of labelled cholic
acid and chenodeoxycholic acid, and normal conjugation of bile
salts(38). In this disorder, hepatic cell nuclei, mitochondria,
rough endoplasmic reticulum, agranular reticulum, Golgi, peroxisomes,
and other cytoplasmic organelles are all normal. Secondary lysosomes and intracytoplasmic vacuoles are found in a small number of
liver cells. Widespread changes are present involving all bile
canaliculi. Canalicular microvilli are variously absent, short,
swollen, elongated, branched or fused. Canaliculi are dilated and
the pericanalicular ectoplasmic zone greatly widened. The canaliculi are filled with retained biliary material which is coarsely
particulate and appears to be derived from the canalicular wall
and microvilli (Fig. 4). Hence, in Byler disease, severe cholestasis exists, and both the biochemical data and morphological
findings suggest a transport defect in the bile canalicular
membrane as the primary abnormality.

Lithocholic acid induced cholestasis is another disorder in
which the early lesion appears to be localized to the bile canaliculus. In this condition, a highly characteristic lesion occurs
with transformation and lamellar changes involving the canalicular
membranes and microvilli (45,46). Canalicular changes are present
within 30 minutes of lithocholic acid infusion. In freeze-fractured
replicas, the intramembranous granules of the canalicular membrane
appear to have become redistributed, being few or absent in transformed regions. Crystalline precipitates of lithocholic acid in
the canaliculus accompany these alterations. It is extremely likely therefore that the bile canaliculus is involved early in the
pathogenesis of cholestasis in this disorder also.

## BILE CANALICULI, MICROFILAMENTS AND CHOLESTASIS

The demonstration of a rich network of microfilaments around
bile canaliculi and the burgeoning evidence that microfilaments in
many cell types have contractile functions (see reviews by Pollard
and Weihing(55); Durham(17), Huxley (32))led us to postulate that
the pericanalicular network may not only provide structural
stability to the canaliculus but may also provide tone to the canalicular system within the liver(48,51). The walls of bile canaliculi appear rather flimsy structures to maintain the dynamic flow
of bile, particularly in a system as widespread as the intrahepatic
canalicular network. A smooth muscle or elastic coat is lacking
and hence a mechanism for maintaining tone would be extremely
advantageous for bile flow; the presence of a contractile microfilamentous meshwork might fulfil this requirement. In order to
add credence to this hypothesis, it would be necessary to show that

the pericanalicular microfilaments are contractile and that alteration in microfilament structure or disposition alters bile flow.

The thin filaments in non-muscle cells that are responsible
for contractile functions are $40^{\circ}A$-$70^{\circ}A$ in diameter when measured
in preparations stained with conventional procedures, and have
been shown to contain actin-like contractile protein by chemical
analysis (21,79), by heavy meromyosin binding(9,78,79) and by
immunofluorescent techniques(3).   Microfilament research has
been enhanced further by the recent observation that the cytochalasins, which are fungal alkaloids, alter microfilament
structure and function(1,41,67,73).  The specific mechanism of
action of the cytochalasins is not known (33,44,60,71).  Altered
cellular permeability to hexoses has been observed in some cell
types(18) but there is evidence that this effect is unrelated to
its effects on microfilaments(2,77).   Despite the lack of precise
knowledge of the molecular action of cytochalasin B, the evidence
that microfilaments are effected is overwhelming(2,37,67,73,77 and
others).

In the liver there is substantial evidence that at least
certain of the hepatocellular pericanalicular microfilaments
contain actin.  The thin microfilaments as seen in isolated bile
canalicular preparations are the correct size; they measure $50^{\circ}A$
in diameter with the uranyl acetate en bloc staining method(48).
Holborow et al (27) have recently shown by immunofluorescence and
by immuno electron microscopy using a peroxidase labelled anti-
actin antibody technique, that tight junctions and bile canaliculi
are selectively stained; thus providing strong evidence that actin
is present in these sites.  Isolated plasma membrane fractions from
rat liver which include bile canaliculi have been shown to contain
actin-like protein (47).  In rat liver preparations, actin or
actin-like protein has been demonstrated by heavy meromyosin
binding (23).  Using similar techniques we have demonstrated heavy
meromyosin binding in microfilaments of isolated bile canalicular
fractions(53).  The thin microfilaments showed decoration with
heavy meromyosin similar to that described by Spooner et al(70)
since there was an overall impression of periodicity in the binding pattern.   Further, cytochalasin B administration produced
morphological and functional evidence of cholestasis in in vivo
infused rat liver(54).   In this study, cytochalasin B in a concentration of 100 ug/ml with 0.2% dimethyl sulfoxide in 0.9% NaCl
was infused for 3 hours using a Harvard infusion pump, following
cannulation of the common bile duct, controls were treated similarly but the cytochalasin B was omitted from the infusate.  After
one hour of cytochalasin B infusion, wide dilation of bile
canaliculi was found and was accompanied by marked reduction in
canalicular microvilli(Fig.5).  Fibrillar material and/or electron
dense amorphous materials were noted in vesicles in the peri-

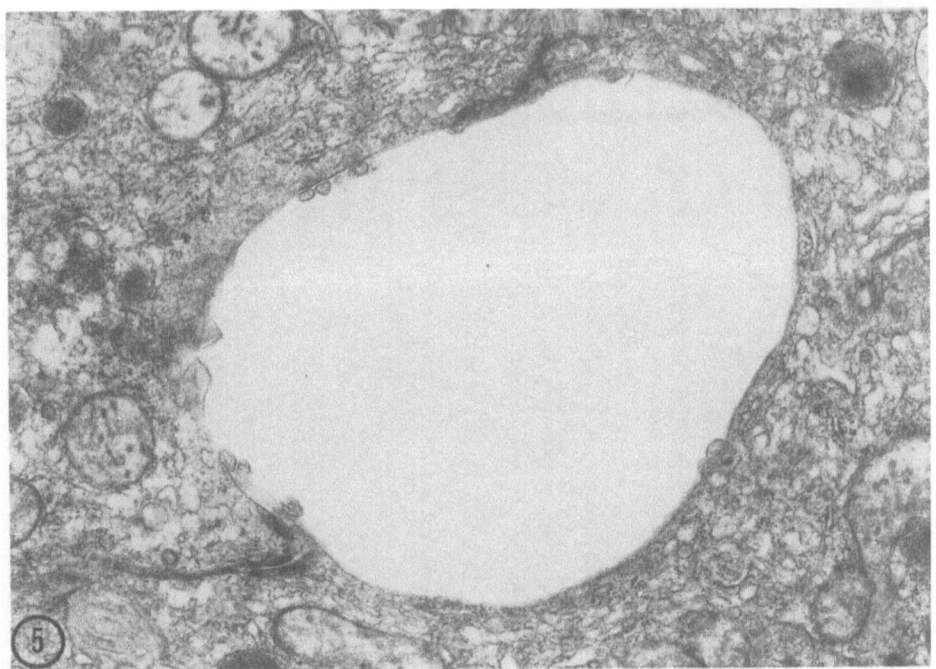

Fig. 5. Bile canaliculus from in vivo cytochalasin B infused liver. Note marked canalicular extasia, loss of microvilli, and absence of normal microfilaments (compare with Fig. 6). Uranyl acetate - en bloc stain  X 25,000

canalicular region and sometimes in dilated canaliculi.  Following two and three hours of infusion, these ultrastructural changes were more advanced; most of the bile canaliculi were devoid of microvilli and markedly dilated.  Smooth surfaced vesicles were prominent and cisternae of the rough endoplasmic reticulum widely dilated.  Large vacuoles containing granular amorphous material was observed in some liver cells.  Other cytoplasmic organelles appeared normal.  In uranyl acetate-en bloc stained preparations, hepatic ultrastructure of controls was normal and pericanalicular microfilaments were easily identified(Fig. 6).   In the cytochalasin B treated animals, microfilaments were not identified, but the pericanalicular ectoplasm appeared thickened and granular. Similar effects of cytochalasin B on microfilaments have been noted by others (72, 73) and it is presumed that the granular material represents altered microfilaments.  Concomittant with these

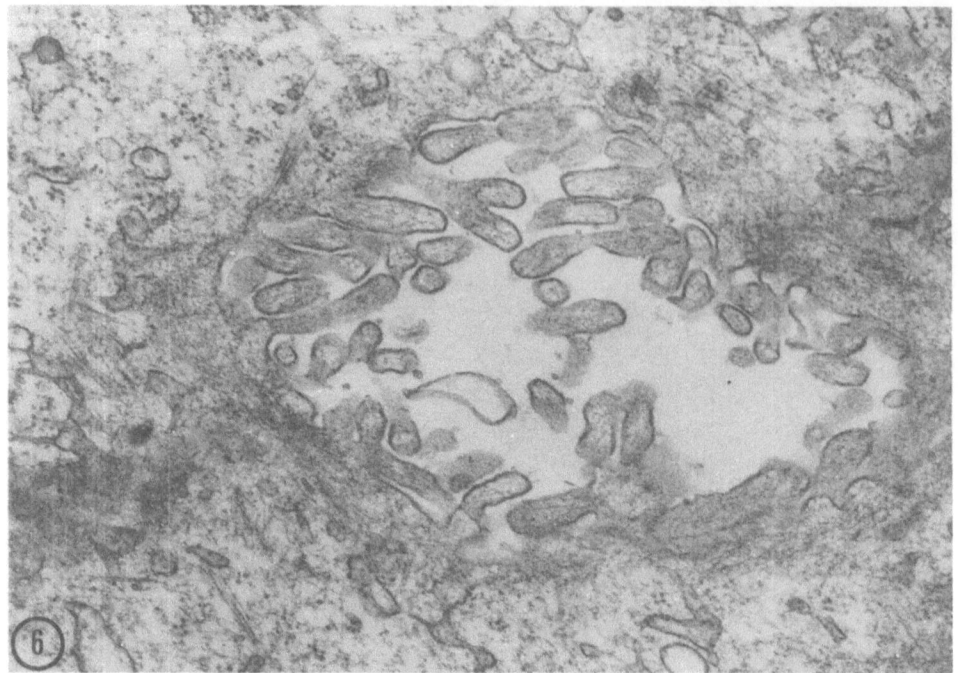

Fig. 6.   Bile canaliculus from a control animal.   Note microfilaments in pericanalicular ectoplasm and in canalicular microvilli.
Uranyl acetate - en bloc   X 38,000

morphological changes, bile flow was reduced more than 50% after
one hour of cytochalasin B infusion, and was totally arrested in all
animals after three hours.   In controls, bile flow was normal
Cytochalasin B produced similar morphological results in isolated
liver cells in suspension; marked bile canalicular dilation and
loss of microvilli were uniformly noted within one hour of the
addition of this agent to the culture medium.    In a recent study
we have isolated bile canaliculi from rat liver previously infused
in vivo with cytochalasin B as used in the previously cited experiment.    The isolated bile canaliculi from cytochalasin B treated
animals were highly abnormal structurally (50).

From all these data, there is substantial evidence that the
pericanalicular microfilaments may contain actin and subserve a
contractile function.   It is suggested that by maintaining the

canaliculi in a contracted or partly contracted state, they may
provide tone to the canalicular system and hence facilitate bile
flow.   Removal of microfilament function would be expected to
result in functional and morphological cholestasis, as was found
with cytochalasin B.   It has been shown previously that the
manifestations of experimental and human cholestasis ultrastructurally are not very specific (57).   Cytochalasin B induced
virtually the entire spectrum of fine structural pathology described
in cholestasis.   It is premature to suggest that microfilament
alterations underlie a wide variety of cholestatic disorders
regardless of aetiology, however, in experimental cholestasis
caused by cytochalasin B, it is extremely likely that microfilament
dysfunction is the primary mechanism involved.   The possible
involvement of microfilaments in other forms of cholestasis remains
to be investigated.

### SUMMARY

The first part of this paper deals with the fine structure of
the normal biliary tree.   Additional information on bile canalicular structure has been achieved by scanning electron microscopy
since the plane of cleavage in teased preparations exposes the
canalicular network.   The problem of whether the canalicular
tight junctions are an impermeable seal under all conditions
remains unsettled.   The consensus of opinion is that in biliary
tract obstruction, there is transcellular passage of biliary
material, and that there are no communications between the bile
canaliculus and the perisinusoidal space or if such communications
occur, they are rare.   Using the ruthenium red stain, a thick
surface coat is present on bile canalicular and microvillous
membranes;   this is especially well demonstrated in isolated liver
cell preparations.   The pericanalicular ectoplasm has been shown
to consist of a microfilamentous network which attach to the canalicular membrane, enter the cores of microvilli and are especially
numerous near the junctional complexes.   Smooth surfaced vesicles
in the canalicular region appear entrapped within this network.

The second part of this paper deals with the pathology of bile
canaliculi.   Emphasis is placed on the possible role of the bile
canaliculus in the pathogenesis of cholestasis.   In virtually all
forms of experimental and human cholestasis, bile canalicular
changes are present.   Most prominent are canalicular ectasia,
alterations in microvilli, widening of the pericanalicular ectoplasmic zone, prominence of the Golgi apparatus, cytolysosome
formation, and retention of biliary pigment within canaliculi,
hepatocytes and Kupffer cells.   The problem is whether the
canalicular changes are the cause or the result of the cholestasis.
It is apparent that there is no single cause or mechanism of
cholestasis.   In certain conditions there is much evidence to
suggest that the bile canaliculus is the primary site of injury;

two such conditions are Byler's disease and acute lithocholic acid induced liver disease.

The final section is more speculative and deals with the possible involvement of pericanalicular microfilaments in normal bile flow and in cholestasis. Since certain microfilaments in many cells are associated with contractile functions, the authors have suggested that the pericanalicular microfilamentous network may provide tone to the canalicular system and hence facilitate bile flow. Evidence from the size of microfilaments, from immuno-electron microscopy using anti-actin antibodies and also from heavy meromyosin binding, all tend to indicate the presence of actin in pericanalicular microfilaments. Cytochalasin B, an agent widely acclaimed to alter microfilament structure and function alters the appearance of the microfilaments, causes canalicular morphological changes of cholestatic type and reduces bile flow. These findings support the view that microfilaments might have a contractile function and influence intrahepatic bile flow.

## ACKNOWLEDGEMENTS

This research was supported by a Grant-in-Aid of the Medical Research Council of Canada (MT-785). Mrs. Ellen Mak, 3rd year Medical Student, University of Toronto, was supported by a summer Student Scholarship of the Canadian Hepatic Foundation. The authors wish to thank Drs. Dinah Yu, K.N. Jeejeebhoy and M.M. Fisher, Departments of Pathology and Medicine, University of Toronto for their collaboration and helpful comments. We also thank Mrs. Janet Rowley and Mr. Vern Edwards for excellent technical assistance.

## REFERENCES

1.    ALLISON,A.C., DAVIES,P., DEPETRIS,S. Role of contractile microfilaments in macrophage movement and endocytosis. Nature (New Biol.) 232: 153-155, 1971.
2.    AXLINE, G.G., REAVEN,E.P. Inhibition of phagocytosis and plasma membrane motility of the cultivated macrophage by cytochalasin B role of subplasma membrane microfilaments. J. Cell Biol. 62: 647-659,1974.
3.    BECKER, C.G., NACHMANN,R.L. Contractile proteins of endo-thelial cells, platelets and smooth muscle. Amer.J.Path.71: 1-22, 1973.
4.    BERRY, M.N., FRIEND,D.S. High yield preparation of isolated rat liver parenchymal cells. A biochemical and fine structural study. J. Cell Biol. 43; 506-520, 1969.
5.    BIAVA, C. Studies on cholestasis. A re-evaluation of the fine structure of normal human bile canaliculi. Lab. Invest. 13: 840-864, 1964.

6.   BIAVA, C.  Studies on cholestasis. The fine structure and morphogenesis of hepatocellular and canalicular bile pigment. Lab.Invest. 13: 1099-1123, 1964.

7.   BILLING, B.H., MAGGIORE,W., CARTER, M.A.  Hepatic transport of bilirubin. Ann.N.Y.Acad.Sci. 111: 319-325, 1963.

8.   BROOKS, S.E.H., HAGGIS,G.H.  Scanning electron microscopy of rat's liver. Application of freeze-fracture and freeze-drying techniques. Lab.Invest. 29: 60-64, 1973.

9.   CHANG, C.M., GOLDMANN, R.D.  The localization of actin-like fibers in cultured neuroblastoma cells as revealed by heavy meromyosin binding. J. Cell Biol. 57: 867-874,1973.

10.  CLAYTON, R.J., IBER, F.K., REUBNER, B.H., McKUSICK,V.A.  Byler disease, fatal familial intrahepatic cholestasis in an Amish kindred. Amer.J.Dis.Child. 117: 112-124, 1969.

11.  COMPAGNO, J., GRISHAM, J.W.  Scanning electron microscopy of extrahepatic biliary obstruction. Arch.Path. 97: 348-351,1974.

12.  COSSEL,L.  Uber den submikroskopischen Zusammenhaug der inter zellularen Raume und Sinusoide in der Leber   Z. Zellforsch Mikroskop.Anat. 58: 76-93, 1962.

13.  COSSEL,L., WEIDENBACH,H., SCHULZ, B.  Elekronemikroskopische Befunde au der Leber bei Anwendung von Ruthenivmrot. Beitr. Pathol. Anat. 139: 381-408, 1969.

14.  DAEMS, W.R.  The micro-anatomy of the smallest biliary pathways in mouse liver tissue. Acta. Anat. 46: 1-24, 1961.

15.  DENK, H., SHENKMAN,J.B., BACCHIN,P.G., HUTTERER,F., SCHAFFNER, F., POPPER,H.  Mechanism of cholestasis. III. Interaction of synthetic detergents with microsomal cytochrome P-450 dependent biotransformation system in vitro. Exper.Molec.Path.14: 263-276, 1971.

16.  DUBIN, I.N.  Intrahepatic bile stasis in acute non-fatal viral hepatitis: its incidence, pathogenesis and correlation with jaundice. Gastroent. 36: 645-660, 1959.

17.  DURHAM, A.C.H.  A unified theory of the control of actin and myosin in non-muscle movements. Cell 2: 123-136, 1974.

18.  ESTENSEN,R.D. , PLAGEMANN,P.G.W.  Cytochalasin B.  Inhibition of glucose and glucosamine transport. Proc.Nat.Acad.Sci.69: 1430-1434, 1972.

19.  FARQUHAR, M., PALADE, G.  Junctional complexes in various epithelia. J. Cell Biol. 17: 375-412, 1963.

20.  FAWCETT,D.W.  Observations on the cytology and electron microscopy of hepatic cells. J. Natl.Cancer Inst.15: Suppl. 1475-1503, 1955.

21.  FINE, R.E., BRAY, D.  Actin in growing nerve cells. Nature (New Biol.) 234: 115-118, 1971.

22.  FISHER, M.M., MAGNUSSON,R., MIYAI,K.  Bile acid metabolism in mammals. I. Bile acid induced intrahepatic cholestasis. Lab.Invest.25: 88-91, 1971.

23.    FRENCH,S.W., DAVIES,P.L.  Ultrastructural localization of actin-like filaments in rat hepatocytes.  Gastroent.68:765-774,1975.

24.    GOODENOUGH,D.A., REVEL,J.P.  The permeability of isolated and in situ mouse hepatic gap junctions studied with enzymatic tracers. J.Cell Biol.50:81-91,1971.

25.    HAMPTON,J.C.  Electron microscopic study of extrahepatic biliary obstruction in the mouse. Lab.Invest.10: 502-513, 1961.

26.    HOFFBAUER,F.W.  Clinical aspects of jaundice resulting from intrahepatic obstruction. J.Amer.Med.Assoc.169:1453-1461, 1959.

27.    HOLBOROW,E.J.,TRENCHEV,P.S.,DORLING,J.,WEBB,Janet. Demonstration of smooth muscle contractile protein antigens in liver and epithelial cells. Annals N.Y.Acad.Sci.254:489-504,1975.

28.    HOLSTI,P.  Cirrhosis of the liver induced in rabbits by gastric instillation of 3-monohydroxycholanic acid. Nature (London)186: 250,1960.

29.    HOPWOOD,D., READ,E.A.,WILLIAMS,R.  Ultrastructural findings in idiopathic recurrent cholestasis. Gut 13:986-995,1972.

30.    HUNT,R.D.,LEVEILLE,G.A.,SAULBERLICH,H.E.  Dietary bile acids and lipid metabolism. III. Effects of lithocholic acid in mammalian species. Proc.Soc.Exper.Biol.Med.115: 277-280,1964.

31.    HUTTERER,F., DENK,H., BACCHIN,P.C., SCHENKMAN,J.B., SCHAFFNER,F.,POPPER,H.  Mechanism of cholestasis.I. Effect of bile acids on microsomal cytochrome P-450 dependent bio-transformation system in vitro. Life Sci.9: 877-887,1970.

32.    HUXLEY,H.E.  Muscular contraction and cell motility. Nature 243:445-449,1973.

33.    JAHN,W.  Similarity between the effect of experimental congestion of the isolated perfused rat liver and the action of cytochalasin B. Naunyn-Schmiedeberg's Arch. Pharmacol.278:431-434,1973.

34.    JAVITT,N.B., EMERMAN,S.  Effect of sodium taurolithocholate on bile flow and bile acid excretion. J. Clin.Invest.47: 1002-1014,1968.

35.    JEEJEEBHOY,K.N., HO,J., GREENBERG,G.R.,PHILLIPS,M.J.,BRUCE-ROBERTSON,A.,SODTKE,U.  Albumin and fibrinogen synthesis in isolated rat hepatocyte suspensions. A model for the study of plasma protein synthesis in the rat. Biochem.J. 146:141-155, 1975.

36.    LACY,P.E., HOWELL,S.L.,YOUNG,D.A.,FINK,C.J.  New hypothesis of insulin secretion.  Nature 219:1177-117-,1968.

37.    LIN,S., SANTI,D.W.,SPUDICH,J.A. Biochemical studies on the model of action of cytochalasin B. J.Biol.Chem.249: 2269-2274,1974.

38. LINARELLI,L.G., WILLIAMS,C.N., PHILLIPS,M.J. Byler's disease Fatal intrahepatic cholestasis. J.Pedial.81:484-492,1972.

39. LUFT,J.H. Ruthenium red and violet. I. Chemistry purification, methods for use for electron microscopy and mechanism of action. Anat.Rec. 171: 347-368, 1971.

40. LUFT, J.H. Ruthenium red and violet. II. Fine structural localization in animal tissues. Anat.Rec. 171:369-415,1971.

41. MANASEK,F.J., BURNSIDE,B., STROMAN,J. Sensitivity of developing cardiac myofibrils to cytochalasin B. Proc.Nat. Acad.Sci.69: 308-312, 1972.

42. MATTER,A., ORCI,L., ROUILLER,C. A study on the permeability barriers between Disse's space and the bile canaliculus. J. Ultrastruct.Res. Supplement 11, 1-71, 1969.

43. McGUIRE,J., MOELLMANN,G. Cytochalasin B: effects on microfilaments and movement of melanin granules within melanocytes. Science 175: 642-644, 1972.

44. MIRANDA,A.F., GODMAN,G.C., DEITCH,A.D., TANENBAUM,S.W. Action of cytochalasin D on cells of established lines. I. Early events. J. Cell Biol. 61: 481-500, 1974.

45. MIYAI,K., MAYR,W.W.,RICHARDSON,A.L. Acute cholestasis induced by lithocholic acid in the rat. A freeze-fracture replica and thin section study. Lab.Invest.32:527-535,1975.

46. MIYAI, K., PRICE,V.M.,FISHER,M.M. Bile acid metabolism in mammals. Ultrastructural studies on the intrahepatic cholestasis induced by lithocholic and chenodeoxycholic acids in the rat. Lab.Invest.24: 292-320,1971.

47. NEIFAKH,S.A., VASILETS,I.M. Actomyosin-like protein in outer membrane of liver cells.Fed.Proc.24:T561,1965.

48. ODA,M., PRICE,V.M., FISHER,M.M.,PHILLIPS,M.J. Ultrastructure of bile canaliculi with special reference to the surface coat and the pericanalicular web. Lab.Invest.31:314-323,1974.

49. ODA,M.,YOUSEF,J.M., PHILLIPS,M.J. Isolation of bile ducts from rat liver.Technique and preliminary ultrastructural characterization. Exper.Molec.Path.(1975). In press.

50. ODA,M., PHILLIPS,M.J. Unpublished observations.

51. PHILLIPS,M.J.,ODA,M. The bile canalicular web. Fed.Proc. 33: 626,1974.

52. PHILLIPS,M.J.,ODA,M.,EDWARDS,V.D.,GREENBERG,G.R., JEEJEEBHOY, K.N. Ultrastructural and functional studies of cultured hepatocytes. Lab.Invest.31: 533-542,1974.

53. PHILLIPS,M.J.,ODA,M., MAK,E., FISHER,M.M. Bile canalicular structure and function in: Jaundice. Goresky,C. and Fisher, M.M. Eds. Plenum Publishing Corp.New York 1975.pp.367-382.

54. PHILLIPS,M.J.,ODA,M.,MAK,E.,FISHER,M.M.,JEEJEEBHOY,K.N. Microfilament dysfunction as a possible cause of intrahepatic cholestasis.Gastroent.69: 48-58,1975.

55. POLLARD,T.D.,WEIHING,R.R. Actin and myosin and cell movement. Chemical Rubber Co. Critical Reviews in Biochemistry 2: 1-65,1974.

56.    POPPER,H.,SCHAFFNER,F.  Pathology of jaundice resulting
       from intrahepatic cholestasis. J.Amer.Med.Assoc.169: 1447-1453,
       1959.
57.    POPPER,H., SCHAFFNER,F. Pathophysiology of cholestasis. Human
       Path.1: 1-24,1970.
58.    REVEL,J.,KARNOVSKY,M.  Hexagonal array of subunits in inter-
       cellular junctions of the mouse heart and liver. J. Cell
       Biol.33: C7-C12,1967.
59.    ROUILLER,C.  Les Canalicules biliares: étude au microscope
       électronique. Acta.Anat.26: 94-109, 1956.
60.    SANGER,J.W., HOLTZER,H.  Cytochalasin B effects on cell
       morphology, cell adhesion and mucopolysaccharide synthesis.
       Proc.Natl.Acad.Sci.USA 69: 253-257,1972.
61.    SASAKI,H., SCHAFFNER,F., POPPER,H.  Bile ductules in
       cholestasis.  Morphologic evidence for secretion and
       absorption in man. Lab.Invest.16: 84-95, 1967.
62.    SCHAFFNER,F., JAVITT,N.B.  Morphological changes in hamster
       liver during intrahepatic cholestasis induced by tauro-
       lithocholate. Lab.Invest.15: 1783-1792, 1966.
63.    SCHAFFNER,F., POPPER,H.  Morphological studies in cholesta-
       sis. Gastroent.37: 565-573,1959.
64.    SCHAFFNER,F., POPPER,H. Cholestasis is the result of hypo-
       active hypertrophic smooth endoplasmic reticulum in the
       hepatocyte. Lancet 2: 355-359,1969.
65.    SCHAFFNER,F.,POPPER,H.,PEREZ,V. Changes in bile canaliculi
       produced by norethandrolone, electron microscopic study of
       human and rat liver. J. Lab.Clin.Med. 56: 623-628,1960.
66.    SCHATZKI,P.F.  Bile canaliculus and space of Disse. Electron
       microscopic relationships as delineated by Lanthanum. Lab.
       Invest.20: 87-93, 1969.
67.    SHEPRO,D., BELAMARICH,F.A.,ROBBLEE,L.,CHAO,F.C. Anti-
       motility effect of cytochalasin B observed on mammalian
       clot retraction. J. Cell Biol.47: 544-547,1970.
68.    SONG,C.S.,RUBIN,W., RIFKIND,A.B.,KAPPAS,A.  Plasma
       membranes of the rat liver. Isolation and enzymatic
       characterization of a fraction rich in bile canaliculi.
       J. Cell Biol.41: 124-132,1969.
69.    SPERBER,I.  Secretion of organic anions in the formation of
       urine and bile. Pharmacol.Rev. 11: 109-134,1959.
70.    SPOONER,B.S., ASH,J.F., WRENN,F.T., FRATER,R.B.,WESSELLS,N.
       K.  Heavy meromyosin binding to microfilaments involved in
       cell and morphogenetic movements.  Tissue and Cell 5: 37-
       46, 1973.
71.    SPOONER,B.S., CONRAD,G.W.  The role of extracellular
       materials in cell movement. I. Inhibition of mucopoly-
       saccharide synthesis does not stop ruffling membrane
       activity or cell movement.J. Cell Biol.65: 286-297,1975.

72.     SPOONER,B.S., YAMADA,K.M., WESSELLS,N.K.  Microfilaments
        and cell locomotion. J. Cell Biol. 49: 595-613,1971.
73.     SPUDICH,J.A.  Effects of cytochalasin B on actin filaments.
        Cold Spring Harbor Symposia on Quantitative Biology 37:585-
        593,1972.
74.     STEINER,J.W., CARRUTHERS,J.S.  Studies on the fine structure
        of the terminal branches of the biliary tree. II. Observa-
        tions of pathologically altered bile canaliculi. Amer.J.Path.
        39: 41-63,1961.
75.     STEINER,J.W., JEZEQUEL,A.M.,PHILLIPS,M.,MIYAI, K., ARAKAWA,K.
        Some aspects of the ultrastructural pathology of the liver.
        In: Progress in Liver Disease,edited by Popper,H. and
        Schaffner,F. Ed.2.New York,Grune and Stratton,Inc. 1965.
        pp.303-372.
76.     STERNLIEB,I.  Functional implications of human portal and
        bile ductular ultrastructure. Gastroent.63:321-327,1972.
77.     TAYLOR,E.L., WESSELLS,N.K.  Cytochalasin B.  Alterations in
        salivary gland morphogenesis not due to glucose depletion.
        Develop.Biol.31: 421-425,1973.
78.     TILNEY,L.G., CARDELL,R.R.  Factors controlling the reassembly
        of the microvillous border of the small intestine of the
        salamander.J.Cell Biol.47: 408-422,1970.
79.     TILNEY,L.G., MOSSEKER,M.  Actin in the brush-border of
        epithelial cells of the chicken intestine. Proc.Natl.Acad.
        Sci.USA 68: 2611-2615,1971.
80.     WACHSTEIN,M., MEISEL,E.  Histochemistry of hepatic
        phosphates at physiologic pH with special reference to the
        demonstration of bile canaliculi. Amer.J.Clin.Path.27:13-23,
        1957.
81.     WESSELLS,N.K., SPOONER,B.S., ASH,J.F., BRADLEY,M.O.,
        LUDUENA,M.A.,TAYLOR,E.L.,WRENN,J.T.,YAMADA,K.M. Microfila-
        ments and cell locomotion. J.Cell Biol.49: 595-613,1971.
82.     WHEELER,H.O.,ROSS,E.D.,BRADLEY,S.E.  Canalicular bile
        production in dogs. Amer.J.Physiol.214:866-8-4.1968.
83.     WITZLEBEN,C.L.  Physiologic and morphological natural
        history of a model of intrahepatic cholestasis.(manganese-
        bilirubin overload). Amer.J.Path.66:577-582,1972
84.     WOOD, R.L.  Some structural features of the bile canaliculus
        in calf liver. Anat.Rec. 140; 207-216,1961.
85.     YODAIKEN,R.  The use of lead as a tracer in ultrastructural
        research. Lab.Invest.15: 403-411, 1966.
86.     ZAKI,F.G.  Ultrastructure of hepatic cholestasis. Med.45:
        537-545,1966.
87.     ZAKI,F.G.,CAREY,J.B.,HOFFBAUER,F.W.,NWOKOLO,C.  Biliary
        reaction and choledocholithiasis induced in the rat by
        lithocholic acid. J.Lab.Clin.Med.69:737-748,1967.

DISCUSSION OF LECTURE BY M.J. PHILLIPS

Boyer:   How do you explain the fact that treatment with cytochalasin will lead to dilatation rather than, say, collapse or
constriction of the canaliculus?

Phillips:   This boils down to the question of what is cytochalasin
actually doing.   About 15 hypotheses could be put forward as to
how cytochalasin works.   All of these hypotheses involve microfilaments, although hexose transport and other things could be
brought in.   I do not want to try to simplify what is obviously
a very complex matter.   The way in which it works is not known,
but the consensus of opinion is that it does have an effect on
microfilaments by altering their morphology and contractility.
What we are dealing with is a preparation in which normally there
is a closed canaliculus with microfilaments around it.   The contractile process is energy-requiring and the way I see it is that
normally the canaliculi are held in this state by what I call
"contraction-tone" of the canalicular system.   When you destroy
this situation by dissociation, detachment or disassembly of the
filament from the membrane bile stasis then occurs.   So it seems
to me that when you remove the contractile function this is the
cause of the stasis.

Boyer:   It appears from your pictures of the canalicular rich
fractions that the microvilli are contained within a closed space,
and you could only see microvilli at small points of rupture.
The openings, which must occur in vivo to enter the microvilli
from the cell, appeared to be closed over.   Have you tried to
disrupt this preparation to open these, or do you think that the
fixation procedure is responsible for this apparent closure?

Phillips:   When you look at the ruptured preparations you wonder
how all the microvilli can be packed back.   What I think happens
is that during the isolation procedure they are not structurally
held in their normal anatomical position:   these are probably
altered by the centrifugation and sedimentation process and
flattened out.   I suspect that the microvilli are lying flat
instead of sticking up.   We would like to do what you suggest;
that is to cut across the appropriate part and look inside, but
we have not done that.   As for the openings you mentioned, we

have not seen any signs of these;  or putting it another way, we cannot distinguish an opening from a disruption.

Erlinger:   As far as we know the main driving forces for bile formation are derived from chemical rather than mechanical energy. On this basis, one doubts whether simple dilatation of canaliculi could explain the reduction in bile flow.   Has cytochalasin any effects on other processes within the cell which might explain the effect on bile flow?

Phillips:   I would like to answer this question by using the analogy of the heart and the blood capillaries and blood pressure. There is more than one thing involved in maintaining blood pressure and blood flow.   One is the contractile force and pumping of the heart, and the other is the maintenance of the peripheral circulation.   I visualise that in the canaliculus you need both mechanical and chemical energy.   It is not a question of just one or the other.   Presumably the excretion of solutes is the active part resulting in bile flow, but I still think you have to have structural elements through which you can get normal flow.

# BILE DUCT FUNCTION IN BILIARY SECRETION

J. CHENDEROVITCH

Unité de Recherches d'Hépatologie - I.N.S.E.R.M. U-9

184, rue du Faubourg St-Antoine - 75012 PARIS - France

For a long time the only site of bile secretion was located at the canalicular level and all the proposed mechanisms were devoted to the activity of the hepatocytes. Bile salts, whose choleretic power had been recognized since the observations of Schiff (22), were known to be the only physiological agent of the hepatic secretion. During this period, when the physiology of bile secretion was restrained to the measurement of the bile flow and of the concentrations of different substances secreted with or into the bile, no other mechanisms were suggested. New methods, mainly derived from those used in renal physiology, allowed a more precise analysis of the mechanisms and of the anatomic sites of the biliary secretion.

Estimation of the canalicular bile flow, calculated by the biliary clearance of lipid insoluble substances such as mannitol or erythritol led to recognize that the bile secreted by hepatocytes into the canaliculi was formed by two fractions : 1) a fraction tightly correlated to the bile salt secretion, the output of water and major electrolytes being directly proportional to the bile salt excretion rate ; that is the canalicular bile salt dependent fraction. The usually proposed mechanism for the secretion of this fraction is that the active secretion of bile salts into the canalicular lumen creates an osmotic gradient which provides an osmotic driving force for water towards the lumen (24) ; 2) a fraction secreted independently of the bile salt secretion, persisting even when bile salt excretion is minimal or absent ; that is the canalicular bile salt independent fraction. The mechanism of secretion of this fraction is unknown ; the role of the active sodium secretion mediated by the sodium-potassium-dependent adenosine triphosphatase was postulated (10) but discrepancies in the results of different experiments do not allow definite conclusions. Besides hepatic cells and canaliculi, the share of bile ducts and ductules in the adjustment of bile composition was progressively suspected.


## ABSORPTION

Absorption by bile ducts was suggested in different circumstances. In cholecystectomized, fasting dogs, the bile stored in the common bile duct and withdrawn at the beginning of the canulation was similar in composition to the concentrated canine gall bladder bile (28) ; likewise, in cholecystectomized dogs, mannitol clearance, which was shown to be a reasonable estimate of canalicular flow, was significantly higher than bile flow, indicating a water reabsorption at a locus of the biliary tree distal to the canaliculi (30). It is not known whether these absorption processes are artefacts due to the cholecystectomy. The same observations were made in functionnally cholecystectomized rhesus monkey (25). In the rabbit, erythritol clearance was found to be higher than the bile flow, suggesting also water reabsorption in the biliary tree (10). This function was not found in all species. In the rat, erythritol clearance is usually identical to the bile flow, when measured in vivo (3) or in isolated perfused liver (4), and bile to plasma concentration ratio of mannitol was only occasionnally above unity (21). In the guinea pig, mannitol and even erythritol clearances were significantly lower than bile flow (11) ; this may be due either to a secretion at the ductal level or to a restricted diffusion of these compounds through the liver cells ; in man, the same fact was observed (18).


## SECRETION

A secretory function of the bile ducts was also demonstrated and a third fraction, the ductular and/or ductal bile salt independent fraction was added to the two previous canalicular fractions.


### Secretin Stimulated Secretion

The first direct demonstration of a secretory activity of the ducts was brought by the use of the hormone secretin. The choleretic activity of secretin was known since its discovery in 1902 by Bayliss and Starling (2) and this activity was demonstrated in many species including man (14), pig (15), dog (19), cat (23), guinea pig (11) and rhesus monkey (25) ; rabbit and rat appear to be insensitive to secretin stimulation so far as bile secretion is concerned (9, 12, 23). It has been shown that the

choleretic effect of secretin results in the addition of an
aqueous solution of inorganic electrolytes, specially chloride
and bicarbonate, to the basal bile flow without modifying bile
salt excretion (19). It was then suggested that the site of
secretion of this electrolyte bile salt independent fraction
was probably the ductal and/or ductular systems and not the
hepatocytes. This view was supported by the following experiments :

1) When secretin was infused, in the dog, into the hepatic
artery, which provides the main blood supply to the bile ducts,
the increment in bile flow was greater than during splenic venous
infusion (29).

2) During constant rate infusions of sulphobromophthalein,
the biliary "wash out volume" was less during secretin than
during taurocholate induced choleresis ; the proposed explanation
was that secretin must have increased in the bile flow by a net
addition of fluid at a locus distal to the point at which fluid
is secreted during taurocholate choleresis (29).

3) Sulphobromophthalein transport maximum was not modified
by secretin infusion, while it was increased during taurocholate
infusion (17).

4) And principally, canalicular bile flow estimated by the
clearance of erythritol or mannitol, compounds which are neither secreted nor reabsorbed by the ductules or ducts, was increased by bile salt induced choleresis and was not modified
when bile flow was increased by secretin infusion (11, 30).

All these experiments were consistent with the hypothesis
that the bile ducts or ductules must be the site of action of
secretin.

## Secretion Without Secretin Stimulation

In the absence of injected secretin stimulation a secretory function of the bile  ducts was not accurately  known,
though a secretion was suggested by  different lines of
evidence :

1) In man, a marked hydrocholeresis was noted in congenital
cystic dilatations of intra hepatic bile ducts (Caroli's disease)
(26).

2) The high rate of bile flow which was described in cirrhosis of the liver might also be related to the secretion of
an additional fluid by the proliferated  bile ductules (5, 27).

3) Chronic intoxication of rats with ethionine or alpha-naphtylisothiocyanate results in a hydrocholeresis and simultaneously was observed a proliferation of bile ductules (13) ; an increased capacity of the biliary tree was also observed in ethionine intoxication (1).

4) Rous and McMaster have shown that isolated canine bile duct can secrete a clear alkaline fluid (20).

During last years we have studied the secretory function of bile ducts without secretin stimulation by different methods. The rabbit was chosen for these experiments because of the great dimension of its extra hepatic bile ducts, which allows easy operations upon these bile segments ; moreover this species is not sensitive to secretin stimulation and thus, it was possible to study bile ducts functions in the absence of secretin influence. It must be outlined that most of these experiments have been carried out on extra hepatic bile ducts, assuming that the functions might be identical in the intra hepatic and the extra hepatic segments. It has been shown that these two segments have the same ultrastructural components : microvilli spread over the luminal side, basement membrane on the serosal side and more or less enlarged intercellular spaces filled with microvilli, all feathers usually related to transport of fluid and solutes.

## STOP FLOW ANALYSIS

The first method we have used was the Stop Flow Analysis derived from the method proposed for renal physiology.

Male rabbits were anesthetized with intravenous sodium pentobarbital ; the cystic duct and all the accessory bile ducts along the common duct were tied ; thus it was possible to isolate a single biliary channel without close relationship with hepatic cells all along its course. A catheter was inserted into the end of the common duct and stop flow analysis was performed in the following manner : after free flow control samples were collected, the catheter was clamped for 15 minutes ; then the clamp was opened and 50 serial samples (3 drops each) were collected ; the volume of each sample was measured by weighing along with the concentration of test substances ; the modifications of the concentration were usually expressed as the ratio of concentration in post-occlusive sample to concentration in control sample and plotted against post-occlusive serial samples.

The whole bile tract may be considered as composed of two segments : a proximal segment including the bile canaliculi surrounded by hepatocytes and a distal segment formed by the intra-hepatic bile ductules and ducts and the extra hepatic ducts, all

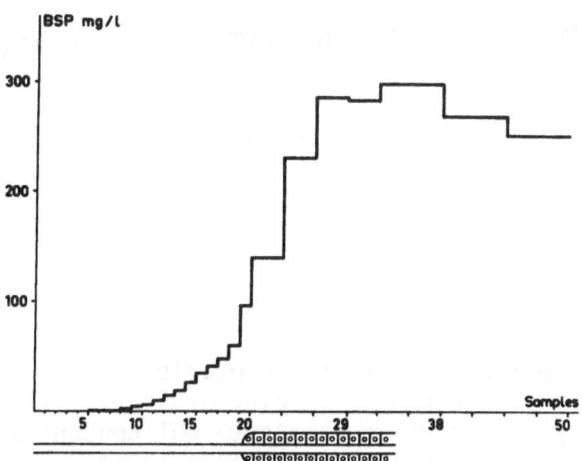

Figure 1. Stop flow pattern for BSP. Occlusion period :
15 min. BSP 15 mg/kg given iv 5 min before clamp release. The
schematic drawing at lower part of the figure indicates that the
calculated distal segment spreads from sample 1 to sample 20.
(Reproduced  from Am. J. Physiol. 214 : 86-93, 1968).


surrounded by biliary cells. In order to distinguish these two
segments, sulphobromophthalein was injected intravenously at the
10th minute of the occlusion period. It was assumed that the dye,
secreted into the proximal segment during the last 5 minutes of
the occlusion period, forms a flat wave front down the bile ducts
when the bile flow resumes ; thus, the volume of the dye-free bile
pushed out ahead of the dye-stained bile will be equal to the
volume accumulated in the distal segment. It must be assumed also
that the dye does not diffuse down the bile channels during occlusion and that the bile secretion is completely stopped during
this period, what is not strictly exact as it has been verified
during this study ; but if the experiments are carried out in
standardized conditions, the results are constantly reproducible.

    Figure 1 shows a typical stop flow pattern for sulphobromoph-
thalein excretion : the first appearance of the dye was usually
noted in the 5th or 7th sample ; then the concentration rises progressively in a S-shaped curve, till a maximum which was always
reached at the 30th sample. It is easy to calculate the biliary
volume accumulated before the dye-stained front ; it is proportional to the surface limited by the curve, the ordinate and a
line parallel to the abscissa drawn through the maximum of the
curve. When calculated by this method, the dye-free biliary volume corresponding to the distal segment plus a small instrumen-
tal dead space, was represented by the first 20 samples.

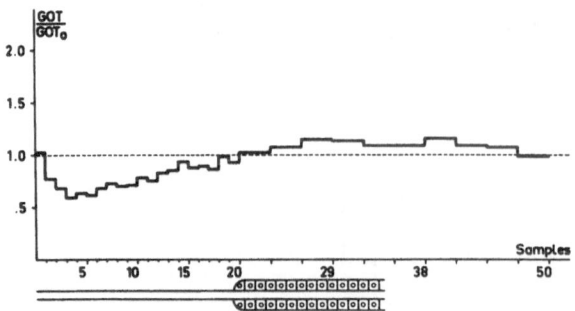

Figure 2. Stop flow pattern for glutamic oxalacetic transaminase (GOT). Occlusion period : 15 min. Ordinate : ratio of GOT concentration in post-occlusive sample to GOT concentration in free flow pre-occlusive sample. Dotted line indicates the 1.0 ratio. Each value is mean of 6 experiments.  (Reproduced from Am. J. Physiol. 214 : 86-93, 1968).


Water movements across bile ducts walls were detected by modifications of the concentration of a non-diffusing solute ; glutamic oxalacetic transaminase was chosen because it fits two necessary conditions : 1) it is secreted in the proximal segment by hepatocytes and a constant rate of secretion may be assumed for the short period of the experiment ; 2) bile ducts walls are impermeable to the transaminase. This was verified by perfusing, in vivo, a known amount of bile containing transaminases through the lumen of an isolated common bile duct segment ; the recovery of transaminases after perfusion was $100.3 \pm 3.7$ per cent.

Figure 2 shows the stop flow pattern for the variations of glutamic oxalacetic transaminase concentration. The ratio of the concentration in post occlusive samples to the concentration in free flow control sample falls rapidly under value 1.00, reaches the value 0.60 and remains below unity during the first 20 samples, that is in the distal segment of the biliary channels. This imply that, in the distal segment, there is, during the stop flow period, a secretion of water towards the lumen. The mean calculated volume of distal fluid before occlusion (6 experiments) was $1,127.71 \pm 35.71 \, \mu l$, and the mean value of the volume of water added during the stop flow period was $287.38 \pm 43.70 \, \mu l$ that is about 25 per cent of the volume of the distal segment.

Figure 3 shows that during stop flow the concentration of the major electrolytes, sodium, potassium and chloride are practically unchanged all along the bile channel ; the slight changes in distal chloride concentration and potassium proximal concentration are not significant ; the increase of potassium concen-

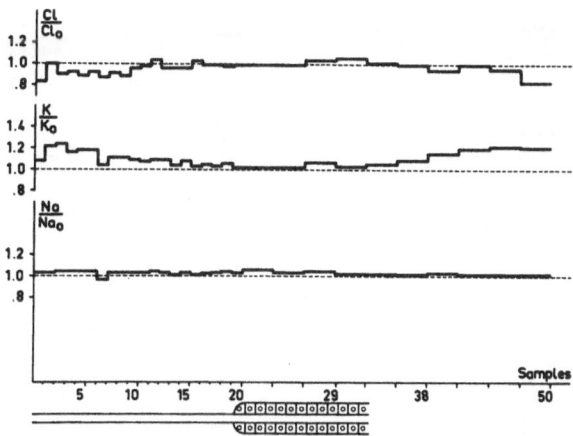

Figure 3. Stop flow pattern for sodium, potassium and chloride. Occlusion period : 15 min. Ordinate : ratios of concentration in post-occlusive sample to concentration in free-flow pre-occlusive sample. Dotted lines indicate the 1.0 ratios (Reproduced from Am. J. Physiol. 214 : 86-93, 1968).

tration in the very first samples has found no explanation. The movements of electrolytes may be considered as correlated to the movements of water. Sodium, potassium and chloride are transported towards the lumen along with water so that the electrolyte composition of the transported solution is close to that of canalicular bile.

Besides this secretion of an electrolyte solution added to the basal bile, bile ducts might have other secretory activities as it is suggested by stop flow analysis of biliary alkaline phosphatase. Figure 4 shows a typical pattern for one of these experiments. Here the ordinate represents the ratio of variations of alkaline phosphatase concentration to variations of transaminase concentration, that is the net transport of alkaline phosphatase after correction for water movements. This ratio begin to rise from the third sample on and reaches a somewhat steady state at the 10th sample ; this might suggest that the alkaline phosphatase is introduced into bile during bile duct occlusion not only at the proximal segment by hepatic cells but also at the distal segment by the biliary cells of bile duct epithelium. The amount of alkaline phosphatase present in the bile channels at the end of the stop flow period (1,678 King-Armstrong Units) is significantly greater than the amount present in the calculated volume of the equivalent bile channel during free flow (508 King-Armstrong Units) ; thus the secretion rate of alkaline phosphatase is increased by hepatic and biliary cells during bile ducts occlusion.

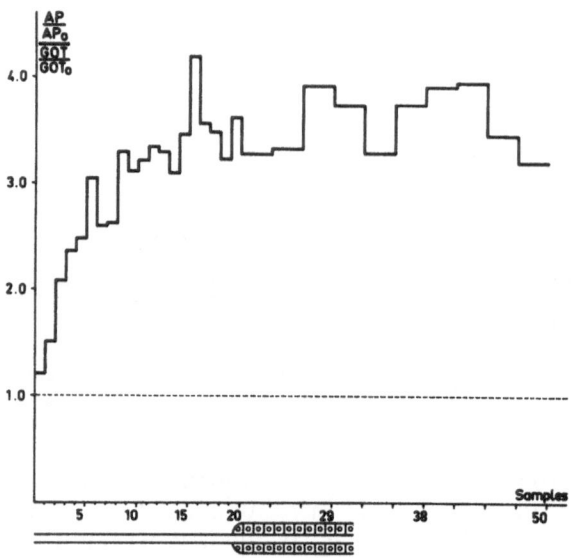

Figure 4. Stop flow pattern for alkaline phosphatase (AP).
Occlusion period : 15 min. Ordinate : ratio of (the ratio of AP
concentration in post-occlusive sample to AP concentration in
free-flow pre-occlusive sample)to (the ratio of GOT concentration in post-occlusive sample to GOT concentration in free-flow
pre-occlusive sample). AP and GOT concentrations measured in the
same sample. Dotted line indicates the 1.0 ratio.  (Reproduced
from Am. J. Physiol. 214 : 86-93, 1968).

## IN VIVO BILE DUCTS PERFUSION

The secretion of an electrolyte solution by the bile ducts,
demonstrated by the stop flow technic, was also verified by in
vivo experiments, using perfusions through the lumen of the common bile duct.

Common bile ducts of rabbits were prepared in the same fashion as in the stop flow experiments but, in addition, the main
right hepatic branch of the bile ducts was tied and a catheter
was inserted downwards into the left hepatic branch. Thus was
obtained an isolated bile channel whose blood supply was carefully
preserved and it was possible to perfuse different solutions
through the lumen of this channel and to study the changes observed in the solutions after perfusion. Three different solutions
were studied : one standard Krebs-Henseleit bicarbonate buffer and

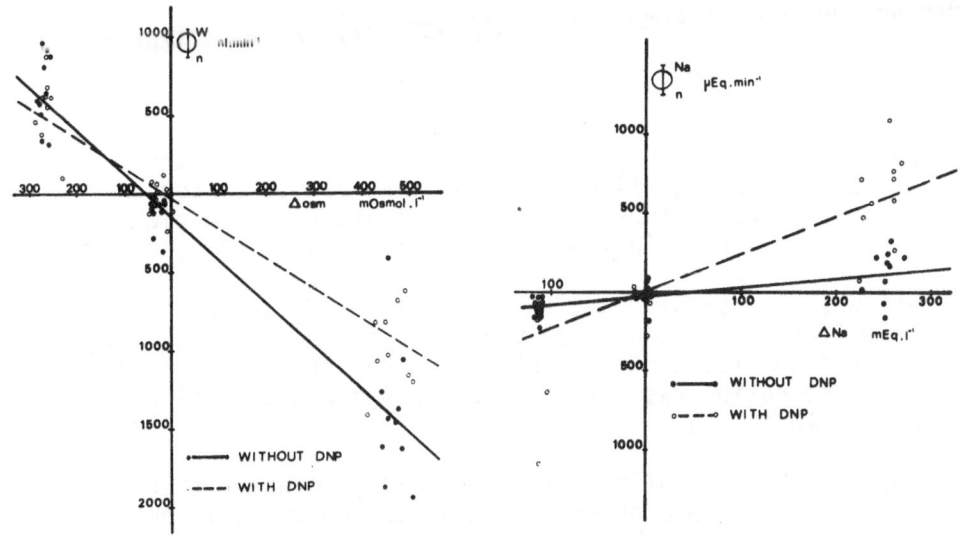

Figure 5. In vivo perfusion of common bile duct without and with 2-4-dinitrophenol (DNP). Left : effect of osmolality gradient on net waterflux across bile duct walls ; the equations of the regression lines are respectively, without DNP : $\Phi_n^W$ (µl/min) = - 0.139 - 2.68 $\Delta$mOsM and with DNP : $\Phi$ (µl/min) = - 0.024 - 1.92 $\Delta$mOsM. Right : effect of sodium concentration gradient on net sodium flux across bile duct walls ; the equations of the regression lines are respectively, without DNP : $\Phi$(µEq/min) = - 0.026 + 0.58 $\Delta$mEq and with DNP :$\Phi$(µ Eq/min) = - 0.011 + 2.42 $\Delta$mEq.

two Krebs-Henseleit solutions modified so that one solution had a low sodium concentration (24.8 mEq/liter) and a low osmolality (70.9 mOsM) and the other a high sodium concentration (401.7 mEq/liter) and a high osmolality (771.9 mOsM). In the same animal, 2 or 3 different solutions were perfused at random and were followed by the perfusion of the same solutions to which was added 2-4 dinitrophenol (3 mM). The perfusions were accomplished by gravity from an inlet weighed vial to an outlet weighed empty vial. The volume of fluid introduced into the bile duct and collected after perfusion were accurately measured and their difference indicated net water movement. The measure of sodium concentrations in the two vials allowed the calculation of net sodium movement.

Figure 5 (left side) shows net water fluxes plotted againts the osmotic gradient, that is solution osmolality minus plasma osmolality, for the 3 solutions. Water fluxes have a linear relationship with the osmotic gradient and the intercept with the ordinate was significantly negative. This indicates that when

there was no osmotic gradient, a secretion of water occured
towards the lumen at a rate of 139 nl/min ;it was inhibited by
addition of dinitrophenol ; the secretion towards the lumen was
effective against an osmotic gradient up to 50 mOsM.

Figure 5 (right side) shows sodium net fluxes plotted
against sodium concentration gradient, that is sodium concentration in the lumen minus sodium concentration in the plasma
of the animal. Here again the fluxes were linearly correlated
to sodium concentration gradient and the intercept with the
ordinate was also significantly negative. In conditions of
ionic equilibrium between lumen and blood there was a net sodium
flux towards the lumen of 25.5 nEq/min, inhibited by dinitrophenol.
The sodium secretion was effective against a concentration
gradient up to 44 mEq.

Thus, in absence of osmotic and ionic gradients, there is a
secretion of water towards the lumen of the common bile duct of
the rabbit, together with a secretion of sodium in the same direction. The inhibition of these transports by dinitrophenol and
the persistence of the secretions against osmotic and ionic gradients suggested some active mechanisms.


### IN VITRO BILE DUCT PERFUSION

A more precise study of these mechanisms was made by a  in
vitro perfusion technic of isolated common bile ducts of rabbits
which allowed a better apprehension of the different parameters.

The experiments were performed by means of a perfusion apparatus composed of a rectangular Lucite chamber containing about
20 ml of the serosal solution and a mucosal perfusing circuit to
which was connected an isolated bile duct, rapidly excised from
a rabbit, containing about 5 ml of the mucosal solution. The circulation and oxygenation of these solutions were accomplished by
the introduction of gas, usually 5 % $CO_2$- 95 % $O_2$. Agar bridges
connected by way of saturated KCl solutions and calomel cells to
a voltmeter were placed into the two bathing solutions in order
to measure transmembrane potentials.

Net movement of water across the bile duct wall was measured
by the variations of $^{14}C$-inuline concentration introduced into
the mucosal solution. Net movements of sodium, potassium, chloride and bicarbonate were calculated from their concentrations
in the mucosal compartment. Unidirectional fluxes of sodium were
estimated by the use of $^{22}Na$. The solutions were usually Krebs-
Henseleit bicarbonate buffer, modified when necessary.

When the two sides of the common bile duct were bathed with

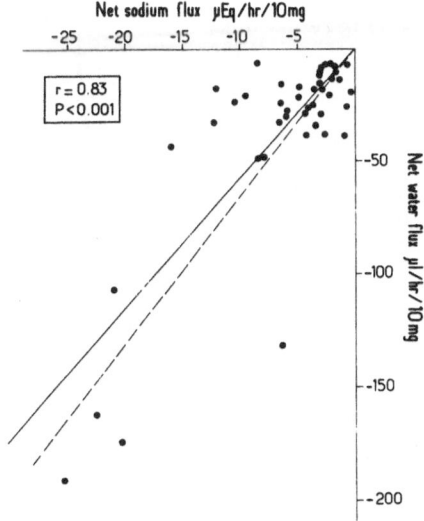

Figure 6. In vitro perfusion of common bile duct. Relation-ship between net water flux and net sodium flux. Equation of the regression line : $\phi$w($\mu$l/hr/10 mg dry wt) = + 0.53 + 5.77 $\phi$Na ($\mu$Eq/hr/10 mg dry wt). Dashed line is that for a transported so-lution of 154 mEq/liter sodium. (Reproduced from Am. J. Physiol. 223 : 695-706, 1972).

identical Krebs-Henseleit solutions there was a net movement of water from serosa to mucosa of 37.71 ± 6.54 (SE) $\mu$l/hr per 10 mg dry weight. Along with water, electrolytes were transported to-wards the same direction, respectively  sodium : 6.628 ± 0.929 (SE), potassium : 1.115 ± 0.364 (SE), chloride : 6.422 ± 1.092 (SE), bicarbonate : 4.186 ± 0.514 (SE) $\mu$ Eq/hr per 10 mg dry weight. A potential difference of 5.59 ± 0.42 (SE) mV, mucosa always nega-tive,was registered.

When osmolality of the serosal bath was progressively in-creased by the addition of sucrose, the net serosal to mucosal water flux decreased as the osmotic gradient increased and fi-nally was reversed when the osmotic gradient was above 50 mOsM. The common bile duct was able to transport water towards the lu-men against an osmotic gradient up to 50 mOsM.

When 2-4 dinitrophenol (3 mM) was added to the serosal or the mucosal bath, the net fluxes of water, sodium and chloride were inhibited and the potential difference fell to zero. The same inhibition was observed when ouabain (3 mM) was added to the serosal bath.

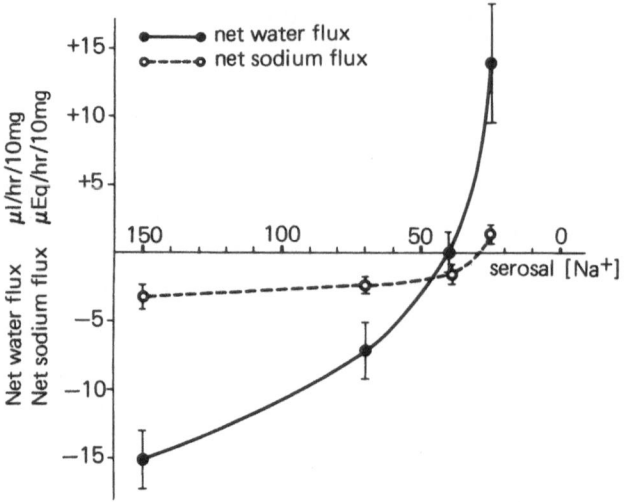

Figure 7. In vitro perfusion of common bile duct. Net water and sodium fluxes as functions of serosal sodium concentration, mucosal concentration being always 150 mEq/liter sodium (Krebs-Henseleit bicarbonate buffer). Bars are means ± SE. (Reproduced from Am. J. Physiol. 223 : 695-706, 1972).

When net water flux was plotted against net sodium flux (Figure 6), there was a linear relationship between the two fluxes and there was no water transport when there was no sodium transport. The regression coefficient of the regression line, 5.77, is slightly lower than the 6.49 value predicted if an isotonic solution of 154 mM sodium chloride was crossing the bile duct wall, indicating that the transported solution was slightly hypertonic and thus that solute transport must be the primary event.

The linkage of water transport to solute transport was also evident when the serosal sodium was progressively replaced with sucrose, thus creating a progressively increasing sodium concentration gradient across the bile duct wall (Figure 7). When this gradient increased, water flux was reduced until the sodium serosal concentration reached the level of 40 mEq/liter ; at this point there was no more net water flux. The sodium transport was also from serosa to mucosa until the same concentration and water and sodium movements were always simultaneously in the same direction. All this points to the fact that water transport is probably passive and secondary to solute transport. The bile duct epithelium was able to transport water and sodium from serosa to mucosa against a concentration gradient up to 100 mEq, suggesting an active transport. But it must be noted that the mucosal potential being negative with respect to the serosal potential, sodium transport occured in a "downhill" direction as far as electrical forces were concerned.

The observed ratio of unidirectional sodium influx to sodium outflux ($0.4637 \pm 0.0686$ SE) was significantly lower than the calculated ratio ($0.8097 \pm 0.0154$ SE) if the ions are supposed to cross the membrane independently and under the influence of concentration gradient and electrical potential only. As there was a net water flux in the same direction, the effect of solvent drag on the difference between observed and calculated flux ratios must be ruled out ; when water flux was near zero or even reversed by addition of 50 mM sucrose to the serosal bath the observed ratio ($0.4000 \pm 0.1121$ SE) was unchanged and always significantly lower than the calculated ratio ($0.9221 \pm 0.1069$ SE). Moreover, when dinitrophenol or ouabain were added to the bathing solutions, the observed flux ratios ( respectively $1.0653 \pm 0.0640$ SE and $0.9055 \pm 0.1134$ SE) became equal to the flux ratios predicted for passive diffusion (respectively $1.0133 \pm 0.0573$ SE and $0.9238 \pm 0.0153$ SE). All these facts provide strong evidence for active sodium transport.

Chloride movements were always effective against an electrochemical potential, even when water flux was reversed by addition of sucrose to serosal bath ; dinitrophenol and ouabain inhibited chloride transport ; so, it may be thought that chloride, as sodium, is transported by an active energy requiring process. An interdependence between active sodium and chloride transports was observed : when all sodium was omitted from the bathing solutions, sodium chloride being replaced with choline chloride and sodium bicarbonate with potassium bicarbonate, there was no water transport and the same inhibition of water transport together with inhibition of sodium transport were observed when chloride was omitted and replaced with equivalent amounts of sulphate salts, plus sufficient sucrose to maintain osmolality. In both groups of experiments, potential differences were only slightly reduced.

Potassium was transported towards lumen, that is down the electrochemical potential, with a magnitude independent of experimental conditions, even in presence of dinitrophenol or ouabain, suggesting that potassium transport is passive, secondary to electrochemical forces.

The net movement of bicarbonate was always from serosa to mucosa, that is against an electrochemical potential, even when water flux was reversed by osmotic forces, ruling out a dominant influcence of solvent drag. It was inhibited by acetazolamide but not by dinitrophenol or ouabain. Moreover when bicarbonate was omitted from bathing solutions, the observed potential difference fell to zero. These features are consistent with the hypothesis that bicarbonate transport is mediated by some active ion transport process. The exact mechanism of this transport is not clear ; in our experiments acetazolamide inhibited not only bicarbonate transport but also the transport of other ions, potassium excepted ; it must be recalled also that there is no carbonic anhydrase in extra hepatic bile ducts epithelium. Different possibilities may be considered : acetazolamide may inhibit the secretory activity of the bile duct by an effect on another enzyme than carbonic anhydrase ; bicarbonate may be secreted by a mechanism independent of carbonic anhydrase, possibly the uncatalyzed hydration reaction ; bicarbonate transport may be linked, in some manner to the transport of other ions. It must be noted also that the active transport of bicarbonate ions cannot be distinguished from the transport of hydrogen ions in the opposite direction.

When the two sides of the bile duct were bathed with the same Krebs-Henseleit bicarbonate buffer, solute and solvent transport was associated with a potential difference about 6 mV the mucosa being always negative with respect to the serosa. In most of the epithelial membranes, except in the gall bladder, active sodium transport is associated with the production of potential differences and the side towards which sodium is transported becomes positively charged. In the bile ducts the situation is different since the same side, that is the mucosal side, becomes negative.

Different transmural potential differences in the isolated bile duct may result from experimental conditions (Figure 8). Streaming potentials were observed when both sides of the bile duct were bathed with identical Krebs-Henseleit bicarbonate solutions and one of the solutions, mucosal or serosal, was made hyperosmotic to the other by addition of sucrose ; the side towards which the water was osmotically transported, the side made hypertonic, becomes more and more positive as the osmotic gradient increased, indicating that the fixed charges of the membrane matrix must be negative ; these streaming potentials were added to, or substracted from, the basal potential observed in equilibrium conditions. Diffusion potentials were observed when, the osmolality of the two bathing solutions being kept constant, an ionic gradient was established across the membrane. Using pure NaCl or KCl solutions instead of Krebs-Henseleit bicarbonate solutions and so having no basal potential in absence of bicarbonate ions, when the ionic concentration of the mucosal solution was progressively decreased, the mucosal potential became increasingly positive and the potential difference was proportional to the logarithm of serosal to mucosal ionic concentration. These diffusion potentials have allowed the calculation of relative permeability coefficient for

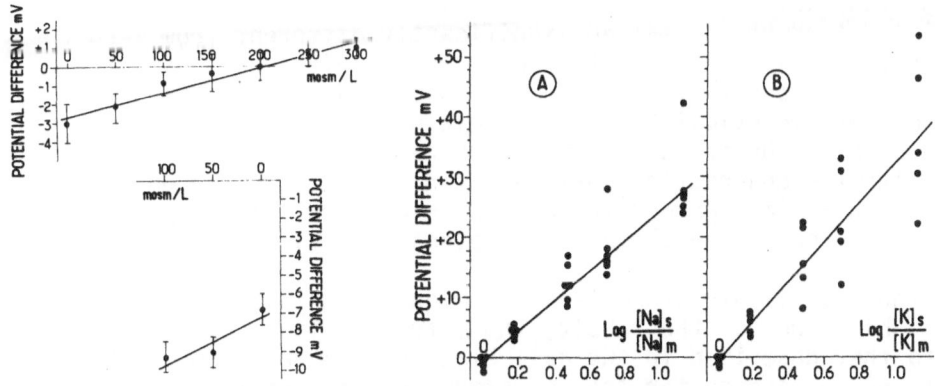

Figure 8. In vitro perfusion of common bile duct. Left : streaming potentials ; potential difference as a function of osmotic gradient ; upper graph, sucrose added to mucosal bath ; lower graph, sucrose added to serosal bath. Bars are means ± SE. Right : diffusion potentials ; potential difference as a function of ionic concentration gradient ; serosal bath is 150 mM NaCl (in A) or 150 mM KCl (in B) ;in mucosal bathes the electrolyte is progressively replaced with isoosmotic amounts of sucrose ; the regression coefficients are respectively 25.0 for NaCl and 32.2 for KCl ; the difference is highly significant. (Reproduced from Am.J. Physiol. 223 : 695-706, 1972).

the univalent ions by means of the Goldman-Hodgkin-Katz equation. Sodium permeability being taken arbitrarily as 1.00, it was found that the permeability coefficients have the following average values : potassium 1.56, chloride 0.33, bicarbonate 0.33 and taurocholate 0.00.

When complete Krebs-Henseleit bicarbonate solution was introduced on mucosal side and the same solution but with varied NaCl concentrations on serosal side, the transmembrane ionic activity gradients resulted in the production of potential differences. If they were related only to diffusion potentials, the Hodgkin-Katz equation should predict the magnitude of these potentials ; but for all tested solutions the observed potential differences were always higher than those predicted, using the permeability coefficient previously estimated. Diffusion potentials appear to be added to a basic potential of other origin. The observed potential differences seems to be related to an active process since they fell to zero by the effect of dinitrophenol while all transports are inhibited. If bicarbonate ions were removed from the solutions, the potential difference fell also to zero while NaCl and water transport were only slightly reduced ;

on the contrary, when sodium or chloride were omitted, the potential differences remained significantly different from zero
though the ionic and water transport were inhibited. Thus, it
appears that the potential difference observed when the two solutions were identical Krebs-Henseleit bicarbonate buffer may
be related to the transport of bicarbonate ions. This is consistent with the observation that secretin activity in the dog
results in a simultaneous increase of bicarbonate biliary output
and in bile duct mucosal negative potential (16).

The experiments presented here might suggest that, in the
common bile duct of the rabbit, the situation is somewhat similar to that described in the gall bladder, and we  propose the
following mechanisms for the secretory function of the bile duct :

1) In absence of injected secretin stimulation, there is a
water transport towards the lumen following the active transport of solutes.

2) Sodium and chloride active transport involves a coupled
cation-anion pump, electrically neutral which develops no potential difference across the bile duct wall.

3) To this transport is added an active bicarbonate transport which is related to the development of the negative mucosal
potential.

## REFERENCES

1) BARBEY-RILEY G. Biliary capacity in rats following ethionine
   ingestion. Am. J. Physiol. 214 : 133-138, 1968
2) BAYLISS WM, STARLING EH. The mechanism of pancreatic secretion.
   J. Physiol. (London). 28 : 325-335, 1902
3) BERTHELOT P, ERLINGER S, DHUMEAUX D, PREAUX AM.  Mechanism of
   phenobarbital-induced hypercholeresis in the rat. Am. J.
   Physiol. 219 : 809-813, 1970
4) BOYER JL.  Canalicular bile formation in the isolated perfused
   rat liver.  Am. J. Physiol. 221 : 1156-1163, 1971
5) CAROLI J, TANASOGLU Y.  Le temps d'apparition de la brome sul-
   fone phtaléine dans la bile. Nouveau test pour le diagnostic
   des ictères incomplets par rétention et les blocages anicté-
   riques. Sem. Hop. (Paris). 29 : 591-606, 1953
6) CHENDEROVITCH J. Stop flow analysis of bile secretion.
   Am. J. Physiol. 214 : 86-93, 1968
7) CHENDEROVITCH J. Transport d'eau et d'électrolytes dans le
   cholédoque de lapin "in vivo". Rev. Eur. Etudes Clin. Biol.
   16 : 591-595, 1971

8) CHENDEROVITCH J. Secretory function of the rabbit common bile duct. Am.J. Physiol. 223 : 695-706, 1972

9) DEBRAY Ch, VAILLE Ch, de la TOUR J, ROZE C, SOUCHARD M. Action des sécrétines du commerce sur la sécrétion pancréatique externe du rat. J. Physiol. (Paris). 54 : 549-577, 1962

10) ERLINGER S, DHUMEAUX D, BERTHELOT P, DUMONT M. Effect of inhibitors of sodium transport on bile formation in the rabbit. Am. J. Physiol. 219 : 416-422, 1970

11) FORKER EL. Two sites of bile formation as determined by mannitol and erythritol clearance in the guinea pig. J. Clin. Invest. 46 : 1189-1195, 1967

12) FORKER EL, HICKLIN T, SORNSON H. The clearance of mannitol and erythritol in rat bile. Proc. Soc. Exp. Biol. Med. 126 : 115-119, 1967

13) GOLDFARB S, SINGER EJ, POPPER H. Biliary ductules and bile secretion. J. Lab. Clin . Med. 62 : 608-615, 1963

14) GROSSMAN MI, JANOWITZ HD, RALSTON H, KIM KS. The effect of secretin on bile formation in man. Gastroenterology 12 : 133-138, 1949

15) HARDISON WG, NORMAL JC. Effect of bile salt and secretin upon bile flow from the isolated perfused pig liver. Gastroenterology 53 : 412-417, 1967

16) LONDON CD, DIAMOND JM, BROOKS FP. Electrical potential differences in the biliary tree. Biochem. Biophys. Acta 150 : 509-517, 1968

17) O'MAILLE ERC, RICHARDS TG, SHORT AH. Factors determining the maximal rate of organic anion secretion by the liver and further evidence on the hepatic site of action of the hormone secretin. J. Physiol. (London). 186 : 424-438, 1966

18) PRANDI D, ERLINGER S, GLASINOVIC JC, DUMONT M. Canalicular bile production in man. Europ. J. Clin. Invest. 5 : 1-6, 1975

19) PREISIG R, COOPER HL, WHEELER HO. The relationship between taurocholate secretion rate and bile production in the unanesthetized dog during cholinergic blockade and during secretin administration. J. Clin. Invest. 41 : 1152-1162, 1962

20) ROUS P, McMASTER PD. Physiological causes for the varied character of stasis bile. J. Exp. Med. 34 : 75-96, 1921

21) SCHANKER LS, HOGBEN CAM. Biliary excretion of inulin, sucrose and mannitol : analysis of bile formation. Am. J. Physiol. 200 : 1087-1090, 1961

22) SCHIFF M. Gallenbildung, abhängig von des Aufsaugung der Gallenstoffe. Archiv für die gesamte Physiologie des Menschen und der Thiere. 3 : 598-613, 1870.

23) SCRATCHERD T. Electrolyte composition and control of biliary secretion in the cat and rabbit. The Biliary System. Edited by W. Taylor, Oxford Blackwell, p. 515-529, 1965

24) SPERBER I. Secretion of organic anions in the formation of urine and bile. Pharmacol. Rev. 11 : 109-134, 1959

25) STRASBERG SM, ILSON RG, SIMIONOVITCH KA, BREMER D, PALAHEIMO JE. Analysis of the components of bile flow in the rhesus

monkey.  Am. J. Physiol. 228 : 115-121, 1975
26)TURNBERG LA, JONES CA, SHERLOCK S.  Biliary secretion in a
   patient with cystic dilatation of the intra hepatic biliary
   tree. Gastroenterology 54 : 1155-1161, 1968
27)TURNBERG LA, GRAHAM G. Bile salt secretion in cirrhosis of
   the liver.  Gut 11 : 126-133, 1970
28)WHEELER HO, RAMOS OL.  Determinants of flow and composition
   of bile in the unanesthetized dog during constant infusion
   of sodium taurocholate. J. Clin. Invest. 39 : 161-170, 1960
29)WHEELER HO, MANCUSI-UNGARO PL. Role of bile ducts during
   secretin choleresis in the dog. Am. J. Physiol. 210 : 1153-1159,
   1966
30)WHEELER HO, ROSS ED, BRADLEY SE.  Canalicular bile production
   in dog. Am.J. Physiol. 214 : 866-874, 1968

DISCUSSION OF LECTURE OF J. CHENDEROVITCH

Taylor:   Have you any explanation for the ability of the rabbit to produce such a copious flow of bile?

Chenderovitch:   No, I cannot explain this only on the basis of the properties of the bile duct.

Brooks:   In the dog at least there is good evidence that response to a meal involves a bile acid independent secretion. Does this come from the ducts or from the canaliculi?

Chenderovitch:   I simply do not know.

Boyer:   When you perfused the ducts _in situ_ did you look to see if the addition of the substances which we traditionally use as markers for canalicular flow, such as mannitol and erythritol, can cross into the lumen of the perfused segment?

Chenderovitch:   I have not tried those substances you mention. By the stop-flow technique I studied the pattern of B.S.P. simultaneously with erythritol, and the pattern was exactly the same.   So it seems that erythritol does not cross bile ducts.

Boyer:   It would be interesting if you were to try it, because we make a lot of assumptions based on erythritol and mannitol clearances.   We have done a few experiments in the rat, and we did find that small amounts of erythritol did cross the bile ducts.

Erlinger:   You mentioned a contradiction between some _in vivo_ experiments supporting the view that there was some reabsorption in the rabbit bile ducts, whereas in the _in vitro_ experiments there was secretion.   Since you have studied segments of common bile duct, have you any morphological or physiological evidence that the distal common bile ducts might have a different function from the proximal intrahepatic bile ducts?

Chenderovitch:   No, there do not seem to be such differences. The ultrastructure of the proximal and distal ducts is the same.

# KINETICS OF HEPATIC UPTAKE AND EXCRETION OF ORGANIC ANIONS

Gustav Paumgartner and Jürg Reichen

Department of Clinical Pharmacology, University

of Berne, Berne, Switzerland

The handling of many organic anions by the liver involves at least three steps, namely hepatic uptake, intracellular transport and biliary excretion. In addition, conjugation and/or other metabolic alterations may occur prior to excretion. Overall hepatic transport from the blood into the bile of a variety of organic anions has been studied in some detail. It has been demonstrated that the overall transport of anionic dyes such as sulfobromophthalein (BSP) (12,25), indocyanine green (ICG)(15) and bilirubin (20,23) as well as of bile acids (10,14,16,22,24) is a saturable process that may be characterized by an excretory transport maximum. Information on the mechanisms responsible for hepatic uptake of organic anions and their relation to overall hepatic transport, however, is still incomplete. Studies of hepatic BSP uptake by Goresky (7) and of taurocholate uptake by Glasinovic et al (6) and by our group (19) have shown that the kinetics of hepatic uptake of anionic dyes as well as of bile acids are consistent with carrier-mediated transport. The nature and location of this hypothetical carrier remain to be elucidated. Furthermore, it is unclear whether a single or multiple transport systems are present for the hepatic uptake of organic anions.

Previous studies of hepatocellular uptake of taurocholate were therefore extended to other bile acids and to the anionic dyes ICG and bilirubin to investi-

287

gate structure transport relationships and competitive
inhibition phenomena. The studies were performed in the
in situ perfused rat liver (11) using the multiple indicator dilution technique and the three compartment
model of Goresky et al (8). The organic anions to be
studied were rapidly injected into the portal vein together with reference indicators. Immediately after the
injection the total hepatic venous outflow was collected
in two second periods up to 40 seconds. [51]Cr-labeled
erythrocytes were used as intravascular and [99]Tcm-
albumin as extravascular reference indicator.

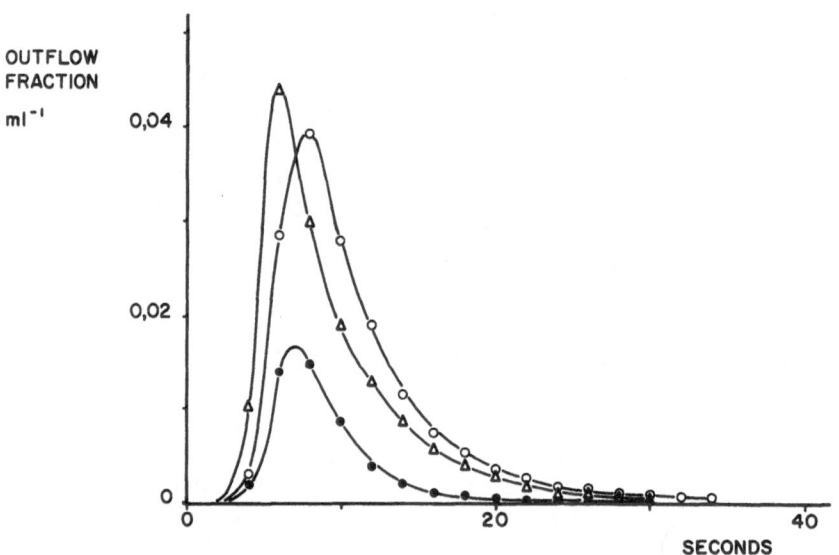

Fig. 1.   Dilution curves of [51]Cr-erythrocytes (trian-
          gles), [99]Tcm-albumin (open circles), and 75
          nmoles [14]C-sodium taurocholate (closed cir-
          cles) in hepatic vein blood after single rapid
          injection of these indicators into the portal
          vein of the in situ perfused rat liver. The
          outflow fraction represents the fraction of
          the injected dose per ml of hepatic vein blood.

Figure 1 shows a set of typical dilution curves of $^{51}$Cr-erythrocytes, $^{99}$Tc$^m$-albumin, and $^{14}$C-taurocholate. Due to a smaller space of distribution the erythrocyte peak occurs earlier and decays more rapidly than that of albumin. The areas under the erythrocyte and the albumin curve, however, are equal since these two reference indicators are not taken up into the hepatocyte. By contrast, the taurocholate curve is contained within the albumin curve but is reduced in magnitude. Its area under the curve is smaller than that of albumin because part of the taurocholate has been taken up into the hepatocyte (19). Similar dilution curves were obtained for other bile acids such as cholate and chenodeoxycholate and for the anionic dyes ICG (17) and unconjugated bilirubin. In the case of bilirubin it must be considered that a fraction of bilirubin rapidly and reversibly binds to erythrocytes (4). This phenomenon may lead to red cell carriage of the label, described by Goresky et al (9), and may influence the results. Since under the conditions of our experiments only about 9 % of bilirubin was bound to erythrocytes and since the mathematical problems associated with the analysis of this effect have not been resolved no correction was attempted.

When the relationship between dose and uptake velocity calculated from these dilution curves was investigated, a qualitatively similar behavior was observed for all organic anions studied. It is exemplified by the dose dependence of taurocholate uptake shown in figure 2. The uptake velocity increased with the dose in a nonlinear fashion, approaching a maximal value asymptotically. Analysis of the data revealed compatibility with Michaelis Menten kinetics and permitted calculation of maximal uptake velocity and apparent half saturation constant. These findings are in accordance with those of Glasinovic et al (6) who studied taurocholate uptake in the dog. They are consistent with the hypothesis that the uptake of taurocholate is carrier-mediated (6,19). Michaelis Menten kinetics were also found for the bile acids cholate and chenodeoxycholate and for the anionic dyes ICG (17) and bilirubin (18). The kinetics of ICG uptake are depicted in figure 3.

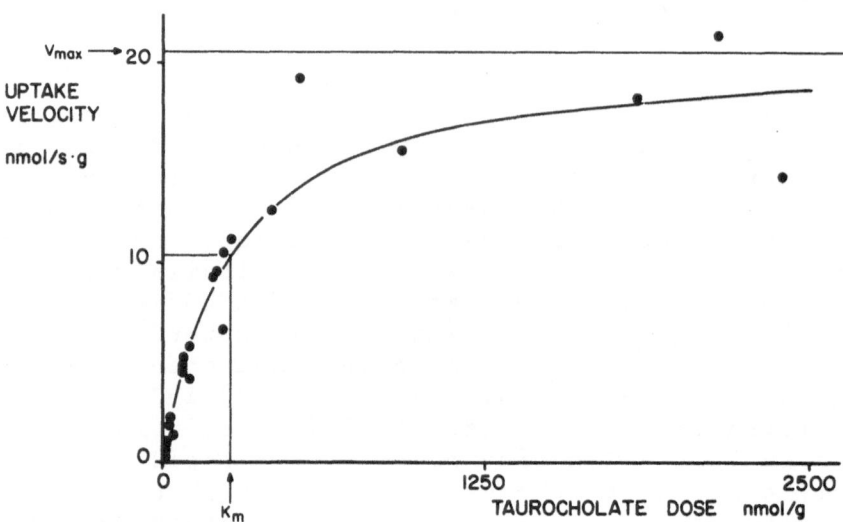

Fig. 2. Relationship between dose and uptake velocity
of taurocholate in the perfused rat liver. The
data in this and the following figures are expressed per gram of liver weight.

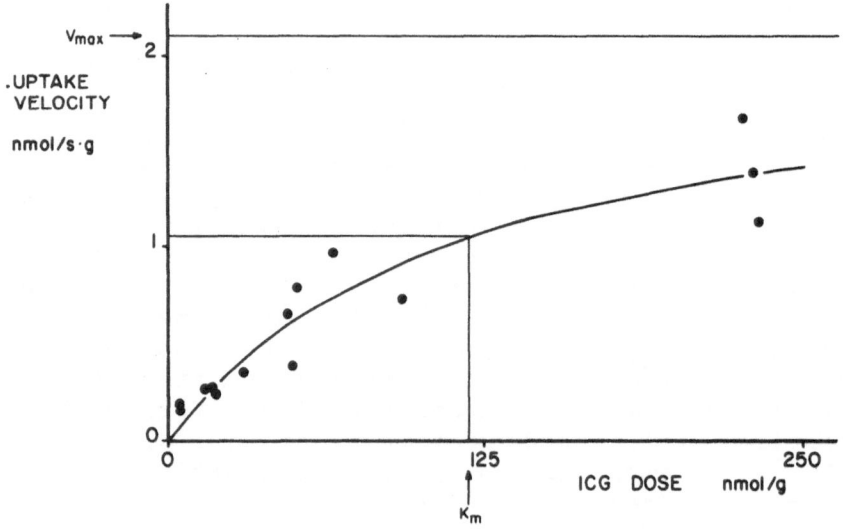

Fig. 3. Relationship between dose and uptake velocity
of indocyanine green in the perfused rat liver.

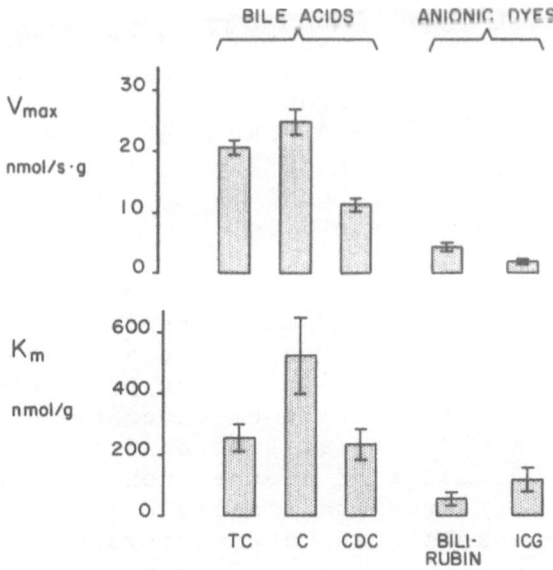

Fig. 4.   Kinetic parameters of hepatic uptake of various organic anions ($\bar{x} \pm$ SD).

As shown in figure 4 the maximal uptake velocity of bile acids markedly exceeded that of bilirubin and ICG. Thus, the maximal uptake velocity of taurocholate was about five times that of bilirubin and about ten times that of ICG. Differences in the maximal uptake velocities and half saturation constants were also noted between individual bile acids. Thus, the maximal uptake velocities of the trihydroxy bile acids, cholate and taurocholate, were not significantly different but were approximately twice that of the dihydroxy bile acid, chenodeoxycholate. These findings suggest that the maximal uptake capacity for bile acids is influenced by the number of hydroxyl groups rather than by conjugation. The apparent half saturation constant, $K_m$, was similar for taurocholate and chenodeoxycholate, whereas it was about 100 % higher for unconjugated cholate.

When the maximal uptake velocities of these anions are compared to their steady state excretory transport maxima measured in the intact rat, it becomes clear that uptake is not the rate limiting step for their overall excretion from the blood into the bile. Thus, the uptake capacity exceeded the reported excretory ca-

pacity about fourfold for taurocholate (16), eightfold
for bilirubin (20,23) and twentyfold for ICG (15).
Goresky has studied this relation for BSP in the dog
and found it to be approximately 60. One may speculate
that the relation between uptake and excretory capacity
represents an important determinant for the accumulation
of substances in the hepatocyte when administered at a
rate exceeding the excretory Tm.

    Since no conclusions can be drawn from these stud-
ies as to whether bile acids and other organic anions
are taken up into the hepatocyte via a common or separate pathways,competitive inhibition phenomena were investigated. In a first series of experiments 250 to
7500 nmoles of a $^{14}$C-labeled bile acid were injected together with 2500 nmoles of another non-labeled, inhibiting bile acid. Between taurocholate and cholate as
well as between cholate and chenodeoxycholate could mutual competitive inhibition be demonstrated when the
effect of the inhibiting bile acid on Vmax and Km of
hepatic bile acid uptake was investigated. It may,
therefore, be assumed that chemically different bile
acids share a common transport system for hepatic uptake.
Furthermore, these findings support the concept that
carrier-mediated transport is responsible for hepatic
uptake of bile acids. The nature of this transport system
as well as the location of the hypothetical carrier remain speculative. Available evidence suggests that Y-
protein does not play a role in bile acid uptake, since
it does not bind bile acids (13). A taurocholate binding
protein has recently been found in isolated liver cell
membranes but awaits further characterization (1).

    To investigate whether anionic dyes and bile acids
enter the hepatocyte via the same or different pathways
the kinetics of bilirubin uptake were studied in the
presence of taurocholate. No significant effect of
taurocholate on Km or Vmax of bilirubin uptake could be
detected by statistical analysis. Vice versa, bilirubin
did not affect taurocholate uptake measured simultaneously (18). Similar to these findings no inhibition of
taurocholate uptake could be demonstrated when indocyanine green was injected together with taurocholate
(17).

    These studies indicate that anionic dyes enter the
hepatocyte by a pathway different from that of bile

acids. The nature of their transfer mechanism from the plasma into the hepatocyte has not been elucidated. Although the role of the Y- and Z-proteins (13) in this first event in the removal of bilirubin remains to be clarified, suggestive evidence is available that the uptake mechanism requires the participation of the plasma membrane (5). In this context, the following arguments appear of importance. No in vitro transfer of [14]C-bilirubin from albumin to the organic anion-binding protein of rat cytosol could be demonstrated. Instead, albumin was shown to strip [14]C-bilirubin from these proteins (5). This behavior can be explained if one considers that the primary binding affinity of Y-protein for bilirubin is less than that of albumin (2,3). It favors the contention that the kinetics of bilirubin uptake, demonstrated in our studies, reflect the existence of a membrane located carrier for bilirubin. Recently, Scharschmidt et al (21) have studied the kinetics of bilirubin uptake in the intact rat. On the basis of Michaelis Menten kinetics, competitive inhibition by ICG and BSP, and countertransport they also suggested that bilirubin uptake is carrier-mediated.


                         CONCLUSIONS

     Available evidence suggests that bile acids and the anionic dyes ICG and bilirubin are taken up into the hepatocyte by different transport systems, the kinetics of which are consistent with carrier-mediated transport. This uptake process is not the rate limiting step in the overall excretion of these anions from the blood into the bile.

     Hepatic transport of organic anions may be regarded as serving mainly two purposes: the generation of bile flow and the elimination of a variety of substances from the circulation. It may offer a biological advantage that these two main functions are not dependent on the same transport mechanism. Thus, under certain conditions the transport of bile acids may be maintained in spite of a disturbance of bilirubin uptake.

ACKNOWLEDGEMENTS

The research in the authors' laboratory was supported by the Swiss National Foundation for Scientific Research. The technical assistance of Mr. H. Sägesser and the secretarial help of Mrs. E. Küttel are gratefully appreciated.

REFERENCES

1.   ACCATINO L, SIMON FR: Characterization of cholic (CA) and taurocholic (TCA) acid binding to a bile acid (BA) receptor in the hepatocyte surface membrane (Abstr.). Gastroenterology 68: 1067, 1975.

2.   ARIAS IM: Transfer of bilirubin from blood to bile. Seminars of Hematology 9: 55-70, 1972.

3.   ARIAS IM, JANSEN P: Protein binding and conjugation of bilirubin in the liver cell, in Jaundice, edited by GORESKY CA, FISHER MM, New York, London, Plenum Press, 1975, p 175-188.

4.   BARNHART JL, CLARENBERG R: Binding of bilirubin to erythrocytes. Proc Soc Biol Med 142: 1101-1103, 1973.

5.   BLOOMER JR, BERK PD, VERGALLA J, BERLIN N: Influence of albumin on the hepatic uptake of unconjugated bilirubin. Clin Science and Molecular Medicine 45: 505-516, 1973.

6.   GLASINOVIC JC, DUMONT M, DUVAL M, ERLINGER S: Hepatic uptake of taurocholate in the dog. J Clin Invest 55: 419-426, 1975.

7.   GORESKY CA: Initial distribution rate of uptake of sulfobromophthaleine in the liver. Am J Physiol 207: 13-26, 1964.

8.   GORESKY CA, BACH GG, NADEAU BE: On the uptake of materials by the intact liver. The transport and net removal of galactose. J Clin Invest 52: 991-998, 1973.

9.  GORESKY CA, BACH GG, NADEAU BE: Red cell carriage of label: its limiting effect on the exchange of materials in the liver. Circ Res 36: 328-351, 1975.

10. HARKAVY M, JAVITT NB: Effect of ethinyl estradiol on hepatic excretory function of the rat, in Metabolic Effects of Gonadal Hormones and Contraceptive Steroids, New York, Plenum Press, 1969, p 11-18.

11. HERZ R, CUENI B, BIRCHER J, PAUMGARTNER G: The excretory capacity of the isolated rat liver. Naunyn-Schmiedebergs Arch Pharmacol 277: 297-304, 1973.

12. KLAASSEN CD, PLAA GL: Determination of sulfobromophthalein storage and excretory rate in small animals. J Appl Physiol 22: 1151-1155, 1967.

13. LEVI AJ, GATMAITAN Z, ARIAS IM: Two hepatic cytoplasmic protein fractions, Y and Z, and their possible role in the hepatic uptake of bilirubin, sulfobromophthalein, and other anions. J Clin Invest 48: 2156-2167, 1969.

14. O'MAILLE ERL, RICHARDS TG, SHORT AH: Conjugation of cholic acid and its uptake and secretion: hepatic extraction of taurocholate and cholate in the dog. J Physiol (Lond) 189: 337-350, 1967.

15. PAUMGARTNER G: The handling of indocyanine green by the liver. Schweiz Med Wschr 105: Supplementum, 1975.

16. PAUMGARTNER G, HERZ R, SAUTER K, SCHWARZ HP: Taurocholate excretion and bile formation in the isolated perfused rat liver. Naunyn-Schmiedebergs Arch Pharmacol 285: 165-174, 1974.

17. PAUMGARTNER G, REICHEN J: Different pathways for hepatic uptake of taurocholate and indocyanine green. Experientia 31: 306-307, 1975.

18.   PAUMGARTNER G, REICHEN J: Separate carrier mediated transport systems for the hepatocellular uptake of bilirubin and bile acids(Abstr.). Digestion. In Press.

19.   REICHEN J, PAUMGARTNER G: Kinetics of taurocholate uptake by the perfused rat liver. Gastroenterology 68: 132-136, 1975.

20.   ROBINSON SH, YANNONI C, NAGASAWA S: Bilirubin excretion in rats with normal and impaired bilirubin conjugation: Effect of phenobarbital. J Clin Invest 50: 2606-2613, 1971.

21.   SCHARSCHMIDT BF, WAGGONER JG, VERGALLA J, BERK PD: Hepatic organic anion uptake in the rat (Abstr.). Gastroenterology 67: 827, 1974.

22.   SPERBER I: Biliary secretion of organic anions and its influence on bile flow, in The Biliary System, edited by TAYLOR W, first edition, Oxford, Blackwell Scientific Publications, 1965, p 457-467.

23.   WEINBREN K, BILLING BH: Hepatic clearance of bilirubin as an index of cellular function in the regenerating rat liver. Brit J Exp Pathol 37: 199-204, 1956.

24.   WHEELER HO, MANCUSI-UNGARO PL, WHITLOCK RT: Bile salt transport in the dog. J Clin Invest 39: 1039-1040, 1960.

25.   WHEELER H, MELTZER J, BRADLEY S: Biliary transport and hepatic storage of sulfobromophthalein sodium in the unanesthetized dog, normal man, and in patients with hepatic disease. J Clin Invest 39: 1131-1144, 1960.

DISCUSSION OF COMMENTARY BY G. PAUMGARTNER

Forker:   It was not clear to me whether the studies you describe
were done by superimposing a tracer injection on a steady-state
background, or whether the whole dose was given at one time.

Paumgartner:   That is an important point.   I thought I had made
it clear by saying that the test substances were injected by single,
rapid injection only.   No infusions were given prior to these
bolus injections.

Forker:   Do you think the results would be different if you had
steady-state conditions?

Paumgartner:   Yes, I think they might be different.

Arias:   Have you made kinetic measurements using similar ligands
in an animal which has been treated with a drug like phenobarbital
for approximately two days?   The basis for suggesting this is that
we have found that the efflux rate of bilirubin from liver back
into plasma is substantially reduced in association with induction
of ligandin.   Can you tell us more of the experiments in which
you replaced sodium with lithium?

Paumgartner:   I have done no studies with phenobarbital, but we
plan to do this, as well as studies of the Gunn rat.   As for your
question about sodium dependence; if you replace 95 per cent of
the sodium by lithium the $V_{max}$ of taurocholate uptake is reduced
by 65 per cent, and the $K_m$ is reduced by 55 per cent.   This is
suggestive that bile acid uptake is a sodium-coupled transport.

Ostrow:   A key point which needs to be emphasized is that you are
really measuring one-way uptake, and that is why you have been
able to measure $T_{max}$ and your data really mean something in terms
of uptake.   Have you studied the effects of albumin on your
kinetics, because your simple kinetics may be affected by binding
in the plasma.

Paumgartner:   Of necessity, there are additional factors influencing our uptake measurements and certainly one of these is albumin
in the perfusate.   That is why I was careful to point out,

especially for the $K_m$, that what we measure are apparent concentrations.   For the highly protein-bound compounds such as
bilirubin and Indocyanin Green, I would agree that what we measure
is the resultant of the kinetics of albumin binding and affinities
to the carrier molecule.   So far, we have not studied the effect
of varying the albumin concentration.   Even so, we feel that the
albumin binding is relatively unimportant in our bile acid studies.

# GENERAL DISCUSSION OF SESSION 2

<u>Graf</u>:   I would like to comment on what happens on the canalicular side of the membrane when stop-flow experiments are done.   The results also have some bearing on what has been found with electron microscopic tracers.   They have been shown to penetrate the tight junctions when injected into the bile duct, but this does not occur when the tracers enter from the sinusoidal side.   Therefore, the junctions may be permeable in only one direction when the biliary pressure increases.   A constant infusion of cholic acid was applied to the isolated, perfused liver.   Bile secretion increases immediately after the start of the cholic acid infusion.   The uptake of bile acid was calculated by measuring the bile acid concentrations in the influent and effluent perfusion media.   When the bile duct cannula was raised to a vertical position the bile secretion pressure gradually rises to a level of about 24-26 centimetres of bile and then gradually decreases.   In this case we find an increase in taurocholate in the effluent medium, and the amount of this is the same as the amount of taurocholate secreted into the bile under control conditions.   This means that we have quantitative regurgitation of bile acids when bile secretion pressure is increased.   This effect is immediately reversible when free bile flow was restored.   These observations indicate that the permeability between bile and perfusion medium increases markedly when pressure in the biliary system rises. This would also explain why lanthanum permeates from the biliary lumen towards the perfusate when injected into the biliary lumen but not in the other direction.

     I have a second comment on tracer fluxes.   It is well known that extracellular space markers used in electron microscopy are taken up by the liver cells by a pincytotic process, and they are then transported by pinocytotic vesicles to the lysosomes into which they become integrated.   But some of these markers also appear in bile in appreciable amounts:  for example, horse radish peroxidase.   We have studied another inert marker, chromium-EDTA and its excretion into bile.   The results are shown in the figure.   After perfusion of an isolated rat liver for one hour with a solution containing $^{51}$Cr-EDTA, the perfusion medium was changed to one without the radioactive compound (Time 0), and the release of radioactivity into the perfusion medium (full triangles)

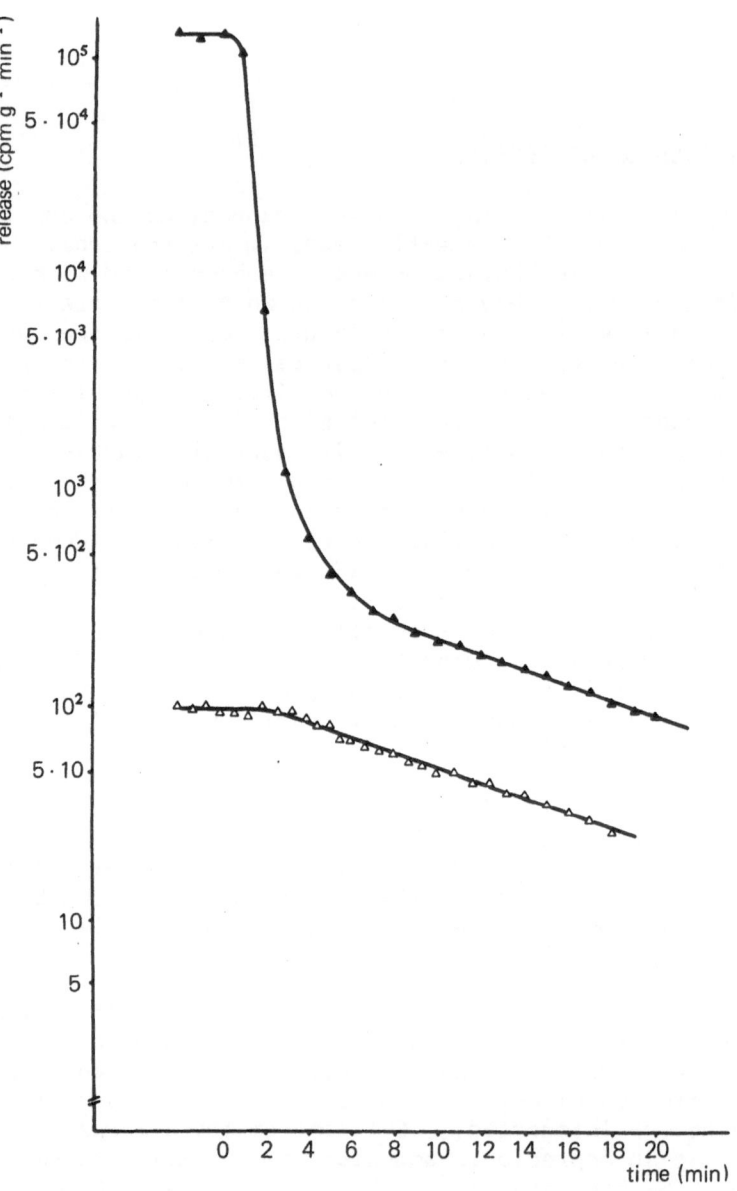

Efflux pattern of $^{51}$Cr-EDTA from rat liver

and bile (open triangles) was followed as a function of time. After the washout of the sinusoidal extracellular space the efflux into the perfusate and bile shows a parallel decrease, indicating release of the isotope from a single small compartment. When we put the chromium-EDTA into the perfusion medium at a constant rate, the concentration in bile gradually rises, and the final concentration is about 30-40 per cent of the amount in the perfusion medium.  If we now apply colchicine or cytochalasin B, there is inhibition of the rate of transport, which indicates that microtubules or microfilaments are involved in this system. Another important observation was that this transport is also calcium dependent.  So we may assume, as a working hypothesis, that there exists an additional transport system in liver cells which transports packaged materials from the sinusoidal space to bile.  I would like to suggest that the vesicles seen on electron micrographs which are connected by actin-containing microfilaments to the canalicular membrane may be important in this type of vesicular transport.

Fisher:  I would like to ask Dr. Phillips a question to which he keeps on giving me the wrong answer.  It is about the origin of the bile canalicular system:  is it intra-hepatocellular?  If the answer is no, how does he explain his findings with the isolated-cell system?  If the answer is yes, why do we see it so infrequently?

Phillips:  Dr. Fisher has discussed this a great deal.  I was very interested in the end-terminal canalicular seen in scanning electron micrographs.  We have been doing scanning-EM for only a short time, so we have only a few hundred pictures of normal livers, and we have not found any canaliculi of the kind Dr. Boyer has shown.  Since I believe that seeing is believing, we must go on looking for these since they must be there.  The problem is that even in those pictures, how do you know that the canaliculus is not going to branch at that point and go out of the plane of the section?  Part of the problem is deciding where the canaliculus begins.  Others have shown intracellular canaliculi in serial sections of normal rat liver, but in all the years I have been doing electron microscopy of human and animal liver, I have never seen a single one.  I think that the canaliculi begin between liver cells rather than inside a liver cell.  I interpret the intracellular canaliculi of isolated cells as being due to reformation and reconstruction of the canaliculus disrupted during the cell separation technique.  Dr. Boyer has good evidence for end-terminal canaliculi which may or may not be intracellular.

Popjak:  I have asked Dr. Phillips the same question.  In the few electron micrographs that we have seen in my own laboratory of isolated hepatocytes we have seen very similar pictures to those

he showed.    But there is the possibility that in the course of
the separation of the cells there is an invagination of the area
of the bile canaliculus.    If that is so, a prolonged search
might reveal a funnel where this invagination occurs.

Boyer:    I just want to clarify a point about the lithocholate-
induced lesions.    Dr. Palmer showed lesions in the end-terminal
cells of the hepatic plates, and I should emphasise that these
are very focal lesions;    they do not occur diffusely throughout
the liver.    Also, they are not intracellular in the sense that
they are continuous with the slightly irregular canaliculus which
one sees more generally in the lithocholate lesion.    But they
are rather severe excavations, if one can use that term, into the
liver substance, causing a space which occupies about half of the
diameter of the cell in these areas.    I do not think that these
lesions necessarily have anything to do with the stasis caused by
lithocholate, because we can give a smaller dose of lithocholate
and not see these lesions yet still have cholestasis.

Popper:    Could we not settle this by using some corrent nomenclature.    Most of us agree that bile canaliculi are diverticular,
so if we use the term "diverticular" then I think even Dr.
Phillips would agree to this.

Berk:    I want to return to the question of hepatic uptake of
organic anions.    Since Dr. Paumgartner has referred to work in
our laboratory, I thought it might be interesting to present some
data which confirm and amplify his studies.    We have looked at
the effect of increasing doses of organic anions on the rate of
hepatic uptake in the whole rat.    Tracer doses of either tritiated
bilirubin, $^{35}$S-B.S.P. or small mass doses of Indocyanin Green were
injected into a jugular vein, and in the syringe used for the
injection there were various mass doses of the same material.
Therefore the rate of disappearance of tracer represents, in fact,
the disappearance of the mass bolus.    In some experiments we had
a potential competitive inhibitor in the same syringe.    Arterial
blood samples were collected at 20 second intervals from the
carotid artery.    Between one minute and, depending on the material,
3 and 4 minutes, the disappearance curves for bilirubin, B.S.P.
and Indocyanin Green are essentially exponential.    In calculating
a fractional disappearance rate for these substances, we have
assumed that the exponential curve represents essentially uptake
of material by the liver from the circulation.    We confirmed that
by doing recovery studies.    At 3 or 4 minutes the animals were
sacrificed, the bile duct was rapidly clamped and the liver was
quickly taken out.    The actual amount of material recovered in
the liver, after correcting for the vascular space, was compared
with that which we calculated had disappeared from the circulation.
When the experiments are confined to this short time scale, the

recovery of bilirubin and B.S.P. in the liver averages between
98-99 per cent; the value for Indocyanin Green is about 90 per
cent.

So we calculate the plasma disappearance rate (or hepatic
uptake rate) V as the fractional disappearance rate times the
dose in micromoles per kilogram for the particular material
injected.  When we injected increasing amounts of bilirubin
along with the tracer doses, we found a typical curve showing
saturation of hepatic uptake similar to that shown by Dr.
Paumgartner.

A Lineweaver-Burk transformation of this data allows us to
calculate the $V_{max}$ and $K_m$ for bilirubin uptake.

In some experiments we pretreated the animals with phenobarbital and examined liver weight, the effect on glucuronyl
transferase activity and on fractional disappearance rate of a
tracer dose of bilirubin.  After pretreatment with 80 mg of
phenobarbital per kilogram for 5 days, there is a 25 per cent
increase in liver weight in both Sprague-Dawley and Gunn rats.
There is appreciable increase in glucuronyl transferase activity
in the former strain, but no change in the Gunn rats.  However,
there is about 25 per cent increase in the fractional hepatic
uptake rate in both strains of rats.  This is just one of the
many lines of evidence which could be cited to show that hepatic
uptake of bilirubin is not driven by conjugation.

We can show that both B.S.P. and Indocyanin Green are
competitive inhibitors of hepatic uptake of bilirubin, and
conversely, bilirubin and Indocyanin Green are competitive
inhibitors of B.S.P. uptake by the liver.  Bilirubin and B.S.P.
competitively inhibit the hepatic uptake of Indocyanin Green.
Very large doses of various bile acids showed no competitive
inhibition of bilirubin, B.S.P. or Indocyanin Green uptake.  So
we confirm Dr. Paumgartner's findings, that the uptake process
for organic anions shows saturability and selective competitive
inhibition.   These are necessary properties to put forward a
hypothesis for a membrane-bound carrier-mediated transport system.
However, the conditions are probably not sufficient to sustain that
hypothesis, since other models can be postulated which would not
involve a carrier-mediated transport system.

We gave various tracer doses of bilirubin and looked at the
effect on the disappearance curves of mass doses of unlabelled
bilirubin, B.S.P. or Indocyanin Green given later in time.   In
each case, such an injection results in the return to the plasma
of labelled bilirubin, which presumably had been in the liver.
The same thing happens when one repeats this type of experiment

with B.S.P. or Indocyanin Green.   So we have shown the additional
property of the "transport system" of counter-transport.   This is
particularly important, because there is no other way to explain
this phenomenon than by invoking some sort of carrier-mediated
system, which almost certainly must reside in the liver-cell
membrane.

Hofmann:   When we measure the plasma disappearance of a hepato-
philic substance in man, we think it necessary to correct the
disappearance curve, or at least interpret the curve, not only
for tissue uptake but also for a mixing factor.   We do this
because any injected substance which is distributed entirely in
the plasma volume also declines exponentially for several minutes
in man.   Can you ignore this in a small animal like the rat, or
do you take it into account?

Berk:   We did not take it into account because the rat has a
heart rate of about 300 beats per minute and a relatively high
cardiac output compared to that of man.   Therefore the mixing
time is trivial.

Forker:   There seems to me to be an explanation as to why your
values are lower than those of Dr. Paumgartner.   Your numbers do
not take into account the translobular concentration gradient.
Your K values are calculated as though the transport process was
being driven by the peripheral circulation, but this is not the
case.   It is being driven by a concentration in that early time
phase, which is substantially less, so your values are lower.

    Apropos of what Dr. Hofman was saying, I think a mixing
artefact will be important if one takes into account the gradient
phenomenon.   If you take the translobular gradient into
consideration and then use the assumption of a well-mixed peripheral compartment, the mixing problem quickly becomes apparent.

Berk:   I think our studies would be less likely to be affected
by this than the linear sinusoidal model Dr. Paumgartner uses.
However, I think that the shapes of the curves generated  indicate
that they conform to Michaelis-Menten kinetics, and that the other
factors I mentioned, such as competitive inhibition exist, is
a strong indication that we have a valid model.

Paumgartner:   Could we speculate further on the molecular
mechanism of this carrier, taking into account your preloading
experiments.   The demonstration that unidirectional flow of
bilirubin into the cell increased when the cells were preloaded
might be interpreted in this way:  the mobility of the carrier-
bilirubin complex through the membrane is greater than the
mobility of the carrier alone.   So in the preloaded situation

there would be more carrier available on the outside of the membrane, which would result in speeding up the process.

Berk:   Certainly that is a possibility.   Basically, there are three different models to explain why the uptake processes are not saturated.   But whatever model you choose, you must postulate that a carrier-mediated process is involved.

Arias:   In general, a hypothesis is only worthwhile if you can design an experiment to prove or destroy it.   With this particular problem we have been discussing, we find it very difficult to design experiments to establish what sort of carrier mechanism we are dealing with.   It could be in the membrane, or indeed within the cell.   That is why I asked Dr. Paumgartner to elaborate on his studies on replacement of sodium by lithium, because it seems to me that this is approaching a more direct identification with the plasma membrane.   I am troubled, due to my own ignorance, about why the preloading experiments need to be interpreted in terms of a plasma-membrane carrier mediated system.   I would add this word of caution that these experiments do not prove the existence of such a plasma membrane system.   For instance, has anyone thought of a model which involves an intracellular, high-affinity protein which would facilitate non-ionic diffusion?

Berk:   As far as I am concerned, there are models, based on a carrier-mediated system, which will explain the data.   Nobody has suggested a model which will withstand rigorous scrutiny based on any other hypothesis which will explain the data.   There is no way that one can explain the data on the basis of a hypothesis that ligandin, or an intracellular protein, is responsible for this sort of phenomenon, because, in fact, it would work in the opposite direction.   For instance, if ligandin were involved the preloaded cell would have decreased ability to withstand further loads.

Arias:   It seems to me that the subsequent fate of the substance within the cell is important here.

Berk:   No.   The phenomenon can be shown in the Gunn rat, in which the bilirubin does not go anywhere once it is inside the cell.   The initial entry rates for bilirubin into the liver of the Gunn rat are virtually identical to those of the Sprague-Dawley strain despite the fact that there is no rapid conjugation and removal of bilirubin in the Gunn rat.   So, in a sense, we have a situation in which the bilirubin is entering a sort of static pool which eventually becomes saturated and then equilibrates with plasma.

Ostrow:   I want to comment on a previous statement that uptake is influenced by subsequent conjugation and excretion.   Therefore, we must specify exactly what we mean by uptake.   The previous statements were referring to net uptake by directional fluxes. In a steady-state situation the first statement may be correct, because once the material has entered the cell it may either go down into the canaliculus via conjugation, or it can go back into the plasma, as you have shown in your kinetic models. If you block off conjugation, and therefore excretion into the bile, the effective net uptake would be impaired.

<u>Javitt</u>:    I do not disagree with these interpretations in any way, but when considering organic anions one has to be rather cautious about a counter-transport type of mechanism.   You may get different information, depending on the type of anion you are using, and the results cannot be interpreted in the same way. When you preload with Indocyanin Green, you can actually see the liver turning green, and maybe the same thing happens with bilirubin.   But with B.S.P. the situation is very different: it is very difficult to say what the subcellular distribution is. Also, B.S.P. and bilirubin are conjugated.   So when you see an increase in radioactivity in serum you do not know if it is conjugated or unconjugated and how the derivatives may affect the counter-transport.   I think we need to know more about the bio-chemical processes involved before we make too many interpret-ations of data obtained from just the plasma side.

<u>Arias</u>:    I think part of the answer to that is in the recovery experiments over the time period of these experiments:   that is partly why we chose those particular times.   We know that the material which has left the plasma is in the liver cells.   Also, from separate experiments we know that, within the time scale we use, most of it is in the cytosol.   In the first 3 minutes there is very little conjugation of bilirubin, and nothing coming down the biliary tract.   So we are aware of the problems you mention, and chose time scales to minimise or avoid them.

# Bilirubin Conjugates

# BILIRUBIN CONJUGATES IN BILE

Clive C. Kuenzle

Dept. of Pharmacology and Biochemistry, School of
Veterinary Medicine, University of Zürich,
Winterthurerstrasse 260, CH-8057 Zürich, Switzerland

In this communication I intend to review the occurrence and
structures of the various conjugates of bilirubin in bile. Although
I cannot promise to clarify all points that in the past have led to
controversies I nevertheless hope that this review will help straigh-
tening out matters at least partially.

I shall divide this paper into two parts. Part 1 will deal with
the question of whether truly monoconjugated bilirubin compounds
exist in bile, and Part 2 will be devoted to the structures of the
various bilirubin conjugates and will give details of the chemistry
of their conjugating moieties.

## THE MONOGLUCURONIDE CONTROVERSY

The monoglucuronide controversy was born concurrent with the
original description by Cole, Lathe and Billing (1954) that the yellow pigments extracted from jaundiced sera could be separated into
three fractions designated bilirubin, pigment I and pigment II. Pigments I and II later came to be known as bilirubin mono- and diglucuronide respectively (Billing, Cole and Lathe, 1957). The early
finding that the monoglucuronide upon warming and evaporation could
be converted to bilirubin and the diglucuronide led these authors to
suspect that the monoglucuronide might be a 1:1-complex between bilirubin and the diglucuronide rather than being a true chemical entity.
This view was nurtured by subsequent investigations, in which it was
shown that rechromatography of isolated monoglucuronide resulted in
its partial dissociation yielding bilirubin and diglucuronide along

309

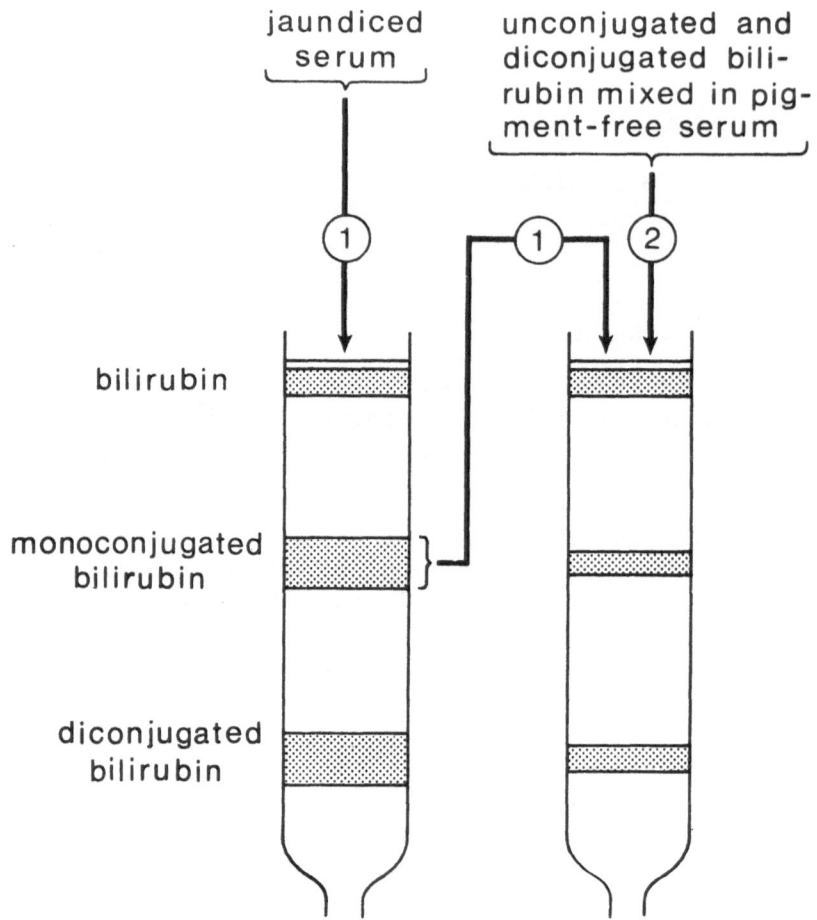

Fig. 1. Two experiments designed to show that monoconjugated bilirubin may be a complex of unconjugated and diconjugated bilirubin. In experiment 1 the bile pigments from jaundiced serum were separated into unconjugated, monoconjugated and diconjugated bilirubin by reverse-phase partition chromatography and the isolated monoconjugate fraction was rechromatographed on a second solumn. This again yielded all three bilirubin fractions suggesting partial dissociation of a complex into its constituents. In experiment 2 unconjugated and diconjugated bilirubin were mixed in pigment-free serum and chromatographed. Some monoconjugated bilirubin appeared along with remainders of untransformed starting materials suggesting reconstitution of a complex from its components.

with a remainder of untransformed starting material (Fig. 1; Nosslin, 1960; Gregory, 1963; Weber et al., 1963). Moreover, Nosslin (1960) succeeded in bringing about the reverse reaction by adding unconjugated bilirubin and diglucuronide from jaundiced urine to pigment-free serum. Chromatography of the resultant mixture not only gave the two bands corresponding to the starting materials but also showed a small but nevertheless distinct band with a mobility similar to that of the monoconjugate. Weber et al. (1963) confirmed these results in principle although their experiments succeeded only when diconjugates isolated from bile were used but not with material obtained from jaundiced urine. On the other hand, Schoenfield & Bollman (1963) were unable to duplicate this reconstitution experiment, and these authors also failed to dissociate isolated monoconjugate into unconjugated and diconjugated material. Later, Ostrow & Murphy (1970) approached the problem by attempting to exchange bilirubin in the putative complex by equilibrating $|^{14}C|$bilirubin with a preparation of conjugated pigments. Upon chromatography less than 2 per cent of the $^{14}$C-radioactivity migrated with the monoglucuronide fraction indicating that appreciable exchange of bilirubin had not taken place.

It thus became clear that more rigorous analyses were required if a solution to the monoglucuronide problem was to be expected. The first success in the direction of a breakthrough was achieved by Jansen & Billing (1971) who exploited the fact that the majority of bilirubin conjugates occur as bilirubin esters. In a search for an ester-specific test that could be used to probe for the number and location of ester-linked substituents their choice fell on ammonolysis. This proved to be an acceptable procedure since the ester functions of bilirubin conjugates not only reacted smoothly with ammonia but the resulting amides were also sufficiently volatile to allow their analysis by high-resolution mass spectrometry. Using this technique it was possible to identify two monoamides each resulting from ammonolysis of the corresponding monoconjugate (Fig.2). Unfortunately, owing to a slight deficiency in experimental design this result could not be taken at face value to reflect the natural occurrence of the monoconjugated form. Since ammonolysis was performed in aqueous solution one could argue that alkaline hydrolysis might have occurred concomitant with substitution thus generating the monoconjugates as in vitro side products.

A similar strategy, though avoiding the drawbacks of the earlier study, was employed by Salmon et al. (1974). These authors converted conjugated bilirubin isolated from rat bile into methyl esters simply by dissolving the mixture of conjugates in methanol and keeping the solution for 2 hours at room temperature. During this time the conjugating moieties attached to the propionic acid side chains of bilirubin were almost completely replaced by methyl groups,

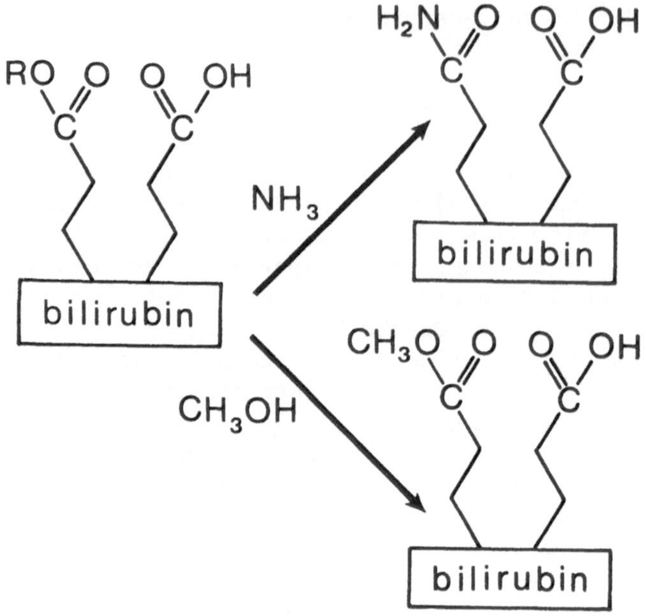

Fig. 2. Two reaction schemes devised for transforming monoconjugated bilirubin (left; R designates any glycosyl residue that might be involved in bilirubin conjugation) into volatile derivatives suitable for mass spectrometry (monoamide at the upper right and monomethyl ester at the lower right). These techniques have yielded unambiguous proof for the occurrence of true monoconjugates of bilirubin.

whereas no reaction occurred at unsubstituted carboxyl functions (Fig. 2). Since the reaction was carried out in the absence of water and base the possibility of interfering side reactions was minimized and the problems encountered with ammonolysis were avoided. The products of this transesterification reaction were then isolated by thinlayer chromatography, and any remaining free carboxyl group (corresponding to a carboxyl group already present in the native conjugate) was trimethylsilylated. The resulting derivatives were then analyzed by mass spectrometry. Using this strategy, it was possible to unambiguously show the presence of derivatives silylated at only one carboxyl group and therefore to prove the natural occurrence of monoconjugates in rat bile. Thus it is now firmly established that monoconjugates exist as true chemical entities.

What, then, is the reason for the earlier findings indicating a complex between bilirubin and its diglucuronide? An answer to this

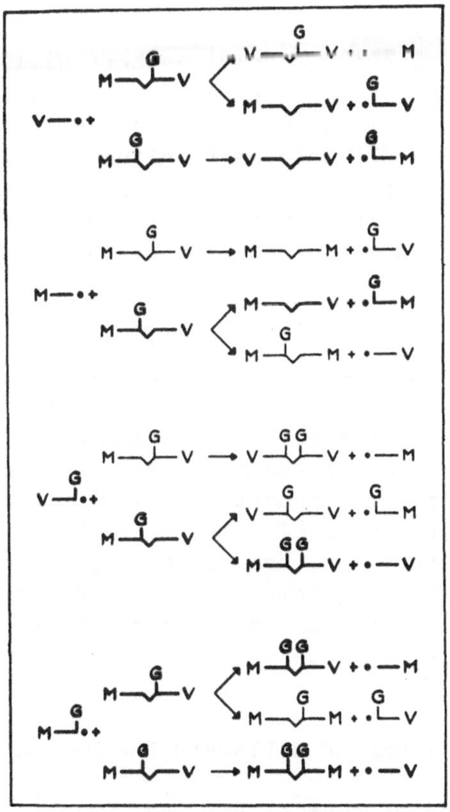

Fig. 3. Isomerisation of bilirubin monoglucuronide by means of a free radical mechanism. The propagation of the reaction.

M $\overset{G}{\sim}$ V    isovinyl isomer of bilirubin-IXα-monoglucuronide

M $\overset{G}{\sim}$ V    vinyl isomer of bilirubin-IXα-monoglucuronide

V $\sim$ V, M $\sim$ V, M $\sim$ M  represent bilirubin IIIα, IXα and XIIIα respectively. The mono- and diglucuronide derivatives of these bilirubin isomers are represented by the attachment of one or two glucuronyl groups ( $\overset{G}{|}$ ) to these structures.

V−., M−., V$\overset{G}{\dashv}$., M$\overset{G}{\dashv}$. represent free radicals with either a dipyrrole or a dipyrrole-methylene structure. (Reproduced from Jansen, 1973, by courtesy of Clinica Chimica Acta.)

question was provided by Jansen (1973) who showed that bilirubin nonoglucuronide prepared enzymically in vitro undergoes rapid isomerisation to yield, apart from the natural isomer IXα, the symmetrical isomers IIIα and XIIIα. This reaction proceeds by cleavage of the bilirubin moiety at the central methylene bridge followed by recombina-

tion of the dipyrrole fragments generated. Thus, if fragments from
two monoglucuronide molecules recombine there will not only be isomerisation of the type described above but in addition this may be
accompanied by disproportionation to yield one molecule of unconjugated and diconjugated bilirubin each. Alternatively, two new mono-
glucuronides may arise (Fig. 3). The isomerisation proceeds most readily at pH 6.5, and in this connection it should be remembered that
the earlier disproportionation and reconstitution experiments with
monoconjugates were carried out at very similar pH values, the latter
ranging from pH 6 to 7.4. Also, the reaction is rapid at room temperature and is already evident after 45 minutes. Oxygen and light catalyze the process, and this suggests the involvement of free radicals. It is very probable that the results of previous experiments,
in which monoconjugates were rechromatographed to give rise to a mixture of bilirubin, monoconjugates and diconjugates or in which bilirubin and diconjugates were incubated to yield monoconjugates, can
all be explained on the basis of this isomerisation-disproportiona-
tion reaction. Thus, they no longer lend support to the once popular
view that monoconjugates are complexes composed of free bilirubin and
its diconjugate. Rather, as already pointed out above, the monoconjugates are true chemical entities.


## STRUCTURES OF BILIRUBIN CONJUGATES

Ever since the appearance of Billing, Cole & Lathe's (1957)
classical paper on the bilirubin conjugates, it has been known that
two types of conjugates occur in bile. These can be distinguished by
their susceptibility to alkaline hydrolysis. The bulk of the pigments
are markedly alkali-labile, to the point of being quantitatively hydrolysed upon treatment with 0.1 M aqueous ammonia for 30 minutes at
room  temperature. As far as has been found all conjugates of this
group contain carbohydrate residues linked to the propionic acide side chains of bilirubin by way of glycosyl ester bonds.

Aside from the alkali-labile conjugates varying amounts of alkali-stable pigments occur in bile. They usually account for not more
than 10-15% of the total. In the minds of many they are associated
with the structure of bilirubin sulphate but we shall see later whether this assignment is really warranted. In contrast, an alkali-
stable pigment has recently been isolated to a high degree of homogeneity and found to contain a polypeptide of molecular weight approximately 7000, covalently linked to the chromophore.

I shall now first discuss the structures of the alkali-labile
conjugates and then proceed to deal with the chemistry of the alkali-
stable pigments.

## Alkali-labile Conjugates of Bilirubin

As already mentioned above the pronounced alkali-lability of the bulk of the bilirubin conjugates occurring in human bile was an early finding (Billing et al., 1957; Schmid, 1957). Together with the demonstration that these conjugates were susceptible to the action of β-glucuronidase and that upon hydrolysis they yielded glucuronic acid this indicated that they were acyl glucuronides of bilirubin. (The compounds should correctly be called bilirubinoyl or acyl glucosiduronates, but the shorter acyl glucuronide is usually preferred. In this paper the two terms will be used interchangeably). Thus a structure was proposed in which the propionic acid side chains of bilirubin were involved in ester linkage with the C(1) hydroxyl group of glucuronic acid. The ester function was later confirmed by Schachter (1957) who, by an ester specific reaction, converted the conjugates into easily identifiable hydroxamates. It thus seemed that the major conjugates of bilirubin were clearly established as bilirubin glucuronides.

However, in 1970 two groups, that of Heirwegh in Belgium and my own, independently published reports indicating that bilirubin conjugation was much more complex than hitherto suspected (Heirwegh et al., 1970; Compernolle et al., 1970; Kuenzle, 1970a,b,c). In both instances a multitude of pigments were separated by chromatography. This complexity has recently augmented as a result of refined separation techniques and the number of conjugates described by both groups is now on the order of 20 pigments (Heirwegh et al., 1975; Kuenzle, 1975).

Both groups performed their structural analyses not on the native bilirubin pigments but rather on their azo derivatives. The rationale for studying the azo derivatives lies in the fact that the native pigments are highly susceptible to oxidative degradation but are converted to more stable compounds upon azo coupling. During the reaction the tetrapyrrole chromophore of bilirubin is cleaved at the central methylene bridge giving rise to two isomeric azo pigments (Fig. 4). This may, in some cases, complicate analysis but may also be exploited as a means of determining which side of the bilirubin molecule carries a particular substituent.

It should perhaps be noted at this point that the two groups employed different diazonium salts for azo coupling. Whereas Heirwegh's group conducted their work with the diazonium salt of ethyl anthranilate the diazonium salt of aniline was preferred in my laboratory. This is, as will become more evident later, one of the reasons why it is presently so difficult to relate the results of the two groups to each other.

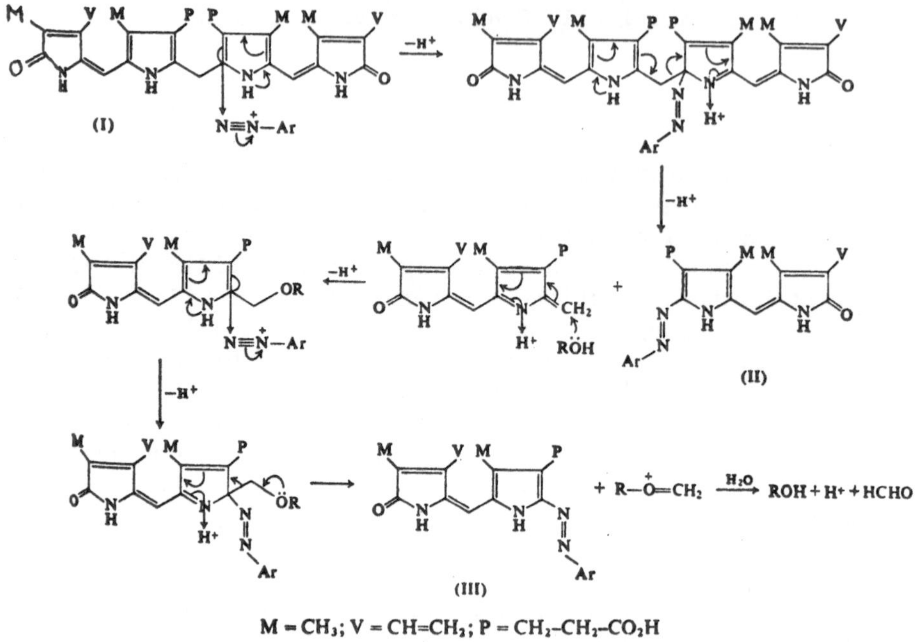

M = CH$_3$; V = CH=CH$_2$; P = CH$_2$-CH$_2$-CO$_2$H

Fig. 4. The azo coupling reaction of bilirubin. Reaction of bilirubin (I) with 2 mole equivalents of a diazotized aromatic amine (such as diazotized ethyl anthranilate or aniline, represented by N≡N-Ar) proceeds sequentially to yield two isomeric azo pigments. The isovinyl isomer is represented by structure (II) and the vinyl isomer by structure (III). (Reproduced from Hutchinson & Johnson, 1972, by courtesy of the Biochemical Journal.)

　　　　Heirwegh's studies were performed on the biles of humans, dogs and rats. He converted the native compounds to ethyl anthranilate azo pigments, which, following extraction with 2-pentanone, were applied to silica gel thin-layer plates. Development with chloroform-methanol-water (65 : 25 : 3, by vol) followed by a second development in the same dimension using chloroform-methanol (17 : 3, v/v) gave the patterns shown in Figs. 5 and 6. Azo pigments were separated into groups of bands denoted by the greek letters α to δ. Depending on the resolution of a particular plate the following individual bands could be recognized : $\alpha_0$, $\alpha_1$ (usually badly resolved from the $\alpha_0$ band), $\alpha_2$, and $\alpha_3$; $\beta_1$ and $\beta_2$; $\gamma_1$ and $\gamma_2$; and finally δ. The relative proportions of the various bands are seen (Fig. 6) to vary considerably between species, $\alpha_3$ being the dominant pigment in dogs,

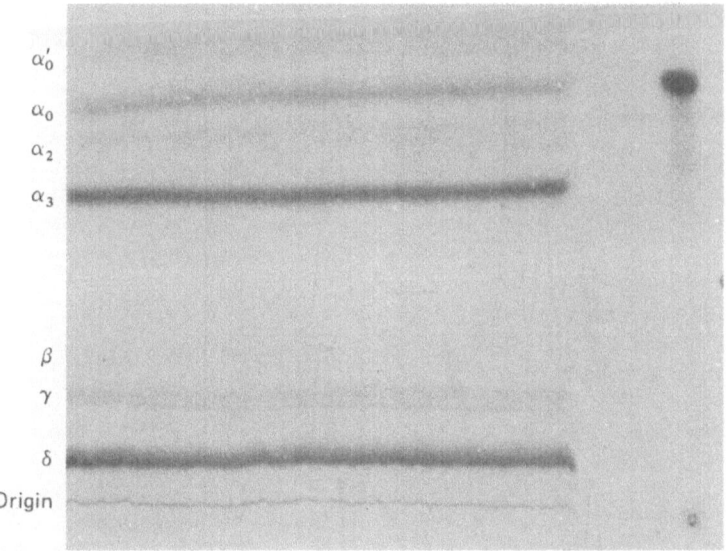

Fig. 5. Thin-layer chromatogram showing ethyl anthranilate azo pigments obtained from dog bile. The $\alpha_3$-and $\delta$-pigments are preponderant in this species. Authentic unconjugated azo pigment was run as a marker (right lane). Silica gel plates were developed with chloroform-methanol-water (65 : 25 : 3, by vol). (Reproduced from Gordon et al., 1974, by courtesy of the Biochemical Journal.)

whereas $\delta$ is preponderant in humans and rats. Rats furthermore have a low percentage of $\beta$ and $\gamma$ pigments. The pigment pattern moreover is dependent on the hydrostatic pressure prevailing in the biliary system. In rats obstruction of the common bile duct causes a pronounced increase in the relative amounts of $\beta$ and $\gamma$ pigments, together accounting for as much as 35%. Upon relieving the obstruction the pigment composition reverts within 6 hours to normal values, with $\beta$ and $\gamma$ pigments falling to a few percent of the total (Van Damme et al., 1971).

Structural analyses were performed on the separated pigments. A word of caution must be put in right here to warn against pigment identification from various sources solely on the basis of the greek letter notation. Heirwegh has pointed out that common symbols merely reflect similar chromatographic behaviour and should not be taken indiscriminately as a proof of structural identity (Fevery et al., 1971). Thus, identification of a particular pigment in one species is not sufficient evidence for concluding that the same compound also occurs in the bile of other animals.

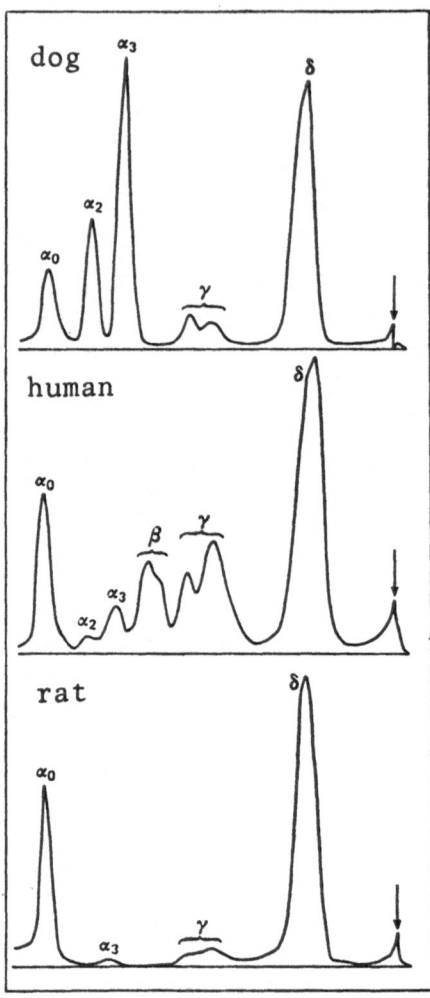

Fig. 6. Thin-layer chromatograms of ethyl anthranilate azo pigments obtained from dog, human and rat bile. Densitometric scans are shown. Chromatography was as in Fig. 5. Note species dependent chromatographic patterns. (Reproduced from Fevery et al., 1971, by courtesy of the Biochemical Journal.)


     A compilation of the techniques employed for structural analysis and of the data obtained by Heirwegh's group (Heirwegh et al., 1970, 1972, 1975; Compernolle et al., 1970, 1971; Fevery et al., 1971, 1972 a,b), Gordon and co-workers (1974) and Jansen & Stoll (1971) is presented in Tables 1 and 2. All pigments were found to be alkali-labile, which indicates that in each case the conjugating moiety is linked to the azodipyrrole chromophore by way of an ester bond.

It will be noted that of the many pigments obtained only $\alpha_0$ from human, dog and rat bile, $\alpha_2$ and $\alpha_3$ from dog bile and $\delta$ from rat bile have been analysed in some detail. The most thoroughly investigated compounds are the $\alpha_0$, $\alpha_2$ and $\alpha_3$ pigments. They have been identified as unconjugated azodipyrrole ($\alpha_0$ from all sources), azodipyrrole $\beta$-D-xylopyranoside ($\alpha_2$, dog) and azodipyrrole $\beta$-D-glucopyranoside ($\alpha_3$, dog), and there can be virtually no doubt that the structures assigned to them are correct. The situation is less clear with regard to the $\delta$-pigment from rat bile. This has been identified as an azodipyrrole $\beta$-D-glucosiduronate mainly on the basis of its susceptibility to $\beta$-glucuronidase and the observation that upon trimethylsilylation the pigment revealed mass spectral properties consistent with an acyl hexosiduronate structure. Although at the time of the identification these results provided accepted arguments for the proposed structure the situation has now changed as a result of observations made in my laboratory (Kuenzle, 1970 c). These indicated that $\beta$-glucuronidase may not only attack terminal glucosiduronate residues but may also act on glucuronic acid residues further substituted at one hydroxyl group. Moreover, evidence has been obtained suggesting that under certain circumstances trimethylsilylation may result in the removal of such substituents giving rise to a fully trimethylsilylated glucuronic acid residue. Mass spectrometry would then reveal the presence of a simple glucuronide although this would have been derived from a more complex structure. As long as these points are not clarified it will be impossible to reach a final conclusion with regard to the structure of this pigment.

The structure of the $\delta$-fraction in humans is even less well established. It is undoubtedly of major interest in view of the abundance of this pigment in man. According to earlier investigations (Billing et al., 1957; Schmid, 1957) this should conform with an acyl $\beta$-D-glucosiduronate. However, its behaviour toward $\beta$-glucuronidase is not totally in accord with this proposal. Heirwegh noted that, depending on the preparations investigated, between 5 to 30% of the fraction resisted prolonged incubation with this enzyme (Heirwegh et al., 1970). This indicated that the $\delta$-pigment in humans is heterogeneous and must be composed of at least two subfractions, i.e. one, $\beta$-glucuronidase resistant, that contains hexuronic acid but not necessarily glucuronic acid, and another, $\beta$-glucuronidase sensitive, that has D-glucuronic acid in $\beta$-glycosidic linkage with the propionic acid side chain of the azodipyrrole chromophore. Whether the latter subfraction represents the glucuronide previously proposed must remain open to question in view of the argument presented above doubting the specificity of $\beta$-glucuronidase for terminal glucuronic acid residues.

The uncertainty about the structure of the $\delta$-pigments is even

Table 1. Properties of ethylanthranilate azo pigments from various sources of bile. Data compiled from the works of Heirwegh et al., Gordon et al. (in the case of the $\alpha_3$-pigment from dog bile) and Jansen & Stoll. The data are listed as +, positive result; -, negative result; no entry, experiment not done.

(1) Azo pigment

(2) Species

(3) Identification by MS and comparison with authentic unconjugated azo pigment

(4) Identification by co-chromatography (TLC) with authentic unconjugated azo pigment or with reference samples obtained enzymatically from bilirubin and UDP-glucuronic acid, UDP-glucose and UDP-xylose

(5) Treatment with dilute alkali yields unconjugated pigment (identified by TLC) and conjugating moiety

(6) Ammonolysis/methanolysis transforms pigment into amide/methyl ester (identified by MS and TLC) and releases conjugating moiety

(7) Treatment with formic acid converts pigment into more polar compound with TLC-mobility similar to that of δ-pigment

(8) Contains free carboxyl groups as evidenced by reaction with $CH_2N_2$

(9) Contains neutral sugar

(10) Contains hexuronic acid

(11) Percentage cleaved by β-glucuronidase (cleavage being inhibited by saccharo-$(1\rightarrow4)$-lactone

(12) Percentage cleaved by β-glucosidase (cleavage being inhibited by glucono-$(1\rightarrow5)$-lactone

(13) Cleavage by β-xylosidase

(14) Uncleaved conjugate identified by MS after treatment with $CH_2N_2$ followed by trimethylsilylation

(15) Conjugating moiety identified by glucose oxidase test

(16) Conjugating moiety identified by TLC (3 systems)

(17) Conjugating moiety identified by ion-exchange chromatography in borate buffer

(18) Conjugating moiety identified by MS following trimethylsilylation or acetylation

(19) Conjugating moiety identified by GLC-MS following (a) borohydride reduction and acetylation
                                                        (b) $CH_2N_2$-treatment and acetylation
                                                        (c) trimethylsilylation

(20) Conjugating moiety identified by NMR

(21) Sugar ring size established by complex sequence of reactions followed by GLC-MS

| | (1) | (2) | (3) | (4) | (5) | (6) | (7) | (8) | (9) | (10) | (11) | (12) | (13) | (14) | (15) | (16) | (17) | (18) | (19) | (20) | (21) |
|---|---|---|---|---|---|---|---|---|---|---|---|---|---|---|---|---|---|---|---|---|---|
| $\alpha_0$ human | | | + | + | − | − | + | | | − | | | | | | | | | | | |
| dog | | | + | + | − | − | + | | | | | | | | | | | | | | |
| rat | | | + | + | − | − | + | | | | | | | | | | | | | | |
| $\alpha_2$ human | | | + | + | | | + | | − | − | − | − | | | | | | | | | |
| dog | | | | + | | + | | | + | | | | + | | | xyl | xyl | pent | | | pyr |
| $\alpha_3$ human | | | + | + | | | + | | − | − | − | − | | | | | | | | | |
| dog | | | | + | | + | | + | + | | − | 70-95% | − | | + | glc | glc | hex | glc | glc | pyr |
| $\beta_1$ human | | | + | + | + | + | + | + | + | + | − | | | | | | | | | | |
| $\beta_2$ human | | | + | + | + | + | + | + | + | + | − | | | | | | | | | | |
| $\gamma_1$ human | | | + | + | + | + | + | + | + | + | − | | | | | | | | | | |
| $\gamma_2$ human | | | + | + | + | + | + | + | + | + | − | | | | | | | | | | |
| $\delta_1$ human | | | + | + | + | − | + | + | + | + | 70-95% | | | | | | | | | | |
| $\delta_2$ rat | | | + | + | + | − | + | + | + | + | 90-100% | | | * | | | | | | | |

* = azodipyrrole hexosiduronate, xyl = xylose, glc = glucose, pent = pentose, pyr = pyranose

Table 2. Structures of ethylanthranilate azo pigments from various sources of bile. Structures based on the data given in Table 1.

| Azo pigment | Species | Structure *) |
|---|---|---|
| $\alpha_0$ | human | unconjugated azodipyrrole |
|  | dog | unconjugated azodipyrrole |
|  | rat | unconjugated azodipyrrole |
| $\alpha_2$ | dog | azodipyrrole (acyl) $\beta$-D-xylopyranoside |
| $\alpha_3$ | dog | azodipyrrole (acyl) $\beta$-D-glucopyranoside |
| $\beta_1$ | human | alkali-labile, hexuronic acid containing azodipyrrole conjugates, which are converted into more polar compounds upon treatment with formic acid |
| $\beta_2$ | human | |
| $\gamma_1$ | human | |
| $\gamma_2$ | human | |
| $\delta$ | human | Probably a group of alkali-labile, hexuronic acid containing azodipyrrole conjugates. In some of these the presence of $\beta$-D-glucuronic acid residues is suggested by the partial susceptibility of the $\delta$-fraction to $\beta$-glucuronidase. |
|  | rat | azodipyrrole (acyl) $\beta$-D-glucosiduronate (?) |

*) The occurrence of both the vinyl and isovinyl azo pigment isomers has been established for groups $\alpha$, $\beta$, $\gamma$ and $\delta$ obtained from human and rat bile (Jansen & Stoll, 1971).

surpassed by the lack of knowledge about the pigments of the β and
γ-group. They share a pronounced alkali-lability with all other pigments detected and therefore are acyl glycosides in all probability.
Hexuronic acids seem to be involved in conjugation but their identity and their mode of attachment is obscure. Of particular interest
appears to be the finding that treatment with 30% formic acid at 37°
overnight converts these pigments into more polar compounds (Heirwegh et al., 1970). This may indicate that lipophilic substituents
are split off during acid treatment rendering the compounds more water-soluble. However, since presently no further data are available
on these pigments this conclusion remains purely speculative.

Summarizing Heirwegh's line of research it can be concluded
that of the many azo pigments separable on thin-layer plates only
three, namely $\alpha_0$ from all sources as well as $\alpha_2$ and $\alpha_3$ from dog bile,
have been unambiguously identified (for their structures, see Table
2). The structure of the δ-pigment from rat bile must be regarded
as controversial, and all other pigments remain largely uninvestiga-
ged. Recently, Heirwegh has presented evidence to show that mixed
conjugates occur in dog bile, with various combinations of substituents being possible at the two carboxyl groups of bilirubin (Heirwegh et al., 1975), but their final identification awaits the elucidation of structure of the component azo pigments.

In contrast to Heirwegh's group, which employed an essentially
one step purification technique of high resolving power but low capacity (thin-layer chromatography) my own approach was to develop a
multistage procedure compensating for a limited resolving power at
each step but having a high capacity (column chromatography). Up to
6 litres of human postoperative T-tube bile could thus be processed
in a single run (Kuenzle, 1970 a). However, the procedure had the
disadvantage of being laborious and time consuming and further that
it did not lend itself to quantitative analysis. As in Heirwegh's
work the conjugates of bilirubin were not isolated in their native
form but as their azo derivatives. However, azo coupling differed
from Heirwegh's in that it was carried out with diazotized aniline
rather than with diazotized ethyl anthranilate.

The original scheme for the isolation of the bilirubin conjugates comprised three column chromatographic steps (Kuenzle, 1970 a),
but recently a fourth step involving thin-layer chromatography on
polyamide sheets has been added (Kuenzle, 1975). This is shown in
Fig. 7. Clearly, a high degree of complexity exists in human bile
with respect to the bilirubin conjugates. On the one hand, conjugates can be grouped into monoconjugated and diconjugates forms (bilirubin fractions 2 and 3, respectively), and on the other, both groups
give rise to at least 12 conjugated azo pigments (azo pigments $B_1$ to

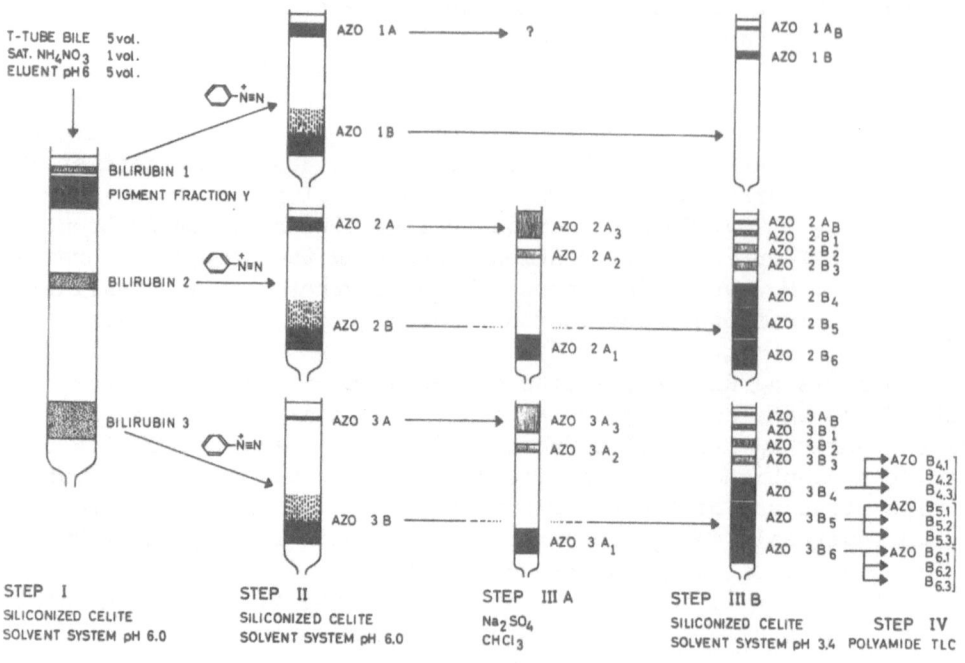

Fig. 7. Separation scheme used for the isolation of phenylazo derivatives of bilirubin from human bile. Monoconjugated and diconjugated bilirubin (bilirubin fractions 2 and 3, respectively) were separated in a first step and were then subjected to azo coupling. Further chromatography on reverse-phase partition columns (steps II and
IIIB) followed by thin-layer chromatography on polyamide sheets yielded a number of conjugated azo pigments, which were labelled azo pig-
ments $B_1$, $B_2$, $B_3$, $B_{4.1}$ – $B_{4.3}$, $B_{5.1}$ – $B_{5.3}$ and $B_{6.1}$ – $B_{6.3}$. (Modified from Kuenzle, 1970 a, by courtesy of the Biochemical Journal.)

$B_3$, $B_{4.1}$ to $_{4.3}$, $B_{5.1}$ to $B_{5.3}$, and $B_{6.1}$ to $B_{6.3}$). Since it is probable that, along with summetrically conjugated bilirubins, there
exist in bile diconjugates of bilirubin carrying different substituents at the two carboxylic positions (see Heirwegh's work cited
above), the complexity may be even greater than appears from the
chromatographic pattern shown in Fig. 7.

So far, structural work has only been performed on the azo pigment fractions $B_4$, $B_5$ and $B_6$ (Kuenzle, 1970 c). In retrospect, the
conclusions reached must be regarded with caution since, as shown
by polyamide chromatography, the fractions analyzed were heterogeneous in composition (Fig. 7). Despite this shortcoming, the results

obtained permit some valid interpretations.

Each of the three fractions proved to be alkali-labile and spectral data indicated that substitution was by ester linkage to the
propionic acid side chains of bilirubin. In each case the naphthare-
sorcinol-sulphuric acid test showed the presence of 1 mole uronic
acid per mole of azo pigment. However, the first indication that
neither pigment was a simple glucuronide came from molecular weight
determinations, which gave values of 720 to 810 as opposed to 566
expected for a simple glucuronide. Further, mild alkaline hydrolysis followed by paper chromatography of the released substituents
showed the presence of reducing substances that were much more polar
than reference glucuronic acid. No spot was observed in the region
of this latter compound. This made the occurrence of a simple glucuronide very unlikely. After many further analyses it was finally concluded that the pigments were linked to various disaccharides with
the structures shown in Fig. 8.

The most thorough investigation was made of azo pigment $B_4$, and
early it was realised that this fraction was heterogeneous in composition. First, treatment with β-glucuronidase converted only about
one third of the material into a pigment of reduced polarity, which
on column chromatography using the solvent system pH 3.4 (Fig. 7)
travelled comparable with azo pigments $B_2$ or $B_3$. Second, when the
polar substituents were isolated as a mixture and were fully methy-
lated, ensueing gas-liquid chromatography showed the presence of
three components in the approximate ratio 3 : 60 : 37, and coupled
mass spectrometry revealed that these were disaccharides of an aldobiouronic acid type (for a definition of aldobiouronic acids, see
the legend to Fig. 8). Since β-glucuronidase treatment of the isolated mixture of substituents followed by trimethylsilylation and gas-
liquid chromatography showed the occurrence of glucuronic acid and
glucose it was concluded that at least one of the three aldobiouronic acids consisted of these carbohydrate components.

With azo pigment $B_5$ β-glucuronidase treatment converted all of
the material into unconjugated azo pigment indicating that β-glucosiduronic acid residues linked directly to the chromophore were present in all three subfractions. When the conjugating carbohydrates
were isolated as a mixture, subjected to acid hydrolysis and trimethylsilylated, a combination of gas-liquid chromatography and mass
spectrometry showed the presence of glucuronic acid along with some
other compounds. These exhibited mass spectra consistent with the
structures of hexuronic acid lactones. Arguments were presented to
suggest that these were derived from a branched-chain uronic acid
(3-C-hydroxymethyl-D-riburonic acid). However, when the proposed
structure was synthesised and compared with the natural material it

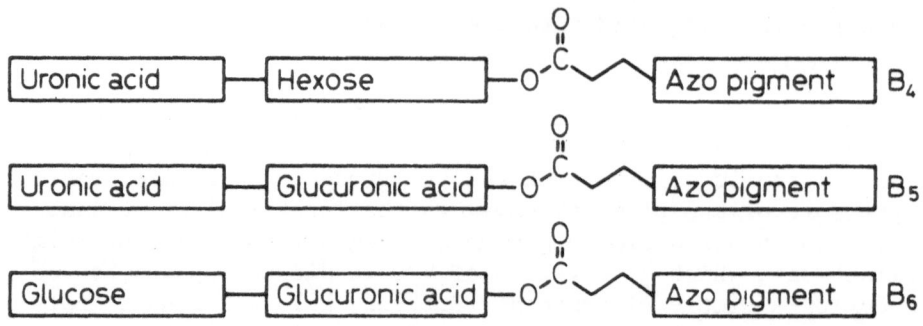

Fig. 8. Schematized structures of the major azo pigments obtained
from human bile by the method shown in Fig. 7. All compounds contain
a disaccharide bound to the propionic acid side chain of azobilirubin. The non-reducing termini of the various disaccharides are at
the left, and each reducing terminus is shown to be involved in an
acyl glycoside linkage with the pigment moiety. Azo pigments $B_4$, $B_5$
and $B_6$ each consist of three subfractions differing in the composition of the conjugating carbohydrates. In azo pigment $B_4$, the disaccharides are aldobiouronic acids (uronic acid → neutral sugar), at
least one of which contains glucuronic acid and glucose; in azo pigment $B_5$, the disaccharides are hexuronosylhexuronic acids (uronic
acid → uronic acid) with glucuronic acid at the reducing terminus;
and in azo pigment $B_6$, the disaccharides are pseudoaldobiouronic
acids (neutral sugar → uronic acid) composed of glucose and glucuronic acid. The pigment moieties of azo pigments $B_4$ and $B_5$ consist
of both isomers obtained upon azo coupling of bilirubin IXα (vinyl-
and isovinyl-isomer) whereas azo pigment $B_6$ contains the vinyl isomer exclusively.


became evident that this structural assignment was incorrect (Blackstock et al., 1974). Thus, apart from the mass spectrometric evidence
for a hexuronic acid, the identity of the second carbohydrate component in azo pigment $B_5$ is still open to question, and, in view of
the heterogeneity of the material analyzed, it is probable that several compounds will ultimately be found. At present the best interpretation possible is that of azo pigment $B_5$ representing a group of
three hexuronosylhexuronides (Fig. 8).

    Azo pigment $B_6$ was also fully cleaved by β-glucuronidase yiel-
ding unconjugated azo pigment. This again suggested that in all subfractions β-glucosiduronic acid residues were directly linked to the
pigment moiety. As with azo pigment $B_5$, the substituents were subjected to a sequence of acid hydrolysis, trimethylsilylation and gas-

liquid chromatography. Since glucuronic acid and glucose were the only compounds detected it was concluded that these represent the components present in all three subfractions. Azo pigment B6 thus stands as a mixture of three isomeric pseudoaldobiouronides containing glucose and glucuronic acid linked to the pigment moiety in this sequence (Fig. 8).

It seems difficult to reconcile the results of my studies with those of Heirwegh's group and earlier investigators. Of particular concern to researchers working in this field was my failure to extract from human bile a simple glucuronide, long thought to be the major conjugate of bilirubin in many species. Various explanations for this puzzling finding have been put forward (Billing & Jansen, 1971; Kuenzle, 1973, and the discussion by Billing therein). It has, for instance, been proposed that in my studies the glucuronide might have been either lost or degraded during isolation. Such a loss seems unlikely in view of the tendency of my scheme to select for non-polar compounds rather than for polar ones, a tendency that would result in the accumulation of the simple glucuronide and not of the disaccharide-containing conjugates of greater polarity. Also, the structural similarity between the simple glucuronide and the complex glycosides rules against their differential susceptibility to degradation. On the other hand, the discrepant results might also be explained by postulating that Heirwegh's group might have isolated the disaccharide conjugates with their δ-fraction but might have missed their identification because of loss of the terminal sugar unit during work-up for analysis. Support for this hypothesis comes from my observation that trimethylsilylation prior to mass spectrometry in fact results in an elimination of the terminal residue. Another possible explanation is that of species difference, the argument being that Heirwegh's work has centered on the bile of dogs and rats whereas my studies were conducted on human T-tube bile. The latter bile specimens have also led to speculations invoking preoperative incidences of bile obstruction and resultant quantitative changes in bile composition as causes of the missing glucuronide. This, together with the suggestion that Heirwegh's pigments β and γ might represent the disaccharide-containing conjugates would seem an attractive way of overcoming the dilemma. However, I seriously doubt that on thin-layer chromatograms these very polar derivatives would travel with the mobility of the β- and γ-pigments while the less polar glucuronide would occupy the δ-position. We have recently tested this contention by running our disaccharide-containing conjugates on Heirwegh's thin-layer system and have found that the compounds moved at a rate comparable with the δ-fraction. However, this result should not be overemphasized taking into account that the compounds investigated were phenylazo derivatives as opposed to the ethyl anthranilate azo pigments employed by Heirwegh. Nevertheless, I personally favour the view that disaccharide-containing conjugates of types $B_4$, $B_5$ and $B_6$ should be sought in Heirwegh's $\delta$-fraction (where they might possibly occur along with some simple glucuronide) whereas the minor conjugates of type $B_1$ to $B_3$ might correspond to Heirwegh's fractions $\alpha$ to $\gamma$. Further work is certainly needed to finally settle this matter of controversy.

## Alkali-stable Conjugates of Bilirubin

Relatively little is known about the alkali-stable conjugates present in bile, one of the reasons being that they occur to a minor extent only. In human bile, for instance, they usually account for not more than 10 - 15% of the total although values of up to 40% seem to occur occasionally (Billing et al., 1957). Early studies have suggested that they may represent sulphates (Isselbacher & McCarthy, 1958, 1959; Schoenfield et al., 1962; Vegas, 1963; Tenhunen, 1965; Noir et al., 1966), phosphates (Tenhunen, 1965), ethereal and N-glucuronides (Gregory & Watson, 1962) and derivatives involving glycine (Jirsa & Večerek, 1958; Jirsa et al., 1958; Isselbacher & McCarthy, 1959), taurine (Jirsa & al., 1956, 1958; Jirsa & Večerek, 1958) and methyl residues (Isselbacher & McCarthy, 1959). However, such identifications must seriously be doubted in light of the low degree of purity of the materials analysed and the limited specificity of the analytical techniques employed. In fact, claims for these structures have not been renewed in the following with the exception of bilirubin sulphate, which has repeatedly cropped up in the literature (Noir et al., 1970; Noir & Nanet, 1974). However, the data presented, when critically evaluated, are not convincing proof for a sulphate and more sophisticated methods of purification and analysis are required to substantiate this claim.

An alkali-stable conjugate with spectral properties indicative of a mesobilirubin structure (i.e., one with reduced vinyl groups) has been isolated in small quantities from human bile and labelled azo pigment $B_1$ (Fig. 7; Kuenzle, 1970 c). However, severe lack of material has prevented its structural analysis. An unknown alkali-stable component has also been detected in some specimens of the $\delta$-azo-pigment obtained from the most polar conjugates of dog bile (Heirwegh et al., 1975) but so far its structure has not been elucidated.

In contrast, we have recently isolated from human bile an alkali-stable conjugate, which, following purification to a high degree of homogeneity, was shown to contain a polypeptide covalently attached to the chromophore (Etter-Kjelsaas & Kuenzle, 1975). A conjugate of this type has formerly been postulated to occur in jaundiced plasma (Fulop et al., 1964, 1965) and normal bile (Gent et al., 1971)

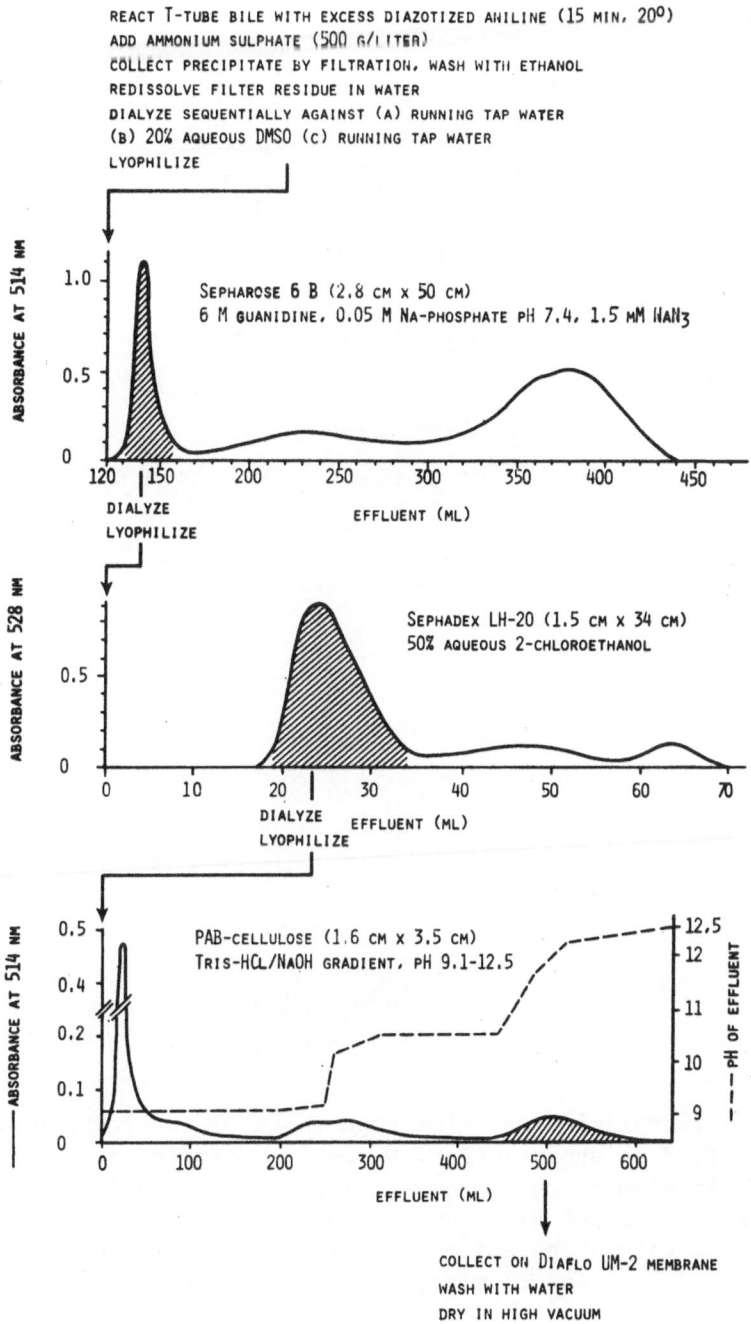

Fig. 9. Flow diagram showing the procedure for isolating a polypeptide conjugate of bilirubin from human bile. Hatched areas represent fractions collected.

Fig. 10. Polyacrylamide gel electrophoresis of the polypeptide conjugate purified as shown in Fig. 9. Left, unstained gel showing position of azo pigment chromophore; right, gel stained for protein
by Coomassie Brilliant Blue. Note mutually corresponding single
bands on both gels. Separation by microdisc electrophoresis was in
30% gels at pH 8.4. Anodal migration was from top to bottom.

but its existence has never been proved conclusively. To settle this question we have developed an essentially three-stage purification scheme (Fig. 9) and have isolated small amounts of a macromolecular azo pigment from 50 litres of human T-tube bile. Upon polyacrylamide electrophoresis the final preparation gave a single band, which in its native form had the pink colour typical of the azobilirubin chromophore whereas with Coomassie Blue showed staining properties indicative of a polypeptide (Fig. 10). The peptide character of the conjugate was substantiated by amino acid analysis. This revealed the presence of all 20 common amino acids with the possible exception of tryptophan and half-cystine, which were not determined. The relative abundance of the various amino acids combined with results from ultrafiltration studies then showed that the best fit was for a polypeptide of molecular weight approximately 7000. Covalent attachment of the chromophore to the peptide was indicated by the observation that strongly denaturing conditions, such as exposure to guanidine, sodium dodecyl sulphate and solvents of high pH (see e.g. Fig. 9), did not release the chromophore from its macromolecular carrier. Moreover, the alkali-stability of the conjugate together with its absorption spectrum suggested that the linkage between chromophore and polypeptide was through an amide bond involving the propionic acid side chains of bilirubin and amino groups of the protein. More detailed analysis was prevented by lack of material but despite this short-coming the polypeptide conjugate can be said to be the best investigated alkali-stable conjugate of bilirubin isolated so far.

## CONCLUSION

I should like to summarize this review by pointing out that conclusive structural data exist for only a limited number of bilirubin conjugates.

1. Alkali-labile conjugates comprise xylosides and glucosides of bilirubin identified in dog bile, and disaccharide-containing conjugates present in human bile. The existence of a simple glucuronide in either human or rat bile is controversial.

2. Alkali-stable conjugates have been found in human, dog and rat bile. Neither of these has been reliably identified with the exception of a polypeptide conjugate isolated from humans. Evidence for the existence of bilirubin sulphate in human, dog and rat bile is not convincing.

3. It is now generally accepted that true monoconjugates of bilirubin occur in bile.

Work performed in the author's laboratory was supported by the Fritz
Hoffmann-La Roche Stiftung and the Swiss National Science Foundation,
Grant 3.518.71.

REFERENCES

Billing, B.H. & Jansen, F.H. (1971) Enigma of bilirubin conjugation.
Gastroenterology 61, 258-260

Billing, B.H., Cole, P.G. & Lathe, G.H. (1957) The excretion of bilirubin as a diglucuronide giving the direct van den Bergh reaction.
Biochem. J. 65, 774-784

Blackstock, W.P., Kuenzle, C.C. & Eugster, C.H. (1974) 3-C-Hydroxy-
methyl-D-riburonic acid synthesis of the branched-chain uronic acid &
comparison with a carbohydrate component of a naturally occurring
bilirubin conjugate. Helv. Chim. Acta 57, 1003-1009

Cole, P.G., Lathe, G.H. & Billing, B.H. (1954) Separation of the bile pigments of serum, bile and urine. Biochem. J. 57, 514-518

Compernolle, F., Jansen, F.H. & Heirwegh, K.P.M. (1970) Mass-spectrometric study of the azopigments obtained from bile pigments with
diazotized ethyl anthranilate. Biochem. J. 120, 891-894

Compernolle, F., van Hees, G.P., Fevery, J. & Heirwegh, K.P.M. (1971)
Mass-spectrometric structure elucidation of dog bile azopigments as
the acyl glycosides of glucopyranose and xylopyranose. Biochem. J.
125, 811-819

Etter-Kjelsaas, H. & Kuenzle, C.C. (1975) A polypeptide conjugate
of bilirubin from human bile. Biochim. Biophys. Acta 400, 83-94

Fevery, J., van Hees, G.P., Leroy, P., Compernolle, F. & Heirwegh,
K.P.M. (1971) Excretion in dog bile of glucose and xylose conjugates
of bilirubin. Biochem. J. 125, 803-810

Fevery, J., Leroy, P. & Heirwegh, K.P.M. (1972a) Enzymic transfer of
glucose and xylose from uridine diphosphate glucose and uridine diphosphate xylose to bilirubin by untreated and digitonin-activated
preparations from rat liver. Biochem. J. 129, 619-633

Fevery, J., Leroy, P., van de Vijver, M. & Heirwegh, K.P.M. (1972b)
Structures of bilirubin conjugates synthesized in vitro from bilirubin and uridine diphosphate glucuronic acid, uridine diphosphate
glucose or uridine diphosphate xylose by preparations from rat liver.
Biochem. J. 129, 635-644

Fulop, M., Sandson, J. & Brazeau, P. (1964) Dialysability of conjugated bilirubin from plasma of jaundiced dogs and patients. Lancet 1964 I, 1017-1019

Fulop, M., Sandson, J. & Brazeau, P. (1965) Dialysability, protein binding and renal excretion of plasma conjugated bilirubin. J. Clin. Invest. 44, 666-680

Gent, W.L., Haslewood, G.A.D. & Montesdeoca, G. (1971) Macromolecular compounds of bilirubin in human bile. Biochem. J. 122, 15-16P

Gordon, E.R., Dadoun, M., Goresky, C.A., Chan, T.-H. & Perlin, A.S. (1974) The isolation of an azobilirubin β-D-monoglucoside from dog gall-bladder bile. Biochem. J. 143, 97-105

Gregory, C.H. (1963) Studies on conjugates bilirubin. III. Pigment I, a complex of conjugated and free bilirubin. J. Lab. Clin. Med. 61, 917-925

Gregory, C.H. & Watson, C.J. (1962) Studies of conjugated bilirubin. II. Problem of sulfates of bilirubin in vivo and in vitro. J. Lab. Clin. Med. 60, 17-30

Heirwegh, K.P.M., van Hees, G.P., Leroy, P., van Roy, F.P. & Jansen, F.H. (1970) Heterogeneity of bile pigment conjugates as revealed by chromatography of their ethyl anthranilate azopigments. Biochem. J. 120, 877-890

Heirwegh, K.P.M., van de Vijver, M. & Fevery, J. (1972) Assay and properties of digitonin-activated bilirubin uridine diphosphate glucuronyltransferase from rat liver. Biochem. J. 129, 605-618

Heirwegh, K.P.M., Fevery, J., Michiels, R., van Hees, G.P. & Compernolle, F. (1975) Separation by thin-layer chromatography and structure elucidation of bilirubin conjugates isolated from dog bile. Biochem. J. 145, 185-199

Hutchinson, D.W. & Johnson, B. (1972) The reaction between bilirubin and aromatic diazo compounds. Biochem. J. 127, 907-908

Isselbacher, K.J. & McCarthy, E.A. (1958) Identification of a sulfate conjugate of bilirubin in bile. Biochim. Biophys. Acta 29, 658-659

Isselbacher, K.J. & McCarthy, E.A. (1959) Studies on bilirubin sulfate and other nonglucuronide conjugates of bilirubin. J. Clin. Invest. 38, 645-651

Jansen, P.L.M. (1973) The isomerisation of bilirubin monoglucuronide. Clin. Chim. Acta 49, 233-240

Jansen, F.H. & Billing, B.H. (1971) The identification of monoconjugates of bilirubin in bile as amide derivatives. Biochem. J. 125, 917-919

Jansen, F.H. & Stoll, M.S. (1971) Separation and structural analysis of vinyl- and isovinyl-azobilirubin derivatives. Biochem. J. 125, 585-597

Jirsa, M. & Večerek, B. (1958) Neue Bilirubinderivate. I. Ihr Vergleich mit Gallen- und Serumbilirubin. Hoppe-Seyler's Z. Physiol. Chem. 311, 87-92

Jirsa, M., Večerek, B. & Ledvina, M. (1956) Di- and mono-taurobilirubin similar to a directly reacting form of bilirubin in serum. Nature 177, 895

Jirsa, M., Ledvina, M. & Večerek, B. (1958) Neue Bilirubinderivate. II. Chromatographie der Azofarbstoffe des direkten Bilirubins und des Taurobilirubins mit inversen Phasen. Hoppe-Seyler's Z. Physiol. Chem. 311, 93-95

Kuenzle, C.C. (1970a) Bilirubin conjugates of human bile. Isolation of phenylazo derivatives of bile bilirubin. Biochem. J. 119, 387-394

Kuenzle, C.C. (1970b) Bilirubin conjugates of human bile. Nuclear-magnetic-resonance, infrared and optical spectra of model compounds. Biochem. J. 119, 395-409

Kuenzle, C.C. (1970c) Bilirubin conjugates of human bile. The excretion of bilirubin as the acyl glycosides of aldobiouronic acid, pseudoaldobiouronic acid and hexuronosylhexuronic acid, with a branched-chain hexuronic acid as one of the components of the hexuronosylhexuronide. Biochem. J. 119, 411-435

Kuenzle, C.C. (1973) in The liver. Quantitative aspects of structure and function. (Paumgartner, G. & Preisig, R., eds.), pp. 215-219, Karger, Basel

Kuenzle, C.C. (1975) Microheterogeneity of complex glycosides of bilirubin from human bile. Experientia 31, 626-627

Noir, B.A. & Nanet, H. (1974) A study of the ethyl anthranilate azo derivatives of bilirubin sulphate. Confirmation of the existence of bilirubin sulphate conjugates in bile. Biochim. Biophys. Acta 372, 230-236

Noir, B.A., Groszman, R.J. & De Walz, A.T. (1966) Studies on bilirubin sulphate. Biochim. Biophys. Acta 117, 297-304

Noir, B.A., De Walz, A.T. & Rodriguez Garay, E.A. (1970) Studies on
the bilirubin sulphate conjugate excreted in human bile. Biochim.
Biophys. Acta 222, 15-27

Nosslin, B. (1960) The direct diazo reaction of bile pigments in
serum. Experimental and clinical studies. Scand. J. Clin. Lab. Invest. 12, Suppl. 49

Ostrow, J.D. & Murphy, N.H. (1970) Isolation and properties of conjugated bilirubin from bile. Biochem. J. 120, 311-327

Salmon, M., Fenselau, C., Cukier, J.O. & Odell, G.B. (1974) Rapid
transesterification of bilirubin glucuronides in methanol. Life Sci.
15, 2069-2078

Schachter, D. (1957) The nature of the glucuronide in direct-reacting bilirubin. Science 126, 507-508

Schmid, R. (1957) The identification of "direct-reacting" bilirubin
as bilirubin glucuronide. J. Biol. Chem. 229, 881-888

Schoenfield, L.J. & Bollman, J.L. (1963) Further studies on the nature and source of the conjugated bile pigments. Proc. Soc. Exp.
Biol. Med. 112, 929-932

Schoenfield, L.J., Bollman, J.L. & Hoffman, H.N. (1962) Sulfate and
glucuronide conjugates of bilirubin in experimental liver injury.
J. Clin. Invest. 41, 133-140

Tenhunen, R. (1965) Studies on bilirubin and its metabolism. Ann.
Med. Exp. Biol. Fenn. 43, Suppl. 6

van Damme, B., Fevery, J. & Heirwegh, K.P.M. (1971) Altered composition of bilirubin conjugates in rat bile after obstruction of the
common bile duct. Experientia 27, 27-28

Vegas, F.R. (1963) Chromatographic behavior on ion-exchange paper
of bilirubin conjugated with sulfate and glucuronide. Anal. Biochem.
5, 465-470

Weber, A.P., Schalm, L. & Witmans, J. (1963) Bilirubin monoglucuronide (pigment I): A complex. Acta Med. Scand. 173, 19-24

DISCUSSION OF LECTURE BY C.C. KUENZLE

Haslewood:    I was interested to hear that you had identified the
macromolecule.    The substance which we described in a crude form
was very strongly associated with the mucin of the bile.    What
do you think is the possibility of the existence of a compound
formed by covalent linkage of bilirubin and the mucilaginous
fraction of bile?

Kuenzle:    It is possible that biliary mucins do contribute to
binding of bilirubin in bile, but I have no real evidence for
that.    We have found it very difficult to remove these contaminat-
ing mucins from our polypeptide conjugate.    We were interested
in trying to isolate one single, pure compound rather than trying
to evaluate all the possible structures of compounds which may
occur in bile.

Ostrow:    The essence of the controversy between you and Dr.
Heirwegh seems to revolve around two things; one is that you
suggest that he does not find your disaccharides because he is
breaking them down to single sugar conjugates during the
diazotisation procedure.    On the other hand, he is concerned,
as some other people are, by the fact you find no glucuronide,
and say it is not present.    However, your total recovery of
material is of the order of one per cent.    It seems to me that
the way to resolve this controversy would be to take a
disaccharide conjugate, treat it with ethyl anthranilate and
see if it does hydrolyse.    I got the impression that you have
indeed done this.    Could you give us a little more detail on
your evidence about this?

Kuenzle:    Do you mean with the azo derivatives?

Ostrow:    No, with the conjugates before diazotisation.    Dr.
Heirwegh has a method for isolating a whole variety of different
conjugates - perhaps 18 or 20 types - by a thin-layer system
without diazotisation.    Then he diazotised the fractions and
showed that monoconjugates were clearly present.    There is
another problem which comes into this: there is a type of
exchange which can occur with conjugates, which is a variation
of aminolysis or methanolysis reaction which you describe.    If

you take conjugated bilirubin isolated from bile and you put it in a solution which is weakly alkaline and contains other sugars, then the side-chains switch around very readily.  So, in your isolation procedure, if your columns contained different sugar moieties you might put sugars onto the side-chains and you would get false conjugates.  This would be unlikely to happen with Dr. Heirwegh's silica gel technique.

Kuenzle:  I do not know where the sugars would come from in my siliconised silica gel columns, so I cannot visualise how such an exchange could occur.  Our conditions are not alkaline, which would be necessary for aminolysis to occur.

Hofmann:  Is there any precedent in other biological systems for the formation of aldobiuronic or pseudoaldobiuronic acids in, say, hepatic transformation of other xenobiotics?

Kuenzle:  I am not aware of any studies which show that such structures can be formed.

Arias:  The material found in jaundiced urine and serum is easily dialyzable, filtratable and of low molecular weight with no peptide reaction.  Has this compound any relationship to those you have been talking about?  Would you restate the evidence for the covalent binding of bilirubin to this polypeptide?  Is it possible that B4 and B5 could be galacturonic conjugates? Finally, what is the biosynthetic mechanism and biological function of these complex sugar conjugates, particularly from the standpoint of disorders characterised by deficiency of UDP-glucuronyl transferases?

Kuenzle:  The evidence for covalent linkage has been obtained by showing that treatment with various strong denaturing conditions, such as 6-molar guanidine, solvents with highly alkaline pH and so on, does not release the chromophore from the pigment.  The pigment always remained attached to the protein.  The uronic acid in B5 is definitely not galacturonic acid, because we know that this unspecified acid forms a lactone, which galacturonic acid cannot do.  In fact it cannot be any of the normal, straight-chain hexuronic acids, such as mannuronic acid, etc.  So it is something new, but I do not know what it is.

As for the biosynthesis question;  B5 and B6 are the most prominent pigments in our studies, and would account for about 70 per cent of the total conjugates.  Since, in B5 and B6 the glucuronic acid moiety is attached directly to the propionic acid side-chain, I think the disaccharide is synthesized in two steps.  First the attachment of glucuronic acid by the usual pathway via UDPGA, and then attachment of a second sugar residue to the already covalently bound glucuronic acid.

# COMPARATIVE STUDIES ON THE STRUCTURES OF CONJUGATED

# BILIRUBIN-IXα AND CHANGES IN CHOLESTASIS

K.P.M. Heirwegh, G.P. Van Hees, N. Blanckaert,
J. Fevery, and F. Compernolle

Katholieke Universiteit te Leuven
Rega Instituut
B-3000 Leuven, Belgium

It is classically admitted that the major bile pigment resulting from heme catabolism in mammals is bilirubin-IXα (Lathe, 1972;
Gray et al., 1972). The IIIα- and XIIIα-isomers that could arise
from bilirubin-IXα by dipyrrole exchange occurring in aqueous solution at about neutral pH (McDonagh and Assisi, 1972) could not be
detected in bile from man, cat, dog and rat (McDonagh and Assisi,
1972; Kuenzle, 1970a; Jansen, 1974; Heirwegh et al., 1975). Small
amounts of non-α isomers such as bilirubin-IXβ have been found in
bile from dog and pig (Petryka, 1966; O'Carra and Colleran, 1970;
Tipton and Gray, 1971), but only a few species were examined. According to a recent screening study bilirubin-IXβ and/or -IXδ is
widely distributed in the animal kingdom, and even the IXγ-isomer
has been detected in some species (our unpublished work).

Except under special conditions (see below) bilirubin-IXα is
excreted nearly exclusively in the conjugated form. For all practical purposes the fraction of bile pigment excreted as unconjugated bilirubin-IXα can be ignored entirely. Its concentration in
normal urine is insignificant (Fevery et al., 1968) in contrast to
earlier reports (for references see, With, 1968). In bile from normal adults and from liver patients bilirubin-IXα represents less
than 1% of total bile pigment (Fevery et al., 1972; our unpublished
work). Most claims to the contrary are ill-founded as they rely on
uncritical application of chloroform extraction procedures or on the
assumption that the difference between total and direct-reacting bilirubin equals unconjugated bilirubin (for an evaluation of these
methods see, Heirwegh et al., 1974). In a number of animal species
the concentration of bilirubin-IXα , estimated by t.l.c., is very

low in bile (Thompson and Hofmann, 1973). In contrast, in bile of amphibia diazo-positive material yielding azodipyrrole but no conjugated azopigment has been detected (Lester and Schmid, 1961). The results suggest that bilirubin-IXα is excreted in such species but its relative importance with respect to heme turn-over is not known. Relatively high amounts of bilirubin-IXα, compared to total bile pigment, present in bile of species that conjugate  bilirubin-IXα very poorly (Crigler-Najjar syndrome of man) or not at all (Gunn rat) represent only a small fraction of heme turn-over (Schmid and Hammaker, 1963). In both species phototherapy increases the biliary output of bilirubin-IXα (Ostrow, 1971; Lund and Jacobsen, 1974; Thaler et al., 1973). A similar increase in the Gunn rat occurring after intravenous administration of bile from normal rats has been explained by the excretion of a complex of bilirubin-IXα and bilirubin-IXα diglucuronide (Callahan and Schmid, 1969). However, no stimulation was found when purified conjugated bilirubin was used instead of bile (Billing et al., 1973).

The non-α isomers, in contrast to bilirubin-IXα, apparently do not require conjugation in order to be excreted (our unpublished work). For species that excrete biliverdin such as the chicken (Lin et al., 1974) and some amphibia (Lester and Schmid, 1961), it would be of great interest to investigate the isomeric composition of the bile pigment and to establish whether conjugation is needed for excretion or not.

In general, it would appear that investigations of the conjugative metabolism of bile pigments in man and currently used laboratory animals can be focussed on the formation of conjugated bilirubin-IXα. It is expected, however, that comparative biochemical studies may reveal interesting deviations from this tentative rule (Lester and Schmid, 1961; Cornelius et al., 1975). Methodology for the direct separation and structure elucidation of conjugated bilirubins is forthcoming (Brodersen and Jacobsen, 1969; Thompson and Hofmann, 1971; Salmon et al., 1974; Heirwegh et al., 1974, 1975). These studies (Heirwegh et al., 1975) and previous work with dipyrrolic azo-derivatives (Compernolle et al., 1970, 1971; Fevery et al. 1971, 1972; Gordon et al., 1974; Heirwegh et al., 1970, 1973-1975; Kuenzle, 1970b) indicate that bilirubin conjugation may follow either  a simple or a complex course depending on species and pathological state. In particular, various types of mono- and diconjugates containing either one or two of several conjugating groups have been detected (Heirwegh et al., 1975) analogous to the biological fate of some steroids (Layne, 1970). Obstruction of the common bile duct in experimental animals and various pathological conditions in man induce a typical change from a relatively simple to a more complex pattern of conjugation of bilirubin-IXα (Van Damme et al., 1971; Fevery et al., 1972). In contrast, glycosidic conjugation of xenobiotics seems to be restricted to the formation of monoconjugates of glucuronic acid (Dutton, 1966, 1971). Therefore,

studies with bilirubin-IXα and/or with steroids provide more powerful tools to probe the conjugative metabolism of endogenous compounds.

In the present paper, the conjugation of bilirubin-IXα in vivo
is reviewed in so far as it is reflected in the nature of the end
products found in bile. Recent development of methods for the separation and structure elucidation of conjugated bilirubins is expected to open new areas of research and to stimulate efforts to further elucidate at the molecular level the mechanisms of conjugation
and excretion of bilirubin. Some aspects of mechanisms of formation of conjugated bilirubin-IXα have been reviewed elswhere (Heirwegh et al., 1973).

## STRUCTURE ELUCIDATION OF CONJUGATED BILIRUBINS

The concepts about the structure of conjugated bilirubin have
been  changed a number of times since Talafant (1956), Billing et
al. (1957) and Schmid (1957) postulated that bilirubin-IXα is excreted as a simple glucuronide in human bile and in icteric urine. Structure assignment was based on analyses of dipyrrolic azo-derivatives.
By submitting preparations of bile pigment to reversed-phase column
chromatography Billing et al. (1957) achieved separation into bilirubin-IXα and two more hydrophilic tetrapyrroles called pigment I
and II. Azopigment analysis showed that the structures of pigment
I and II were compatible, respectively, with mono- and diglucuronides of bilirubin-IXα. As heating of pigment-I produced mixtures of
bilirubin-IXα and pigment-II alternative identification of pigment-I
as a bilirubin-IXα : bilirubin-IXα diglucuronide molecular 1:1 complex was considered possible, though less likely (Billing et al.,
1957). Confirmation of the observation (Nosslin, 1960) and the
apparent impossibility to rechromatograph pigment-I (Gregory, 1963;
Weber et al., 1963) strengthened the hypothesis of complex formation. The conjugative metabolism of bilirubin-IXα thus appeared to
be reducible to the unique transformation: bilirubin-IXα → bilirubin-IXα diglucuronide. However, successful rechromatography of pigment-I was achieved subsequently by Schoenfield and Bollman (1963)
and by Heirwegh et al. (1970). Also, Ostrow and Murphy (1970) could
not demonstrate exchange of radioactive bilirubin-IXα. Furthermore,
the preparation and characterization of stable monoamide derivatives
seems to prove unequivocally that monoconjugated bilirubin-IXα exists (Jansen and Billing, 1971). Several animal species are predominant, and some even exclusive, monoconjugate excretors (Our unpublished work). In dog bile a variety of monoglycosides of bilirubin-IXα have been detected (Heirwegh et al., 1975).

The conversion of pigment-I into two bile pigments that was observed by some authors but not by others deserves some comment. Recently, Jansen (1973) showed that in aqueous solution bilirubin-IXα

monoglucuronide may isomerize into a mixture of bilirubin-IXα and
its diglucuronide. Determination of the isomeric composition of
the reaction products (the ratio IIIα- : IXα- : XIIIα-isomers) indicated that the conversion was due to dipyrrole exchange (McDonagh
and Assisi, 1972; Jansen, 1973). Differences in the treatments (pH,
solvent composition) to which pigment-I had been submitted probably
explain the contradictory results obtained with regard to its stability (see above). The reaction is inhibited by binding protein
(McDonagh and Assisi, 1972; Jansen, 1974).

Since the formulation of the complex-formation hypothesis in
1963 many observations in the bilirubin field have been interpreted
on this basis. This has led to some completely invalid results; in
most cases, however, re-interpretation on the basis of the existence
of both mono- and diconjugated bilirubin is possible (for some examples see, Heirwegh et al., 1973). Obviously, demonstration that
monoconjugated bilirubin exists does not exclude per se the possible occurrence of the mentioned complex in vivo. Spectral studies
of Jacobsen (1970) indicate that in aqueous solution at pH 8.2 bilirubin-IXα and its diglucuronide form a complex with an association
constant of $5 \times 10^5$ M$^{-1}$. Complex formation is inhibited by urea, ethanol and Tween-80, and probably also by binding of the bile pigments
to protein. Evidence supporting complex formation in vivo (Callahan and Schmid, 1969) has been refuted (Billing et al., 1973).

The initial concept of the formation of simple glucuronides
from bilirubin-IXα (Talafant, 1956; Billing et al., 1957; Schmid,
1957) has recently been challenged in two apparently contradictory
ways (1) by Kuenzle (1970b, 1973), and (2) by Gordon et al. (1974)
and our group (Compernolle et al., 1970, 1971; Fevery et al., 1971,
1972; Heirwegh et al., 1970, 1973-1975). As we feel that the conjugative metabolism of bilirubin-IXα in animal species with cholestatic syndromes differs significantly from that in the normal state we will discuss these topics separately.

Conjugated Bilirubin-IXα in Normal Animals

In the present context it is of importance to define clearly
what is understood by a normal animal. In most previous studies
human bile was obtained by T-tube drainage from patients on whom
cholecystectomy had been performed. Even if clinical symptoms of
jaundice are absent the bile pigment metabolism could be perturbed
to some extent. Indeed, deposits of conjugated bilirubin can sometimes be observed by histochemical methods (Desmet et al., 1968) in
human liver cells even when bilirubin concentrations in serum are
normal (Desmet et al., 1970) and probably more so when cholelithiasis is present (Naccarato et al., 1974). By studying bile from
patients i.a. with cholelithiasis Fevery et al. (1972) demonstrated
the formation of so-called β-azopigments whereas these derivatives

were not detected when bile from healthy volunteers was analysed. Therefore, for the present work bile was obtained in normal situations in the following ways. (1) It was obtained from healthy, adult volunteers before and after MgSO4 instillation by duodenal intubation (Fevery et al.,1972). (2) Rats were provided with a catheter brought into the common bile duct and were placed in restraining cages. The catheters should be of sufficiently wide internal diameter to permit free flow. After the animals had reached their normal body temperature and had recovered from the anaesthesia bile collection was started. These precautions are imperative as even partial hindrance to bile flow and/or the anaesthesia may cause alterations of the bile pigment composition (Van Damme et al., 1971; Fevery et al., 1972). Similar changes have been noted in studies with Guinea pigs (Our unpublished work). (3) The other animal species tested had no obvious illnesses. In particular, the dogs were selected by a veterinary doctor. Whenever possible both hepatic bile and gall bladder bile were analysed.

Studies of dipyrrolic azo-derivatives. On treatment of 1 mole of a diazo-positive tetrapyrrolic bile pigment with a diazo-reagent 2 moles of dipyrrolic azopigment(s) are obtained (Fischer and Orth, 1968; Overbeek et al., 1955; Kuenzle, 1970a; Compernolle et al., 1970, 1971; Jansen and Stoll, 1971; Salmon et al., 1974). The azo-derivatives, and in particular those obtained with diazotized ethyl anthranilate (Van Roy and Heirwegh, 1968), are more stable than the parent tetrapyrrolic pigments. For this reason nearly all structural studies on bile pigments have been done, so far, after azopigment formation. Unfortunately, in general, calculation of the composition of the parent pigments from the relative amounts of dipyrrolic azo-derivatives is impossible. Information can still be obtained about the following: (1) provided certain conditions are met (Fevery et al., 1972; Heirwegh et al., 1973) determination of the fraction of unconjugated azodipyrrole allows one to calculate the ratio of monoconjugated to diconjugated bilirubin-IXα; (2) separation and structure identification of the azopigments (Brodersen and Jacobsen, 1969; Heirwegh et al., 1974) yields information about dipyrrolic moieties, with or without conjugating groups, that are present in tetrapyrrolic bile pigments.

The use of diazo-reagents that bear no charged activating group facilitates extraction and subsequent separation and structure elucidation of the azo-derivatives (Heirwegh et al., 1974). Separation and purification of azopigment glycosides before sugar analysis has the advantage that the sugars are protected at C1 which, in general, is the most vulnerable site of reducing sugars.

The azopigments obtained from normal bile can be separated by t.l.c. into several components. They have been denoted by Greek letters (Heirwegh et al., 1970). From bile of man and the rat two major derivatives were obtained: azopigment-$\alpha_0$ (azodipyrrole) and

azopigment-δ (azodipyrrole β-D-glucopyranuronoside). Dog bile yielded, in addition, two azopigments: azopigment-$\alpha_2$ (azodipyrrole β-D-
xylopyranoside) and azopigment-$\alpha_3$ (azodipyrrole β-D-glucopyranoside). A screening study done with laboratory animals and commercial
species revealed considerable species variation with respect to the
four derivatives mentioned (Our unpublished work). Some animal species even seem to excrete predominantly diazo-positive bile pigments
that yield conjugated azopigments of unknown structures (Cornelius
et al., 1975). The subsequent discussion will be restricted to the
components $\alpha_2$, $\alpha_3$ and δ. For reasons that will become clear the
azopigments studied by Kuenzle (1970b) will be discussed below under
'Conjugated bilirubin-IXα in animals with cholestatic syndromes'.

     (A) The identification of azopigments $\alpha_2$ and $\alpha_3$ (derived from
dog bile) as azodipyrrole β-D-xylopyranoside and azodipyrrole β-D-
glucopyranoside, respectively, is based on the following evidence.
Treatment of purified preparations of azopigments $\alpha_2$ and $\alpha_3$ with
acetic anhydride and pyridine produced acetylated derivatives that
were separated by t.l.c. into mixtures of vinyl and isovinyl isomers of conjugated azodipyrroles. The fragmentation patterns and
molecular ions found in the mass spectra of acetylated azopigments
$\alpha_2$ and $\alpha_3$ were consistent, respectively, with a pentose and a hexose conjugated to azodipyrrole (Compernolle et al., 1971). The nature of the sugar moieties, their pyranose ring structures and their
attachment at C1 to the aglcyone were demonstrated by the isolation
of the 1-bromides of xylopyranose tri-acetate and glucopyranose te-
tra-acetate after reaction of the acetylated azopigments with hydrogen bromide and acetic acid. The 1-bromides and further derivatives
were identified by g.l.c.-m.s. (Compernolle et al., 1971). These
studies establish unequivocally the structures of the acetylated
azopigments $\alpha_2$ and $\alpha_3$ as the fully acetylated xylopyranoside and
glucopyranoside of azodipyrrole, respectively.

     In view of Kuenzle's claim (Kuenzle, 1970b, 1973) that human
bile contains exclusively disaccharidic conjugates of bilirubin-IXα
the question may be raised whether acetylation of conjugated azopigments could have removed completely and furthermore have destroyed
any terminal sugar residues. It may be noted first that acetylation with acetic anhydride in pyridine solution has been used by
Kuenzle (1970b) in his studies of disaccharidic conjugates obtained
from human bile. Further, various attempts to demonstrate oligo-
saccharidic structures for azopigments $\alpha_2$ and $\alpha_3$ have failed completely. (1) Treatment of azopigments $\alpha_2$ and $\alpha_3$, on thin-layer plates, with ammonia vapour followed by sugar chromatography detected
only xylose and glucose, respectively (Fevery et al., 1971; Gordon
et al., 1974). Note that in this procedure the risk of loosing any
sugar is virtually non-existent as between application of azopigment and final t.l.c. of sugar no material ever leaves the plate.
Formation of the carboxylic acid amide of azodipyrrole proved ester
linkage of the sugars to the propionic acid side chain of the agly-

cone (Compernolle et al., 1970, 1971; Fevery et al., 1971). The same conclusions were reached when azopigments $\alpha_2$ and $\alpha_3$, obtained from human bile, were analysed (Our unpublished work). (2) Ammonolysis of the conjugated azopigments followed by isolation of the sugars and separation by anion-exchange chromatography in boric acid confirmed the previous conclusions (Fevery et al., 1971). (3) The sensitivity of the ester linkages to attack by β-xylosidase and β-glucosidase (Fevery et al., 1971; Gordon et al., 1974) and, in particular, inhibition of the latter enzymic process (Fevery et al. 1971) by glucono-1,5-lactone (Conchie et al., 1967) strongly supported β-D-monoglycosidic structures and confirmed binding at C1. From azopigment $\alpha_3$, glucose (assayed with glucose oxidase) and azodipyrrole were formed in a 1:1 ratio (Gordon et al., 1974). Doubts raised against the diagnostic value of tests with a related glycosidase, β-glucuronidase (Kuenzle, 1973) will be commented upon below. (4) Methanolysis with water-free sodium methoxide (2 h, room temperature, pH 8-9) of azopigment $\alpha_3$ liberated only glucose in an azodipyrrole:sugar ratio equal to one. The nature of the sugar was verified by applying g.l.c.-m.s. to various derivatives (Gordon et al., 1974).

We therefore conclude that not only the acetylated derivatives of azopigments $\alpha_2$ and $\alpha_3$ but also the unsubstituted azopigments are simple glycosides of β-D-xylopyranose and β-D-glucopyranose, respectively.

(B) With a few modifications structure assignment to azopigment-δ (obtained from normal bile of man, the dog and the rat and from synthetic bilirubin-IXα glucuronide) followed essentially the same course as adopted for structure elucidation of azopigments $\alpha_2$ and $\alpha_3$. The diazo-reagent was prepared from stoichiometric amounts of $NaNO_2$ (at the same concentration as used in the standard procedure of Van Roy and Heirwegh, 1968) and ethyl anthranilate; coupling of conjugated bile pigment in diluted bile (pH 6, 0°C, 1 h) is complete (Our unpublished work). Amongst other advantages the present procedure operates under much milder conditions than the routine assay (pH 2.7, 25°C, 30 min) and avoids the use of an excess of aromatic amine. Synthetic reference δ-azopigment was prepared from enzymic incubation mixtures containing microsomal material from rat liver, bilirubin-IXα and UDP-glucuronic acid (Heirwegh et al., 1972).

In 1970 Compernolle et al. submitted the trimethylsilyl derivative of the methyl ester of δ-azopigment from normal rat bile to mass spectrometric analysis. The fragmentation pattern and the molecular ion were compatible with a derivative of a simple hexuronide of azodipyrrole. Loss of a terminal sugar residue was suggested by Kuenzle (1973) as this author (Kuenzle, 1970b) showed that sylilation of isolated aldobiuronic acids, pseudoaldobiuronic acids and hexuronosylhexuronic acid (obtained from conjugated azopigments derived from post-operative human T-tube bile) caused complete degra-

dation of the sugar at the non-reducing terminus. We have now further investigated this controversy (our unpublished work). The fully acetylated methyl esters of δ-azopigment from the biological
sources mentioned and synthetic material were analysed by mass spectrometry. Their fragmentation patterns and molecular ions were
compatible again with simple hexuronoside structures. Formation
and analysis of 1-bromide derivatives of the acetylated sugar moieties, done essentially as outlined above for azopigments $\alpha_2$ and $\alpha_3$
established the pyranose ring structure for glucuronic acid and attachment at C1 to the aglycone. These studies demonstrate beyond
doubt that the fully acetylated methyl ester of δ-azopigment from
normal bile (man, dog, rat) and of synthetic reference material is
a derivative of azodipyrrole glucopyranuronoside.

      Does this conclusion also apply to the underivatized δ-azopig-
ments? The following observations and comments support a positive
answer. (1) Both after silylation and acetylation of the methylester
of δ-azopigments, derivatives of a simple hexuronide were demonstrated. The acetylation procedure used by us has also been applied by
Kuenzle (1970b) in preparing acetylated derivatives of hexuronic
acid-containing disaccharides. It is highly unlikely that the free
disaccharides would resist acetylation whereas the terminal sugar
residue would be lost when the same treatment is applied to the same sugar groups  connected to azodipyrrole at C1. (2) The δ-azopigments from the biological sources  mentioned  and synthetic
azodipyrrole β-D-glucopyranuronoside showed identical t.l.c. mo-
bilities. Identity persisted after formation of the methyl esters (treatment with diazomethane) and further, after acetylation.
The fully acetylated methyl esters separated each into identical
pairs of vinyl and isovinyl isomers. Monosaccharide (reference
δ-azopigment) and hypothetical disaccharides (other δ-azopigments),
would be expected to be separable by t.l.c., both in the derivatized and underivatized forms. Loss of terminal sugar residues as
a consequence of methylation is unlikely as a methylation procedure
similar to that used by us has been applied by Kuenzle (1970b). (3)
The t.l.c. procedure used for separation of sugars liberated by ammonolysis allowed a clear distinction between glucuronic acid and
galacturonic acid. A single spot moving as glucuronic acid was observed. Hexuronic acid-containing disaccharides are expected to
show smaller $R_F$ values, as observed by Kuenzle (1970b) for paper
chromatography. The formation of the carboxylic acid amide of azodipyrrole indicated binding of sugar in ester linkage to the propionic acid side chain of azodipyrrole. (4) β-Glucuronidase has
been shown to attack specifically terminal β-D-glucuronyl and β-D-
galacturonyl residues leaving structures with hexuronic acid at
non-terminal positions intact (Levvy and Conchie, 1966). Critical
application of the test requires parallel demonstration of inhibition of hydrolysis by saccharo-1,4-lactone (Conchie et al., 1967),
as β-glycosidase preparations are frequently contaminated by related hydrolases. The value of the test has been put in doubt by

Kuenzle (1973) as treatment of azopigments B5 and B6 (disaccharidic conjugates of azodipyrrole containing glucuronic acid at the reducing terminus) liberated azodipyrrole. This observation was interpreted to demonstrate endoglycosidase activity for β-glucuronidase. However, the nature of the sugar(s) liberated was not established. Also, no controls were made with saccharo-1,4-lactone. Therefore, Kuenzle's observations (Kuenzle, 1970b) do not invalidate the admitted specificity of β-glucuronidase.

We conclude that not only the derivatized δ-azopigments but also the parent azopigments correspond to azodipyrrole β-D-glucopyranuronoside. This applies to δ-azopigment obtained from synthetic bilirubin glucuronide and from normal bile of man, the dog and the rat.

Bile pigment composition and structures of tetrapyrrolic conjugated pigments. Structural studies of azo-derivatives, in particular those obtained with diazo-reagents that do not bear a charged activating group, are valuable to elucidate the structures of dipyrrolic moieties of diazo-positive bile pigments (Heirwegh et al., 1974). However, in general, to establish the composition and structures of the parent tetrapyrrolic pigments separation before analysis is required (Heirwegh et al., 1975).

In 1957 Billing et al. developed a reversed-phase column chromatographic technique allowing separation of bile pigments from human bile into bilirubin-IXα and two bands of conjugated pigment(s). In our opinion the potential of this method has not been fully exploited. If, in the future, reversed-phase chromatography is used due attention should be given to temperature control, and to factors such as speed of elution that affect resolution of components. Possible changes due to dipyrrole exchange (McDonagh and Assisi, 1972; Jansen, 1973) should also be kept in mind. Several other methods for direct separation of conjugated bilirubin have been reviewed by Brodersen and Jacobsen (1969).

Thin-layer chromatography has great potential for separating complex mixtures of conjugated bile pigments (Tenhunen, 1965). A technique developed by Thompson and Hofmann (1971, 1973) avoids potential losses due to pre-extraction of biological samples but in its present state has insufficient resolving power. A succint description of a t.l.c. system applicable to extracted bile pigment has been given by Salmon et al. (1974). Similar separation procedures have been developed independently by Heirwegh et al. (1975) and micro-methods for elucidating the structures of the separated pigments have been established. Extraction from slightly acidified bile and development of thin-layer plates with neutral solvent systems did not induce dipyrrole exchange to any significant extent. Occasional finding of very small amounts of bilirubin-IXα methyl ester(s) (Heirwegh et al., 1975) indicates that in some experiments methanolysis (Salmon et al., 1974) may have occurred to a small extent. The technique is useful mainly for qualitative studies (Heirwegh et al., 1975). Depending on the biological sample analysed, procedures allowing nearly quantitative or quantitative extraction have now been developed (Our unpublished work). A full qualitative and quantitative exploration of the bile pigments of some representative animal species has still to be done.

In general, conjugated bilirubin-IXα consists of mono- and diconjugates. Based on determination of the azodipyrrole fraction estimates of monoconjugated bilirubin-IXα amounted to 20-100% of total conjugated bile pigment depending on the species examined (Our unpublished work).

Normal bile of man and the rat is expected to show a relatively simple composition as after treatment with diazo-reagent azodipyrrole β-D-glucopyranuronoside was the predominant conjugated azopigment (Fevery et al., 1972). In contrast, normal dog bile yielded three relatively important simple glycosides: the β-D-xylopyranoside, the β-D-glucopyranoside and the β-D-glucopyranuronoside of azodipyrrole (Compernolle et al., 1970, 1971; Fevery et al., 1971; our unpublished work). The expected complex composition of the parent bile pigments was born out by t.l.c. (Heirwegh et al., 1975). The separated pigments contained predominantly monoconjugates of xylose, glucose and glucuronic acid, and homogeneous diconjugates (e.g. the diglucuronide of bilirubin-IXα) and mixed diconjugates (e.g. the monoglucose monoglucuronic acid diester of bilirubin-IXα).

## Conjugates in Animals with Cholestatic Syndromes

Cholestasis is defined here as any condition that is characterized by impaired biliary secretion of bilirubin-IXα. In most species with the exception of the rat conjugated bilirubin accumulates in the hepatocytes. Usually there is conjugated hyperbilirubinaemia although its importance may differ strikingly in the increasing and decreasing phases of the cholestasis (Desmet et al., 1970; Naccarato et al., 1974). In such cases (pancreatic or hepatic duct carcinoma, obstruction of the bile duct by gall stones, primary biliary cirrhosis, benign recurrent cholestasis, Dubin-Johnson and Rotor syndromes, etc.) analysis of azopigments obtained by treating bile with diazotized ethyl anthranilate at pH 2.7 revealed typical deviations from the normal azopigment pattern (Fevery et al., 1972). Bile from normal adults yielded 11.1% of azodipyrrole, 9.4% of γ-azopigment and 75.4% of δ-azopigment (expressed as percentages of total azopigment). In the  patients, so-called β-azopigments (2-15% of total azo-colour) that were not obtained from normal bile, were detected; the γ-azopigment group was increased (12-35% of total azocolour). The changes were highly significant. The β- and γ-azopigments contain 1 mole of naphthoresorcinol-reactive hexuronic acid per 1 mole of azodipyrrole (Heirwegh et al., 1970).

Experimental mechanical and hydrostatic obstruction of the common bile duct in the rat (Van Damme et al., 1971; Fevery et al.,
1972) and in the Guinea pig (Our unpublished work) induces a rapid
change from the normal, simple azopigment pattern to one that is essentially the same as that found in patients with cholestatic syndromes. Releave of obstruction causes gradual return to normal
over 6 h. The increased complexity has now been demonstrated in
several other ways. For example, if 'cholestatic' bile is reacted
at pH 6 with diazotized ethyl anthranilate not containing an excess
of aromatic amine the β-azopigments are not formed and the γ-azopigments are not noticeably increased. However, the δ-material now
contains a mixture of conjugated azodipyrroles. Methyl ester formation, in general, showed at least three derivatives moving more rapidly than reference methyl ester prepared either from normal bile
(man, dog, rat) or from synthetic bilirubin glucuronide. For some
patients, material moving as the reference compound (methyl ester
of azodipyrrole β-D-glucopyranuronoside) was even lacking completely. Structure elucidation of the derivatives is under way.

Can the present studies be reconciled with Kuenzle's demonstration of disaccharidic bilirubin-IXα conjugates in human bile?
We must first explain why we prefer to discuss Kuenzle's work here
and not in the section on normal bile pigments. (1) Kuenzle (1970b)
obtained human bile by T-tube drainage from patients on whom cholecystectomy had been performed. Sensu stricto this is an abnormal
condition, although the patients were said to be clinically normal
at the time of surgical intervention (Kuenzle, 1973a). However,
in a discussion to the latter paper Dr. J. Fevery noted that bile
from some anicteric patients operated for cholelithiasis also yielded a typical 'cholestatic' azopigment pattern. It is difficult to
exclude the occurrence of a period of slight cholestasis before
removal of a gall bladder stone and accumulation of bile pigment in
the hepatocytes has been demonstrated in these patients, even with
serum bilirubin concentrations within the normal range (Desmet et
al., 1970; Naccarato et al., 1974). Further, anaesthesia is known
to decrease bile secretion and can even lead to post-operative hyperbilirubinaemia, especially when blood transfusions are given at
operation (Schmid et al., 1965; La Mont and Isselbacher, 1973). Also, the use of drainage tubes of a diameter that is insufficient to
allow free flow of bile induces cholestatic features (Our unpublished work). (2) Detailed studies of bile of healthy volunteers only demonstrated simple glycosides of bilirubin-IXα (this work).
Doubtlessly, Kuenzle's studies (1970b, 1973, 1973a) demonstrate a
complex bile pigment composition that is mirrored in some sense
by our findings for 'cholestatic' bile.

The disaccharidic conjugates detected by Kuenzle (1970b) have
not yet been confirmed independently in another laboratory. Some

aspects of Kuenzle's work may need further examination.  In particular, the validity of the proposed disaccharidic structures relies
heavily on rigorous exclusion of the possibility that rearrangement
or recombination of sugars would have occurred in the course of li-
berating the glycosidic moieties by ammonolysis in aqueous medium.

The authors express their gratitude to Professors G. Smets, J.
Vandenbroucke and J. De Groote for their encouragement and to Dr.
M.T. Campbell for linguistic help and critical remarks on the text.
Research done by the authors was supported in part by the Founda-
tion for Medical Scientific Research and the Foundation for Collec-
tive Research of Belgium.

## REFERENCES

Billing, B.H., P.G. Cole, and G.H. Lathe.  1957.  The excretion of
      bilirubin as a diglucuronide giving the direct van den Bergh
      reaction.  Biochem. J. 65:774-784.
Billing, B.H., F.H. Jansen, and E. Bilton.  1973.  The effect of
      bile depletion on the biliary excretion of unconjugated bili-
      rubin and bilirubin conjugates, p. 386-391.  In The liver.
      Quantitative aspects of structure and function (G. Paumgart-
      ner and R. Preisig, eds.). Karger, Basel.
Brodersen, R., and J. Jacobsen.  1969.  Separation and determina-
      tion of bile pigments.  Methods Biochem. Anal. 17:31-54.
Callahan, E.W., Jr., and R. Schmid.  1969.  Excretion of unconjuga-
      ted bilirubin in the bile of Gunn rats.  Gastroenterol.
      57:134-137.
Compernolle, F., F.H. Jansen, and K.P.M. Heirwegh.  1970.  Mass-
      spectrometric study of the azopigments obtained from bile
      pigments with diazotized ethyl anthranilate.  Biochem. J.
      120:891-894.
Compernolle, F., G.P. Van Hees, J. Fevery, and K.P.M. Heirwegh.1971.
      Mass-spectrometric structure elucidation of dog bile azopig-
      ments as the acyl glycosides of glucopyranose and xylopyra-
      nose.  Biochem. J. 125:811-819.
Conchie, J., A.L. Gelman, and G.A. Levvy.  1967.  Inhibition of gly-
      cosidases by aldonolactones of corresponding configuration. The
      C-4- and C-6-specificity of β-glucosidase and β-galactosidase.
      Biochem. J. 103:609-615.
Cornelius, C.E., K.C. Kelley, and J.A. Himes.  1975.  Heterogeneity
      of bilirubin conjugates in several animal species.  Cornell
      Veterinarian 65:90-99.
Desmet, V.J., A.-M. Bullens, J. De Groote, and K.P.M. Heirwegh.  A
      new diazo reagent for specific staining of conjugated biliru-
      bin in tissue sections.  J. Histochem. Cytochem. 16:419-427.
Desmet, V.J., A.-M. Bullens, and J. De Groote.  1970.  A clinical
      and histochemical study of cholestasis.  Gut 11:516-523.
Dutton, G.J.  1966.  The biosynthesis of glucuronides, p. 185-299.

In Glucuronic acid: free and combined (G.J. Dutton, ed.). Academic Press, New York and London.

Dutton, G.J. 1971. Glucuronide-forming enzymes, Handb. Exp. Pharmacol. 28 (part 2):378-400.

Fevery, J., F.H. Jansen, J.A.T.P. Meuwissen, and K.P.M. Heirwegh. 1968. Bilirubin-like material in urine of normal adults. Clin. Chim. Acta 21:401-410.

Fevery, J., G.P. Van Hees, P. Leroy, F. Compernolle, and K.P.M. Heirwegh. 1971. Excretion in dog bile of glucose and xylose conjugates of bilirubin. Biochem. J. 125:803-810.

Fevery, J., B. Van Damme, R. Michiels, J. De Groote, and K.P.M. Heirwegh. 1972. Bilirubin conjugates in bile of man and rat in the normal state and in liver disease. J. Clin. Invest. 51:2482-2492.

Fischer, H., and H. Orth. 1968. Die Diazoreaktion, p. 717-723. In Die Chemie des Pyrrols, vol. 2 (part 1) (Akademische Verlagsgesellschaft, Leipzig, 1937). Johnson Reprint Corp., New York.

Gordon, E.R., M. Dadoun, C.A. Goresky, T.-H. Chan, and A.S. Perlin. 1974. The isolation of an azobilirubin β-D-monoglucoside from gall-bladder bile. Biochem. J. 143:97-105.

Gray, C.H., D.C. Nicholson, and G. Tipton. 1972. Degradation of haem compounds to bile pigments. Nature New Biology 239:5-8.

Gregory, C.H. 1963. Studies on conjugated bilirubin. III. Pigment I, a complex of conjugated and free bilirubin. J. Lab. Clin. Med. 61:917-925.

Heirwegh, K.P.M., G.P. Van Hees, P. Leroy, F.P. Van Roy, and F.H. Jansen. 1970. Heterogeneity of bile pigment conjugates as revealed by chromatography of their ethyl anthranilate azopigments. Biochem. J. 120:877-890.

Heirwegh, K.P.M., M. Van de Vijver, and J. Fevery. 1972. Assay and properties of digitonin-activated bilirubin uridine diphosphate glucuronyltransferase from rat liver. Biochem. J. 129:605-618.

Heirwegh, K.P.M., J.A.T.P. Meuwissen, and J. Fevery. 1973. Critique of the assay and significance of bilirubin conjugation. Advances Clin. Chem. 16:239-289.

Heirwegh, K.P.M., J. Fevery, J.A.T.P. Meuwissen, J. De Groote, F. Compernolle, V. Desmet, and F.P. Van Roy. 1974. Recent advances in separation and analysis of diazo-positive bile pigments. Methods Biochem. Anal. 22:205-250.

Heirwegh, K.P.M., J. Fevery, R. Michiels, G.P. Van Hees, and F. Compernolle. 1975. Separation by thin-layer chromatography and structure elucidation of bilirubin conjugates from dog bile. Biochem. J. 145:185-199.

Jacobsen, J. 1970. Dimerisation of bilirubin diglucuronide and formation of a complex of bilirubin and the diglucuronide. Scand. J. Clin. Lab. Invest. 26:395-398.

Jansen, F.H., and B.H. Billing. 1971. The identification of monoconjugates of bilirubin in bile as amide derivatives. Biochem.

J. 125:917-919.

Jansen, F.H., and M.S. Stoll. 1971. Separation and structural an-
    alysis of vinyl- and isovinyl-azobilirubin derivatives. Bio-
    chem. J. 125:585-597.

Jansen, P.L.M. 1973. The isomerisation of bilirubin monoglucuro-
    nide. Clin. Chim. Acta 49:233-240.

Jansen, P.L.M. 1974. The enzyme-catalysed formation of bilirubin
    diglucuronide by a solubilized preparation from cat liver mi-
    crosomes. Biochim. Biophys. Acta 338:170-182.

Kuenzle, C.C. 1970a. Bilirubin conjugates of human bile. Nuclear-
    magnetic-resonance, infrared and optical spectra of model com-
    pounds. Biochem. J. 119:395-409.

Kuenzle, C.C. 1970b. Bilirubin conjugates of human bile. The ex-
    cretion of bilirubin as the acyl glycosides of aldobiouronic
    acid, pseudoaldobiouronic acid and hexuronosylhexuronic acid,
    with a branched-chain hexuronic acid as one of the components
    of the hexuronosylhexuronide. Biochem. J. 119:411-435.

Kuenzle, C.C. 1973a. How can the novel report of disaccharide-
    containing bilirubin conjugates be reconciled with the gene-
    rally accepted view that bilirubin is excreted as a simple glu-
    curonide? p. 215-219. In The liver. Quantitative aspects of
    structure and function (G. Paumgartner and R. Preisig, eds.).
    Karger, Basel.

Kuenzle, C.C. 1973. Bilirubin conjugates of human bile, p. 351-
    386. In Metabolic conjugation and metabolic hydrolysis, vol.
    3 (W.H. Fishman, ed.). Academic Press, New York and London.

La Mont, J.T., and Isselbacher, K.J. 1973. Current concepts:
    post-operative jaundice. New Engl. J. Med. 288:305-307.

Lathe, G.H. 1972. The degradation of haem by mammals and its ex-
    cretion as conjugated bilirubin. Essays Biochem. 7:107-148.

Layne, D.S. 1970. New metabolic conjugates of steroids, p. 21-52.
    In Metabolic conjugation and metabolic hydrolysis, vol. 1 (W.
    H. Fishman, ed.). Academic Press, New York and London.

Lester, R., and R. Schmid. 1961. Bile pigment excretion in amphi-
    bia. Nature, Lond. 190:452.

Levvy, G.A., and J. Conchie. 1966. β-Glucuronidase and the hydroly-
    sis of glucuronides, p. 320-364. In Glucuronic acid: free and
    combined (G.J. Dutton, ed.). Academic Press, New York and Lon-
    don.

Lin, G.L., J.A. Himes, and C.E. Cornelius. 1974. Excretion of bi-
    lirubin and biliverdin in the chicken. Am. J. Physiol. 226:
    881-885.

Lund, H.T., and J. Jacobsen. 1972. Influence of phototherapy on
    unconjugated bilirubin in duodenal bile of newborn infants with
    hyperbilirubinemia. Acta Paediat. Scand. 61:693-696.

McDonagh, A.F., and F. Assisi. 1972. The ready isomerization of
    bilirubin-IXα in aqueous solution. Biochem. J. 129:797-800.

Naccarato, R., A. Rizzo, R. Farini, M. Chiaramonte, S. Pedrazzoli,
    G.F. Zanon, L. Okolicsanyi, and R. Polin. 1974. Liver his-
    tology, biochemical and immunochemical data in patients with

gallstones. Digestion 10:372.

Nosslin, B. 1960. The direct diazo reaction of bile pigments in serum. Scand. J. Clin. Lab. Invest. 12 (suppl. 49):1-176.

O'Carra, P., and E. Colleran. 1970. Separation and identification of biliverdin isomers and isomer analysis of phycobilins and bilirubin. J. Chromatog. 50:458-468.

Ostrow, J.D. 1971. Photocatabolism of labeled bilirubin in the congenitally jaundiced (Gunn) rat. J. Clin. Invest. 50:707-718.

Ostrow, J.D., and N.H. Murphy. 1970. Isolation and properties of conjugated bilirubin from bile. Biochem. J. 120:311-327.

Overbeek, J.T.G., C.L.J. Vink, and H. Deenstra. 1955. Kinetics of the formation of azobilirubin. Rec. Trav. Chim. Pays-Bas 74:85-97.

Salmon, M., C. Fenselau, J.O. Cukier, and G.B. Odell. 1974. Rapid transesterification of bilirubin glucuronides in methanol. Life Sciences 15:2069-2078.

Schmid, M., M.L. Hefti, R. Gattiker, H.J. Kistler, and A. Senning. 1965. Benign postoperative intrahepatic cholestasis. New Engl. J. Med. 272:545-550.

Schmid, R. 1957. The identification of direct-reacting bilirubin as bilirubin glucuronide. J. Biol. Chem. 229:881-888.

Schmid, R., and L. Hammaker. 1963. Metabolism and disposition of $^{14}$C-bilirubin in congenital nonhemolytic jaundice. J. Clin. Invest. 42:1720-1734.

Schoenfield, L.J., and J.L. Bollman. 1963. Further studies on the nature and source of the conjugated bile pigments. Proc. Soc. Exp. Biol. Med. 112:929-932

Talafant, E. 1956. Properties and composition of the bile pigment giving a direct diazo reaction. Nature, Lond. 178:312.

Tenhunen, R. 1965. Studies on bilirubin and its metabolism. Annls Med. Exp. Biol. Fenn. 43 (suppl. 6):1-45.

Thaler, M.M., N.H. Dawber, J. Krasner, S.J. Yaffe, and L. Mosovich. 1973. Effects of phototherapy on bilirubin (B) metabolism and sulphobromophthalein (BSP) excretion in unconjugated hyperbilirubinemia. Pediat. Res. 7:334.

Thompson, R.P.H., and A.F. Hofmann. 1971. Separation of bilirubin and its conjugates by thin layer chromatography. Clin. Chim. Acta 35:517-520.

Thompson, R.P.H., and A.F. Hofmann. 1973. Free and conjugated bile pigments of body fluids: qualitative analysis by thin-layer chromatography. J. Lab. Clin. Med. 82:483-489.

Tipton, G., and C.H. Gray. 1971. Gas chromatographic analysis of pyrrolic acid esters from the potassium permanganate oxidation of bile pigments. J. Chromatog. 59:29-43.

Van Roy, F.P., and K.P.M. Heirwegh. 1968. Determination of bilirubin glucuronide and assay of glucuronyltransferase with bilirubin as acceptor. Biochem. J. 107:507-518.

Van Damme, B., J. Fevery, and K.P.M. Heirwegh. 1971.Altered composition of bilirubin conjugates in rat bile after obstruction of the common bile duct. Experientia 26:27-28.

Weber, A.P., L. Schalm, and J. Witmans. 1963. Bilirubin monoglucu-
    ronide (pigment I): a complex. Acta Med. Scand. 173:19-24.

With, T.K. 1968. The bile pigments. Chemical, biological and cli-
    nical aspects. Academic Press, New York. 830 pp.


## DISCUSSION OF COMMENTARY BY K.P.M. HEIRWEGH

Taylor:   A minor part of this controversy seems to arise from
the inference that glucuronic acid is present because the conjugate
is cleaved enzymically by β-glucuronidase and inhibition of the
hydrolysis by saccharolactone.   I wonder if Drs. Heirwegh and
Kuenzle are using the same preparation of this enzyme, because
commercial preparations of so-called β-glucuronidase do not have
consistent properties from batch to batch.   Some enzyme
preparations will hydrolyse uronic acid conjugates other than
glucuronides, and even the purest preparations contain a few per
cent of sulphatase.   So we should not get into the habit of
thinking that commercial β-glucuronidase is a single, pure enzyme
and draw final conclusions on the basis of what the enzyme
preparations will hydrolyse.

Heirwegh:   I quite agree.   Some of the preparations also contain
β-glucosidases also, and that varies from batch to batch too.

Bergan:   Does the occurrence of these pigments in post-
obstructive bile reflect some hepatic dysfunction or is it just
a result of changes occurring within the stagnant bile in the
ducts?   I have been doing studies involving injection of labelled
bilirubin and delta-laevulinic acid in dogs, and I have never
found the beta and gamma fractions elevated in serum.

Heirwegh:   Were you using bile fistula animals?

Bergan:   No, the material was injected intravenously.

Heirwegh:   Well, if you make a bile fistula in your animals and
you have narrow catheters to hinder bile flow, I predict that you
will get a cholestatic situation.

Bergan:   You misunderstand my point.   I inject unconjugated
labelled bilirubin intravenously and find all your azo pigments,
in the normal situation, but there is no beta or gamma in serum
in the cholestatic condition.

Heirwegh:   That is because they are excreted in urine;   certainly
in rats and man, but I do not know about dogs.

Fevery:    One should keep species differences in mind here.  The dog has a fantastic renal excretion.   I am sure that in a dog with biliary obstruction, even the serum bilirubin will be low. In our experience with man, we find these beta and gamma pigments in serum, bile, liver and in urine.   The fact that they are found in liver suggests that they are not formed in stagnant bile in the biliary tract.

Erlinger:    Could you briefly summarise the data you got in patients with glucuronyl transferase deficiency and comment on any conclusions you can derive from this data?

Heirwegh:    In Gunn rats we do not find any evidence for glycosyl transferase, and we could not find any conjugated bilirubin in the bile.   In Crigler-Najjar patients in all 12 cases, we found alpha 3, and we are reasonably sure that it is a glucoside, and this is excreted in bile and urine.   We also found in some cases a small amount of material moving on our chromatograms with the delta fraction.   I do not know what this means biologically.

Erlinger:    Do you define "cholestatic bile" as bile from patients with any kind of bilirubin excretion.

Heirwegh:    I would prefer to leave it in the classical sense. Patients with Rotor's syndrome have these complex azo patterns. Hindrance to bilirubin excretion alone would be sufficient to give these complex patterns, but we must analyse many more samples before coming to any firm conclusions.

Hofmann:    Where do people who do not work in this field get reference compounds and standards from?

Heirwegh:    For the azo pigments, dog bile is the best source, and it is quite easy.   But they are not commercially available. We need more experience in handling and stabilising these compounds, before we could send them out to other people.

Palmer:    Have Drs. Heirwegh or Kuenzle had the opportunity to analyse bile concurrently obtained by duodenal aspiration and from a patient with a T-tube with obstructive jaundice.

Heirwegh:    Yes, Dr. Fevery has done this.

Fevery:    Just to be sure we were getting good bile, we obtained duodenal bile the day before the operation and followed this up by studying the T-tube bile.   The results were essentially the same. After about 7 days post-operatively you begin to see a decrease in the complex conjugates, but in our hospital usually on the ninth or tenth day the T-tube is removed.   No patient showed a

normal pattern at that time, so it seems to take a long time for
the normal pattern to be restored.    The rat differs from man in
this respect, in that this animal cannot store bilirubin conjugates
in the liver, so obstructed rats spill the bilirubin conjugates
back into the blood, whereas man has a huge storage capacity and
so this spill-over does not occur.

GENERAL DISCUSSION OF SESSION 3

Heirwegh:   I wish to refer to criticisms of our pH 2.7 method.
Of course, dilution of bile is quite important.   If we treat
Gunn rat bile a large fraction of the unconjugated bilirubin
reacts in our diazo system.   This is not unexpected, since bile
salts may accelerate the reaction, and when we demonstrate
selectivity of reaction of conjugated bilirubins, we dilute the
biles considerably.   This may explain why Dr. Ostrow's group
find such acceleration.

Ostrow:   I think that this is so.   Even if you do get a
significant reaction with unconjugated bilirubin, the fact that
this fraction is so small means that the error by the method is
very small.   So the method is an accurate one.

Heirwegh:   Of course it is important to use fresh bile, otherwise
the unconjugated bilirubin will apparently increase, and the
results will be falsified.

Hofmann:   Yes, but we must not assume that the absence of
unconjugated bilirubin in bile reflects anything at all about
what is going into the canaliculus, because the entire biliary
tract may be extracting unconjugated bilirubin from the bile as
it moves along.   Is that not true?

Heirwegh:   That is quite true.

Haslewood:   I wanted to add a word about this macromolecular
fraction of conjugates.   We found in spectroscopic assay,
without diazotisation, that this fraction must represent about
20 per cent of the total bile pigments.   However, the human
bile we used was partly obtained at post mortem and also from
patients with T-tube drainage, and we can safely assume that it
was highly abnormal.   However, at the same time I was working
with germ-free pigs and I obtained some fresh bile immediately
after the death of these animals and immediately preserved it
in ethanol.   I found in the mucin of this pig bile a very
similar fraction to that found in the human bile.   So I think
we ought to pay more attention to the mucin content of bile.
Perhaps the proportion of mucin bound to bilirubin might be a

useful lead into this problem.

Billing:    I wish to raise the problem of alkali-stable conjugates.
Fifteen years ago it was pointed out that about 40 per cent of the
serum bile pigments could be alkali-stable.   Dr. Kuenzle found
only a small proportion of this type of conjugate in bile.   There
have been a number of reports about the possible existence of
sulphates, but I would agree that the evidence is not very
conclusive.   The sulphate derivative which Dr. Kuenzle formed
as a model for demonstrating that it was not present in his
isolated azo-pigments, does not eliminate the possibility.   I
would be interested to hear the views of Drs. Heirwegh and Kuenzle
what they feel about this question of sulphates and other alkali-
stable compounds.

Kuenzle:    First, the significance of the macromolecular conjugate
in bile;  we designed a technique for isolation and not for
quantitation, since we were interested in the elucidation of the
structure.   So I cannot say anything about the amount which is
present in bile, and whether it is important or not.   As for the
second question about the sulphates, neither Dr. Heirwegh nor
myself have been able to find anything which resembles a sulphate,
which does not prove anything, of course, because we have conflicting views even about the glucuronide.   The work on sulphates you
mentioned is not very convincing.

Heirwegh:    We have never really looked for the alkali-stable
conjugates as our interest is in the glycosides.   But in a lot
of bile samples, in the delta area, we find an alkali-stable
portion, and it would be reasonable to assume that the $R_f$ would
be in that region.   We think that a few per cent of sulphate
may be present, but we cannot say more than that.   In most bile
samples we find a few per cent of alkali-stable unconjugated
pigment, which we call beta-X.   We find it contains two
carboxylic acid groups and is exactly the fragment you would
obtain if you treat bilirubin beta, or bilirubin delta.   We
have good evidence that in dog bile this fragment is derived
from bilirubin 9-beta, which would account for a few per cent
of an alkali-stable, unconjugated pigment in bile.

# Bile Acids and Lipids I

SOME NEW ASPECTS OF THE REGULATION OF CHOLESTEROL BIOSYNTHESIS

AND METABOLISM OF MEVALONATE[1]

G. Popják, Alan M. Fogelman, John Edmond and Peter Edwards[2]

School of Medicine, University of California Los Angeles

Los Angeles, California, 90024

The intermediary steps of cholesterol biosynthesis are now well understood with the possible exception of the details of the transformations of the animal protosterol, lanosterol, into cholesterol. A knowledge of these latter transformations is still of very great interest because we do not know how, or whether, these transformations are regulated.

During the early days of research on cholesterol biosynthesis investigators were content at defining qualitatively the reaction sequences that led from acetate to the characteristic substituted tetracyclic ring structure. The reaction sequences having been defined, the interest has shifted to an understanding of control mechanisms that regulate the metabolism of cholesterol in the hope that a scourge of Western man, hypercholesterolaemia associated with atherosclerosis, responsible for too many premature deaths, may be eliminated.

We have not yet reached our goal, but there seem to be chinks of blue sky above us suggesting that the fulfillment of our hopes may not be too far away. Before I turn to a discussion of specific

---

[1]
Work supported by United States Public Health Service Research Grants HL-12745, HL-18016 and RR-865, and by the Edna and George Castera and the Occidental Life of California funds at UCLA.

[2]
Senior Research Fellow of the American Heart Association Greater Los Angeles Affiliate.

information, I should like to present a very broad question worthy
of contemplation.  Why did eukaryotic life need sterols from the
start, about 2.5 x 10$^9$ years ago, and how did sterols and their
derivatives become regulators of many metabolic processes?  Why
are some species, such as insects, doomed to death, or imperfect
development, if sterols are not provided in their diet, and why
this apparent elixir of life, sterol, augurs premature death to
man if present in the body in amounts that we have come to regard
as abnormally high?

It is an interesting fact that although there are many enzyme
deficiency diseases in man, many of them crippling, yet there is
not one in which synthesis of cholesterol is blocked.  Such a genetic mutation is, presumably, lethal.  In contrast we have genetic
mutations, the various forms of familial hypercholesterolaemia, in
which amounts of sterol accumulate in the body far above those we
have come to regard as normal.  Thus, it became of paramount importance to learn of the processes that regulate synthesis and degradation of cholesterol in man and animals.

The synthesis of cholesterol begins with acetyl-CoA and, after
two further steps, arrives at the intermediate of 3-hydroxy-3-
methylglutaryl-CoA (HMG-CoA).  This intermediate is at a branching
point in metabolism:  it is a substrate for HMG-CoA lyase in ketogenic organs, the liver, kidneys and intestine, and is the substrate
for HMG-CoA reductase which yields mevalonate, the key intermediate
in sterol biosynthesis.  From here on the chain of reactions rolls
on freely, through two phosphorylated derivatives of mevalonate,
to isopentenyl and 3,3-dimethylallyl pyrophosphate, the condensa-
tions of which with one another lead to farnesyl pyrophosphate,
the last water soluble intermediate in cholesterol biosynthesis.
The condensation of two farnesyl pyrophosphate molecules gives
first presqualene pyrophosphate which is, in turn, converted reduc-
tively into squalene.  All these reactions are now part of textbook
knowledge including the cyclization of squalene-2,3-oxide to lanosterol and the degradation of the latter to cholesterol.

One intriguing step in this long chain of reactions is the one
catalyzed by HMG-CoA reductase.  The substrate for this reaction,
HMG-CoA, is at a branching point in metabolism:  it is either
cleaved to free acetoacetate and acetyl-CoA, or it is reduced to
mevalonate.  It is almost axiomatic now that, at such a branching
point in metabolism, one or other reaction of the common substrate
is severely controlled.  In this instance it is the reaction catalyzed by HMG-CoA reductase that is limiting in respect of cholesterol biosynthesis.

It is well known that suppression of cholesterol synthesis in
the liver from acetate by dietary cholesterol (1-3), or by fasting
(4) is related to the suppression of HMG-CoA reductase (5-7); at

Table 1

Incorporation of $[2-^{14}C]$acetate and $[2-^{14}C]$mevalonate
into digitonin precipitable sterols by human leukocytes
(Data from Fogelman et al. (16))

Leukocytes, prepared aseptically, were incubated for 6 hours
in media containing either normal or lipid-free AB negative serum
diluted with Krebs-Ringer phosphate buffer, pH 7.4, containing
0.03 M glucose, and either 44.05 µCi of $[2-^{14}C]$acetate (56 Ci per
mol) or 9.46 µCi of $[2-^{14}C]$mevalonate (10.3 Ci per mol).

| Substrate and addition | Medium | |
|---|---|---|
| | Full serum | Lipid-free serum |
| | (dpm/$10^8$ cells)X$10^{-3}$ | |
| $[2-^{14}C]$Acetate | 26.7+3.5 | 60.0+9.8 |
| $[2-^{14}C]$Acetate + 2 µM CHX* | 26.5+4.0 | 43.4+2.0 |
| $[2-^{14}C]$Acetate + 10 µM CHX* | 26.1+5.0 | 27.5+5.0 |
| $[2-^{14}C]$Mevalonate | 8.8±0.8 | 9.7±1.1 |

*CHX = cycloheximide

the same time synthesis of cholesterol from mevalonate, or production of ketone bodies and synthesis of HMG-CoA from acetate remain
unchanged (8-11). The truly regulatory role of this reductase in
cholesterol biosynthesis was further emphasized on the discovery
of the large diurnal variations in the hepatic levels of this enzyme which could be related also to changes in rates of cholesterol
synthesis from acetate (5,12-14).

These background facts prompted us to explore the possibility
that familial hypercholesterolaemia in man might result from some
abnormality of the regulation of HMG-CoA reductase. For our
studies we chose human leukocytes, in which many of the genetically
determined metabolic abnormalities of man are expressed. No doubt,
similar considerations led Goldstein and Brown, whose work will be
discussed later, to choose cultured human fibroblasts, for similar
studies. We have begun recently studies on freshly isolated hepatocytes also.

In our very earliest experiments with human leukocytes we
could readily confirm the original observations of Marks, Gellhorn
and Kidson (15) that human leukocytes contained all the enzymes
needed for the synthesis of cholesterol from acetate (16). The
method of Coulson and Chalmers (17), we chose for the isolation of
the leukocytes, caused no detectable impairment in the synthetic

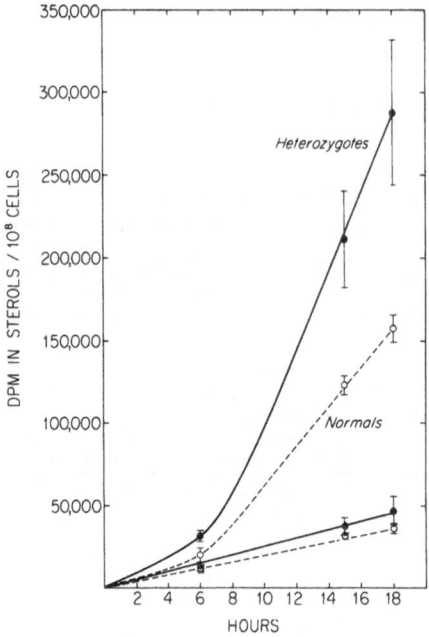

Fig. 1.  Comparison of sterol synthesis from [2-$^{14}$C]acetate in
leukocytes of five heterozygous familial hypercholesterolaemics
and of their age- and sex-matched controls incubated in full serum
and lipid-free serum.  The two lower curves are data from experiments made in full serum, and the upper curves are data from experiments in lipid-free serum.  The cells were incubated with
44.05 µCi of [2-$^{14}$C]acetate (18.67 Ci/mol), penicillin, 100 units/
ml, and streptomycin, 100 µg/ml, for the times shown.  From
Fogelman et al. (22).  Reproduced with the permission of the
Editor, J. Biological Chemistry.


ability of the cells, unlike the procedure of Marks et al. (15).

     Our first major observation was (16) that when human leuko-
cytes were incubated for 6 hours in a lipid-free serum, diluted
with buffer, the incorporation of [$^{14}$C]acetate into sterols rose
two- to three-fold over the incorporation of this substrate in
control cells incubated in a medium containing full serum (Table
1).  The utilization of mevalonate for sterol synthesis was not
affected at all by the choice of the medium.  Subsequently we
made comparisons between the behavior of leukocytes of normocho-
lesterolaemic individuals and the cells of those, who, by well-
established criteria (18-21), were deemed heterozygous for familial
hypercholesterolaemia.  There was a very clear-cut difference
between the two groups (Fig. 1).  Even at 6 hours from the start

of the incubation, the cells of heterozygotes could be distinguished from those of the normal controls. The control cells,
incubated for 6 hours in a lipid-free medium, incorporated usually
twice as much [$^{14}$C]acetate into sterols as the cells incubated in
full serum. In the cells of heterozygotes this incorporation rose
three-fold under identical conditions. The difference became even
more exaggerated beyond the 6th hour of incubation in that the
cells of the heterozygotes kept in a lipid-free medium incorporated much more [$^{14}$C]acetate into sterols than did the cells of
their age-matched controls (22). There was no statistically significant difference between normal and heterozygous cells incubated
in full serum, even though the cells of all heterozygotes incorporated a little more acetate into sterols than the cells of nor-
mocholesterolaemic individuals. The activation of sterol synthesis
from acetate in lipid-free serum was biphasic: a slow rise up to
6 hours followed by a steep increase. Since acetate was not limiting in any of the experiments, and since the effect of lipid-free
serum was to induce an enzyme, or enzymes, preceding the formation
of mevalonate, we can consider that the acetate incorporated into
sterols in lipid-free medium minus that incorporated into sterols
in full serum was the amount attributable to the activity of the
induced enzyme. The calculated values for the cells of normals
and hypercholesterolaemics are set out in Table 2 and show a
nearly twice as large activation of acetate utilization in the
hypercholesterolaemics as in the normals both in the early and in
the later period of incubation.

We have examined then (22) whether the activation of sterol
synthesis from acetate in the leukocytes could be correlated with
levels of HMG-CoA reductase in the cells. In every instance we
have found a perfect match between acetate utilization for sterol
synthesis and levels of HMG-CoA reductase (Table 3). We have
found also that the induction of HMG-CoA reductase in leukocytes
of normal and heterozygous individuals, by incubation in a lipid-

Table 2

Average amounts of [2-$^{14}$C]acetate incorporated into sterols
by induced enzyme in leukocytes of normal and heterozygous
familial hypercholesterolaemic individuals
(Data of Fogelman et al. (16,22))

| | Time period | | | |
|---|---|---|---|---|
| | 0-6 hrs | | 6-15 hrs | |
| | Normals | Hetero-zygotes | Normals | Hetero-zygotes |
| | pmol acetate/(hr X 10$^8$ cells) | | | |
| Mean + S.E. | 41+4 | 76+6 | 202+13 | 392+53 |
| No. of cases | 13 | 11 | 5 | 5 |
| Significance | p < 0.001 | | p < 0.01 | |

Table 3

Comparison of HMG-CoA reductase activity in extracts
of leukocytes incubated for 9 hours in full serum and
lipid-free serum, and endogenous synthesis of
mevalonate from [2-$^{14}$C]acetate by whole cells

(The endogenous synthesis of mevalonate was calculated from
the incorporation of [2-$^{14}$C]acetate, added to the medium after a
preliminary 8-hour incubation in the media.)
(Data from Fogelman et al. (22))

| Product formed by | Medium | | Ratio B:A |
| --- | --- | --- | --- |
| | A Full serum | B Lipid-free serum | |
| | pmol mevalonate formed/ (hr X $10^8$ cells) | | |
| HMG-CoA reductase from [$^{14}$C]HMG-CoA in cell extracts | 20 | 252 | 12.6 |
| Whole cells from [$^{14}$C]-acetate | 11 | 126 | 11.5 |

free serum, followed a very similar course to that we have noted
for the activation of sterol synthesis from acetate (Fig. 2).
This activation could be prevented completely by as little as
10 μM cycloheximide (see Table 1) without any impairment to the
ability of the leukocytes to utilize either acetate or mevalonate
for sterol synthesis at the basal level (16).

Next, we have inquired as to the possible mechanism for the
induction of HMG-CoA reductase in the leukocytes during incubation
in a medium containing lipid-free serum.  The most obvious possibility was that the phenomenon was related to a loss of sterol
from the cells.  There is now overwhelming evidence showing that
induction of HMG-CoA reductase is related, in more than one system,
to loss of sterol from the cells.

In our first experiments, probing this question, we have preincubated normal and heterozygous leukocytes in full serum for 3
hours with [5-$^3$H]mevalonate (22).  The cells were then sedimented
by centrifuging, and the medium was decanted.  The cells were
washed and were transferred to a medium containing lipid-free
serum.  We followed then the release of [$^3$H]sterol and [$^3$H]squalene
into the medium and determined also the labelled sterol and
squalene content of the cells.  At the end of the preliminary
labelling period the cells contained 25- to 30-times more [$^3$H]-

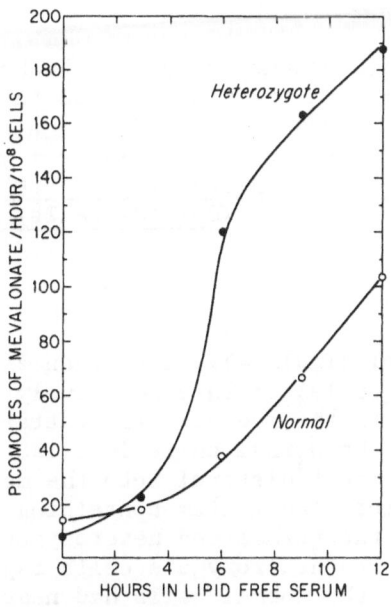

Fig. 2.  Time course of the induction of HMG-CoA reductase in leukocytes incubated in lipid-free serum.  From Fogelman et al. (22).
Reproduced with the permission of the Editor, J. Biological Chemistry.

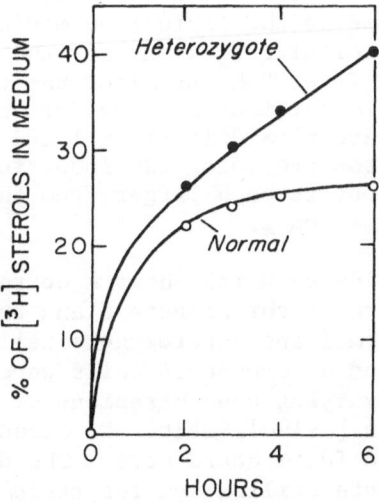

Fig. 3.  Release of [3H]sterols by leukocytes of a normal and a
heterozygous familial hypercholesterolaemic into lipid-free medium.
From Fogelman et al. (22).  Reproduced with the permission of the
Editor, J. Biological Chemistry.

Table 4

[$^3$H]Sterol and [$^3$H]squalene content of leukocytes after
3 hours incubation with [5-$^3$H]mevalonate in full serum

| Cell type | [$^3$H]Sterol | [$^3$H]Squalene |
|-----------|---------------|-----------------|
|           | (dpm/10$^8$ cells) X 10-$^3$ | |
| Normal | 4.2 | 144 |
| Heterozygous | 4.0 | 112 |

squalene than [$^3$H]sterol (Table 4). Less than 2% (2080 dpm/10$^8$
normal or heterozygous cells) of this relatively large amount of
[$^3$H]squalene was found in the medium. In contrast, after the first
3 hours in full serum, the normal cells lost 13% and the heterozygous cells lost 21% of the [$^3$H]sterol into the medium. After the
transfer of the cells into the medium containing lipid-free serum,
the difference between the normal and heterozygous cells continued
(Fig. 3). Both normal and heterozygous cells rapidly lost sterol
upon this transfer, but the normal cells had nearly reached by 2
hours on the lipid-free medium a new steady state without losing
much more sterol during subsequent hours, whereas the heterozygous
cells continued to lose an ever-increasing amount of their cellular
sterol into the medium, reaching 40% of the total [$^3$H]sterol after
6 hours as compared to only 26% loss by the normal cells. The
continued transfer of sterols from the heterozygous cells over 6
hours was contrasted by the very small loss of [$^3$H]squalene after
the transfer of the cells to the lipid-free medium. This amounted
to only 3% of the intracellular squalene for the normal and heterozygous cells during the first 2 hours after the transfer to the
lipid-free medium and did not increase any further afterwards.
Thus it appears that there is a differential and specific loss of
sterol from the leukocytes preceding the induction of HMG-CoA reductase and that this loss is much larger from the heterozygous
cells than from the normal ones.

We have further evidence which shows a correlation between
sterol loss and induction of the reductase and the difference in
this respect between normal and heterozygous cells. In a series
of experiments normal and heterozygous cells were preincubated for
5 hours in mixtures of varying concentrations of normal and lipid-
free sera (Fig. 4), then [2-$^{14}$C]acetate was added to the media and
the incubation continued for 2 hours more. The data of Fig. 4 show
that activation of acetate utilization for sterol synthesis, which
is equivalent to induction of HMG-CoA reductase, did not occur in
the normal cells before the concentration of the normal serum in
the medium had been reduced to 20%, at which point the medium
contained 70 μg of total cholesterol. Induction in the heterozygous cells was apparent already when the proportion of normal serum

Fig. 4. Effect of varying proportions of full serum (100 ⟶ 0%) and lipid-free serum (0 ⟶ 100%) in the incubation medium on the induction of HMG-CoA reductase in leukocytes of a normal individual and of a heterozygous familial hypercholesterolaemic. (The data presented at the Conference cannot be reported here on account of their pending publication elsewhere.)

in the medium was reduced to 40% and, once again, the induction reached much higher levels in the heterozygous than in the normal cells. The induction was parallelled exactly by the release of radioactive sterol into the medium (Fig. 5). From a large number of experiments made with normal and heterozygous leukocytes, under a variety of conditions, a very close correlation could be established between acetate utilization for sterol synthesis, which in

Fig. 5. Effect of varying proportions of full serum (100 ⟶ 0%) and lipid-free serum (0 ⟶ 100%) in the incubation medium on the release of sterols into the medium. (The data presented at the Conference cannot be reported here on account of their pending publication elsewhere.)

the leukocytes is a good measure of the activity of HMG-CoA reductase, and the amount of sterol lost to the medium (Fig. 6). Thus it seems to us that the abnormally high induction of HMG-CoA reductase in cells of individuals heterozygous for familial hypercholesterolaemia may be attributed to a greater than normal propensity of these cells to lose sterol to their environment.

Fig. 6. Correlation between conversion of [14C]acetate into sterols by leukocytes of various origins, and under various conditions, and sterol released to the medium. A linear correlation is demonstrated. (The data presented at the Conference are withheld here on account of their pending publication elsewhere.)

Jakoi and Quarfordt (23) have shown recently that a 4-hour intravenous infusion of egg-lecithin in the rat produced acute hypercholesterolaemia, associated with a lowering of the cholesterol content of liver microsomes and the induction of liver HMG-CoA reductase to levels above the normal, parallelled by an increased conversion of acetate to cholesterol. Recent experiments in our laboratory with freshly isolated hepatocytes demonstrated (P. Edwards, unpublished results) that incubation of the hepatocytes in Swim's S-77 medium with added serum albumin and increasing

Fig. 7.  Correlations between concentrations of lecithin in the
incubation medium and release of cholesterol into the medium,
shown on the left, and between increase in HMG-CoA reductase and
cholesterol released to the medium by isolated rat liver hepatocytes.  A linear proportionality between sterol loss and induction of HMG-CoA reductase is shown.  (The data presented at the
Conference are withheld here pending their publication elsewhere.)

concentrations of egg-lecithin dispersions caused an efflux of
cholesterol from the cells into the medium that could be correlated with the concentrations of lecithin.  At the same time there
was an induction of HMG-CoA reductase which was linearly proportional to the amount of sterol lost to the medium (Fig. 7), sub-
stantiating again the hypothesis that induction of HMG-CoA reductase results from the loss of intracellular sterol.

Does then the hyperlipaemia in familial hypercholesterolaemia
result from an excessive loss of intracellular sterol?  Our hypothesis is that it does.  The question then arises what are the
factors that regulate the movement of sterols in and out of the
cells.  There is no information of any kind available to suggest
what these factors might be in vivo in the whole animal.  So we
need to resort to experiments made in vitro with cultured cells.
An elegant study by Bates and Rothblat (24) with mouse L-cell
fibroblasts suggests that this is regulated by the high- and low-
density lipoproteins of plasma.

It is pertinent to discuss at this point the observation of
Goldstein and Brown and their associates (25-29) made on cultured
human skin fibroblasts derived from normal individuals and from
individuals homozygous and heterozygous for familial hypercholesterolaemia.  These workers have studied the repression of HMG-CoA
reductase in the fibroblasts by serum lipoproteins and have found
that the high levels of HMG-CoA reductase, induced in normal fibroblasts and fibroblasts of heterozygous familial hypercholesterolaemics by growth in a lipoprotein-deficient medium, could be repressed by low density lipoproteins (LDL).  However, higher concentrations of LDL-cholesterol were needed for the repression of
the enzyme in the heterozygous than in the normal fibroblasts.
The fibroblasts of homozygous familial hypercholesterolaemics,
grown in 10% foetal calf serum had HMG-CoA reductase levels that
were 40 to 60 times higher than those of normal cells similarly
grown and, in contrast to the normal and heterozygous cells, the
HMG-CoA reductase levels in the homozygous fibroblasts did not
increase upon transfer to a lipoprotein-free medium, neither could
the enzyme be repressed by as much as 2 mg of LDL-cholesterol per
ml, whereas 25 to 40 μg were sufficient to repress the enzyme in
normal cells.  Goldstein and Brown attributed the cellular defect
in familial hypercholesterolaemia to a defect of LDL binding to

the cells and of LDL degradation which they have demonstrated with the aid of $^{125}$I-labelled LDL (29). They attribute the abnormality to a genetic mutation that results in a failure of the synthesis of specific LDL receptors on the cell surface and a failure of degradation of LDL and hence transport of cholesterol into the cell.

There is a fundamental difference between the concepts of Goldstein and Brown and our own. Their postulate is, unless we misinterpret their writings, that the control of cholesterol synthesis in the cells is exercised from the outside of the cell, by extracellular LDL and by the uptake of LDL-cholesterol into the cells. We hold that the control of cholesterol synthesis, exercised by levels of HMG-CoA reductase, is determined by the cell's ability to retain sterol synthesized within the cell. The fundamental difference between the two concepts is that one postulates a control from without and the other from within the cell. We think that the high levels of LDL found in familial hypercholesterolaemia are secondary to an excessive loss of intracellular sterol rather than a primary defect.

In support of our idea that intracellular sterol regulates HMG-CoA reductase is the experimental observation (P. Edwards and G. Popják, unpublished) that the induction of HMG-CoA reductase in freshly isolated hepatocytes by incubation in a medium containing lecithin is completely suppressed by the inclusion of 0.5 mM RS-mevalonate in the medium. The presumption is that the free availability of mevalonate and its conversion within the cells into sterols compensates adequately for the loss of intracellular sterol. It behoves us, at this moment, to weigh dispassionately the available evidence, which is as yet very young: the first indications as to the existence of a biochemical abnormality related to the control of HMG-CoA reductase in familial hypercholesterolaemia appeared within a few weeks of one another (16,25) as recently as October 1973. It will be necessary to ascertain to what extent conclusions drawn from the study of cultured human fibroblasts or of freshly prepared human leukocytes are applicable to the behavior of liver cells which are thought to be the primary source of blood plasma sterols and lipoproteins.

A startling new twist has been given to the whole story in two recent papers by Goldstein, Dana and Brown (30,31). These workers have discovered that when in normal human fibroblasts HMG-CoA reductase is repressed by the addition of LDL to the medium there is a great rise in the activity of an intracellular membrane bound fattyacyl-CoA:cholesteryl acyl transferase, which is not observed with fibroblasts of homozygous familial hypercholesterolaemics. An effect similar to that of LDL can be produced by the incubation of cultured human fibroblasts for 5 hours with 7-keto-cholesterol, 6-hydroxycholestanol or 25-hydroxycholesterol. These oxygenated sterols are known to be more potent repressors of HMG-CoA reductase in cultured mouse cells and human fibroblasts than free cholesterol itself (32-35). It is not clear at present whether LDL-cholesterol, free cholesterol and the oxygenated sterols achieve their effect through the activation of the fattyacyl-CoA: cholesteryl acyl transferase, or through the induction of this enzyme. Goldstein and his colleagues infer that the activity of this enzyme and the levels of intracellular esterified cholesterol may be regulatory factors in determining the levels of HMG-CoA reductase in the cells. These are important observations, but their validity as to the regulation of HMG-CoA reductase has not been established yet in an unambiguous way. For example, 7-keto-cholesterol reduces dramatically, in less than 2 hours, HMG-CoA reductase levels of cultured human fibroblasts (35), but the activation of the fattyacyl-CoA: cholesteryl acyl transferase was demonstrated only after a 5-hour incubation. It would be of the utmost importance to establish a timed relationship between activation of this enzyme esterifying cholesterol and induction or repression of HMG-CoA reductase. This is yet to be done. Nevertheless, the role of the fattyacyl-CoA: cholesteryl acyl transferase in the possible regulation of HMG-CoA reductase deserves very close attention.

It has been generally assumed for nearly 20 years now that once the product of HMG-CoA reductase, mevalonate, has been formed, that product had no fate other than to be converted into polyisoprenoids and, in mammals, specifically to sterols. Christophe and Popják (36) reported in 1961 that in liver homogenates the allylic pyrophosphates, derived from mevalonate, were hydrolysed by a microsomal phosphatase to the free allylic alcohols and that these were irreversibly dehydrogenated in two steps to the corresponding carboxylic acids. Not much attention was paid to that observation, perhaps because it was thought that the phenomena observed were not pertinent to in vivo conditions.

Based on those old observations, Popják (37) produced a hypothesis suggesting that cholesterol synthesis in vivo might be reduced by substances inhibiting prenyl transferase (the enzyme that synthesizes farnesyl pyrophosphate from dimethylallyl and isopentenyl pyrophosphate) without toxic effects because there might exist a pathway for the metabolism of dimethylallyl pyrophosphate through dimethylacrylyl-CoA back to HMG-CoA (Fig. 8). The hypothesis postulated the existence of a bridge between intermediates derived from mevalonate on the one hand, and from leucine on the other. The main consequence of such a metabolic pathway, if it exists, is that carbon atoms 2,3, and 3' of mevalonate may end up in acetoacetate, and carbon atoms 4 and 5 will be found in acetyl-CoA in ketogenic organs. We have now strong evidence from many experiments, some reported (38,39), that there is a metabolic pathway whereby these five carbon atoms of mevalonate indeed end up in $C_2$-units and ketone bodies. The experimental evidence for

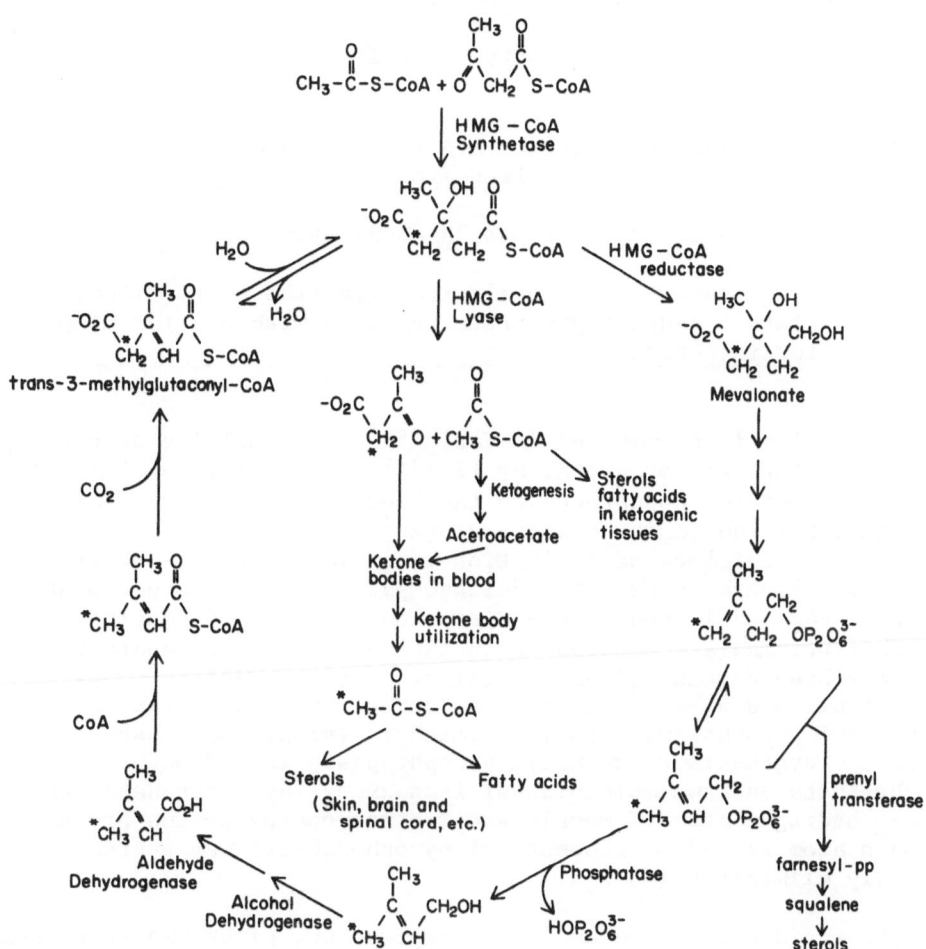

Fig. 8.  Hypothetical scheme for metabolism of mevalonate and not leading to sterols (37,38).

## Table 5

### Evidence for metabolism of mevalonate
### not leading to sterols

1. Transfer of carbon atoms 2,3',4 and 5 of MVA to n-fatty acids (palmitate and stearate)

2. Transfer of $^3H$ to n-fatty acids from 4R-[4-$^3H$]MVA but not from 4S-[4-$^3H$]MVA

3. Rapid transfer of C-5 of MVA to exhaled $CO_2$ but not of cholesterol biosynthesized from [5-$^{14}C$]MVA

4. Reactions are specific to 3R-Mevalonate

5. [2-$^{14}C$]- and [5-$^{14}C$]Mevalonate give rise to [$^{14}C$]Acetoacetate + β-Hydroxybutyrate in blood within a few minutes after injection

this conclusion is summarized in Table 5. The labelling of n-fatty acids, palmitate and stearate, by [2-$^{14}C$]-, [5-$^{14}C$]-, [3',4-$^{13}C_2$]-mevalonate, and the appearance in the blood of β-hydroxy-[$^{14}C$]-butyrate after the administration of [2-$^{14}C$]- or [5-$^{14}C$]mevalonate furnish clear evidence of derivation of at least acetyl-CoA from mevalonate through an as yet undefined pathway. From experiments made with [4R-4-$^3H$]- and [4S-4-$^3H$]mevalonate we could conclude that the intermediate through which the $C_2$-units were generated must have been beyond 3,3-dimethylallyl pyrophosphate. It has been established some years ago that during the isomerization of isopentenyl pyrophosphate to 3,3-dimethylallyl pyrophosphate, and during the synthesis of farnesyl pyrophosphate from dimethylallyl pyrophosphate and two molecules of isopentenyl pyrophosphate, the 4-pro-S hydrogen atom of mevalonate (corresponding to the pro-R hydrogen atom at C-2 of isopentenyl pyrophosphate) was stereospecifically eliminated (40).

The rapid appearance of $^{14}C$ in expired $CO_2$ after the injection of [5-$^{14}C$]mevalonate is also in accord with our hypothesis, which demands that C-5 of mevalonate should appear as C-1 of acetyl-CoA. In rats and man $^{14}CO_2$ is detectable in the breath within 1 minute after subcutaneous or intravenous injection of [5-$^{14}C$]mevalonate and rises up to about 45 minutes and then declines exponentially. It is well to recall that there are no reactions in the chain of conversion of mevalonate into cholesterol, or in the conversion of cholesterol into bile acids, which could generate $^{14}CO_2$ from [5-$^{14}C$]mevalonate (Fig. 9). The only reaction which could generate a product from cholesterol, biosynthesized from [5-$^{14}C$]mevalonate, and give rise to $^{14}CO_2$ is isocaproyl-CoA from the cleavage of the

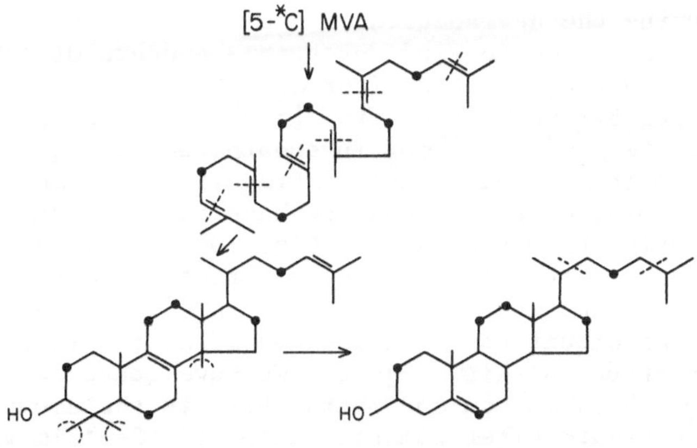

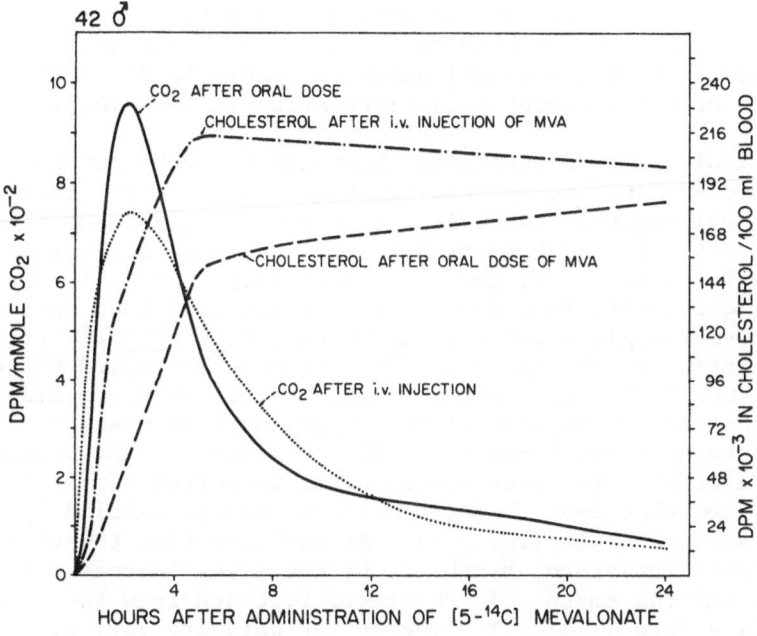

Fig. 9. Labelling pattern of squalene, lanosterol and cholesterol biosynthesized from [5-$^{14}$C]mevalonate.

Fig. 10. Specific activity-time curve of $CO_2$ exhaled by man after intravenous or oral administration of [5-$^{14}$C]mevalonate. From Fogelman et al. (39). Reproduced with the permission of the Editor, J. Biological Chemistry.

side-chain during the degradation of cholesterol into pregnenolone. However, we have failed to find detectable amounts of $^{14}CO_2$ in the breath of a rat during 7 hours after an oral dose of 10 $\mu$Ci of [$^{14}$C]cholesterol biosynthesized from [5-$^{14}$C]mevalonate.  Since S-[5-$^{14}$C]mevalonate gives no $^{14}CO_2$ in breath, we must assume that the $^{14}CO_2$ comes from an alternative metabolism of R-mevalonate not leading to sterols, by the pathway we have called, for convenience, the trans-methylglutaconate shunt.  Fig. 10 illustrates the specific activity-time curve of $^{14}CO_2$ in the breath of man given [5-$^{14}$C]-mevalonate either intravenously or by mouth.  There was no difference between the amount of $^{14}CO_2$ exhaled after the intravenous or oral administration in this subject.  We have found so far a fairly wide variation, both in man and in the rat, in the amount of $^{14}CO_2$ exhaled in the breath after administration of [5-$^{14}$C]mevalonate. In man these have ranged between 7 and 12%, and in rats between 6 and 17% of the dose of R-mevalonate.  We estimate that up to 20 to 25% of the mevalonate might be metabolized on a pathway not leading to sterols.  We have suggested (39) that an impairment in the trans-methylglutaconate shunt might be responsible for the origin of some of the secondary hypercholesterolaemias in man, since such an impairment would leave more mevalonate for sterol biosynthesis. We have calculated (39) that if the "trans-methylglutaconate shunt" were reduced to one-half of the normal, and a normal rate of meva-lonate synthesis were maintained, then an adult man would synthe-size in one year an additional amount of cholesterol equal to twice the amount of total cholesterol circulating in the blood.

We should like to underline this suggestion by our own obser-vations and by experiments recorded by Hellström, and Siperstein and their colleagues.  There is a complete agreement among the investigators that the kidneys utilize mevalonate for sterol bio-synthesis far more avidly than the liver (e.g., 41, 42).  It seems to us, however, more important that somewhat more than one-half of the "trans-methylglutaconate shunt" activity in vivo is attributable to the function of the kidneys.  We have come to regard the genera-tion of $^{14}CO_2$ in breath after an injection of [5-$^{14}$C]mevalonate as to give the minimum measure of the "trans-methylglutaconate shunt". Bilateral nephrectomy resulted in the reduction of the amount of $^{14}CO_2$ exhaled by rats after subcutaneous injection of [5-$^{14}$C]meva-lonate to somewhat less than one-half the amount exhaled by the sham operated controls (Table 6).  At the same time the utilization of mevalonate for sterol synthesis by the liver increased about six-fold, and the amount of $^{14}$C-sterol released into the blood in-creased five-fold (Table 7).  The latter data are very similar to those recorded by Cuzzopoli et al. (43).  In relation to our con-tention that impairments of the "trans-methylglutaconate shunt" might be responsible for some of the as yet unexplained human hypercholesterolaemias is the observation by Edgren and Hellström (44) that in rats, rendered nephrotic by an aminonucleoside [6-dimethyl-9-(3'-amino-3'-deoxy-$\beta$-ribofuranosyl)-purine], there was

Table 6

$^{14}CO_2$ In breath of control and nephrectomized rats
exhaled in 2.5 hours after injection of
2 μmoles of RS-[5-$^{14}$C]MVA

| Experiment Number | $^{14}CO_2$ as % of R-MVA dose | | $\frac{B}{A}$ X 100 |
|---|---|---|---|
| | A* | B** | |
| 1 | 6.08 | 2.64 | 43.5 |
| 2 | 6.31 | 3.02 | 47.8 |
| 3 | 6.76 | 2.58 | 38.0 |
| 4 | 17.88 | 5.60 | 31.3 |
| 5 | 14.35 | 6.28 | 43.8 |

* Sham operated controls; mean body wt 284 + 14 g
**Bilaterally nephrectomized; mean body wt 286 +
   15 g

Table 7

Effect of nephrectomy on conversion of [5-$^{14}$C]MVA
into unsaponifiable lipids in rats*

| | Kidneys (dpm/g) X $10^{-3}$ | Liver | Blood (dpm/ml) X $10^{-3}$ |
|---|---|---|---|
| Controls | 4111 + 120 | 132 + 18 | 25 + 3 |
| Nephrecto-mized | — | 730 + 25 | 96 + 17 |

*Values 2.5 hrs after injection of 2 μmols (20 μCi) of
RS-[5-$^{14}$C]mevalonate. Mean body wt of controls 284 +
14 g, and of nephrectomized rats 286 + 15 g.

a three- to four-fold increase in the conversion of [2-$^{14}$C]meva-
lonate into sterols in the liver and a corresponding increase in
the release of [$^{14}$C]cholesterol into the blood, without a significant change in the utilization of mevalonate for sterol synthesis
by the kidneys themselves. It remains to be determined whether
nephrotoxic agents, such as the aminonucleoside, affect only the
trans-methylglutaconate shunt or enzymes of other metabolic pathways as well.

This conference was titled "the biliary system". Little that
I had to say was directly concerned with the biliary system.
Nevertheless, I believe that the experiments I reported, and discussed, were pertinent to our understanding of the animal, including
man, as a whole. I should like to conclude with some records and

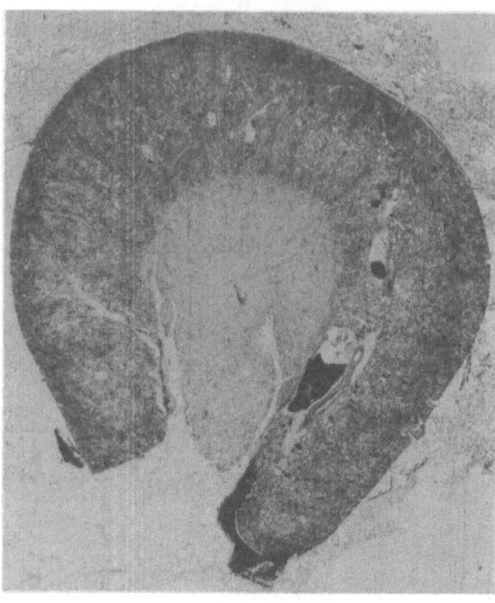

Fig. 11.   Low power view of a radioautograph of kidney of a rat
2.5 hours after injection of [5-$^{14}$C]mevalonate.   The radioactivity
is almost entirely confined to the cortex.   Unstained preparation.


citations to show how fallacious it can be sometimes to try to
understand the workings of a highly coordinated system, such as a
living animal from the study of its parts in artificial systems.

     A group of Danish researchers (45,46) have reported that
slices of renal medulla were quite efficient in converting mevalonate into sterols.   Raskin and Siperstein (47) reported on the
other hand that the renal cortex was the primary site of the utilization of mevalonate by the kidneys for squalene and sterol biosynthesis and that 95% of the activity of the renal cortex in this
respect was attributable to the activity of the glomeruli.   This
conclusion was reached from experiments made in vitro with isolated
glomeruli and tubules made from the cortex of kidneys of dogs.   The
events in vivo are quite different, at least in rats.   Fig. 11 is
a radioautograph from the cross section of the kidney of a rat
injected with [5-$^{14}$C]mevalonate 2.5 hours before the removal of the
kidneys.   All water-soluble radioactivity from the block of the
kidney, fixed in formol-saline, was removed by washing for 24 hours
in running tap water.   The sections, 20 μm thick, were cut after
embedding in gelatin, on a cryostat and were covered with a Kodak
stripping film emulsion.   Exposure of the films for as short a
time as 24 hours showed that only the proximal and distal convoluted tubules of the kidney cortex contained significant amounts of

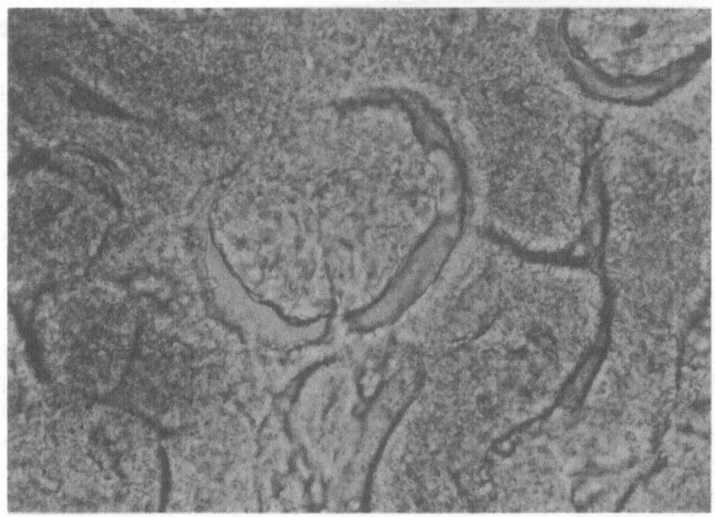

Fig. 12. High power view of kidney cortex from the section shown in Fig. 11. The photograph was taken with lowered condenser in the microscope in order to gain the outlines of cortical structures. A glomerulus is seen in the centre of the picture with very few reduced silver grains over it; the remaining structures are mostly proximal convoluted tubules which contained most of the radioactivity.

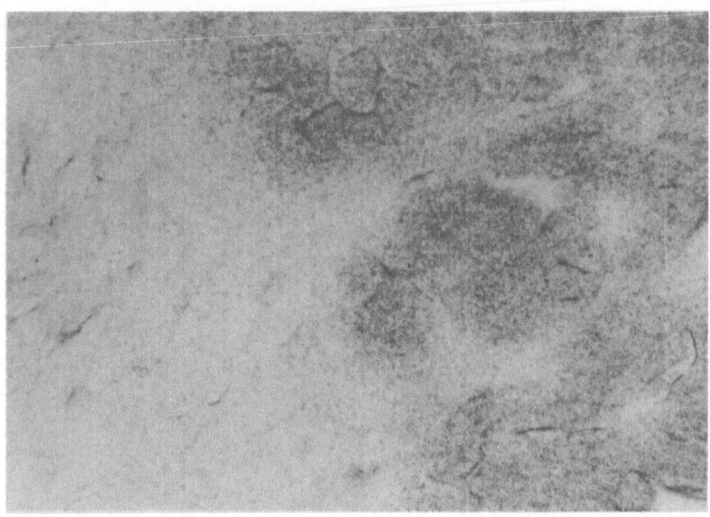

Fig. 13. High power view of kidney radioautograph showing junction of cortex (at the right) and medulla (on the left). Photograph taken from the same section as shown in Fig. 11.

radioactivity. There were no detectable reduced silver grains
above background over the medulla and very few over the glomeruli.
Over 90% of the radioactivity in the sections of the kidneys could
be extracted by the immersion of the sections in chloroform:meth-
anol (2:1, by volume) for 30 min. at room temperature. Exposure
for 3 weeks fully confirmed the impression gained from the 24-hour
radioautographs. In Fig. 11 the sharply defined gray band of the
renal cortex is due entirely to reduced silver grains. Examination under high power (Fig. 12) showed that the glomeruli contained
relatively little radioactivity and that most of the reduced grains
were over proximal and distal convoluted tubules. If Raskin and
Siperstein's (45) conclusions were valid for the living animal, we
would have expected the glomeruli to stand out as black blobs
above a nearly clear background. Fig. 13 is a radioautograph
showing an area at the junction of the renal cortex and medulla.
There are very few silver grains over the tubules of the medulla
in contrast to the thousands seen over the cortical tubules. These,
and other pictures we have, force us to conclude that only the
tubules of the renal cortex contribute significantly to the metabolism of mevalonate by the kidneys in vivo.

The conclusions we offer, from our observations, and from
published experiments of others are (a) that we need to examine
further the mechanisms regulating levels of HMG-CoA reductase,
and (b) that the function of the kidneys in mevalonate metabolism
deserves very close scrutiny.

REFERENCES

1. Gould, R.G., and Taylor, C.B., Fed. Proc. 9, 179 (1950)
2. Langdon, R.G., and Bloch, K., J. Biol. Chem. 202, 77 (1953)
3. Frantz, I. D., Jr., Schneider, H. S., and Hinkelman, B. T., J. Biol. Chem. 206, 465 (1954)
4. Regen, D., Riepertinger, C., Hamprecht, B., and Lynen, F., Biochem. Z. 346, 78 (1966)
5. Shapiro, D.J., and Rodwell, V. W., Biochem. Biophys. Res. Commun. 37, 867 (1969)
6. Linn, T. C., J. Biol. Chem. 242, 990 (1967)
7. Kandutsch, A. A., and Packie, R. M., Arch. Biochem. Biophys., 140, 122 (1970)
8. Gould, R. G., and Popják, G., Biochem. J. 66, 51P (1957)
9. Bucher, N. L. R., McGarrahan, K., Gould E., and Loud, A. V., J. Biol. Chem., 234, 262 (1959)
10. Siperstein, M. D., and Guest, M. J., J. Clin. Invest., 39, 642 (1960)
11. Siperstein, M. D., and Fagan, V. M., J. Biol. Chem., 241, 602 (1966)
12. Kandutsch, A. A., and Saucier, S. E., J. Biol. Chem., 244, 2299 (1969)
13. Hamprecht, B., Nüssler, C., and Lynen, F., Fed. Eur. Biochem. Soc. Lett. 4, 117 (1969)
14. Shapiro, D. J., and Rodwell, V. W., J. Biol. Chem., 246, 3210 (1971)
15. Marks, P. A., Gellhorn, A., and Kidson, D. G. J. Biol. Chem., 235, 2579 (1960)
16. Fogelman, A. M., Edmond, J., Polito, A., and Popják, G., J. Biol. Chem., 248, 6928 (1973)
17. Coulson, A. S., and Chalmers, D. G., Lancet, 1, 468 (1964)
18. Goldstein, J. L., Harrod, M. J. E., and Brown, M. S., Amer. J. Hum. Gen. 26, 199 (1974)
19. Brown, M. S., and Goldstein, J. L., Science, 185, 61 (1974)
20. Goldstein, J. L., Schrott, H. G., Hazzard, W. R., Bierman, E. L., and Motulsky, A. G., J. Clin. Invest., 52, 1544 (1973)
21. Kwiterovich, P. O., Jr., Fredrickson, D. S., and Levy, R. I., J. Clin. Invest., 53, 1237 (1974)
22. Fogelman, A. M., Edmond, J., Seager, J., and Popják, G., J. Biol. Chem., 250, 2045 (1975)
23. Jakoi, L., and Quarfordt, S. H., J. Biol. Chem., 249, 5840 (1974)
24. Bates, S. R., and Rothblat, G. H., Biochim. Biophys. Acta, 360, 38 (1974)
25. Goldstein, J. L., and Brown, M. S., Proc. Nat. Acad. Sci., U.S.A., 70, 2804 (1973)
26. Brown, M. S., Dana, S. E., and Goldstein, J. L., J. Biol. Chem., 249, 789 (1974)
27. Goldstein, J. L., Harrod, M. J. E., and Brown, M. S., Amer. J. Hum. Gen., 26, 199 (1974)

28. Brown, M. S., and Goldstein, J. L., Proc. Nat. Acad., U.S.A., 71, 788 (1974)

29. Brown, M. S., and Goldstein, J. L., Science, 185, 61 (1974)

30. Goldstein, J. L., Dana, S. E., and Brown, M. S., Proc. Nat. Acad. Sci., U.S.A.,71, 4288 (1974)

31. Brown, M. S., Dana, S. E., and Goldstein, J. L., J. Biol. Chem., 250, 4025 (1975)

32. Kandutsch, A. A., and Chen, H. W., J. Biol. Chem., 248, 8408 (1973)

33. Kandutsch, A. A., and Chen, H. W., J. Biol. Chem., 249, 6057 (1974)

34. Chen, H. W., Kandutsch, A. A., and Waymouth, C., Nature, 251, 419 (1974)

35. Brown, M. S., and Goldstein, J. L., J. Biol. Chem., 249, 7306 (1974)

36. Christophe, J., and Popják, G., J. Lipid Res., 2, 244 (1961)

37. Popják, G., Ann. Int. Med., 72, 106 (1970)

38. Edmond, J., and Popják, G., J. Biol. Chem., 249, 66 (1974)

39. Fogelman, A. M., Edmond, J., and Popják, G., J. Biol. Chem., 250, 1771 (1975)

40. Cornforth, J. W., Cornforth, R. H., Donninger, C., and Popják, G., Proc. Roy. Soc., Ser. B., 163, 492 (1966)

41. Hellström, K. H., Siperstein, M. D., Bricker, L. A., and Luby, L. J., J. Clin. Invest., 52, 1303 (1973)

42. Edmond, J., J. Biol. Chem., 249, 72 (1974)

43. Cuzzopoli, M., Hellström, K., and Svensson, B., Metabolism, 21, 1161 (1972)

44. Edgren, B., and Hellström, K., Nutr. Metab. 14, 331 (1972)

45. Bojesen, I., and Roepstorff, P., Biochim. Biophys. Acta, 316, 83 (1973)

46. Bojesen, E., Bojesen, I., and Capito, K., Biochim. Biophys. Acta, 316, 237 (1973)

47. Raskin, P., and Siperstein, M. D., J. Lipid. Res., 15, 20 (1974)

DISCUSSION OF LECTURE BY G. POPJAK

Ostrow:    I wonder if you could comment on which of the various
aspects of cholesterol metabolism account for the hypercholesterolemia seen in patients with obstructive jaundice and hypercholesterolemia seen in patients with acute hepatobiliary diseases.

Popjak:    I cannot at the moment.   We are speculating that this
may be both a combination of changes in levels of HMG CoA-
reductase and possibly also changes in the alternative metabolism
of mevalonate.   We are currently working on a sensitive method
for the estimation of blood mevalonates because it is now known
that mevalonate does circulate in the blood.   We suspect that
in some conditions there may be higher than normal circulating
levels of mevalonate which may be utilized by some organs for
steroid biosynthesis.   But as yet we have no information.
There is no concrete information as yet for the origin of, say,
hypercholesterolemia in hyperlipoproteinemia or in renal disease
or in hepatic disease.   This is an extraordinary situation.

Dam:    How were the lipids removed from the serum?

Popjak:    The method we used is a very old one that was described
in 1942.   It consists of mixing the serum which is chilled down
to zero degrees with about one third volume of diethyl ether, and
then rapidly freezing the mixture to below $-27^{\circ}C$.   Afterwards
you centrifuge and you take off the ether, and by repeating this
process about six times you can reduce the cholesterol content of
the serum to about 2-5 micrograms per ml.   This method does not
remove any of the apoproteins or the lipoproteins which remain
behind.   I examined this many years ago by electrophoretic
methods.   It is a very simple method.

Dam:    So that means that this treatment does not remove other
components from the serum or make other changes.

Popjak:    It removes free and esterified cholesterol, triglycerides
and about 50 per cent of the total phospholipids.

Dam:    So removal of the cholesterol is the most important factor.

383

Popjak:    Yes, we believe so.

Dam:    Are there any ideas about in what way cholesterol influences the synthesis of HMG CoA-reductase?

Popjak:    From the fact that the induction is completely inhibited by cycloheximide, we believe that this true induction requires new protein synthesis but we do not know at what level this induction operates;   that is at the transcription or translational level. We are trying to design the experiments at the moment to look into this question.

Dam:    Yes, and further whether it is cholesterol itself that does the trick.

Popjak:    That is really a 64,000 dollar question.   During the last two years first it has been demonstrated in mouse L-cells that the HMG CoA-reductase can be repressed in these cells much more readily with some oxygenated sterols.   For example, 7-ketocholesterol, 7-hydroxycholesterol, 6-hydroxycholesterol or 25-hydroxycholesterol are far more potent repressors of the induction of HMG CoA-reductase than cholesterol itself.   Now, whether trace amounts of these oxygenated sterols work in the cell or not is not known at the moment.   It is a very difficult point to determine, because after all it is quite easy to get 7-ketocholesterol and 6-hydroxy- or 7-hydroxycholesterol just by auto-oxidation.

Dam:    According to old experiments squalene apparently does the same as cholesterol.

Popjak:    Those experiments were done really before we knew about HMG CoA or HMG CoA-reductase.   I believe that it was noticed that the utilization of acetate in the animals fed squalene was lower than normal.   But that has never been really followed up and nobody has examined yet in detail whether squalene can suppress or not.   I suspect that probably it has some effect.

Dam:    But it was believed that cholesterol formed from squalene did the trick.

Popjak:    That is possible, yes.

Dowling:    I am intrigued by your observations concerning nephrectomy;   having demonstrated that the kidney is capable of incorporating labelled mevalonate into sterols it is not surprising that nephrectomy should reduce incorporation.   What is puzzling is that there should be a corresponding rise in the incorporation in the liver and the plasma, and I am just intrigued by the mechanism involved.   Is it specific?   Have you looked at

the incorporation or the synthetic activity of any other
substances in the liver? Have you looked at apoproteins in the
liver, and have you any ideas on the basic mechanism?

Popjak:   We have not looked at these other systems.   At the
moment we simply interpret the results as meaning that on the
removal of the kidneys or, for that matter, malfunctioning of
the kidneys, there is more mevalonate available for utilization
by the liver.   I could add that we have also some evidence for
this.   For example, if you give nephrotoxic agents like dichromate
at a time when there is no visible morphological change in the
kidney, or when we cannot detect any functional change after
dichromate injection the mevalonate shunt is impaired in the
animals and there is increased utilization of mevalonate for sterol
synthesis in the liver.   So we suspect that if mevalonate is
really released in significant amounts into the circulation, then
the function of kidneys may be quite important.

Mitropoulos:   I would like to ask two questions.   First, do you
have any evidence that mevalonate formed *in situ* comes out of the
liver cell, because if I am right, those calculations about the
shunt came from injected mevalonate.   It is possible that
mevalonate does not go into the liver as readily as it comes out.
The other thing which I wanted to say is that perhaps there is not
so much fundamental difference between your experiments and those
of others because you use a different approach.   You start with
uninduced cells and try to induce them and that means exit of
cholesterol from this cell.   Others start with induced cells and
they try to repress them.   Therefore, they have to have movement
of cholesterol from outside the cell to the inside.   In both
cases it seems to be an abnormality in the membrane, of course.
But now, how does cholesterol get in those experiments, and how
does the cholesterol come out in your system?

Popjak:   In reply to your first question:  of course, it is quite
right that at the moment we are basing our calculations on the
metabolism of exogenous, injected mevalonate.   On the other hand,
there is evidence from other work that mevalonate does circulate
in the blood, and moreover that it has an extraordinarily short
half-life in the blood.   Concentrations of 20-50 nanograms per ml
and with a half-life of, I think, less than five minutes have been
reported.   Now, given a rapid clearance by the kidney there may
be significant amounts of mevalonate that get into the blood during
the day.   It appears that the kidney has a stereospecific
reabsorption mechanism for the R-mevalonate whereas the S-meval-
onate is excreted and the kidneys can utilize both for sterol
synthesis and degradation.   Now, I agree with you that there is
no disagreement between other workers and ourselves.   That is
only a matter of interpretation and certainly it appears from

in vitro experiments that the efflux and entry of sterol into the
cell is regulated by lipoproteins.   But, at first, it was implied
by others that it was the extraneous LDL that was regulating HMG
CoA-reductase by binding onto the cell surface.   Now they are
changing their minds a little, and they are now demonstrating that
indeed there is a sterol loss in the course of induction of HMG
CoA-reductase, and certainly the induction can be prevented by
extraneous LDL and LDL cholesterol certainly enters the cell.   So
we think that the extraneous LDL, as it builds up in familial
hypercholesterolemia really acts like a dam preventing the leakage
of sterol from the cell.   Perhaps just a little twist of thought
is all that exists between us.

Bradley:   Perhaps some experience we have had in the last few
months might be germane to this point.   Workers in our laboratory
have carried out portacaval anastomoses in rats and shown that
even on high fat diets there is a fall in the cholesterol and
triglycerides.   Now, this reduction in serum cholesterol and
triglyceride content is associated with hepatic atrophy but not
with renal atrophy.   If I followed you correctly, is it possible
that there is a balance between liver and kidney so that the
increased kidney activity relative to hepatic activity might play
a role in producing a fall in sterols.

Popjak:   That is a very real possibility.

Hofmann:   As you know chenodeoxycholic acid and the $7\beta$-epimer,
ursodeoxycholic acid, are now being used to treat cholesterol
gallstones and Dr. Dowling will tell us this in detail later.
The mechanism of action involves phenomenologically decreased
cholesterol secretion in bile.   It may involve decreased
hepatic concentrations of cholesterol, and it probably involves
lower HMG CoA-reductase activity.   Since the acute addition of
chenodeoxycholic acid to the perfused liver is not associated
with inhibition of HMG CoA-reductase activity, one proposed
mechanism of action has been inhibition of synthesis of the
enzyme HMG CoA-reductase.   My question is this:  can one, should
one, has one added bile acids to your leucocyte model and looked
at their effect on the induction of HMG CoA-reductase?

Popjak:   We have not done that yet.   These are detergents and
rather badly damage leucocytes, but we will try.   Also, we have
now an excellent isolated hepatocyte system in which we can do
many more experiments than we can do with human leucocytes.   We
are limited to one individual, and if that person is in a very
generous mood giving us 400 ml of blood.   So you can see, our
experimentation with human cells is limited, but with hepatocytes
all those questions could be examined.

Lucy:    I wonder if one might regard the cells that release excess cholesterol into the medium as suffering from some kind of membrane defect and, in that case, is there any evidence that there are abnormalities in composition of the membranes of these cells in particular?    Is there anything wrong with the ratio of saturated to unsaturated fatty acids in the phospholipids of their membranes?

Popjak:    That is a clear possibility, but at the moment there is no information at all.    We are trying to persuade some electro-microscopist colleagues to do scanning electron microscopy with the leucocytes and also we are planning to do some analyses of membranes themselves.

# BILE ACID METABOLISM AND ITS CONTROL

Henry Danielsson

Department of Pharmaceutical Biochemistry
University of Uppsala
S-751 23 Uppsala, Sweden

## SEQUENCE OF REACTIONS IN BILE ACID FORMATION

Formation of bile acids occurs only in the liver and cholesterol is the obligatory precursor of the normal primary bile acids, cholic acid and chenodeoxycholic acid. There is now a considerable amount of information concerning pathways for the biosynthesis of these bile acids, at least in the rat (1-3). The conversion of cholesterol into cholic acid and chenodeoxycholic acid involves some 15 different steps. In the apparently major pathways, the nuclear transformations precede oxidation of the side chain (cf. Fig. 1). The first step is the microsomal 7α-hydroxylation of cholesterol. This reaction is the major rate-limiting step in the overall biosynthesis of bile acids and has been the subject of extensive investigations recently. Oxidation of 7α-hydroxycholesterol yields 7α-hydroxy-4-cholesten-3-one which either can be hydroxylated in the 12α-position by the microsomal fraction to give 7α,12α-dihydroxy-4-cholesten-3-one and ultimately cholic acid or can be converted into 5β-cholestane-3α,7α-diol, primarily a precursor of chenodeoxycholic acid. The conversion of 7α,12α-dihydroxy-4-cholesten-3-one into 5β-cholestane-3α,7α,12α-triol as well as of 7α-hydroxy-4-cholesten-3-one into 5β-cholestane 3α,7α-diol is catalyzed by soluble $\Delta^4$-3-ketosteroid 5β-reductase(s) and 3α-hydroxysteroid dehydrogenase(s). Oxidation of the side chain of 5β-cholestane-3α,7α,12α-triol and 5β-cholestane-3α,7α-diol starts with a 26-hydroxylation catalyzed by the mitochondrial or the microsomal fraction (cf. Fig. 2). Conversion of the 26-hydro-

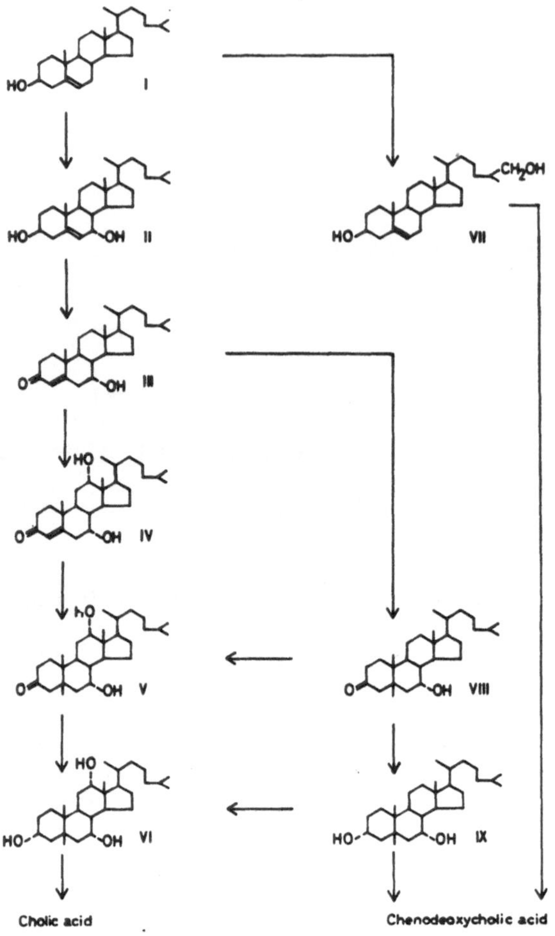

Fig. 1. The steps involving transformations of steroid nucleus in the biosynthesis of cholic acid and chenodeoxycholic acid. I, cholesterol; II, 7α-hydroxycholesterol (5-cholestene-3β,7α-diol); III, 7α-hydroxy-4-cholesten-3-one; IV, 7α,12α-dihydroxy-4-cholesten-3-one; V, 7α,12α-dihydroxy - 5β-cholestan-3-one; VI, 5β-cholestane-3α,7α,12α-triol; VII, 26-hydroxycholesterol (5-cholestene-3β,26-diol); VIII, 7α-hydroxy - 5β-cholestan-3-one; IX, 5β-cholestane-3α,7α-diol.

xy derivatives to the corresponding carboxylic acids is catalyzed by soluble ethanol and acetaldehyde dehydrogenase. Cholic acid and chenodeoxycholic acid arise by β-oxidation of the $C_{27}$-bile acids with release of propionic acid. The formation of propionic acid from choleste-

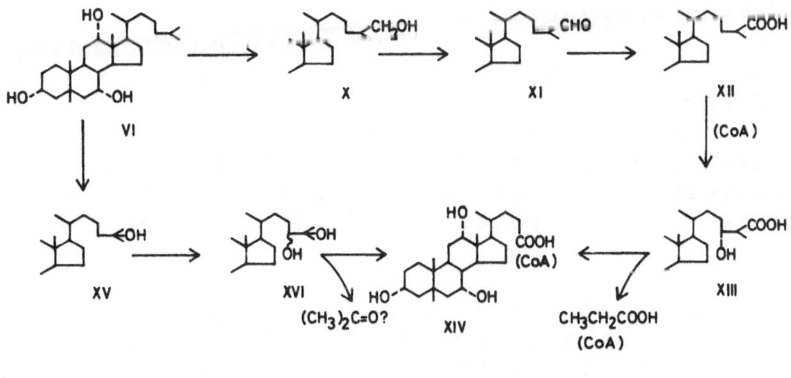

Fig. 2. Oxidation of the side chain. VI, 5β-chole-stane-3α,7α,12α-triol; X, 5β-cholestane-3α,7α,12α,26-te-trol; XI, 3α,7α,12α-trihydroxy-5β-cholestan-26-al; XII, 3α,7α,12α-trihydroxy-5β-cholestanoic acid; XIII, 3α,7α, 12α,24α-tetrahydroxy-5β-cholestanoic acid; XIV, cholic acid; XV, 5α-cholestane-3α,7α,12α,25-tetrol; XVI, 5β-cholestane-3α,7α,12α,24ξ,25-pentol.

rol and 5β-cholestane-3α,7α,12α-triol has been shown in mitochondrial systems (4,5). It has been assumed that the reactions in the oxidation of the $C_{27}$-bile acids to $C_{24}$-bile acids are analogous to those in the β-oxidation of fatty acids and that they occur with the coenzyme A esters of the steroid acids (1,5). No definite evidence for this contention has been reported. The 24-hydroxyla-tion of 3α,7α,12α-trihydroxy-5β-cholestanoic acid has been found to be catalyzed also by the microsomal frac-tion fortified with the 100,000 x g supernatant fluid and ATP (6). In this case, the reaction does not appear to involve the coenzyme A esters. The reaction is the re-sult of the combined action of a dehydrogenase and a hyd-ratase. The role of ATP is not known.

Alternate pathways have been described and yet others can be considered. A mitochondrial pathway for the for-mation of chenodeoxycholic acid has been described by Mitropoulos and Myant (7-9). This pathway involves the intermediate formation of 5-cholestene-3β,26-diol and 3β-hydroxy-5-cholenoic acid (cf. Fig. 1). The quantita-tive role of this pathway has not been established. Under conditions of increased biosynthesis of cholic acid as

well as chenodeoxycholic acid, as for instance in biliary drainage, the rate of 7α-hydroxylation of cholesterol increases manyfold whereas the rate of 26-hydroxy-
lation of cholesterol remains unchanged (10, 11). These
conditions may indicate that the discussed pathway for
chenodeoxycholic acid formation is of minor importance,
quantitatively. Although its bearing on this question
is not immediately apparent, the recent finding by
Mitropoulos et al. (12) of partly different pools of
cholesterol as precursors of cholic acid and chenodeoxycholic acid must be mentioned. According to the foregoing
discussion the pathways to cholic acid and chenodeoxycholic acid separate at the stage of 7α-hydroxy-4-chole-
sten-3-one (cf. Fig. 1). The main finding to support this
contention is that this compound is 12α-hydroxylated in
vitro  at a considerably faster rate than several other
$C_{27}$-steroids (13). However, 5β-cholestane-3α,7α-diol is
also 12α-hydroxylated at an appreciable rate. It is thus
conceivable that 5β-cholestane-3α,7α-diol could be a key
intermediate and that the pathways for cholic acid and
chenodeoxycholic acid formation separate at this stage,
i.e. 5β-cholestane-3α,7α-diol is either 12α-hydroxylated
to yield cholic acid or 26-hydroxylated to yield chenodeoxycholic acid. Other points of separation are also
conceivable (cf. Fig. 1). In any case, the preferrred substrates for microsomal 26-hydroxylation, which may play
a major role in overall side-chain oxidation, are 5β-
cholestane-3α,7α-diol and 5β-cholestane-3α,7α,12α-triol
(11). It should be pointed out that the schemes for bile
acid biosynthesis are based mainly on the results of experiments in vitro and in vivo on the metabolism of a
large number of different steroids. Of the postulated
intermediates, only 3α,7α-dihydroxy-5β-cholestanoic acid
and 3α,7α,12α-trihydroxy-5β-cholestanoic acid have been
isolated from bile, in both cases from human bile (14,
15). No intermediates have been isolated from liver. The
possibility that there may be species differences with
respect to pathways for bile acid biosynthesis is indicated by the results reported by Javitt and associates
(Anderson et al. (16) and Wachtel et al. (17)) and by
Mosbach, Salen and associates (Setoguchi et al. (18) and
Salen et al. (19)). The former authors have suggested that
in man and in the hamster 5-cholestene-3β,26-diol is a
precursor of not only chenodeoxycholic acid but also cholic
acid. On the basis of the finding that patients with the
rare, inherited disease cerebrotendinous xanthomatosis
excrete large amounts of polyhydroxysteroids including 5β-
cholestane-3α,7α,12α,25-tetrol and 5β-cholestane-3α,7α,
12α,24,25-pentol and that the former sterol is converted
efficiently into cholic acid, Mosbach, Salen and associates

have discussed the possibility that the mechanisms of side-chain oxidation in man may differ from those generally accepted to prevail in the rat.

The formation of 5α-cholanoic(allocholanoic) acids has been extensively studied in recent years, primarily by Elliot and associates (cf. ref. 3). Pathways from cholesterol both with and without cholestanol as an intermediate have been described. A noteworthy finding is that in allocholic acid biosynthesis 12α-hydroxylation can occur with 26-hydroxylated $C_{27}$-steroids and even with allochenodeoxycholic acid. Otherwise, the reactions and their sequence appear to resemble those in 5β-bile acid biosynthesis.

## BILE ACID METABOLISM

The pathways of metabolism of bile acids have been established in a number of species (1, 20). Several differences between species exist. As examples may be mentioned the efficient 7α-hydroxylation of taurodeoxycholic acid and the 6β-hydroxylation of taurochenodeoxycholic acid and lithocholic acid in the rat and the mouse. These reactions occur for instance in man at very slow rates. The 6α-hydroxylation has been considered specific for the pig. However, Trülzsch et al. (21) have reported recently that human liver microsomes catalyze 6α-hydroxylation of taurolithocholic acid.

Common features of bile acid metabolism in most species are some reactions occurring during the enterohepatic circulation of bile acids. The primary bile acids, cholic acid and chenodeoxycholic acid, are 7α-dehydroxylated to yield the secondary bile acids deoxycholic acid and lithocholic acid, respectively. Conjugates are split and oxidoreductions of the hydroxyl groups occur to varying extent. The reactions mentioned are catalyzed by enzymes present in the intestinal microorganisms. The main reaction that the bile acids reabsorbed from the intestine undergoes in the liver is reconjugation of any free bile acid with glycine or taurine. In addition, oxireductions of the oxygenated groups occur.

## HYDROXYLATIONS IN BILE ACID FORMATION AND METABOLISM

Many of the individual reactions in the formation and metabolism of bile acids have been studied in detail. Most of the reactions are catalyzed by particulate enzymes

and in these cases many studies have been performed with
whole subcellular fractions. During the last few years
much of the work on individual reactions in the biosynthesis and metabolism of bile acids has focused on the
many hydroxylations involved (22). With the exception
of the 26-hydroxylation, which is catalyzed also by the
mitochondrial fraction, all hydroxylations are catalyzed by the microsomal fraction and require NADPH and
oxygen. The microsomal hydroxylations appear all to involve cytochrome P-450 and have now been shown in reconstituted systems consisting of partially purified cytochrome P-450, NADPH-cytochrome P-450 reductase and a
phospholipid (23-26). Studies with microsomal fraction
and with reconstituted systems have shown that the hydroxylations in the biosynthesis and metabolism of bile acids
differ in one or several respects from each other and
from microsomal hydroxylations of fatty acids, steroid
hormones, drugs and other foreign compounds (cf. Table 1).
Of particular interest are the 7α-hydroxylation of cholesterol, the 12α-hydroxylation and the 26-hydroxylation.
These hydroxylations appear to play important roles in
the regulation of overall bile acid biosynthesis and of
the ratio between cholic acid and chenodeoxycholic acid
formed from cholesterol. The 7α-hydroxylation of cholesterol is the major rate-limiting step in bile acid biosynthesis and is the reaction most intensively studied
(cf. ref. 3). There is evidence to indicate that it is
catalyzed by a specific type of cytochrome P-450. The
cholesterol 7α-hydroxylase system shows considerable
specificity with respect to structure of steroid nucleus
as well as side chain (27-29). The utilization of the
endogenous substrate - microsomal cholesterol - has been
recently investigated. Mitropoulos and Balasubramaniam (30)
and Balasubramaniam et al. (31) have shown that only part
of microsomal cholesterol serves as substrate. The authors have provided evidence to indicate that newly synthesized cholesterol is the preferred substrate. Mitropoulos, Balasubramaniam and Myant (30-32) have also found
that the "substrate pool" varies between 30 and 70% of
total microsomal cholesterol under different conditions.
The findings of Mitropoulos, Balasubramaniam and Myant
have been confirmed by work in this laboratory (33) and
by van Cantfort and Gielen (34). The problem of saturation of cholesterol 7α-hydroxylase with substrate has
been studied by Balasubramaniam et al. (31) and in this
laboratory (33). The results indicate that it is not
possible to achieve substrate saturation. In most studies
on cholesterol 7α-hydroxylase activity under different
physiological and pathological conditions the activity
has been assayed by analyzing conversion of added, labeled

Table 1. Properties of microsomal hydroxylases in biosynthesis and metabolism of bile acids.

| | 7α-OH choleste-role | 12α-OH | 24-OH | 25-OH | 26-OH | 7α-OH taurodeoxy-cholic acid | 6β-OH |
|---|---|---|---|---|---|---|---|
| Inhibition by carbon mono-xide | + | (+) | + | + | + | + | + |
| Hydroxylation by reconsti-tuted system | + | + | + | + | + | + | + |
| Isotope effect | - | - | + | nd | - | + | - |
| Stimulation by phenobarbi-tal | -(+) | - | + | + | - | + | + |
| Stimulation by biliary drain-age | + | + | - | - | - | - | - |
| Stimulation by cholestyramine treatment | + | - | - | - | - | - | - |
| Effect of starvation | inhib | stim | - | - | - | - | - |
| Effect of treatment with thy-roid hormone | stim | inhib | nd | - | stim | nd | nd |
| Effect of hypothyroidism | inhib | stim | nd | nd | inhib | inhib | nd |
| Diurnal variations | + | - | nd | nd | nd | - | nd |

nd = not determined

cholesterol. More recent methods involve measurement of
mass of 7α-hydroxycholesterol formed (30, 35, 36). These
methods are preferable but it should be pointed out that
there is in general good agreement between the results
obtained with the different methods (33). Cholesterol
7α-hydroxylase activity increases severalfold upon biliary drainage, increases markedly upon cholesterol feeding and decreases upon starvation (cf. ref. 3, also 32,
37). Takeuchi et al. (38) have reported that in hyperthyroidism cholesterol 7α-hydroxylase activity is increased
and in hypothyroidism decreased as compared to normal.
However, Story et al. (39) have found that when cholesterol 7α-hydroxylase activity is calculated on a total
liver basis, there is no difference between hyperthyroid
and euthyroid rats but a decrease in hypothyroid rats.
The combined activities of 12α-hydroxylase and microsomal 26-hydroxylase may play a role in the regulation
of the ratio between cholic acid and chenodeoxycholic
acid. In hyperthyroidism in the rat, which is associated
with a reversal of the normal ratio between these bile
acids, 12α-hydroxylase activity is inhibited and 26-hydro-
xylase activity stimulated markedly (40). The reverse is
observed in hypothyroidism. It should be pointed out that
in biliary obstruction, which is also associated with a
proportional increase in formation of chenodeoxycholic
acid and its metabolites, 12α-hydroxylase activity is
not inhibited (41).

Some of the effects of various treatments on cholesterol 7α-hydroxylase, 12α-hydroxylase and 26-hydroxy-
lase have also been studied in reconstituted systems.
Examples of these studies are shown in Tables 2 and 3.
In all cases, the changes in activity have been mainly
associated with the cytochrome P-450 fraction. Some specificity may reside also in the NADPH-cytochrome P-450
reductase fraction.


## REGULATION OF BILE ACID FORMATION

There is now convincing evidence that the formation
of bile acids is regulated homeostatically by bile acids.
Removal of bile acids from the enterohepatic circulation
leads to an increased rate of bile acid biosynthesis and
feeding of bile acids leads to a decreased rate. Changes
in rate of bile acid biosynthesis are parallelled in
many instances by corresponding changes in rate of cholesterol biosynthesis in the liver. These changes are
generally reflected in changes of the activities of the
rate-limiting enzymes in cholesterol and bile acid bio-

Table 2. 7α-Hydroxylation of cholesterol by different reconstituted systems from rat liver microsomes. Irrespective of source, 2 nmoles of cytochrome P-450 and 600 units of NADPH-cytochrome P-450 reductase were used and were incubated with 10 μg of $[4-^{14}C]$ cholesterol (cf. ref. 26).

| System | $[4-^{14}C]$ 5-Cholestene-3β,7α-diol formed |
|---|---|
| | picomoles |
| Cytochrome P-450 from untreated rats + NADPH-cytochrome P-450 reductase from untreated rats | 50 |
| Cytochrome P-450 from untreated rats + NADPH-cytochrome P-450 reductase from phenobarbital-treated rats | 99 |
| Cytochrome P-450 from untreated rats + NADPH-cytochrome P-450 reductase from cholestyramine-treated rats | 74 |
| Cytochrome P-450 from cholestyramine-treated rats + NADPH-cytochrome P-450 reductase from untreated rats | 99 |
| Cytochrome P-450 from cholestyramine-treated rats + NADPH-cytochrome P-450 reductase from phenobarbital-treated rats | 248 |
| Cytochrome P-450 from cholestyramine-treated rats + NADPH-cytochrome P-450 reductase from cholestyramine-treated rats | 174 |

synthesis, hydroxymethylglutaryl coenzyme A reductase (HMG CoA reductase) and cholesterol 7α-hydroxylase, respectively. Such parallel changes are observed in biliary drainage, cholestyramine feeding, and bile acid feeding and both enzyme activities have the same diurnal rhythm. These factors may influence primarily HMG CoA reductase or cholesterol 7α-hydroxylase or they may influence both activities simultaneously. Early work by Myant and Eder (42) indicates that in biliary drainage the increase in cholesterol synthesis in the liver precedes the increase in bile acid synthesis. Hence, the primary site of overall regulation of bile acid biosynthesis could be at the level of HMG CoA. The possibility that a rate-limiting factor in bile acid biosynthesis is the supply of cholesterol, as suggested by Mitropoulos et al. (32), also points to an important role for HMG CoA reductase in the regulation of bile acid biosynthesis. As shown by Balasubramaniam et al. (31) and by work in this laboratory (33), the preferred substrate for cholesterol 7α-hydroxylase

Table 3. 12α-Hydroxylation of 7α-hydroxy-4-cholesten-3-one and 6β-hydroxylation of lithocholic acid by different reconstituted systems from rat liver microsomes. Irrespective of source, 1.5 nmoles of cytochrome P-450 and 500 U of NADPH-cytochrome P-450 reductase were used.

| System | 12α-Hydroxylation of 7α-Hydroxy-4-cholesten-3-one | 6β-Hydroxylation of lithocholic acid |
|---|---|---|
| | % | |
| Cytochrome P-450 from untreated rats | 2.8 | 1.5 |
| Cytochrome P-450 from untreated rats + cytochrome P-450 reductase from untreated rats | 4.6 | |
| Cytochrome P-450 from untreated rats + cytochrome P-450 reductase from starved rats | 5.1 | |
| Cytochrome P-450 from untreated rats + cytochrome P-450 reductase from phenobarbital-treated rats | 4.9 | 3.1 |
| Cytochrome P-450 from starved rats | 6.8 | 1.2 |
| Cytochrome P-450 from starved rats + cytochrome P-450 reductase from untreated rats | 11.8 | |
| Cytochrome P-450 from starved rats + cytochrome P-450 reductase from starved rats | 11.3 | |
| Cytochrome P-450 from starved rats + cytochrome P-450 reductase from phenobarbital-treated rats | 15.2 | 2.8 |
| Cytochrome P-450 from phenobarbital-treated rats | 3.2 | 1.6 |
| Cytochrome P-450 from phenobarbital-treated rats + cytochrome P-450 reductase from untreated rats | 3.9 | |
| Cytochrome P-450 from phenobarbital-treated rats + cytochrome P-450 reductase from starved rats | 4.6 | |
| Cytochrome P-450 from phenobarbital-treated rats + cytochrome P-450 reductase from phenobarbital-treated rats | 5.9 | 7.2 |

is newly synthesized cholesterol. Apparently, this is
not an absolute requirement since increased bile acid
biosynthesis is observed upon cholesterol feeding (37).
Under certain conditions, the activity of HMG CoA reductase is not rate limiting for bile acid biosynthesis.
Feeding cholesterol leads to marked inhibition of HMG
CoA reductase activity and cholesterol synthesis but to
marked stimulation of cholesterol 7α-hydroxylase activity
and bile acid biosynthesis (32, 37). The reverse is seen
upon feeding tomatine (43, 44) or β-sitosterol (37).

The site of action of bile acids in regulating their
own synthesis has not been definitely established. Conceivably, bile acids could influence the rate of cholesterol and bile acid biosynthesis directly in the liver
or they could influence these processes indirectly by
regulating the extent of cholesterol absorption from the
intestine, since bile acids are obligatory for cholesterol absorption. A combination of these alternatives is
also possible. Hamprecht et al. (45) and Shefer et al.
(46) have concluded that the main site of action of bile
acids is in the liver. On the other hand, Weis and Dietschy
(47, 48) maintain that bile acids regulate their own synthesis by influencing synthesis of cholesterol in the
intestine and extent of absorption of cholesterol from
the intestine. The same conclusions can be drawn from the
work of Chevallier, Lutton and associates (49-51) who have
also suggested that the rate of conversion of cholesterol
into bile acids is controlled adaptively by the dynamic
equilibrium of cholesterol. Chevallier and associates
have also concluded that intestinal cholesterol,
not liver cholesterol, plays the major role in overall
cholesterol balance in the rat.

The mechanisms of action of bile acids in regulating cholesterol and bile acid biosynthesis in the liver
have not been defined. Several reports indicate that bile
acids do not regulate the activities of HMG CoA reductase
and cholesterol 7α-hydroxylase in an allosteric fashion
(34, 52-54). There is some information concerning the
specificity of the effect of bile acids on bile acid formation. In rats fed various taurine-conjugated bile acids
at the 1% level in the diet (cf. Table 4), cholesterol 7α-
hydroxylase activity is inhibited by taurocholic acid,
taurochenodeoxycholic acid, and taurodeoxycholic acid,
whereas taurohyodeoxycholic acid and taurolithocholic
acid have no effect (55). Shefer et al. (46) have also
found inhibition by taurocholic acid but no inhition by
taurochenodeoxycholic acid. Shefer et al. (46) analyzed
cholesterol 7α-hydroxylase at its diurnal minimum which

Table 4. Effect of feeding taurine-conjugated bile acids on hydroxylations in bile acid formation and metabolism. Bile acids were fed at the 1% level in the diet for three days.

| Bile acid fed | 7α-Hydroxylation of cholesterol | 12α-Hydroxylation of 7α-hydroxy-4-cholesten-3-one | 7α-Hydroxylation of taurodeoxycholic acid | 6β-Hydroxylation of lithocholic acid | 6β-Hydroxylation of taurochenodeoxycholic acid |
|---|---|---|---|---|---|
| | | nmoles/mg microsomal protein | | | |
| Control | 0.41 ± 0.06 | 1.80 ± 0.10 | 7.4 ± 0.6 | 3.6 ± 0.4 | 6.8 ± 0.5 |
| Taurocholic acid | 0.07 ± 0.01 | 0.30 ± 0.01 | 4.0 ± 0.1 | 7.2 ± 0.4 | 12.3 ± 1.0 |
| Taurochenodeoxycholic acid | 0.13 ± 0.03 | 0.70 ± 0.05 | 6.3 ± 1.0 | 3.2 ± 0.6 | 4.8 ± 0.8 |
| Taurodeoxycholic acid | 0.15 ± 0.02 | 0.40 ± 0.01 | 4.7 ± 0.3 | 9.4 ± 0.4 | 13.8 ± 1.5 |
| Taurohyodeoxycholic acid | 0.27 ± 0.05 | 4.10 ± 0.45 | 9.6 ± 0.4 | 2.0 ± 0.3 | 5.9 ± 0.6 |
| Taurolithocholic acid | 0.20 ± 0.04 | 1.30 ± 0.15 | 0.4 ± 0.2 | 4.4 ± 1.0 | 7.5 ± 1.5 |

may explain the difference in results. In the hamster,
cholesterol 7α-hydroxylase activity is inhibited by
taurochenodeoxycholic acid (56). As shown in Table 4,
feeding of bile acids influences in varying ways also
other enzyme activities involved in the biosynthesis
and metabolism of bile acids. These effects are difficult to explain at present.

Experiments in vivo in the rat have shown that a)
taurocholic acid inhibits taurocholic acid and taurochenodeoxycholic acid synthesis, b) taurochenodeoxycholic
acid inhibits taurocholic acid synthesis, and c) taurodeoxycholic acid inhibits taurochenodeoxycholic acid
synthesis (46, 57-59). In man, chenodeoxycholic acid
inhibits cholic acid synthesis (60) and cholic acid inhibits chenodeoxycholic acid synthesis (61). A recent
communication by Swell et al. (62) reports that in a patient with a biliary fistula, a single dose of 300 mg
of chenodeoxycholic acid orally suppressed within 2 hours
and for 10 hours both cholic acid and chenodeoxycholic
acid synthesis. The rapid onset of the effect is noteworthy and could indicate the presence of an allosteric
type of feedback inhibition as part of the regulatory
mechanisms. With respect to deoxycholic acid, Einarsson
et al. (63) found an inhibition of cholic acid synthesis
by a dose of 0.5 g/day, whereas Pomare and Low-Beer (64)
with doses of 100-150 mg/day obtained inhibition of chenodeoxycholic acid synthesis and no effect on cholic acid
synthesis. Pomare and Low-Beer (64) have suggested that
the synthesis and pool size of chenodeoxycholic acid is
regulated by deoxycholic acid independently of the total
amount of bile acids in the enterohepatic circulation.

A few reports have appeared concerning the presence
in bile of other components than bile acids that may influence cholesterol and bile acid biosynthesis in the
liver. In 1966, Ogilvie and Kaplan (65) reported that
a protein fraction from rat bile with a molecular weight
of about 20,000 inhibited incorporation of labeled acetate but not mevalonate into cholesterol by rat liver
homogenates. Later, Mayer and Petrosilius (66) have found
that addition of dialyzed bile inhibits cholesterol 7α-
hydroxylase activity. Ultrafiltered bile inhibited much
less, indicating that the inhibitory factor is a protein
or peptide. McNamara and Rodwell (67) have reported
recently the purification of a high molecular weight
lipoprotein from bovine bile that inhibits HMG CoA reductase, apparently irreversibly.

REFERENCES

1. Danielsson, H. (1973) in The Bile Acids (Nair, P.P.,
   and Kritchevsky, D., eds) Vol. 2, pp. 1-32 and 305-
   306, Plenum Press, New York
2. Mosbach, F.H. (1974) Digestive Deseases 19, 920-929
3. Danielsson, H., and Sjövall, J. (1975) Ann.Rev.Bio-
   chem. 44, 233-253
4. Mitropoulos, K.A., and Myant, N.B. (1965) Biochem.J.
   97, 26c-28c
5. Staple, E. (1969) in Bile Salt Metabolism (Schiff, L.,
   Carey, J.B. Jr., and Dietschy, J.M., eds) pp. 127-
   139, Charles C. Thomas, Springfield
6. Gustafsson, J. (1975) J.Biol.Chem. in press
7. Mitropoulos, K.A., and Myant, N.B. (1967) Biochem.J.
   103, 472-479
8. Mitropoulos, K.A., and Myant, N.B. (1967) Biochim.
   Biophys.Acta 144, 430-439
9. Mitropoulos, K.A., Avery, M.D., Myant, N.B., and
   Gibbons, G.F. (1972) Biochem.J. 130, 363-371
10. Danielsson, H., Einarsson, K., and Johansson, G. (1967)
    Eur.J.Biochem. 2, 44-49
11. Björkhem, I., and Gustafsson, J. (1973) Eur.J.Biochem.
    36, 201-212
12. Mitropoulos, K.A., Myant, N.B., Gibbons, G.F., Bala-
    subramaniam, S., and Reeves, B.E.A. (1974) J.Biol.Chem.
    249, 6052-6056
13. Einarsson, K. (1968) Eur.J.Biochem. 5, 101-108
14. Carey, J.B. Jr. (1964) J.Clin.Invest. 43, 1443-1448
15. Hanson, R.F. (1971) J.Clin.Invest. 50, 2051-2055
16. Anderson, K.E., Kok, E., and Javitt, N.B. (1972) J.
    Clin.Invest. 51, 112-117
17. Wachtel. N., Emerman, S., and Javitt, N.B. (1968) J.
    Biol.Chem. 243, 5207-5212
18. Setoguchi, T., Salen, G., Tint, G.S., and Mosbach, E.H.
    (1974) J.Clin.Invest. 53, 1393-1401
19. Salen, G., Shefer, S., Setoguchi, T., and Mosbach, E.H.
    (1975) J.Clin.Invest. 56, 226-231
20. Nair, P.P., and Kritchersky, D. Eds. (1971/1973) The
    Bile Acids, Vols. 1/2, Plenum Press, New York
21. Trülzsch, D., Roboz, J., Greim, H., Czygan, P., Rudick,
    J., Hutterer, F. Schaffner, F., and Popper, H. (1974)
    Biochem.Med. 9, 158-166
22. Björkhem, I., and Danielsson, H. (1974) Mol.Cell.Bio-
    chem. 4, 79-95
23. Björkhem, I., Danielsson, H., and Wikvall, K. (1973)
    Biochem.Biophys.Res.Commun. 53, 609-616
24. Bernhardsson, C., Björkhem, I., Danielsson, H., and
    Wikvall, K. (1973) Biochem.Biophys.Res.Commun. 54,
    1030-1038

25. Björkhem, I., Danielsson, H., and Wikvall, K. (1974) J.Biol.Chem. 249, 6439-6445
26. Björkhem, I., Danielsson, H., and Wikvall, K. (1974) Biochem.Biophys.Res.Commun. 61, 934-941
27. Johansson, G. (1971) Eur.J.Biochem. 21, 68-79
28. Boyd, G.S., Brown, M.J.G., Hattersley, N.G., and Suckling, K.E. (1974) Biochim.Biophys.Acta 337, 132-135
29. Brown, M.J.G., and Boyd, G.S. (1974) Eur.J.Biochem. 44, 37-47
30. Mitropoulos, K.A., and Balasubramaniam, S. (1972) Biochem.J. 128, 1-9
31. Balasubramaniam, S., Mitropoulos, K.A., and Myant, N.B. (1973) Eur.J.Biochem. 34, 77-83
32. Mitropoulos, K.A., Balasubramaniam, S., and Myant, N.B. (1973) Biochim.Biophys.Acta 326, 428-438
33. Björkhem, I., and Danielsson, H. (1975) Eur.J.Biochem. 53, 63-70
34. van Cantfort, J., and Gielen, J. (1975) Eur.J.Biochem. 55, 33-40
35. Björkhem, I., and Danielsson, H. (1974) Anal.Biochem. 59, 508-516
36. Shefer, S., Nicolau, G., and Mosbach, E.H. (1975) J.Lipid Res. 16, 92-96
37. Raicht, R.F., Cohen, B.J., Shefer, S., and Mosbach, E.H. (1975) Biochim.Biophys.Acta 388, 374-384
38. Takeuchi, N., Ito, M., Uchida, K., and Yamamura, Y. (1975) Biochem.J. 148, 499-503
39. Story, J.A., Tepper, S.A., and Kritchevsky, D. (1974) Biochem.Med. 10, 214-218
40. Björkhem, I., Danielsson, H., and Gustafsson, J. (1973) FEBS Lett. 31, 20-22
41. Danielsson, H. (1973) Steroids 22, 567-579
42. Myant, N.B., and Eder, H.A. (1961) J.Lipid Res. 2, 363-368
43. Cayen, M.N. (1971) J.Lipid Res. 12, 482-490
44. Boyd, G.S. (1975) Personal communication
45. Hamprecht, B., Roscher, R., Waltinger, G., and Nüssler, C. (1971) Eur.J.Biochem. 18, 15-19
46. Shefer, S., Hauser, S., Lapar, V., and Mosbach, E.H. (1973) J.Lipid Res. 14, 573-580
47. Weis, H.J., and Dietschy, J.M. (1969) J.Clin.Invest. 48, 2398-2408
48. Dietschy, J.M. (1968) J.Clin.Invest. 47, 286-300
49. Chevallier, F., and Lutton, C. (1973) Nature New Biol. 242, 61-62
50. Lutton, C., Mathé, D., and Chevallier, F. (1973) Biochim.Biophys Acta 306, 483-496
51. Chevallier, F., and Magot, T. (1975) Experientia 31, 627-629

52. Shefer, S., Hauser, S., and Mosbach, E.H. (1968) J.Lipid Res. 9, 328-333

53. Hamprecht, B., Nüssler, C., Waltinger, G., and Lynen, F. (1970) Eur.J.Biochem. 18, 10-14

54. Liersch, M.E.A., Barth, A., Hackenschmidt, H.J., Ullman, H.L., and Decker, K.F.A. (1973) Eur.J.Biochem. 32, 365-371

55. Danielsson, H.(1973) Steroids 22, 667-676

56. Schoenfield, L.J., Bonorris, G.G., and Ganz, P. (1973) J.Lab.Clin.Med. 82, 858-868

57. Bergström, S., and Danielsson, H. (1958) Acta Physiol. Scand. 43, 1-7

58. Shefer, S., Hauser, S., Bekersky, I., and Mosbach, E.H. (1969) J.Lipid Res. 10, 646-655

59. Danielsson, H., and Johansson, G. (1974) Gastroenterology 67, 126-134

60. Danzinger, R.G., Hofmann, A.F., Thistle, J.L., and Schoenfield, L.J. (1973) J.Clin.Invest. 52, 2809-2821

61. Einarsson, K., Hellström, K., and Kallner, M. (1973) Metabolism 22, 1477-1483

62. Swell, L., Schwartz, C.C., Halloran, L.G., and Vlahcevic, Z.R. (1975) Biochem.Biophys.Res.Commun. 64, 1083-1089

63. Einarsson, K., Hellström, K., and Kallner, M. (1974) Clin.Sci.Mol.Med. 47, 425-433

64. Pomare, E.W., and Low-Beer, T.S. (1975) Clin.Sci.Mol. Med. 48, 315-321

65. Ogilvie, J.W., and Kaplan, B.H. (1966) J.Biol.Chem. 241, 4722-4730

66. Mayer, D. and Petrosilius, U. (1972) Hoppe-Seyler's Z. Physiol.Chem. 353, 1185-1186

67. McNamara, D.J., and Rodwell, V.W. (1975) Arch.Biochem. Biophys. 168, 378-385

DISCUSSION OF LECTURE BY H. DANIELSSON

Mayer:   First I have a question about the effect of thyroxine on cholesterol 7$\alpha$-hydroxylase.   Can you tell us something further about the experimental design of what you have reported?

Danielsson:   It was not my work.   It was published in Biochemical Journal just a month ago.

Mayer:   When we have done such experiments we found an inhibition in thyroidectomized rats, and addition of thyroxine leads to normal values.   In intact rats we did not find any activation of 7$\alpha$-hydroxylase activity.   Only in the case of cholestyramine treatment, which leads to an increased 7$\alpha$-hydroxylase activity, did we find activation by this hormone.   So, we should like to say that thyroxine affects only the enzyme activity in a state of bile acid deficiency.

Danielsson:   May I comment on that.   As was apparent, I hope, we have not worked on the effect of thyroid hormone on 7$\alpha$-hydroxylase. I am afraid that I will make things a little more complicated.   I did not mention a report in 1974 in which they found a stimulation of 7$\alpha$-hydroxylase activity by thyroxine and an inhibition in hyperthyroidism.   However, when they calculated their value on total liver weight, there was no difference between the two.

Mayer:   And then to the effect of chenodeoxycholic acid:   there is not only a decrease of enzyme activity in the dark period in the time of high enzyme activity but there is also a marked decrease of enzyme activity in the light period.   We found this about 8 hours after treatment with chenodeoxycholic acid in the light period.

Danielsson:   I should say that our rats are somewhat different in this respect.   What we do is to subject them to a reversed schedule of day and night.   That is, we have light during the night and dark during the day.   I can say that these animals are not exactly, so to speak, normal rats.   We do not get exactly as nice diurnal patterns as you do with, so to speak, standard rats.

Mayer:    You cannot change the light-dark period completely.
Our animals have been kept in boxes closed from all daylight and
the light period was from 6 to 18 hours and the dark period was
from 18 to 6 hours.

Mitropoulos:    In the experiment where you fed cholesterol, do you
think in that case the substrate pool was expanded by the cholesterol that was absorbed, and, if so, the increased activity
observed might have been due to increased supply of substrate for
the enzyme.    In that case I cannot understand what you said about
the values obtained by direct measurement of $7\alpha$-hydroxycholesterol
formed are equal to those calculated by the incorporation method.
I thought that an expansion in the size of the substrate pool
could have explained the failure of some people to find the effects
with feeding of cholesterol on $7\alpha$-hydroxylase, when they used
isotope incorporation method, because they did not take into
account the expanded size of the substrate pool.

Danielsson:    First of all, in our experiments we could not detect
a significant increase of cholesterol $7\alpha$-hydroxylase activity.
This, as I said, was intentional.    Secondly, I think today all
people agree on the effect of cholesterol feeding on both $7\alpha$-
hydroxylase activity and bile acid biosynthesis.    Now, when it
comes to substrate pool, this is of course a tricky subject and
the substrate pool is completely unknown.    I think we can agree
on that.    We can, with the experiments with Tween 80, give a
maximum figure for it.    But we do not know how far away the real
figure is from the maximum figure.    We did not pay too much
attention to measuring "substrate pool", because we performed the
experiments not in the interest of finding out about the effect
of cholesterol feeding, but only for comparisons.    May I say
that it turns out that the results are the same, but I tried to
state very clearly that in all instances measurement  of mass of
$7\alpha$-hydroxycholesterol is by far preferable.

Popper:    You just said that the question of allosteric regulation
of bile acids on each other is not quite a clear one.    Would you
extend that to any other regulatory function of bile acid on other
enzyme systems in liver?    There is some evidence that they do and
some that they do not.

Danielsson:    I am not able to comment on that.    As I tried to
say, the report by Drs. Vlahcevic and Swell indicates something
that is different from the generally held opinion, but I do not
think this is the last word, and as also these authors write in
their paper, there is definitely more than this primary effect.
They discuss also a secondary feed-back effect.    I am afraid
that I cannot discuss other enzymes than HMG CoA-reductase and
cholesterol $7\alpha$-hydroxylase.

<u>Dowling</u>:    Dr. Hofmann has already referred to studies on the effect of the 7β-epimer of chenodeoxycholic acid showing that it apparently like chenodeoxycholic acid depresses biliary cholesterol secretion and also dissolves gallstones.   With this in mind, have you looked at the effect of ursodeoxycholic acid on the levels of HMG CoA-reductase and cholesterol 7α-hydroxylase?

<u>Danielsson</u>:    It is on our programme.

<u>Hofmann</u>:    You have stated through many years and there is good experimental evidence in agreement with this general statement, that the synthesis of bile acids is inversely proportional to the amount of bile acids returning to the liver.   The one exception is starvation and my real question is:  what concepts are useful in teaching that exception?   My second question is: would you expand or speculate on non-allosteric mechanisms by which bile acids inhibit either their own synthesis or that of cholesterol?

<u>Danielsson</u>:    I have no comments to your first question that will make much sense right now.   Concerning the second question. As Dr. Popjak said, we do not really know much.   But I would like to point out something that was determined a number of years ago and has been since also done in several other laboratories. The half-life time of rat liver cholesterol 7α-hydroxylase activity is in the order of 2 hours and that checks very nicely with the half-life time of HMG CoA-reductase.   Dr. Mitropoulos will perhaps discuss the effect of diurnal variations.

<u>Fisher</u>:    I just wonder if you have any information of sex differences in bile acid synthesis.

<u>Danielsson</u>:    No.  We have done very little on that.   We have always used male rats.   I know that you published and found differences between female and male rats.   There are some sex differences when one analyses some hydroxylations but there is no correlation, to my knowledge, of these sex differences with bile acid synthesis and bile acid patterns.   One of the most interesting enzymes, the cholesterol 7α-hydroxylase, shows no sex differences in our hands.

# DIURNAL VARIATION IN BILE ACID BIOSYNTHESIS

K.A. MITROPOULOS

Medical Research Council Lipid Metabolism Unit

Hammersmith Hospital, London, England

Cholesterol is a cellular constituent in mammals. The sterol is synthesized in practically all cells of the body in order to provide for the cellular requirements in cholesterol, an important constituent of cell membranes. Furthermore, the synthesis of bile acids from cholesterol in the liver provides an outlet for the elimination of cholesterol from the body together with these metabolites of major physiological role for the absorption of sterols and of triglycerides from the digestive tract. The maintenance of a constant amount of cholesterol in the body seems to be the result of regulation and of balance between many processes. Since hepatic cholesterogenesis is quantitatively the most important source of the endogenous cholesterol and since the excretion of bile acids with the faeces constitutes the major metabolic route for the elimination of cholesterol from the body, the regulation of hepatic cholesterogenesis and of the conversion of cholesterol to bile acids are of major importance for the maintenance of a constant amount of cholesterol in the body. Several factors that influence the rate of synthesis of bile acids have noticeable parallel effects on the activity of cholesterol $7\alpha$-hydroxylase. Factors that influence the rate of hepatic cholesterogenesis are known to do so by modifying the activity of the microsomal enzyme HMG-CoA reductase.

In recent years it has become apparent that the rate of synthesis of certain metabolites in the body varies diurnally and this is achieved by the control of the flow of intermediates along a given pathway exerted on strategic enzymes whose activities vary diurnally. Signals causing a daily rhythm in the rate of synthesis of a metabolite could originate either within the organism or outside. In the first case the rhythm signal could either

originate within the cell itself or elsewhere in the body and
would have to reach the cell via the bloodstream in the form of a
nutrient or a hormone.    Whatever is the signal that controls the
diurnal rhythm in the rate of synthesis of a metabolite, the
physiological significance of diurnal rhythms is either to satisfy
the variable needs of the cell for the metabolite or to synthesize
variable amounts of metabolite needed by another part of the body
during the diurnal cycle.

The activity of cholesterol 7α-hydroxylase of rat-liver microsomes varies considerably according to the time of day that the
liver is removed for the assay.    In intact rats adapted to a
cyclic lighting schedule and given food ad libitum only during the
dark period of the light cycle, enzyme activity is considerably
higher at the middle of the dark period than at the middle of the
light period.    This increase probably reflects a change in the
quantity of enzyme protein controlled at the level of cholesterol
7α-hydroxylase synthesis.    The activity of HMG-CoA reductase
exhibits a similar pattern of variation during the light cycle
that is also controlled at the level of enzyme synthesis and
degradation.    In the present paper we shall see that the diurnal
rhythm in the activity of cholesterol 7α-hydroxylase persists in a
great number of physiological conditions that are associated with
changes in the rate of synthesis of bile acids and it is probably
associated with parallel fluctuations in the rate of biosynthesis
of bile acids in the liver.    In addition, we shall consider the
importance of circulating glucocorticoids as the oscillating
signal controlling the synthesis of HMG-CoA reductase and of cholesterol 7α-hydroxylase and we shall consider the physiological
significance of the variation in the rate of hepatic cholesterogenesis and of bile acid biosynthesis.

## ASSAY OF THE ACTIVITY OF CHOLESTEROL 7α-HYDROXYLASE

The incubation of $[^{14}C]$-cholesterol with liver microsomal
fraction in the presence of NADPH results in incorporation of
radioactivity into the 7α-hydroxycholesterol fraction.    Since,
under these conditions, the only product formed is 7α-hydroxychol-
esterol, this provides an essentially simple system for the assay
of the activity of the enzyme.    However, a radioisotope incorporation method cannot be used to assay the activity of this
enzyme because liver microsomal fraction contains appreciable
amounts of cholesterol and it is now recognized that only a fraction of this cholesterol is available to cholesterol 7α-hydroxy-
lase (1-3).    We have, therefore, used a direct method to assay
the mass of 7α-hydroxycholesterol formed during the incubation
from the endogenous cholesterol in the microsomal preparation (3).
The endogenous cholesterol in microsomes can support a constant
rate of 7α-hydroxycholesterol synthesis with respect to time and

to protein concentration (in the range employed).   Moreover, we
have shown (1) that the addition, under certain conditions, of
tracer amounts of $[^{14}C]$-cholesterol to the incubation mixture
results in a fast and preferential labelling of the part of microsomal cholesterol that acts as substrate for the enzyme (substrate
pool).   A comparison, therefore, of the specific radioactivity of
7α-hydroxycholesterol with that of total cholesterol could give an
estimate of the size of the substrate pool.   Since the size of
the endogenous substrate pool may vary under certain physiological
conditions (see below), and since cholesterol 7α-hydroxylase is
not saturated by endogenous microsomal cholesterol (1,2), a measure of the activity of the endogenous cholesterol concentration
and the estimate of the size of the substrate pool can provide
more relevant information about the activity of the enzyme in the
cell and the influence of the size of the substrate pool on the
observed activity than is provided merely by measurement of enzyme
capacity.

## DIURNAL VARIATION IN THE ACTIVITY OF CHOLESTEROL

## 7α-HYDROXYLASE

The diurnal rhythm in the activity of cholesterol 7α-hydroxy-
lase in rat-liver microsomes was first described by Gielen (4).
Subsequently the results of Gielen were confirmed in reports from
other laboratories (5-7).   For the experiments shown in Fig. 1,
groups of rats that were adapted to a controlled feeding and
lighting schedule were killed every four hours and the activity of
the enzyme was assayed in the microsomal preparation from the combined livers of each group.   Three groups of rats each containing
three rats were killed at each period.   For reasons of comparison
the activity of tyrosine transaminase, an enzyme extensively
studied for its diurnal rhythm, was assayed in the soluble part of
the same liver homogenates.   As may be seen from Fig. 1, the
activity of cholesterol 7α-hydroxylase is maximal during the middle
of the dark period.   The activity then declines to a minimum
around noon, before rising again in the evening.   The activity of
tyrosine transaminase also exhibits a similar pattern of variation.
A similar pattern of variation in the activity of cholesterol 7α-
hydroxylase is also obtained if the activity is expressed per g
of liver.   It is not possible to explain the observed rhythmicity
in the activity of the enzyme on the basis of changes either in
the level of total liver microsomal cholesterol or in the size of
the microsomal substrate pool.   The total cholesterol content of
the microsomal preparation, expressed either per mg of microsomal
protein or per g wet weight of liver, does not change significantly
during the 24-h cycle.   The estimated size of the substrate pool.
however, reaches a minimum around midnight when the activity of

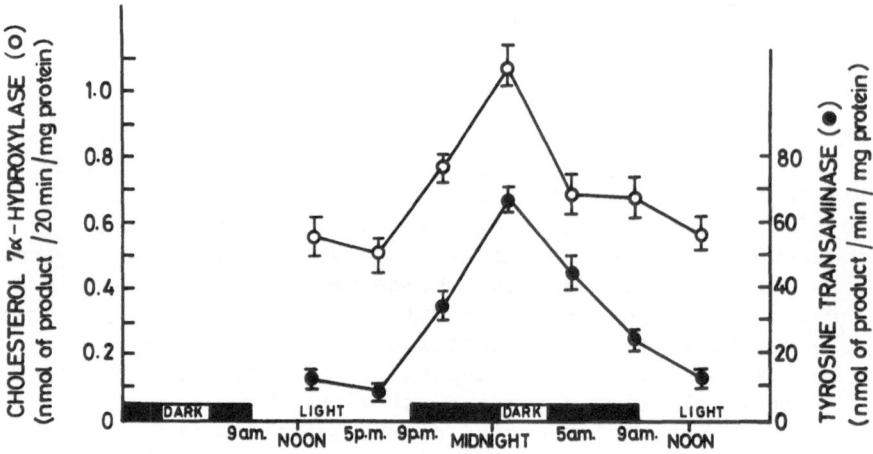

Fig. 1.    Diurnal changes in the activity of hepatic cholesterol
7α-hydroxylase and tyrosine transaminase in rats adapted to controlled lighting and feeding.    The rats were supplied with food
only between 7.0 p.m. and 9.0 a.m.    Each point shows the mean
and SD of values obtained from three groups of rats.    (From
Reference 5, by permission.)

cholesterol 7α-hydroxylase is at its peak value and a maximun
around noon when enzyme activity is minimum (5).    If substrate
availability has any influence on the variation of the activity
of the enzyme, then the amplitude of the oscillation observed
should have been even higher, if the size of the substrate pool
remained constant.

There is strong evidence to suggest that the diurnal rise and
fall in the activity of a number of enzymes is controlled at the
level of enzyme synthesis and degradation.    The results of Table
I suggest that this is the case for the diurnal rise in the activity of cholesterol 7α-hydroxylase.    For this experiment rats were
injected intraperitoneally with a solution of actinomycin D or
cycloheximide at 7.0 p.m. and the animals were killed 4 hours
later.    The control rats were injected with the solvent of the
protein synthesis inhibitors.    In the control rats, the activity
of cholesterol 7α-hydroxylase was twice as high at 11.0 p.m. as at
7.0 p.m.    However, in the rats injected with actinomycin D or
cycloheximide at 7.0 p.m. the activity of the enzyme at 11.0 p.m.
did not rise above that observed 4 hours earlier.    These results
indicate that an increase in enzyme synthesis was responsible for

TABLE I

EFFECT OF ADMINISTRATION OF INHIBITORS OF PROTEIN SYNTHESIS ON THE
DIURNAL VARIATION IN THE ACTIVITY OF CHOLESTEROL 7α-HYDROXYLASE

| Treatment of animals | Activity of cholesterol 7α-hydroxylase (nmole/20 min/mg protein) | |
|---|---|---|
| | 7.0 p.m. | 11.0 p.m. |
| Control | 0.40 | 0.89 |
| Actinomycin D | 0.40 | 0.38 |
| Cycloheximide | 0.40 | 0.25 |

The rats were adapted to controlled feeding (7.0 p.m. - 9.0 a.m.)
and lighting (9.0 a.m. - 7.0 p.m.) for 2 weeks before the experiment.   Actinomycin D (0.5 mg/kg) or cycloheximide (0.5 mg/100 g)
was injected intraperitoneally at 7.0 p.m. and the rats were
killed 4 h later.   Control animals were killed at 7.0 p.m. and
11.0 p.m.   Each value shows the results obtained from a group of
three rats.   (From Reference 5, by permission.)


the rise in the activity of cholesterol 7α-hydroxylase observed
at 11.0 p.m.


## DIURNAL RHYTHM IN THE ACTIVITY OF HMG-CoA REDUCTASE

The activity of HMG-CoA reductase in liver microsomes, measured in vitro, varies markedly according to the time of day the
tissue is taken for assay.   This diurnal variation, which was
first described by Kandutsch and Saucier (8) and confirmed elsewhere (9,10), exhibits a pattern similar to that of cholesterol
7α-hydroxylase, with a maximum at the middle of the dark period
and a minimum around noon.   Puromycin (8) and cycloheximide (9,
11) blocks the rise in activity of HMG-CoA reductase, suggesting
that protein synthesis is required for the rise observed in the
early part of the dark period.   This was confirmed by measuring
the rate of incorporation of [$^3$H]-leucine into HMG-CoA reductase
purified from rats killed at various times (12).   A similar
pattern of variations was observed for the rate of sterol synthesis in the liver (13).

TABLE II

EFFECT OF CHOLESTEROL IN THE DIET ON THE ACTIVITY OF CHOLESTEROL
7α-HYDROXYLASE OF RAT-LIVER MICROSOMAL FRACTION

| 1% Cholesterol (hours fed) | Activity of cholesterol 7α-hydroxylase (nmol/20 min/ mg protein | | Total cholesterol (nmol/mg protein) | | Estimated size of substrate pool (nmol/mg protein) | |
|---|---|---|---|---|---|---|
| | 1 a.m. | 1 p.m. | 1 a.m. | 1 p.m. | 1 a.m. | 1 p.m. |
| 0 | 0.63 | 0.33 | 52.5 | 52.6 | 14.4 | 14.1 |
| 6 | 0.99 | 0.45 | 76.2 | 67.4 | 25.4 | 16.8 |
| 24 | 1.21 | 0.77 | 79.4 | 81.1 | 29.0 | 22.1 |
| 168 | 1.25 | 0.58 | 73.3 | 74.8 | 25.5 | 19.6 |

Cholesterol (1%) was added to the food for various periods before
killing the animals at 1.0 a.m. or 1.0 p.m.   All rats were
adapted to controlled lighting and feeding on the standard diet
for 14 days before the start of the experiment.   Controlled lighting and feeding was maintained throughout the experimental period.
Each value was obtained from the pooled livers of three rats.
(From Reference 17, by permission.)

THE ACTIVITY OF CHOLESTEROL 7α-HYDROXYLASE AND ITS DIURNAL
VARIATION IN VARIOUS CONDITIONS ASSOCIATED WITH CHANGES IN
THE RATE OF SYNTHESIS OF BILE ACIDS

The addition of cholesterol to the food increases bile acid
synthesis in the rat (14,15,16).   Feeding rats with cholesterol
for 12 hours results in increased activity of cholesterol 7α-hyd-
roxylase (Balasubramaniam and Mitropoulos, unpublished results).
This increase is accompanied by an increase in the cholesterol
content of the microsomal preparation and is proportional to the
amount of cholesterol added to the food.   Similar results were
obtained in the experiment shown in Table II.   In this experiment
1% cholesterol in the food was given for various periods before
killing the animals at 1.0 a.m. or 1.0 p.m.   In the absence of any
additional cholesterol in the food, the activity of the enzyme at

TABLE III

ACTIVITY OF CHOLESTEROL 7α-HYDROXYLASE IN LIVER MICROSOMAL PREPARATIONS FROM BILE-FISTULA AND FROM CHOLESTYRAMINE-FED RATS KILLED IN THE DAY AND IN THE NIGHT

| Treatment | Time of day when killed | Activity of cholesterol 7α-hydroxylase (nmol/20 min/ mg protein) | Total cholesterol in incubation flask (nmol/mg protein) | Estimated size of substrate pool (nmol/mg protein) |
|---|---|---|---|---|
| Control | 1.0 a.m. | 1.51 | 52.2 | 27.2 |
| | 1.0 p.m. | 0.88 | 48.0 | 32.0 |
| Cholestyramine | 1.0 a.m. | 3.06 | 65.6 | 22.2 |
| | 1.0 p.m. | 1.91 | 46.7 | 22.3 |
| Control | 1.0 a.m. | 0.86 | 53.5 | 24.9 |
| | 1.0 p.m. | 0.49 | 37.8 | 33.6 |
| Bile-fistula | 1.0 a.m. | 1.96 | 48.0 | 24.6 |
| | 1.0 p.m. | 1.52 | 40.0 | 26.9 |

The rats were adapted to controlled lighting and feeding on the standard diet for 14 days before the start of the experiment. Cholestyramine (5%) was given for 7 days before the animals were killed at 1.0 a.m. or 1.0 p.m.  Bile-duct cannulations or sham operations were carried out 4 days before the experiment.  Each value was obtained from the pooled livers of two rats. (From Reference 17, by permission).


1.0 a.m. was about twice that at 1.0 p.m.  When cholesterol was added to the food, the diurnal rhythm of enzyme activity was maintained, but at higher average levels.  The increase in enzyme activity was accompanied by an increase in the microsomal cholesterol content and in the estimated size of the substrate pool. There is a close parallel between the diurnal rhythm in enzyme activity and the size of the substrate pool, both increasing at night and decreasing during the day.  This correlation raises the possibility that the increase in enzyme activity observed during cholesterol feeding is due to an expansion of the size of the

substrate pool by the cholesterol, rather than to increased capacity of the enzyme.    Hence the increased output of bile acids in
cholesterol-fed rats may be due to an increase in the supply of
cholesterol as substrate for an enzyme that is not saturated under
normal conditions (1).

The interruption of the return of bile acids to the liver,
either by feeding cholestyramine (18) or by making a bile fistula
(19,20), increases the 24-hour output of bile acids in rats.
Table III shows the effect of total interruption of the enterohepatic circulation or of partial diversion of bile acids on the
activity of cholesterol 7α-hydroxylase.    For the experiment of
total diversion of bile, bile fistulas were established in a group
of rats and another group of rats included sham-operated animals.
The rats were killed four days after the operation.    In both
groups of rats the activity of the enzyme was higher at night than
during the day, but the activity in bile-fistula rats was 2-3
times higher than that in the sham-operated animals killed at the
same time of day or night.    The cholestyramine-treated animals
were fed for seven days on a diet that contained 5% cholestyramine.
Again, the activity during the night was higher than during the
day, and the activity in the treated animals was about twice that
in the control animals killed at the corresponding time of day or
night.    Both in the bile-fistula and the cholestyramine-fed rats
the cholesterol content of microsomes was not significantly different from that in the corresponding controls.    Moreover, there
was no increase in the estimated size of the substrate pool in the
treated animals.    The maintenance of a normal diurnal rhythm in
the activity of cholesterol 7α-hydroxylase in cholestyramine-fed
rats has also been described by others (7).

## DIURNAL RHYTHM IN THE RATE OF SYNTHESIS OF BILE ACIDS

If the formation of 7α-hydroxycholesterol is rate-limiting
for the formation of bile acids, the rate of synthesis of bile
acids in the intact rat will be expected to undergo diurnal oscillations with a maximum rate of synthesis during the night and a
minimum rate during the day.    However, for the intact rat we do
not have methods for obtaining information about rapid changes in
the rate of synthesis of bile acids.    In the bile-fistula rat,
once the pools of bile acids in the enterohepatic circulation have
been drained, the output of bile acids in the bile may be assumed
to be equal to their rate of synthesis.    With this assumption and
with the evidence that the diurnal rhythm in the activity of cholesterol 7α-hydroxylase persists in the bile-fistula rat, we have
investigated the rate of bile acid synthesis during the diurnal
cycle.    Fig. 2 shows the rate of excretion of bile acids plotted
against the time of day.    Twenty-four hours from the introduction
of the cannula, when the pools of bile acids were completely

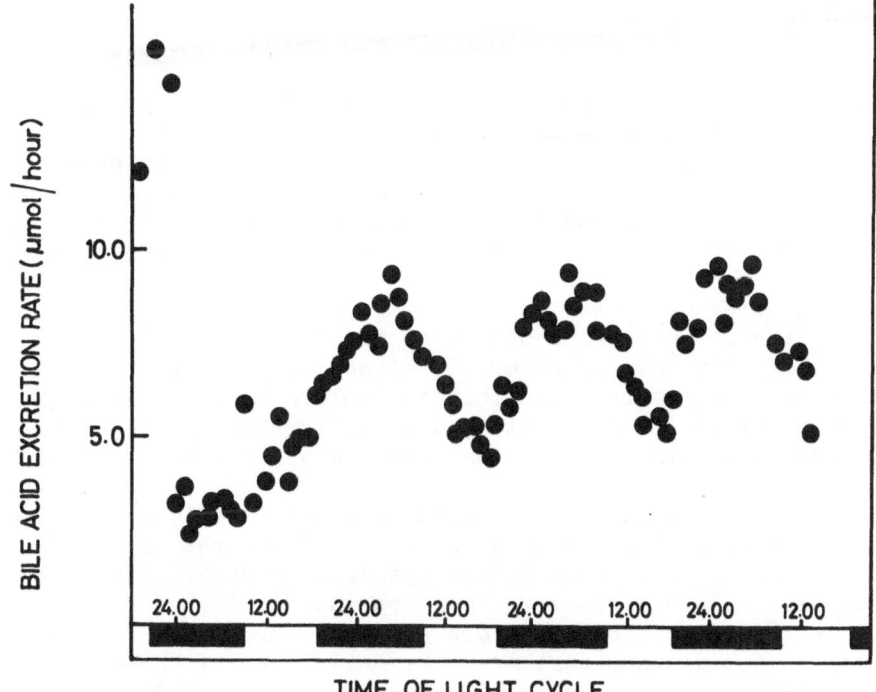

Fig. 2.   Biliary excretion of total bile acids after the introduction of the bile-duct cannula in a rat.   The black rectangles
show dark periods of the light cycle.   (From Reference 17, by
permission.)

washed out, the bile acid excretion rate assumed a diurnal rhythm
with minimum rate of excretion in the afternoon and maximum during
the dark period.   The fact that bile acid excretion and enzyme
activity both rise at night and fall during the day is consistent
with the view that the rate-limiting step in bile acid synthesis
is the formation of 7α-hydroxycholesterol from cholesterol.  Accordingly, the rate of bile acid biosynthesis in the intact rat
undergoes diurnal oscillation in parallel with the activity of
cholesterol 7α-hydroxylase and HMG-CoA reductase.  Analysis of
bile samples obtained during the diurnal cycle from the bile-fistula rat demonstrated that the rate of excretion of the two main
primary bile acids exhibit diurnal variation with maximum rates
of excretion occurring at the same time in the middle of the dark
period and minimum rates occurring at about noon (27).  Cholic
acid is the major of the bile acids excreted, with a rate of excretion that is about four times that of chenic acid.

THE ROLE OF GLUCOCORTICOIDS IN THE EXPRESSION OF THE DIURNAL
RHYTHM OF CHOLESTEROL 7α-HYDROXYLASE AND HMG–CoA REDUCTASE

Any rhythm in the composition or biochemical activity of a
mammalian tissue could have an originating stimulus either from
an endogenous or from an exogenous source.   Since it is never
possible to design experiments with the animals kept in an environment devoid of cyclic inputs it has proven difficult to provide
evidence about the relative contribution of endogenous or exogenous stimuli to the maintenance of a normal diurnal rhythm (21).
Moreover, since experiments designed to investigate the effect of
a single factor of endogenous origin on the diurnal rhythm of a
particular activity have considerable effects on a number of other
factors it is practically impossible to isolate a single factor
that is responsible for originating a daily rhythm and the biochemical events within the cell that mediate a rhythmic process.

Like the rate of hepatic cholesterogenesis, the concentration
of corticosterone in the adrenals and blood of the rat varies diurnally, rising several hours before the maximum activity of HMG-
CoA reductase.   Several workers have considered, therefore, the
possibility that glucocorticoids are of major importance in the
regulation of the diurnal rhythm in the activities of HMG–CoA
reductase (22,23) and cholesterol 7α-hydroxylase (24,25).

We have also, in our laboratory, investigated the effects of
adrenalectomy and of glucocorticoid replacement on the diurnal
rhythm in the activities of HMG–CoA reductase and cholesterol 7α-
hydroxylase.   Fig. 3 summarises the effect of bilateral adrenalectomy on the diurnal rhythm of these enzyme activities.   The
diurnal rhythm in the activity of all enzymes persists after adrenalectomy.   However, the amplitude of variation for the activity
of HMG–CoA reductase and cholesterol 7α-hydroxylase is greatly
reduced after adrenalectomy, since the decrease in the activity of
both enzymes is much higher during the dark period than during the
light period of the light cycle.   As shown earlier by others (26,
21) the effects of adrenalectomy on the diurnal rhythm of tyrosine
transaminase are minor.   Results from other laboratories on the
effect of adrenalectomy on the diurnal rhythm in the rate of hepatic cholesterogenesis or on that of the activity of HMG–CoA reductase are contradictory.   For example, Huber et al.(23) found
that adrenalectomy had no effect on the diurnal variation of HMG-
CoA reductase, whilst Edwards (22) has reported that adrenalectomy
abolishes the diurnal rhythm with enzyme activity at a low level
similar to that observed in the intact rat killed at noon.   With
regard to cholesterol 7α-hydroxylase, the previous findings are
less contradictory (24,25) and agree that the activity of cholesterol 7α-hydroxylase in adrenalectomized rats is low throughout the
diurnal cycle.

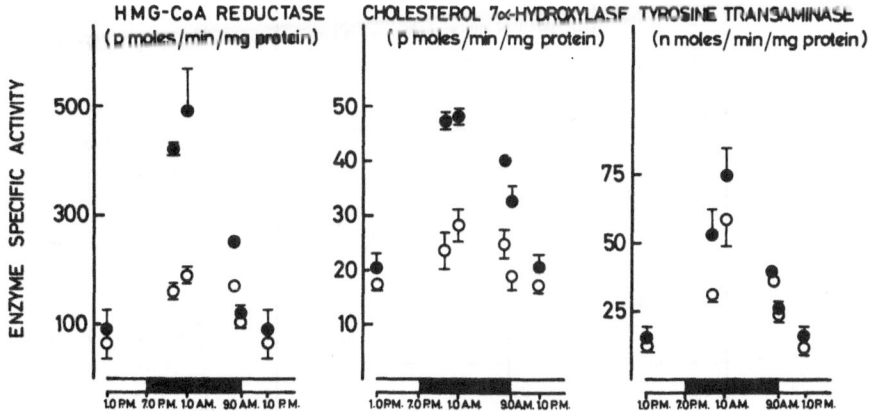

Fig. 3.    Diurnal rhythm in the activity of HMG-CoA reductase, of cholesterol 7α-hydroxylase and of tyrosine transaminase in liver subcellular fractions from adrenalectomized ( O ) and sham-operated ( ● ) rats.    The rats were adapted to controlled lighting and feeding for 2 weeks before they were adrenalectomized or sham-operated.    Ten to fifteen days after the operation, groups of rats were killed at the time designated and the livers were removed to prepare subcellular fractions for the assay of enzyme activity.    Each group contained at least three rats and the results are given as the mean ± SD (vertical line).    (Mitropoulos & Balasubramaniam, unpublished results).

     The effect of a single injection of hydrocortisone into adrenalectomized rats on the activity of cholesterol 7α-hydroxylase and HMG-CoA reductase is variable and depends on the time of day at which the animals are killed (Table IV). Administration of hydrocortisone three hours before the expected maximum in the activity of HMG-CoA reductase and of cholesterol 7α-hydroxylase results in a two-fold increase in the activity of both enzymes three hours later at levels similar to those observed for sham-operated rats killed at the same time.    The administration of hydrocortisone three hours before the expected minimum does not result in significant change in the activity of the enzymes.    However, the activity of tyrosine transaminase is increased both at 1.0 a.m. and at 1.0 p.m., following a single injection of hydrocortisone three hours earlier.    The increase in the activity of HMG-CoA reductase, of cholesterol 7α-hydroxylase and of tyrosine transaminase obtained following the administration of hydrocortisone to adrenalectomized rats is blocked by the simultaneous administration of actinomycin D (Table V).    Since a single injection of hydrocortisone into adrenalectomized rats at the beginning of the

## TABLE IV

EFFECT OF ADRENALECTOMY AND HYDROCORTISONE TREATMENT ON THE ACTIVITY OF HEPATIC HMG-CoA REDUCTASE, CHOLESTEROL 7α-HYDROXYLASE AND TYROSINE TRANSAMINASE

| Treatment | HMG-CoA reductase (pmol/min/mg protein) | | Cholesterol 7α-hydroxylase (pmol/min/mg protein) | | Tyrosine transaminase (nmol/min/mg protein) | |
|---|---|---|---|---|---|---|
| | 1.0 p.m. | 1.0 a.m. | 1.0 p.m. | 1.0 a.m. | 1.0 p.m. | 1.0 a.m. |
| Control | 87 ± 19 | 492 ± 79 | 25.2 ± 4.5 | 48.0 ± 3.1 | 8.0 ± 3.1 | 57.8 ± 3.7 |
| Adrenalectomized | 70 ± 17 | 168 ± 15 | 17.5 ± 2.5 | 28.0 ± 5.5 | 6.7 ± 1.0 | 36.6 ± 3.2 |
| Adrenalectomy + Hydrocortisone | 54 ± 10 | 387 ± 65 | 25.5 ± 6.5 | 44.5 ± 7.5 | 41.2 ± 0.8 | 60.6 ± 13.3 |

The rats were adapted to controlled feeding and lighting for 14 days before adrenalectomy or sham-operation. Adrenalectomized rats received a single intraperitoneal injection of a solution of hydrocortisone phosphate (250 μg/100 g rat) in saline, either at 10.0 a.m. or at 10.0 p.m. Sham-operated controls and adrenalectomized rats received injections of saline at the same time. All rats were killed 3 hours after the injection, either at 1.0 a.m. or at 1.0 p.m. There were three animals in each group and mean values ± SD are given. (Mitropoulos & Balasubramaniam, unpublished results.)

EFFECT OF ACTINOMYCIN D ON THE HYDROCORTISONE-MEDIATED INCREASE IN
THE ACTIVITY OF HMG-CoA REDUCTASE, OF CHOLESTEROL $7\alpha$-HYDROXYLASE
AND TYROSINE TRANSAMINASE

| Treatment | HMG-CoA reductase (pmol/min/ mg protein) | Cholesterol $7\alpha$-hydroxylase (pmol/min/ mg protein) | Tyrosine transaminase (nmol/min/ mg protein) |
|---|---|---|---|
| Control | 431 | 46.5 | 34.1 |
| Adrenalectomy | 195 | 28.3 | 22.8 |
| Adrenalectomy + Hydrocortisone | 371 | 40.8 | 62.4 |
| Adrenalectomy + Hydrocortisone + Actinomycin D | 180 | 23.8 | 17.9 |

The rats were adapted to controlled feeding and lighting for 2
weeks before adrenalectomy or sham-operation.   Each group contained 3 rats.   At 8.0 p.m. on the day of the experiment (14 days
after the operation) adrenalectomized rats received either hydrocortisone (250 ug/100 g rat) or hydrocortisone and actinomycin D
(50 ug/100 g rat).   The rats in the adrenalectomy and control
groups received saline injection.   All rats were killed 3 hours
later at 11.0 p.m. and the livers of the rats in each group were
pooled to prepare subcellular fractions.   (Mitropoulos and Balasubramaniam, unpublished results.)

dark period restored the peak activity of HMG-CoA reductase and
cholesterol $7\alpha$-hydroxylase to the levels observed for intact animals, and since these effects were blocked by actinomycin D, it is
reasonable to assume that an elevated plasma corticosterone concentration is responsible for the induction of synthesis of HMG-CoA
reductase and of cholesterol $7\alpha$-hydroxylase that occurs in the intact rat during the early part of the dark period.   However, the
fact that injection of hydrocortisone into adrenalectomized rats
at 10.0 a.m. did not affect the activity of HMG-CoA reductase or
of cholesterol $7\alpha$-hydroxylase three hours later, and that a diurnal
rhythm with low amplitude persists in adrenalectomized rats, suggests that glucocorticoids are not the only factor triggering induction of the enzymes.

TABLE VI

EFFECT OF ADRENALECTOMY AND HYDROCORTISONE TREATMENT ON THE POOL
SIZE AND THE DAILY SYNTHESIS OF CHOLIC ACID

| Treatment | Weight at end of experiment | Pool size (μmol/100 g rat) | Half-life (days) | Daily synthesis (μmol/day/ 100 g rat) |
|---|---|---|---|---|
| Control | 235 ± 9 | 20.2 ± 1.7 | 2.15 ± 0.17 | 6.55 ± 0.9 |
| Adrenalectomy | 197 ± 39 | 11.2 ± 3.1 | 2.22 ± 0.42 | 3.46 ± 1.1 |
| Adrenalectomy + Hydrocortisone | 200 ± 8 | 18.8 ± 3.0 | 2.63 ± 0.31 | 5.32 ± 0.6 |

The rats were adapted to controlled feeding and lighting for 14
days before the operation.   Each group contained 5 rats that were
housed in individual cages.   All rats received [14C]-cholic acid
on the 10th day after the operation.   Adrenalectomized rats treated with hydrocortisone received a hydrocortisone injection 24
hours before they received [14C]-cholic acid and daily injections
for 7 days thereafter.   At the end of the 7th day all rats were
killed.   Values are expressed as means ± SD for the 5 rats in each
group.   (Mitropoulos and Balasubramaniam, unpublished results.)

     The effects of adrenalectomy and glucocorticoid replacement
on the activity of cholesterol 7α-hydroxylase observed in vitro
suggest measurable effects on the overall rate of synthesis of
cholic acid under these conditions.   We have, therefore, compared
certain parameters related to the metabolism of cholic acid in
adrenalectomized rats, adrenalectomized-hydrocortisone-treated
rats and sham-operated controls (Table VI).   The cholic acid pool
size was considerably reduced in adrenalectomized rats, as compared with that in the sham-operated controls, but the bile acid
pool size in hydrocortisone-treated adrenalectomized rats was not
significantly different from that of the sham-operated animals.
Since there was no considerable difference in the half life and
fractional turnover rate of cholic acid between the three groups
of rats changes in the pool size reflect changes in the daily rate
of synthesis of cholic acid.

The effects of adrenalectomy and glucocorticoid replacement on the in vivo determined daily synthesis of cholic acid are, thus, consistent on the effects on the activity of cholesterol 7α-hydroxylase, observed in vitro under similar conditions of treatment.

## INTERACTION OF THE DIURNAL RHYTHM IN THE RATE OF HEPATIC CHOLESTEROGENESIS AND IN THE RATE OF BILE ACID BIOSYNTHESIS

The diurnal rhythms in the rate of hepatic cholesterogenesis and in the rate of synthesis of bile acids from cholesterol are independently controlled probably through an alternating cycle of repression and derepression of synthesis of HMG-CoA reductase and cholesterol 7α-hydroxylase respectively. Although the rate of hepatic cholesterogenesis varies manyfold between the maximum in the middle of the dark period and the minimum around noon, there is no evidence that the cholesterol content in liver or other pools of exchangeable cholesterol in the body varies diurnally. Since the liver is the site for synthesis of bile acids and since the rate of bile acid biosynthesis undergoes diurnal oscillations it is possible that a major physiological function of the diurnal rhythm in the rate of hepatic cholesterogenesis is the supply of the precursor pool for the synthesis of bile acids with cholesterol at variable rates. If this was the case, we should expect that newly synthesized cholesterol feeds preferentially into the cholesterol pool that acts as substrate for bile acid biosynthesis. Evidence for this was obtained by studying the effect of rapid changes in the rate of cholesterol synthesis (associated with the diurnal rhythm in the rate of hepatic cholesterogenesis) on the specific radioactivity of bile acids during the diurnal cycle in the bile-fistula rat, when cholesterol in different pools was selectively labelled.

Fig. 4 shows the rate of excretion and the specific radioactivity of total bile acids in bile samples obtained during the second diurnal cycle after the introduction of the bile-duct cannula in a rat in which the exchangeable cholesterol throughout the body was uniformly labelled by prolonged feeding with [3H]-cholesterol. The specific radioactivity declined progressively during the first half of the dark period to a minimum value at about the same time as the peak in the excretion of bile acids occurred. Towards the end of the dark period the specific radioactivity began to increase as the rate of excretion of bile acids decreased. Since cholesterol is not absorbed unless bile acids reach the intestine (28), absorption of [3H]-labelled cholesterol must have ceased when the bile fistula was made. This would have led to a progressive fall in the specific radioactivity of exchangeable cholesterol as [3H]-cholesterol was replaced by newly-synthesized cholesterol. However, this does not explain the changes in

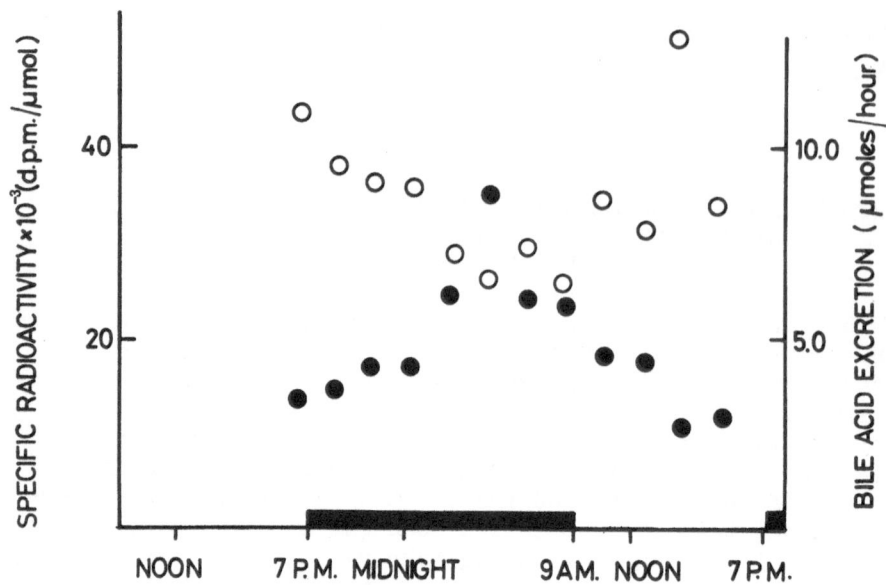

Fig. 4.    Diurnal changes in the rate of excretion ( ● ) and specific radioactivity ( ○ ) of total bile acids in a bile fistula
rat after prolonged feeding with [³H]-cholesterol.    The black
rectangle shows the dark period of the light cycle.    (From Reference 27, by permission.)

specific radioactivity of bile acids observed in Fig. 4.    The
steep decline in specific radioactivity followed by a secondary
rise suggests, rather, that bile acids are derived from a relatively small pool of cholesterol that equilibrates more rapidly
with newly-synthesized cholesterol than  with the exchangeable
cholesterol in other pools.    The rise in the rate of hepatic cholesterogenesis that occurs during the night caused the specific
radioactivity of the precursor pool of bile acids to fall more
rapidly than that of the pools which equilibrate less rapidly
with newly-synthesized cholesterol.    When the rate of hepatic
cholesterogenesis declined from its maximum, the specific radioactivity of the precursor pool rose, as it equilibrated with other
pools in which the specific radioactivity had not fallen so
steeply.

     Similar resluts for the rate of excretion and for the changes
in the specific radioactivity of cholic acid were obtained in another experiment shown in Fig. 5.    This rat was fed with [³H]-
cholesterol for five weeks before the cannulation and was then
infused with trace amounts of [2-C¹⁴]-mevalonic acid at a constant
rate.    The changes in the specific radioactivity of [³H]-cholate

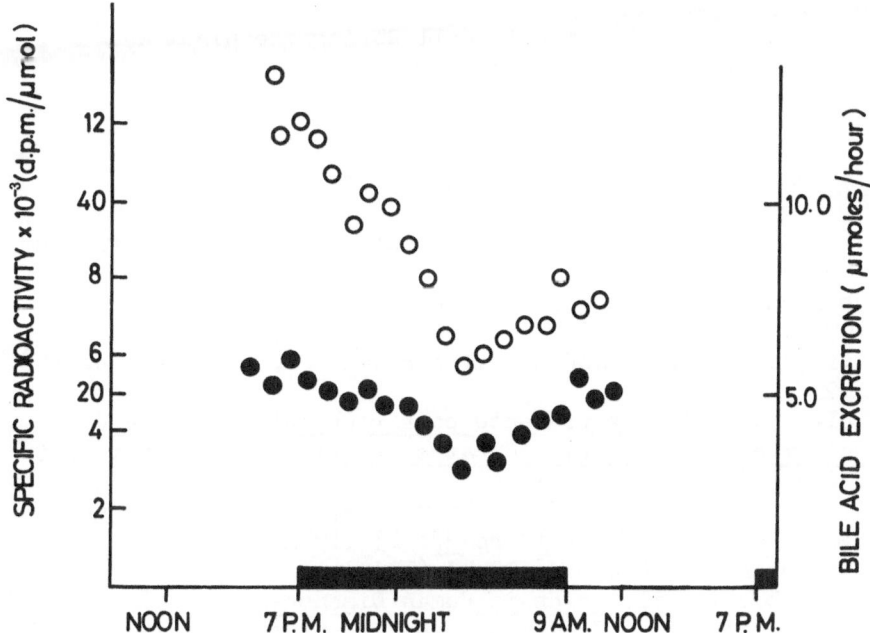

Fig. 5. Diurnal changes in the specific radioactivity of [3H]-cholic acid ( o ) and [14C]-cholic acid ( ● ) during intravenous infusion of [2-14C]-mevalonic acid into a bile-fistula rat after prolonged feeding with [3H]-cholesterol. The black rectangle shows the dark period of the light cycle. (From Reference 27, by permission.)

show a pattern similar to the pattern of changes in the specific radioactivity of [3H]-total bile acids (Fig. 4). Since cholic acid is quantitatively the major bile acid synthesized in the liver, the specific radioactivity of [3H]-cholate excreted after prolonged feeding with [3H]-cholesterol would be expected to follow a pattern similar to that of [3H]-labelled total bile acids. The specific radioactivity of [14C]-cholic acid decreased to a minimum coinciding with the maximum of excretion and then increased to the level observed at the beginning of the dark period (Fig. 5). The changes in the specific radioactivity of [14C]-cholic acid may also be explained in terms of a cholesterol precursor pool for cholic acid that equilibrates preferentially with the newly-synthesized cholesterol. Since mevalonate lies after the rate-limiting step in the hepatic synthesis of cholesterol, [14C] should be incorporated into newly-synthesized cholesterol at a constant rate during a constant infusion of a tracer amount of [14C]-mevalonic acid.

Therefore, the specific [14C]-radioactivity of newly-synthesized cholesterol would be expected to fall during the night and to rise again as cholesterol synthesis declines.

REFERENCES

1.  Balasubramaniam, S., K.A. Mitropoulos, and N.B. Myant. Eur. J. Biochem. 34:77 (1973).
2.  Björkhem, I., and H. Danielsson. Eur. J. Biochem. 53:63 (1975).
3.  Mitropoulos, K.A., and S. Balasubramaniam. Biochem. J. 128:1 (1972).
4.  Gielen, J. Mémoire présenté pour l'obtention du grade de docteur en sciences biomédicales experimentales. Université de Liège (1969).
5.  Mitropoulos, K.A., S. Balasubramaniam, G.F. Gibbons, and B.E.A. Reeves. FEBS Letters 27:203 (1972).
6.  Danielsson, H. Steroids 20:63 (1972).
7.  Mayer, D., in Bile Acids in Human Diseases. (Eds.) P. Back and W. Gerok, F.K. Schattauer Verlag, Stuttgart (1972) p. 103
8.  Kandutsch, A.A., and S.E. Saucier. J. Biol. Chem. 244:2299 (1969).
9.  Shapiro, D.J., and V.W. Rodwell. Biochem. Biophys. Res. Commun. 37:867 (1969).
10. Hamprecht, B., C. Nussler, and F. Lynen. FEBS Letters 4:117 (1969).
11. Edwards, P.A., and R.G. Gould. J. Biol. Chem. 247:1520 (1972).
12. Higgins, M., T. Kawachi, and H. Rudney. Biochem. Biophys. Res. Commun. 45:138 (1971).
13. Edwards, P.A., H. Muroya, and R.G. Gould. J. Lipid Res. 13: 396 (1972).
14. Portman, O.W., G.V. Mann, and A.P. Wysocki. Arch. Biochem. Biophys. 59:224 (1955).
15. Beher, W.T., K.K. Casazza, M.E. Beher, A.M. Filus, and J. Bertasius. Proc. Soc. Exp. Biol. Med. 134:595 (1970).
16. Wilson, J.D. Am. J. Physiol. 202:1073 (1962).
17. Mitropoulos, K.A., S. Balasubramaniam, and N.B. Myant. Biochim. Biophys. Acta. 326:428 (1973).
18. Huff, J.W., J.L. Gilfillan, and V.M. Hunt. Proc. Soc. Exp. Biol Med. 114:352 (1963).
19. Thompson, J.C., and H.M. Vars. Am. J. Physiol. 179:405 (1954).
20. Eriksson, S. Proc. Soc. Exp. Biol. Med. 94:578 (1957).
21. Wurtman, R.J. Life Sciences 15:827 (1974).
22. Edwards, P.A. J. Biol. Chem. 240:2912 (1973).
23. Huber, J., B. Hamprecht, O.-A. Müller, and W. Guder. Hoppe-Seyler's Z. Physiol. Chem. 353:313 (1972).

24. Gielen, J., B. Robaye, J. Van Cantfort, and J. Renson. Arch. int. Pharmocodyn 183:403 (1970).
25. Van Cantfort, J. Biochimie 55:1171 (1973).
26. Wurtman, R.J., and J. Axelrod. Proc. Nat. Acad. Sci. 57:1594 (1967).
27. Mitropoulos, K.A., N.B. Myant, G.F. Gibbons, S. Balasubramaniam, and B.E.A. Reeves. J. Biol. Chem. 249:6052 (1974).
28. Siperstein, M.D., I.L. Chaikoff, and W.O. Reinhardt. J. Biol. Chem. 198:111 (1952).

DISCUSSION OF COMMENTARY BY K. MITROPOULOS

Ostrow:    I have done some studies on the effects of phototherapy
on bile acid metabolism in both Gunn and normal rats.    There are
two things that I am puzzled about.    These rats are put on
biliary drainage for 33 hours before the experiments were conducted
and then they are either kept in the dark or exposed to about 20
times the amount of light that you normally have in a room or the
amount in a sunny day outside.    In both groups of rats there was
no difference in bile acid excretion as compared to those kept in
the dark and those kept in the light, nor was there any difference
in the group that was kept in the dark.    There was another group
where I just let them go through the normal cycle laboratory life
and I did not see any difference in the amount of bile acid
excretion under those conditions.    Now, is this possibly due to
the time at which I am examining them after the enterohepatic
cycle is interrupted, or what?

Mitropoulos:    What was happening to those rats before they were
put under such conditions?    Were they normally fed and housed?

Ostrow:    They were just normally fed and housed.    Yes.

Mitropoulos:    If you try to reverse the light-cycle in a group
of rats, it does take a long time to reach peak activity in the
new dark period and minimum activity in the new light period.
It takes about 3 weeks or something like that.

Taylor:    I just have one comment and a question.    Almost all the
work that one sees on bile acid metabolism is done in rats or man
and I would like to make a plea for investigation with other
animals.    The question I like to ask is based on the didactic
statement that one often hears and reads that the rabbit is
deficient in 7$\alpha$-hydroxylase.    I wonder if any experiments have
been done of this type with rabbits, or indeed with bile acid
biosynthesis.

Mitropoulos:    I would like to ask Dr. Danielsson that.

Danielsson:    Although, to my knowledge, it has not been examined,
this is completely impossible, because certainly rabbit bile

428

consists predominantly of deoxycholic acid and also, for that matter, allodeoxycholic acid, but as soon as you make a fistula it only produces cholic acid.

Coleman:   This is a question relating to the pool size of cholesterol in your experiments.   The enzyme, the hydroxylase, is presumably an endoplasm reticulum enzyme.   When you fractionate liver cells, much of the cholesterol is in the plasma membrane. When you make microsomes, there is a proportion of plasma membrane in the microsomal fraction.   Could it be that the proportion of the pool size that does not appear to equilibrate is that proportion of the microsomes which is related to the plasma membrane and the proportion which is equilibrating with the hydroxylase is that proportion of cholesterol which is in the endoplasmic reticulum?

Mitropoulos:   That is possible.   We never tried to find what you call a substrate pool.   But there is a possibility that plasma membrane which is rich in cholesterol would account for the cholesterol that does not equilibrate with the enzyme.

Coleman:   It would clearly equilibrate in an intact cell, in an in vivo situation, but in an in vitro situation it may not be equilibrating.   That may possibly be tested by taking a purified plasma membrane preparation and adding that to the microsomes in which case you would not increase your pool size.

Mayer:   I have only a short comment.   If you talk about the Circadian rhythm of cholesterol $7\alpha$-hydroxylase you should mention that that has also arisen in animals with a depressed enzyme activity.   That means, in animals fed cholic acid or chenodeoxycholic acid.   So I should say that the Circadian rhythm is concerned with the regulation of $7\alpha$-hydroxylation by the bile acid content of the enterohepatic circulation.   And there is another interesting effect.   The maximum activity of a normal animal is at 24 hours.   In animals with a depressed enzyme activity you find the maximum of enzyme activity shifted to 21, three hours before.

Brooks:   I wonder if there was any evidence of a role of the central nervous system in this phenomenon.   Does the cerebration of chronic stress of some kind modify the diurnal variation?

Mitropoulos:   There is a lot of work done about other enzymes and other metabolic activities.   I do not know of any relevant work on cholesterol $7\alpha$-hydroxylase and HMG CoA-reductase.   Presumably many factors are interrelated and interconnected when they produce this picture which you see there.   There is not a single factor that controls the diurnal rhythm of any activity or metabolite synthesis.

Faergeman:    You feel that the precursor pool for bile acid
synthesis is newly synthesized cholesterol.    However, you also
showed that feeding cholesterol to rats increased the diurnal
variation of the enzymes measured.    Would you care to discuss
this in light of the hypothesis that cholesterol-containing plasma
lipoproteins might be the specific precursor pool for bile acids.

Mitropoulos:    "Pools" is what an experiment defines, and an
experiment defines a "pool" because there is a small difference
in the equilibration time between two different positions in the
cell.    Nobody has said that the precursor pool is a closed system
that accepts newly synthesized cholesterol, and newly synthesized
cholesterol does not go to other pools.    We know that if we
inject cholesterol we get bile acids, and in the same way, if
cholesterol is taken in the food and a lot of cholesterol goes to
the liver, that will be distributed to other pools, and of course
the precursor pool will get its share.

Popjak:    I am just wondering about this differentiation of newly
synthesized cholesterol as the specific pool for the formation of
bile acids.    As I understand it, it is free cholesterol which is
hydroxylated first.    At the same time it is quite true, both
in vitro and in vivo, that newly synthesized cholesterol is there
in the free form.    So, is it not just simply that it is the free
cholesterol pool that is the precursor pool for bile acid synthesis,
not necessarily related to newly synthesized cholesterol?

Mitropoulos:    In the experiment described, cholesterol was fed to
the rat for 5 weeks.    This will be enough for every pool, even
esterified cholesterol, to be uniformly labelled.    Now, the point
is that the newly synthesized cholesterol will have diluted more
the pool from which bile acids were synthesized than the other
pools, and the other pools which retained higher specific activity
just increase the specific radioactivity of the precursor pool as
soon as the rate of cholesterol synthesis declined.    But there is
not only this evidence.    Since we have done this work, work from
other laboratories has shown that this is true, and independent
methods were used.

Borgström:    You have given good evidence why, in the rat, you
increase the formation of bile salts when you feed cholesterol,
that is by increasing the liver pool of cholesterol.    Why does
not this take place in man?    Why do you not have an increased
bile salt production from sterols in man when feeding cholesterol?
Do you have any ideas about this?

Mitropoulos:    I would not like to answer that question.    Perhaps somebody else in the audience would be more qualified to answer it.

Vlahcevic:    You have shown that specific activity of cholic acid
goes down during the nocturnal cycle while bile acid secretion
goes up for cholic acid and total bile acids.    That does not
happen with chenodeoxycholic acid.    Would you like to comment on
that?

Mitropoulos:    Yes, that is true.    I showed the specific radioactivity of $^{14}$C-labelled cholic acid after infusion of trace
amounts of $2-^{14}$C mevalonic acid at a constant rate.    When we
looked at the same thing for chenodeoxycholic acid the specific
radioactivity did not have this gradual fall, the minimum and
the secondary rise.    It was kept rather constant throughout the
diurnal cycle, and we concluded from that that the precursor pool
for the synthesis of cholic acid must be different from that for
the synthesis of chenodeoxycholic acid.    Except for that, and
the fact that there is in rat an alternative pathway for the
synthesis of chenodeoxycholic acid in mitochondria, I cannot add
any more.

Dowling:    In other species than the rat and man, there are
comparable changes.    In the Rhesus monkey there is a diurnal
variation in bile acid synthesis in animals with a complete bile
fistula.    It is also influenced by fasting and feeding.    My
question is about the factors regulating cholesterol $7\alpha$-hydroxylase
activity.    Is it related to the mass of bile acid passing through
the liver cell or the concentration of bile acid?    It has been
suggested that in some situations where there is a small bile acid
pool, the cycling frequency of the pool increases so that the
total mass of bile acid fluxing through the liver cell is no
different from normal.    In such a situation, is it concentration
or mass which is going to influence the synthetic activity?

Mitropoulos:    I cannot answer that question.

Hofmann:    If I understand your presentation you propose that in
the rat substrate is changing with cholesterol synthesis and that
the enzyme is unsaturated.    Is it possible that the opposite is
true in man?    Namely, there is always plenty of substrate and
what is really limiting is the amount of enzyme.

Mitropoulos:    I do not know.    The thing is that we have to do
certain experiments in man to decide the properties of the enzyme
in man.

Boyer:    You have shown that with a persistent biliary fistula
the diurnal variation in bile acid excretion continues for up to
2 or 3 days.    Have you carried this out further, and was this

done under conditions where feeding was also intermittent?   If
so, might you guess what may happen to diurnal variation if you in
some way maintain feeding constantly in those conditions?

Mitropoulos:   What do you mean by feeding constantly?   Do you
mean feeding them throughout the 24-hour cycle?

Boyer:   Yes.   Tube-feeding for example.

Mitropoulos:   The rat, like other species, eats at certain times
during the day.

Boyer:   Correct, but I wonder whether you can do this by constant
infusion or tube-feeding for example.

Mitropoulos:   No, but I can answer your question indirectly.
The activity of cholesterol $7\alpha$-hydroxylase persists if you withdraw
the food from the rat.

Boyer:   For how long?

Mitropoulos:   We were interested in the first diurnal cycle after
having withdrawn the food.   I do not know how long one would have
to withdraw food to produce changes.

# HEPATIC TRANSPORT OF BILE ACIDS

S. Erlinger, J.C. Glasinović, R. Poupon, M. Dumont

Unité de Recherches de Physiopathologie Hépatique

(INSERM), Hôpital Beaujon, F 92110 Clichy, France

The liver is responsible for the secretion of bile acids into bile and for the uptake and reexcretion of bile acids that participate in the enterohepatic circulation. In addition, the secretion of bile acids by the liver is of major importance for the secretion of bile itself and for the secretion of biliary lipids. In this review will be summarised the current concepts on the steps of the hepatic transport of bile acids (uptake, cellular transport, biliary secretion), as well as the views on the mechanisms of bile formation and on biliary lipid secretion.

## HEPATIC TRANSPORT OF BILE ACIDS
### Uptake from Plasma

Most of the bile acid found in normal bile is not newly synthesized, but bile acid that has been reabsorbed by the intestine and returns to the liver. The first step in hepatic transport is therefore the uptake of bile acid from sinusoidal plasma into liver cell.

Bile acids in plasma are bound to plasma protein (44). Other compounds very efficiently taken up by the liver, such as sulfobromophthalein (BSP), indocyanine green or bilirubin, are also tightly bound to plasma proteins. This is possible because the endothelial wall of the sinusoids in the liver is permeable to proteins, so that protein-bound substances can get access to the sinusoidal surface of the hepatic cell plasma membrane.

The hepatic removal of bile acids from the plasma by the liver is extremely efficient. As originally shown by O'Maille et al. (37), the extraction of taurocholate during a single

433

passage through the canine liver may be of the order of 90 % .
Therefore, the hepatic clearance of bile acids approaches the
liver plasma flow. The high removal efficiency of the liver for
bile acids suggests that specific uptake mechanisms are involved.

The hepatic uptake of bile acids has been studied with the
multiple indicator dilution technique (20, 43) previously used
for BSP and other compounds (23, 25). A vascular indicator
(labelled red cells), an extracellular reference substance
(labelled albumin) and a known dose of the labelled bile acid to
be tested are rapidly injected into the portal vein. Hepatic
venous dilution curves are obtained and the analysis of the dilution curves allows to calculate the extraction of the bile acid,
a removal rate constant from plasma to liver, and the "initial"
velocity of uptake (25). In experiments using anesthetized dogs
(20)and isolated rat livers perfused in situ (43), it was found
that the initial velocity of uptake increased in a non-linear
fashion when the dose of taurocholate injected increased (Fig.1).
This finding suggests saturation kinetics. The calculated maximal "initial" velocity of uptake (Vmax) was, in the dog, 4.53
$\mu mol.s^{-1}.100$ g liver$^{-1}$, and the dose yielding half-maximal velocity of uptake ($K_D$) was 7.11 $\mu mol.100$ g liver$^{-1}$ for taurocholate.
Values obtained in the rat were of the same order of magnitude.
Subsequent experiments in the dog showed that the uptake of taurocholate was competitively inhibited by taurochenodeoxycholate (21).
These findings suggest that the uptake of bile acids by the liver
cell is dependent on a carrier-mediated transport system. Whether
this system is located within the cell membrane, the cytoplasm,
or both, is unknown.

It is interesting to note that the maximal capacity of uptake
(Vmax) is about 10 to 20 times higher than the known maximal capacity of biliary excretion (biliary transport maximum or Tm) : the
Tm for taurocholate is of 70-140 $\mu mol. min^{-1}$ (39, 52), i.e. approximately 0.2-0.4 $\mu mol. s^{-1}.100$ g liver$^{-1}$. Therefore, uptake is not
rate-limiting in the overall process of hepatic transport.

It is not known whether the uptake transport system of bile
acids is shared by other organic anions. Some studies have shown
inhibition of BSP uptake by bile acids (22) ; others have not (45) ;
these discrepancies may be due to differences in the experimental
design. Precise answer to this question must await a better cellular characterization of the transport systems. Whatever the mechanisms involved, the maximal capacity of uptake of bile acids is
much higher than that of BSP : the maximal capacity for BSP uptake
has been estimated to 110 mg. min$^{-1}$ per 10 kg b.wt. (24), i.e.
approximately 1 $\mu mol.s^{-1}.100$ g liver$^{-1}$, or about 5 times less than
that of taurocholate.

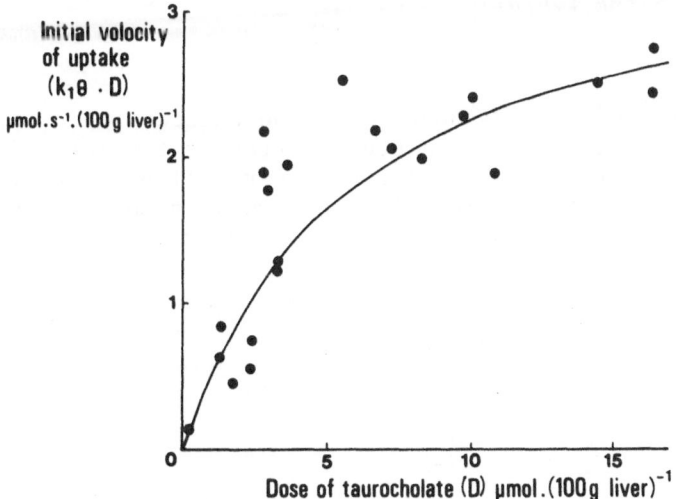

Figure 1. Influence of the dose of taurocholate on the initial velocity of uptake in the anesthetized dog. Each point is derived from an hepatic vein indicator dilution study ; in each study, a known dose of labelled taurocholate is injected into the portal vein together with appropriate indicators. The calculated initial velocity of uptake increases in a non-linear way with the dose. From Glasinović, Dumont, Duval, Erlinger (1975).

## Cellular Transport

The transport pathways of bile acids within the liver cell are poorly known. It is not known whether bile acids are bound to cytoplasmic proteins, such as Y and Z (32) which efficiently bind BSP, bilirubin and other organic anions. These proteins may play a role in the process of storage, well documented for BSP (53). In recent studies, a relative storage capacity for bile acids has been measured in the dog (39) ; the relative storage capacity was of the same order of magnitude as that of BSP ; this finding could imply

that binding sites for bile acids are available within the liver
cell that allow a concentration gradient between the plasma and
the cell to be maintained.

Some of the bile acids undergoing the enterohepatic circulation
and returning to the liver are deconjugated by the intestinal bacteria ; they are reconjugated by the liver cell prior to their
reexcretion into bile. Conjugation, however, is not a prerequisite
for biliary secretion : in an elegant study, O'Maille et al (35)

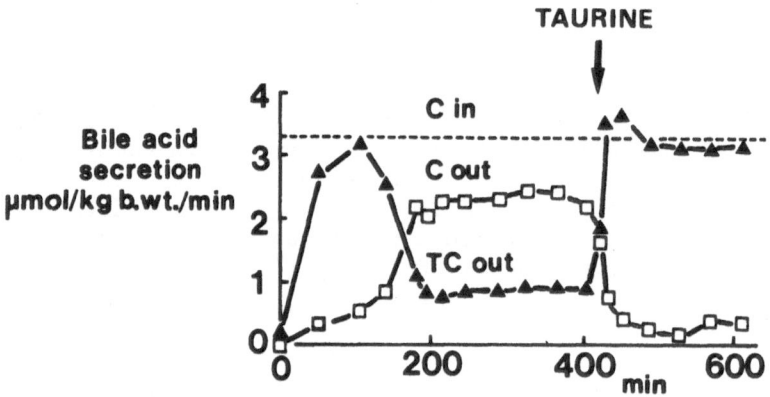

Figure 2. Influence of taurine depletion on bile acid secretion
in bile. Sodium cholate was infused at a rate of 3.3 µmol.min⁻¹.kg⁻¹
(dotted line). As hepatic pool of taurine becomes depleted, secretion of taurocholate falls, whereas secretion of unconjugated cholate increases. When taurine is administered, taurocholate secretion increases again. From O'Maille, Richards, Short (1965).

have shown that in taurine-depleted dogs, infusion of cholate was
followed by the biliary secretion of unconjugated cholate ; taurine
administration was promptly followed by reappearance of taurocholate
in bile (Fig.2).

Some metabolic transformations other than conjugation may occur within the liver cell ; for instance, dehydrocholate, a synthetic triketo bile acid, is secreted into bile after various hydroxylations, in the rabbit (Fig.3), the rat, the dog and in man (8,27,48).

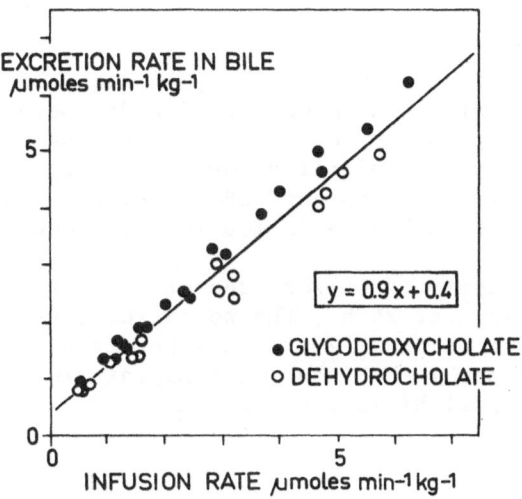

Figure 3. Hepatic hydroxylation of dehydrocholate in the rabbit. Dehydrocholate and glycodeoxycholate were infused intravenously at identical rates (abcissas) in two groups of rabbits. The secretion rates of 3-hydroxylated metabolites (ordinates) into bile were not different with dehydrocholate and glycodeoxycholate. Since dehydrocholate itself is not 3-hydroxylated, the experiment indicates that it has been entirely 3-hydroxylated during its passage through the liver.

## Biliary Secretion

Like BSP and bilirubin, bile acids are secreted into bile where they appear at concentrations much higher than those found in plasma. The secretion of bile acids into bile is probably a carrier-mediated or an active process ; a transport maximum (Tm) for bile acids has been measured ; for taurocholate, it is of the order of 4.75 to 8.50 $\mu mol.min^{-1}.kg^{-1}$ in the dog (35,39) and of 14 $\mu mol.$

$min^{-1}.kg^{-1}$ in the sheep (2) ; for cholate in the dog it is 8 μmol. $min^{-1}.kg^{-1}$ (37).

There is evidence that the transport system responsible for the biliary secretion of bile acids is distinct from that of BSP and bilirubin ; firstly, the Tm values for bile acids are much higher than that of BSP ; Tm for BSP in the dog is of the order of 0.23 $μmol.min^{-1}.kg^{-1}$ (53) ; secondly, in the mutant Corriedale sheep (which closely resembles the Dubin-Johnson syndrome in man), BSP and bilirubin transport are defective, whereas bile acid transport is normal (2) ; finally, no competition is observed between bile acids and BSP secretion into bile ; in fact, administration of taurocholate results in an enhancement of BSP apparent Tm (36) ; this enhancement is probably not ascribable to the increase in canalicular bile flow, as initially postulated (7), but to a specific effect of the bile acid on the BSP transport system (16,19) ; the precise nature of this interaction is not known.

The maximal capacity of biliary secretion corresponds to approximately 6 to 11 mmol per 24 h ; the normal biliary secretion rate of bile acids in man is about 20 to 30 g per 24 h, or approximately 30 to 50 mmol per 24 h ; thus, the biliary Tm is about 5 times in excess of the normal biliary secretion.


INFLUENCE OF BILE ACIDS ON BILE SECRETION

The mechanisms of bile formation have been reviewed recently (10,12,50) and will only be briefly summarized here.


Bile Acid Dependent Bile Formation

Bile acids are potent choleretics in most animal species. A linear relationship has been found between bile flow and bile acid secretion rate in animal experiments (42) and in man (6,40,41,46). The relationship between bile flow and bile acid secretion in man is illustrated on Fig.4, and suggests that, in this species, 10 μl of bile are formed per each μmol of bile acid secreted. Sperber (49) has proposed that the mechanism of the choleretic effect of bile acids was osmotic ; in this widely accepted view, the transport of bile acids into the canalicular lumen is responsible for an osmotic gradient allowing filtration of water and inorganic ions. In support of this hypothesis, it has been repeatedly observed that the choleretic effect of dehydrocholate (which does not form micelles in vitro and has presumably a higher osmotic activity than physiological bile acids) was greater than that of physiological bile acids. However, other explanations may be postulated, for instance stimulation by bile acids of a solute pump (48).

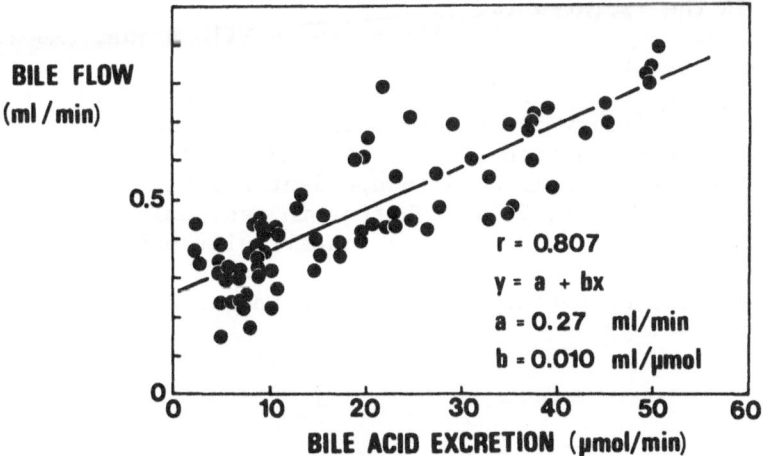

Figure 4. Relationship between bile flow and bile acid secretion in man. Data obtained from patients with T-tubes. There is a
linear relationship between bile flow and bile acid secretion,
with a slope b of 0.010 ml/μmol (10 μl of bile being formed per
each μmol of bile acid secreted) and an intercept for a zero bile
acid secretion a of 0.27 ml.min[-1] (indicating a total bile acid
independent bile flow of 0.27 ml.min[-1]).  From Prandi, Erlinger,
Glasinović, Dumont (1975).

Whatever the precise mechanism, bile acid secretion is associated with choleresis that is directly proportional to the rate of
bile acid secretion.  It is understandable that the magnitude of
bile acid dependent bile formation varies in time with the amount
of bile acids available in the liver.


Bile Acid Independent Bile Formation

Canalicular. In all species studied, extrapolation of the
relationship between bile flow and bile acid secretion for a zero
bile acid secretion yields a positive intercept.  This has generally been interpreted as due to a bile acid independent process

(13,14).   In the isolated rat liver preparation, it has even been
possible to collect bile without detectable bile acids, and its
flow approximated the value extrapolated from the bile flow –
bile acid secretion regression line (5).  Measurement of erythritol or mannitol biliary clearance, which is considered to estimate
canalicular bile production (18,54) has indicated that, in rabbits
and rats, most of the bile acid independent fraction of bile was
of canalicular origin (4,5,14), whereas in man, only part of it
(approximately 0.16 ml.min⁻¹) was of canalicular origin, the remaining being, as will be discussed later, of ductular or ductal
origin (40).  The components of bile flow in man are illustrated
on Fig.5.

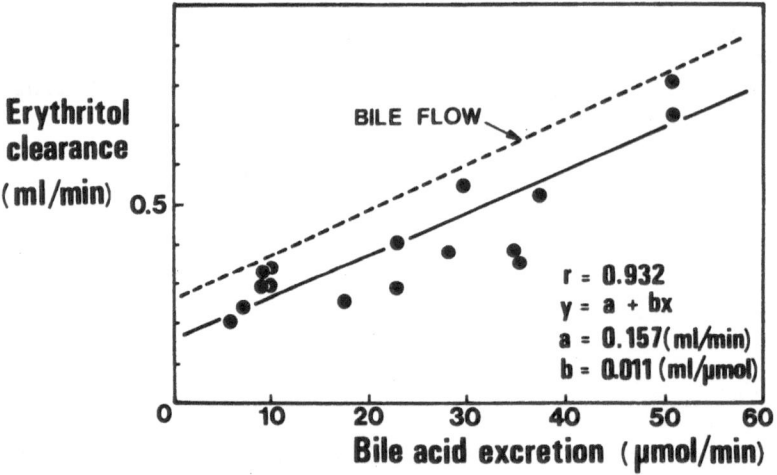

Figure 5.  Relationship between canalicular bile flow and bile
acid secretion in man.  Data obtained from the same patients as
those of Fig.4. Canalicular bile flow is estimated by erythritol
biliary clearance (ordinates).  There is a linear relationship
between canalicular bile flow and bile acid secretion (abcissas) :
the bile acid dependent canalicular bile flow is of 11 µl per µmol
of bile acid secreted ; the canalicular bile acid independent bile
flow (a) is of 0.157 ml.min⁻¹ ; the ductal or ductular bile acid
independent bile flow is of 0.11 ml.min⁻¹. From Prandi et al. (1975).

The canalicular bile acid independent bile flow has been shown
to be decreased by inhibitors of sodium transport (5,14), by various dyes, such as rose bengale or indocyanine green (9,28), by
estrogens (26) ; it is increased by acute administration of theophylline, glucagon or hydrocortisone (17,30,34) and chronic administration of microsomal enzyme inducers, such as phenobarbital
(4,31,38). Its mechanism of elaboration is yet unknown ; the most
currently accepted view is that it could be the result of active
sodium transport into bile canaliculi (14).

Ductular/Ductal. As seen in Fig.5, part of the bile acid independent bile flow is not reflected in erythritol clearance ; therefore, presumably it does not originate in the canaliculi but probably at a site distal within the biliary system, i.e. the bile
ductules or ducts. Studies in guinea-pigs and dogs have clearly
shown that choleresis induced by the hormone secretin was not associated with increases in erythritol or mannitol clearance, and was,
therefore, presumably of ductular or ductal origin (18,54). Ductal
or ductular choleresis (such as secretin choleresis) is usually
associated with an increase in bicarbonate concentration in bile
(42). Its mechanism of elaboration and its physiological role are,
at present, unknown.

## INFLUENCE OF BILE ACIDS ON BILIARY LIPIDS

Bile acid secretion appears to be the most important determinant of biliary cholesterol and phospholipid secretion. Kay and
Entenman originally demonstrated that in the isolated rat liver
the biliary secretion of phospholipids is enhanced by taurocholate
secretion (29). This observation has been repeatedly confirmed
and extended to cholesterol secretion (27,51). In general, the
relationship between bile acid secretion rate on the one hand,
and cholesterol or phospholipid secretion rate has been found to
be not linear (27,51), so that the amount of lipid secreted per
each mole of bile acid decreases at high bile acid secretion rates.
In recent studies, however, both in man (33), and in dogs ( R.Pou-
pon, R. Poupon, M. Duval, M. Dumont, S. Erlinger, unpublished observations), when only one molecular species of bile acid is secreted into bile, there is a linear relationship between bile acid
secretion and cholesterol or phospholipid secretion.

The cellular mechanism by which bile acids stimulate cholesterol or phospholipid secretion is not known. It is, however, highly likely that it is related to the ability of bile acids to form
micelles, i.e. polymolecular aggregates with lipid solubilizing
properties. It has been suggested that cholesterol and phospholipids may be directly derived from the canalicular membrane (47).
Consistent with the view that micelle formation has a key role in
biliary lipid secretion, it has been noted that dehydrocholate

(whose metabolites in vivo are apparently poor micelle-formers)
is unable to stimulate cholesterol or phospholipid secretion
(8,27,51) ; conversely, secretion of taurochenodeoxycholate, a
dihydroxy conjugated bile acid whose micellar weight and size are
higher than those of taurocholate, is associated with much more
cholesterol or phospholipid than taurocholate secretion in dogs
(3, R. Poupon et al., unpublished observations) ; its ability to
decrease cholesterol secretion in man (1) and to dissolve cholesterol gallstones appears to be specific and has not yet been
explained.

Finally, it is noteworthy that acetylsalicylate, a bile acid-
independent choleretic, was able to decrease biliary cholesterol
and phospholipid secretion (11). This may be due to dilution of
intracanalicular bile acids and decreased micelle formation ; similar observations have been made with SC 2644, another bile acid-
independent choleretic (51) and suggest that bile acid independent
canalicular choleresis may play a role in regulating biliary lipid
secretion. In the search of agents decreasing biliary cholesterol
content and potentially useful in the treatment of cholesterol
gallstones, these observations may be of interest.


## REFERENCES

1.  ADLER RD, BENNION LJ, DUANE WC, GRUNDY SM (1975) Effects of
        low dose chenodeoxycholic acid feeding on biliary lipid
        metabolism. Gastroenterology 68 : 326-334.

2.  ALPERT S, MOSHER M, SHANSKE A, ARIAS IM (1969) Multiplicity of
        hepatic excretory mechanisms for organic anions. J Gen
        Physiol 53 : 238-247.

3.  BERGMANN K Von, PAUMGARTNER G, PREISIG R (1973) Increased cho-
        lesterol saturation in dog bile induced by chenodeoxy-
        cholic acid. Digestion 8 : 440. (abstract).

4.  BERTHELOT P, ERLINGER S, DHUMEAUX D, PREAUX AM (1970) Mechanism
        of phenobarbital-induced hypercholeresis in the rat.
        Am J Physiol 219 : 809-813.

5.  BOYER JL, KLATSKIN G (1970) Canalicular bile flow and bile
        secretory pressure : evidence for a non-bile salt depen-
        dent fraction in the isolated perfused rat liver.
        Gastroenterology 59 : 853-859.

6.  BOYER JL, BLOOMER JR (1974) Canalicular bile secretion in man. Studies utilizing the biliary clearance of $^{14}$C mannitol. J Clin Invest 54 : 773-781.

7.  BOYER JL, SCHEIG RL, KLATSKIN G (1970) The effect of sodium taurocholate on the hepatic metabolism of sulfobromophthalein sodium (BSP) : the role of bile flow. J Clin Invest 49 : 206-215.

8.  DESJEUX JF, ERLINGER S, DUMONT M (1973) Métabolisme et influence sur la sécrétion biliaire du déhydrocholate chez le chien. Biol Gastroentérol (Paris) 6 : 9-18.

9.  DHUMEAUX D, ERLINGER S, BENHAMOU JP, FAUVERT R (1970) Effects of rose bengal on bile secretion in the rabbit : inhibition of a bile salt-independent fraction. Gut 11 : 134-140.

10. ERLINGER S (1972) Physiology of bile flow. In : Progress in Liver Diseases. Ed. by H Popper, F Schaffner. Grune and Stratton, New York. pp. 63-82.

11. ERLINGER S, BIENFAIT D, POUPON R, DUMONT M, DUVAL M (1975) Effect of lysine acetylsalicylate on biliary lipid secretion in dogs. Clin Sci Mol Med (in press).

12. ERLINGER S, DHUMEAUX D (1974) Mechanisms and control of secretion of bile water and electrolytes. Gastroenterology 66 : 281-304.

13. ERLINGER S, DHUMEAUX D, BENHAMOU JP, FAUVERT R (1969) La sécrétion biliaire du lapin : preuves en faveur d'une importante fraction indépendante des sels biliaires. Rev Fr Etud Clin Biol 14 : 144-150.

14. ERLINGER S, DHUMEAUX D, BERTHELOT P, DUMONT M (1970) Effect of inhibitors of sodium transport on bile formation in the rabbit. Am J Physiol 219 :416-422.

15. ERLINGER S, DUMONT M (1971) Metabolism of dehydrocholate in the rabbit liver : influence of micelle formation on choleresis. Eur J Clin Invest 1 : 371. (abstract).

16. ERLINGER S, DUMONT M (1973) Influence of canalicular bile flow on sulfobromophthalein transport maximum in bile in the dog. In : The Liver. Quantitative Aspects of Structure and Function. Ed. by G Paumgartner and R Preisig. Karger, Basel. pp. 306-313.

17. ERLINGER S, DUMONT M (1973) Influence of theophylline on bile formation in the dog. Biomedicine 19 : 27-32.

18. FORKER EL (1967) Two sites of bile formation as determined by mannitol and erythritol clearance in the guinea pig. J Clin Invest 46 : 1189-1195.

19. FORKER EL, GIBSON G (1973) Interaction between sulfobromoph-thalein (BSP) and taurocholate. The kinetics of transport from liver cells to bile in rats. In : The Liver. Quantitative Aspects of Structure and Function. Ed. by G Paumgartner and R Preisig. Karger, Basel. pp. 326-335.

20. GLASINOVIC JC, DUMONT M, DUVAL M, ERLINGER S (1975) Hepatoce-llular uptake of taurocholate in the dog. J Clin Invest 55 : 419-426.

21. GLASINOVIC JC, DUMONT M, DUVAL M, ERLINGER S (1975) Hepatoce-llular uptake of bile acids in the dog : evidence for a common carrier-mediated transport system. An indicator dilution study. Gastroenterology (in press).

22. GLASINOVIC JC, DUMONT M, DUVAL M, ERLINGER S (1975) Captation hépatique du taurocholate (TC) et de la bromesulfonephta-léine (BSP) : preuves en faveur d'un système de transport commun. Biol Gastroenterol (Paris) 8 : 173. (abstract).

23. GORESKY CA (1964) Initial distribution and rate of uptake of sulfobromophthalein in the liver. Am J Physiol 207 : 13-26.

24. GORESKY CA (1965) The hepatic uptake and excretion of sulfobro-mophthalein and bilirubin. Can Med Ass J 92 : 851-857.

25. GORESKY CA, BACH GG, NADEAU BE (1973) On the uptake of materials by the intact liver. The transport and net removal of galactose. J Clin Invest 52 : 991-1009.

26. GUMUCIO JJ, VALDIVIESO VD (1971) Studies on the mechanism of ethynylestradiol impairment of bile flow in the rat. Gastroenterology 61 : 339-344.

27. HARDISON WGM, APTER JT (1972) Micellar theory of biliary cho-lesterol excretion. Am J Physiol 222 : 61-67.

28. HORAK W, GRABNER G, PAUMGARTNER G (1973) Inhibition of bile salt-independent bile formation by indocyanine green. Gastroenterology 64 : 1005-1012.

29. KAY RE, ENTENMAN C (1961) Stimulation of taurocholic acid synthesis and biliary excretion of lipids. Am J Physiol 200 : 855-859.

30. KHEDIS A, DUMONT M, DUVAL M, ERLINGER S (1974) Influence of glucagon on canalicular bile production in the dog. Biomedicine 21 : 176-181.

31. KLAASSEN CD (1971) Studies on the increased biliary flow produced by phenobarbital in rats. J Pharmacol Exp Ther 176 : 743-751.

32. LEVI AJ, GATMAITAN Z, ARIAS IM (1969) Two hepatic cytoplasmic protein fractions, Y and Z, and their possible role in the hepatic uptake of bilirubin, sulfobromophthalein and other anions. J Clin Invest 48 : 2156-2167.

33. LINDBLAD L, LUNDHOLM K, SCHERSTEN T (1975) Mannitol clearance and biliary lipid secretion. Influence of cholic and chenic acid. Digestion (in press). (abstract).

34. MACAROL V, MORRIS TQ, BAKER KJ, BRADLEY SE (1970) Hydrocortisone choleresis in the dog. J Clin Invest 49 : 1714-1723.

35. O'MAILLE ERL, RICHARDS TG, SHORT AH (1965) Acute taurine depletion and maximal rates of hepatic conjugation and secretion of cholic acid in the dog. J Physiol (London) 180 : 67-79.

36. O'MAILLE ERL, RICHARDS TG, SHORT AH (1966) Factors determining the maximal rate of organic anion secretion by the liver and further evidence on the hepatic site of action of the hormone secretin. J Physiol (London) 186 : 424-438.

37. O'MAILLE ERL, RICHARDS TG, SHORT AH (1967) The influence of conjugation of cholic acid on its uptake and secretion : hepatic extraction of taurocholate and cholate in the dog. J Physiol (London) 189 : 337-350.

38. PAUMGARTNER G, HORAK W, PROBST P, GRABNER G (1971) Effect of phenobarbital on bile flow and bile salt excretion in the rat. Naunyn-Schmiedebergs Arch Pharmak 270 : 98-101.

39. POUPON R, POUPON R, DUMONT M, DUVAL M, ERLINGER S (1975) Hepatic storage and biliary transport maximum of sodium taurocholate in the dog. Digestion (in press). (abstract).

40. PRANDI D, ERLINGER S, GLASINOVIC JC, DUMONT M (1975) Canali-
    cular bile production in man. Eur J Clin Invest 5 : 1-6.

41. PREISIG R, BUCHER H, STIRNEMANN H, TAUBER J (1969) Postopera-
    tive choleresis following bile duct obstruction in man.
    Rev Fr Etud Clin Biol 14 : 151-158.

42. PREISIG R, COOPER HL, WHEELER HO (1962) The relationship bet-
    ween taurocholate secretion rate and bile production in
    the unanesthetized dog during cholinergic blockade and
    during secretin  administration. J Clin Invest 41 : 1152-
    1162.

43. REICHEN J, PAUMGARTNER G (1975) Kinetics of taurocholate uptake
    by the perfused rat liver. Gastroenterology 68 : 132-136.

44. RUDMAN D, KENDALL FE (1957) Bile acid content of human serum :
    II. The binding of cholanic acids by human plasma pro-
    teins. J Clin Invest 36 : 538-542.

45. SCHARSCHMIDT BF, WAGGONER JG, BERK PD (1975) Hepatic organic
    anion uptake in the rat. 2nd International Gstaad Sympo-
    sium. The liver. Quantitative Aspects of Structure and
    Function. Gstaad, September 2-4, 1975.

46. SCHERSTEN T, NILSON S, CAHLIN E, FILIPSON M, BRODIN-PERSSON G
    (1971) Relationship between the biliary excretion of bile
    acids and the excretion of water, lecithin, and choleste-
    rol in man. Eur J Clin Invest 1 : 242-247.

47. SMALL DM (1970) The formation of gallstones. Adv Intern Med
    16 : 243-264.

48. SOLOWAY RD, HOFMANN AF, THOMAS PJ, SCHOENFIELD LJ, KLEIN PD
    (1973) Triketocholanoic (dehydrocholic) acid. Hepatic
    metabolism and effect on bile flow and biliary ·lipid
    secretion in man. J Clin Invest 52 : 715-724.

49. SPERBER I (1959) Secretion of organic anions in the formation
    of urine and bile. Pharmacol Rev 11 : 109-134.

50. WHEELER HO (1968) Water and electrolytes in bile. In : Hand-
    book of Physiology. Section 6 : Alimentary Canal, vol.5.
    Ed. by CF Code. American Physiological Society, Washing-
    ton D.C. pp. 2409-2431.

51. WHEELER HO, KING KK (1972) Biliary excretion of lecithin and
    cholesterol in the dog. J Clin Invest 51 : 1337-1350.

52. WHEELER HO, MANCUSI-UNGARO PL, WHITLOCK RT (1960) Bile salt
    transport in the dog. J Clin Invest 39 : 1039-1040.
    (abstract).

53. WHEELER HO, MELTZER JI, BRADLEY SE (1960) Biliary transport
    and hepatic storage of sulfobromophthalein sodium·in
    the unanesthetized dog, in normal man, and in patients
    with hepatic disease. J Clin Invest 39 : 1131-1141.

54. WHEELER HO, ROSS ED, BRADLEY SE (1968) Canalicular bile pro-
    duction in dogs. Am J Physiol 214 : 866-874.

DISCUSSION OF LECTURE BY S. ERLINGER

Forker:   I want to ask you just one question about the Goresky technique for measuring hepatic uptake.   As you know, in an intact dog the steady-state extraction fraction for taurocholic is usually reported to be very high, in the neighbourhood of 90 per cent or so.   Just looking at your curves, it looks as though your single pass extraction, which, if anything, might be expected to be higher, looks appreciably lower than that.   Is there a reasonable explanation for that?

Erlinger:   The extraction, of course, is markedly dependent on the dose, and in some of the lower doses, we got an extraction which was higher than 95 per cent.   Of course, when you increase the dose the extraction decreases, and in some of the curves you have seen the extraction was lower.

Combes:   It is now becoming apparent that organic anion secretion, regardless of whether it is bile acids or other anions, markedly stimulates canalicular bile flow by a mechanism in addition to the osmotic driving force of the organic anion secreted into canalicular bile.   I think a number of people have shown that taurocholate generates about an average of 10 microlitres of bile per micromole of taurocholate excreted in the bile.   For cholecystographic agents values of 20 microlitres per micromole have been found.   For B.S.P. we found values of 39 microlitres per micromole.   At an earlier point in the discussion in this conference someone asked what might be the teleologic reason for stimulating bile flow in addition to the osmotic activity of the organic anions.   Since these are compounds that are actively secreted, and can be secreted in extremely high concentration, it makes sense to try to dilute them, because some of these compounds approach precipitability at the concentrations that can be generated in bile if there were not an additional inorganic electrolyte solution which accompanies them into bile.   This, perhaps, is a teleological explanation.   But it is interesting that the inorganic bile secretion that goes along with the organic acid osmotic drive is almost coupled in some way.   There seems to be a proportional increment in the inorganic bile secretion as well as in that which is osmotically induced.

Erlinger:    I think this is reasonable.

Dowling:    When you were referring to studies both in rats and in
dogs, you suggested that there was a difference in aggregation
number and micelle size between the trihydroxy and dihydroxy bile
salts, and this is certainly true if we are talking about isolated
bile salt micelles.    You are looking at the effects of these
things in bile in the presence of phospholipids and cholesterol,
therefore there are mixed micelles.    Do you have any information
about aggregation and micelle size in this situation as opposed
to the isolated bile salt situation?

Erlinger:    No, I have not of course.    You are the expert.

Schwarz:    We did some studies with isolated liver cells and
taurocholate uptake, and we did kinetic analyses of pH-dependence
and temperature-dependence.    Then we tried inhibition studies
with B.S.P. and we found just the same as Dr. Erlinger.    It
inhibited the taurocholate uptake in a non-competitive way.

Erlinger:    Our preliminary results are indeed compatible with
non-competitive inhibition.

Hofmann:    I would like to ask two questions.    When you did your
multiple-infusion techniques and estimated the storage capacity,
did you attempt, admittedly, with making some assumptions, to
calculate the intracellular concentration of bile acids?    Is it
possible to do that?

Erlinger:    We did not attempt to measure intracellular concentrations.    It is quite difficult to make reasonable assumptions
from the storage capacity.

Hofmann:    I have one other question.    You have found, as Dr.
Paumgartner and ourselves have also found, that the extraction
efficiency for taurocholate is greater than that for taurochenodeoxycholate.    I guess this means that the cells in the distal
sinusoid then are perfused by different bile acid composition in
the cells in the proximal part of the sinusoid.    I wonder if
that is correct and what you think the significance of it is?

Erlinger:    I do not know if you really need to infer from that
that there is a different perfusion of the lobular regions.    I
am not really sure of that.    I would like to think about it a
little more.

Paumgartner:    We have found that when you give dehydrocholate,
an hydroxy group is introduced into the 3α-position.    You can
measure it by the enzymatic method.    Did you only use free de-

hydrocholic acid, unconjugated dehydrocholic acid or did you also try taurine or glycine conjugated dehydrocholic acid?  Does this alter the metabolic transformation of dehydrocholic acid in the liver?

Erlinger:   We used also taurodehydrocholic acid with the same results.

Paumgartner:   When you did your Tm studies on bile acids, what was the percentage of bile acids excreted in the urine?  Could you comment on that?

Erlinger:   In some experiments we measured the urinary secretion which was on the average in the range of 5-10 micromoles per minute, which is at most 10 per cent of the biliary secretion measured simultaneously.

Paumgartner:   Did you also study the effect of sodium salicylate on biliary lipid excretion.  The reason I ask this is that Dr. Preisig and myself have studied, in some pilot studies, biliary lipid excretion after infusion of sodium salicylate and we could not find these marked effects on lipid excretion you have shown.

Erlinger:   No, we did not use sodium salicylate itself.  We wanted to test the most commonly used drug in therapeutics; so we used acetyl salicylate, but not sodium salicylate.

Tygstrup:   This is more a comment than a question, but perhaps you can help me anyway.  I have some doubts about the interpretation of the kinetic curves you obtain with this Goresky technique. The unfamiliar thing for me is that the $K_m$ is expressed as a dose rather than as a concentration which we used to do.  It is a little difficult to see what difference it makes.  I know that you have no other possibility at the moment, but what are the physiological conclusions we can draw from this?  I think that as long as you compare different substances with the technique, there is no problem.  You can do it on a comparable basis. But when you want to compare it with other processes, such as excretion processes, later on, which have been measured by other methods I would have some doubt about the comparability of the results.  Also, it is an uncommon situation which both you and Dr. Paumgartner described previously.  It is the last step in a sequence which is really rate-limiting.  The normal situation is that it is the first step, and in this situation you could easily have an accumulation of the intermediates in the liver cells.  This would be the physiological significance of your data, that you could have an accumulation of bile acids for instance in the cells, which might be harmful.  On the other hand, the method you use, as far as I can see, does not include back-diffusion and this may alter the physiological consequence completely. You may have a very rapid uptake process but if it goes back just as rapidly then it is not very interesting, at least from the pathogenetic point of view. The other point I would like to raise again, which was raised yesterday, is influence of flow on these determinations. The flow must be one of the given conditions, and before you compare results from different people you must know that they use the same flow. Because if you have a higher flow you will have a lower mean concentration and probably a lower uptake. So I would just say one word of warning against over-interpretation of the method and ask if you have any comments on this.

Erlinger:    Thank you. I think I would agree with most of your comments, especially as far as the comparison of data obtained with this method with other data regarding biliary secretion for instance. This is a very important point. However, at the moment I think it is the best we can really do. And, as far as flow is concerned, I think it is reassuring to see that in Dr. Paumgartner's preparation, in which flow is maintained at a constant level, similar qualitative as well as quantitative results are obtained.

Coleman:    Early on in your talk you said that you had used theo-pholin. Which fraction of the bile flow does theopholin increase?

Erlinger:    It increases the canalicular bile salt independent bile flow.

Coleman:    Is anything known about any inhibitors or stimulators of the bile salt dependent flow?

Erlinger:    I think any agent that would decrease bile salt secretion would, of course, decrease the bile salt associated choleresis. I do not know of any agent that would actually decrease the osmotic activity of a given bile salt, at a given bile salt secretion rate.

Fisher:    Did you do biliary Tm with taurocholic and either chenodeoxycholic or lithocholic at the same time? I ask this in the hope that you might be able to shed light on the fact that the simultaneous perfusion of cholic acid along with lithocholic or chenodeoxycholate prevents the cholestasis induced by those latter two agents.

Erlinger:    No, we did not do simultaneous measurements.

Low-Beer:    Did you find the same thing with theopholin as you did with acetyl salicylic acid in terms of biliary lipid excretion?

Erlinger:    We are at the moment studying this.    However, we
found the same with another bile salt independent cholerectic,
methyl umbellipherone, which I think increases bile flow by a
mechanism which is different from acetyl salicylate, with the
same qualitative results.

Forker:    I would just like to reassure Dr. Tygstrup about the
flow problem.    I believe it is fair to say that, with the
exception of whatever changes there may be in the blood flow
distribution relative to the rate of blood flow, the calculation
of the unidirectional transfer coefficient by Goresky's model is
really quite independent of the flow.    The rate of flow is an
intrinsic part of the model, and if things work the way they
should one ought to get the same transfer coefficient independent
of the flow.

# FORMATION, METABOLISM, AND EXCRETION OF BILE SALT SULFATES IN MAN

A. Stiehl, E. Ast, P. Czygan, and M. Liersch

University of Heidelberg, Dept. of Medicine

6900 Heidelberg, Bergheimerstr.58, Germany

Bile acids are formed in the liver from cholesterol and are conjugated with taurine or glycine before their excretion into the bile. In healthy man essentially all the bile acids are present within the enterohepatic circulation (fig.1). In patients with cholestasis the biliary excretion of bile acids is diminished and increased concentrations are found in the peripheral blood leading to an increased excretion into the urine. Elevated bile acid concentrations can also be found in the skin and can cause pruritus.

Besides the formation of taurine and glycine conjugates at their carboxyl group bile acids also can form sulfate esters with their hydroxyl groups. Sulfate esters of lithocholic acid were first identified in human bile by PALMER in 1967 (1). Subsequently we identified sulfate esters of cholate and chenodeoxycholate in the urine of a patient with intrahepatic biliary atresia (4,5). In this patient with severe cholestasis 46% of cholate and 23% of chenodeoxycholate synthesized daily

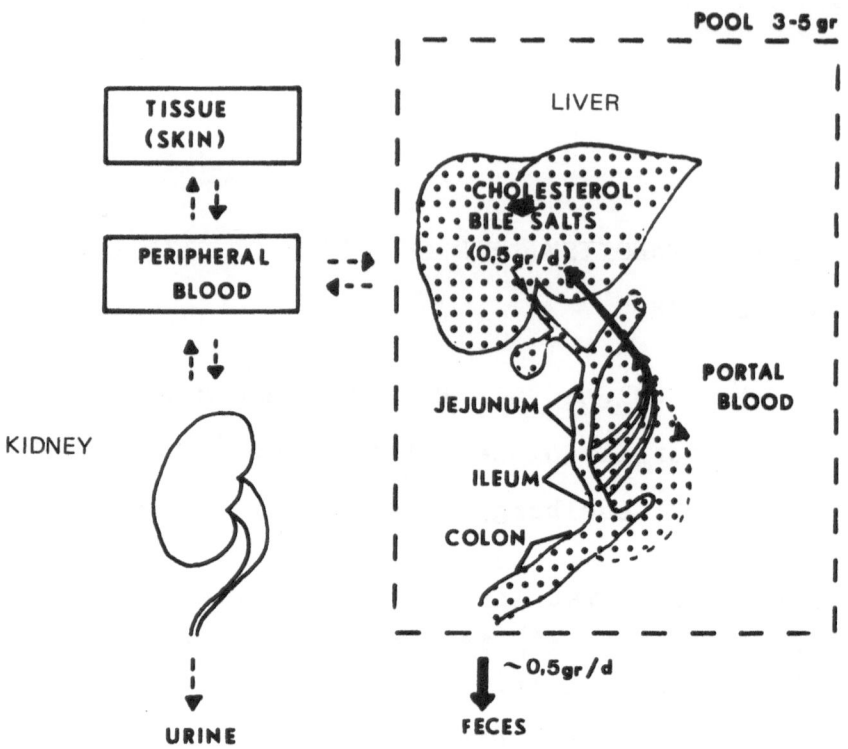

Fig.1: Bile salt metabolism in man. Bile salts are
present in liver, biliary system, intestine, and portal
blood. In patients with cholestasis increased bile salt
concentrations are found in the peripheral blood, in
urine and skin.


were excreted by the urine. More than 75% of the bile
acids excreted were sulfate esters. In patients with
cholestasis due to extrahepatic obstruction, hepatitis or
cirrhosis 20-40 mg/ 24h of bile salts were excreted,
more than 50% of which were sulfated (11). Thus
substantial amounts of bile salts are excreted in the
urine in the sulfated form (6-14). In patients with
cirrhosis and renal insufficiency bile salt excretion
rates of up to 150 mg/24h have been observed. In these

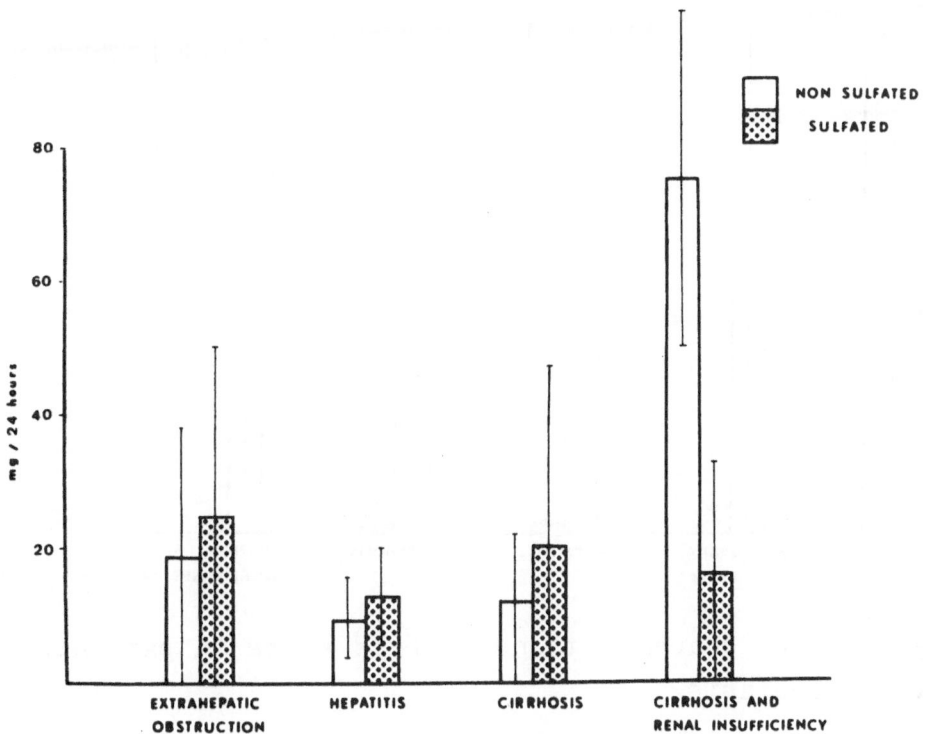

Fig.2: Urinary excretion of bile salts in patients with cholestasis.

patients the major part of bile salts excreted by the urine was non-sulfated.

Column chromatography on Sephadex LH-20 was used to separate mono-, di- and tri-sulfates of bile acids. In our patients studied 76.9% of bile acid sulfates in urine were mono-sulfates, 21.3% di-sulfates and 1.8% tri-sulfates (11).

In the serum of these patients less than 10% of cholate and chenodeoxycholate were sulfated (11). Therefore the the renal clearance of sulfated bile acids calculated on the basis of urinary excretion per 24h divided by

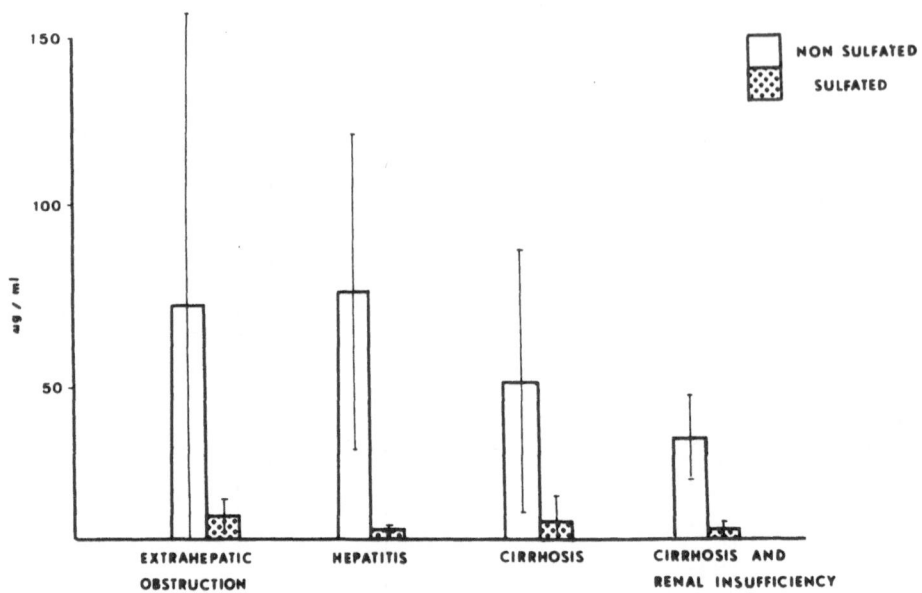

Fig.3: Serum concentrations of bile salts in patients
with cholestasis.

serum concentrations were on average more than 10 times
greater than those of non-sulfated bile acids (11).

The hepatic uptake of 14C-cholate in patients with
cholestasis is considerably slower than in healthy
subjects. Four hours after injection of a tracer dose
of 14C-cholate to healthy subjects essentially all the
radioactivity is eliminated from the serum. In patients
with cholestasis however the serum clearance of bile
salts takes much longer and after 4 hours radioactivity
is still present in the serum (fig.4). The hepatic
uptake of 14C-cholate and 14C-cholate sulfate is almost
identical (fig.4). In contrast 14C-cholate sulfate is
much more rapidly excreted by the kidneys than non-
sulfated 14C-cholate (fig.5). Similar results were
obtained for chenodeoxycholate and chenodeoxycholate

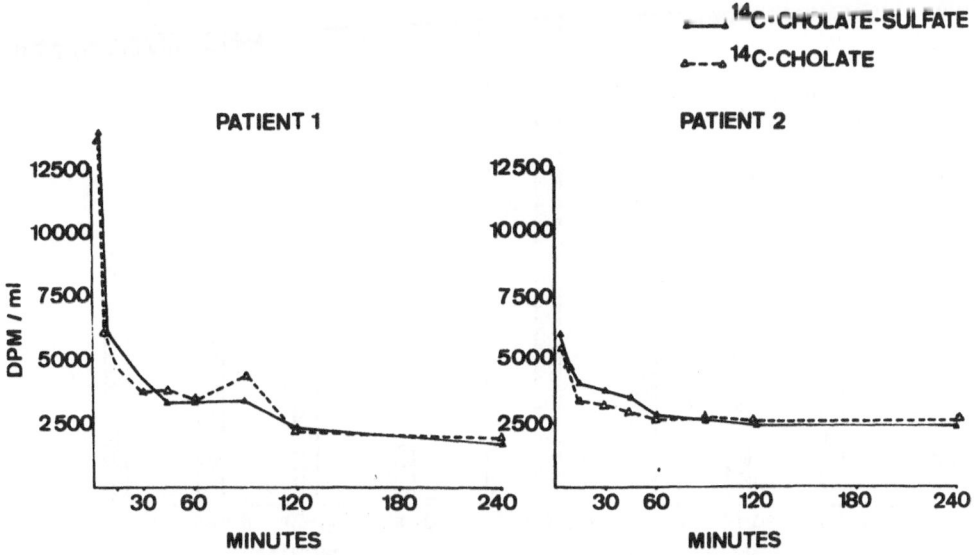

Fig.4: Serum clearance of sulfated and non-sulfated
14C-cholate in two patients with cholestasis.

sulfate. Clearance rates calculated on the basis of
these experiments confirmed previous findings that the
renal clearance rates of sulfated bile salts are
approximately 10 times greater than the clearance rates
of non-sulfated bile salts.

In patients with cholestasis the turnover of bile acids
can be decreased (fig.6). In the patient studied the
$t_{1/2}$ of 14C-cholate was 50 hours. In contrast $t_{1/2}$
for cholate sulfate was only 8 hours. Increased renal
elimination and decreased reabsorption in the intestine
as has been described so far only for lithocholate (16)
are probably the factors contributing to this rapid
turnover of sulfated bile salts.

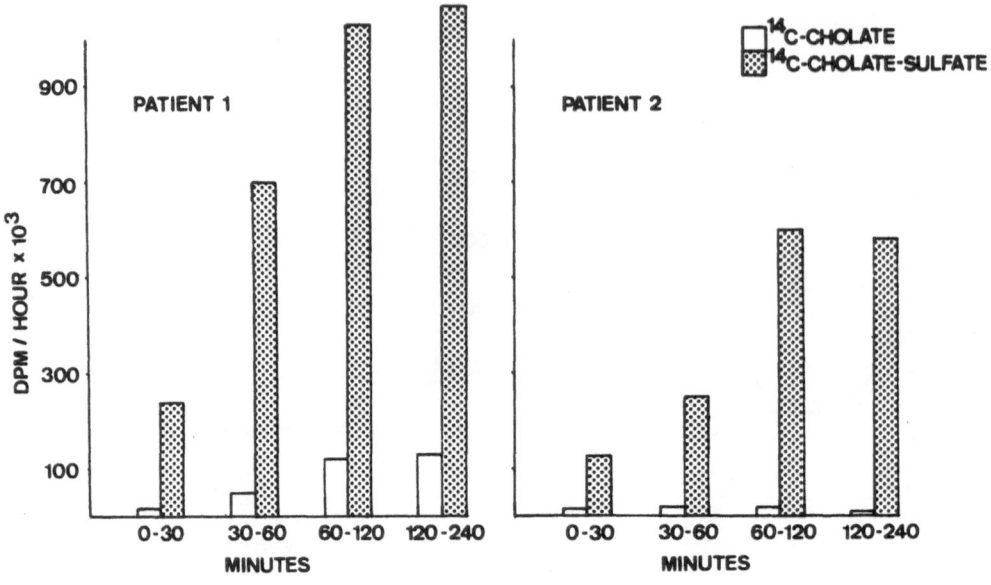

Fig.5: Urinary excretion of sulfated and non-sulfated
14C-cholate in two patients with cholestasis.

Patients with cholestasis and pruritus have significantly
higher bile salt concentrations in their skin than
patients without pruritus. Sulfate esters however
constituted only less than 5% of the total bile acids
( 19). No significant differences were found between
patients with and without pruritus (fig.7). It is
unlikely therefore that sulfated bile acids are
responsible for the pruritus in patients with cholestasis.

Cholate and chenodeoxycholate are sulfated in greater
amounts only in patients with cholestasis and not in
healthy subjects in whom less than 10% of these bile
acids in bile are present as sulfate esters. In contrast

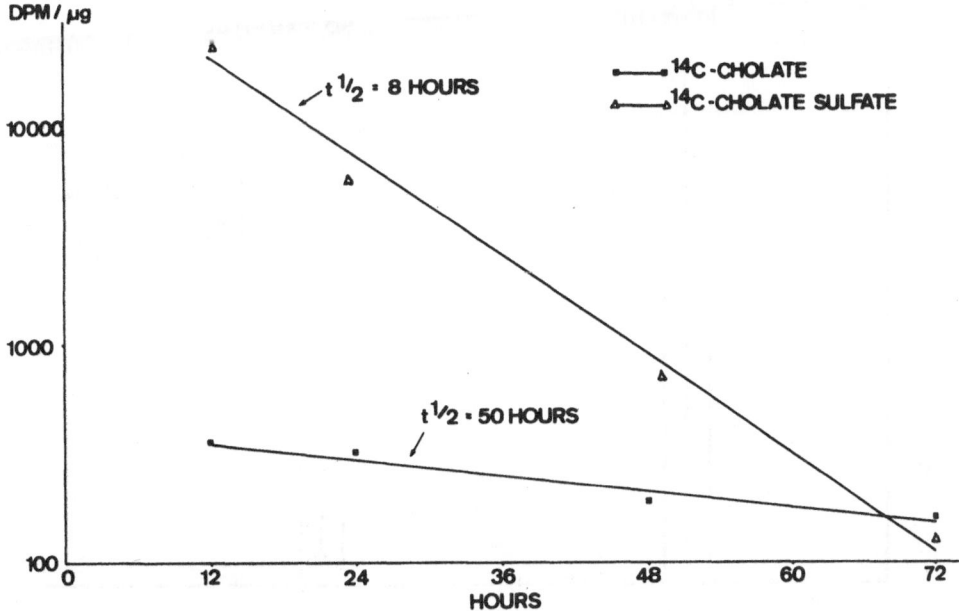

Fig.6: Turnover of 14C-cholate and 14C-cholate sulfate in a patient with cholestasis.

up to more than 90% of lithocholate in bile are present as sulfate esters in healthy man (2,20). This extensive sulfation of lithocholate leads to a very rapid turnover of this bile acid in normal man with a biological halflife of only 0.7 days (17,18).

Under normal conditions only small amounts of litho-cholate are found in bile ( approximately 1% of total bile acids). However in patients with cholesterol gallstones treated with chenodeoxycholate increased amounts of lithocholate are formed ( in mean 3.5% of total bile acids). In these patients the sulfation

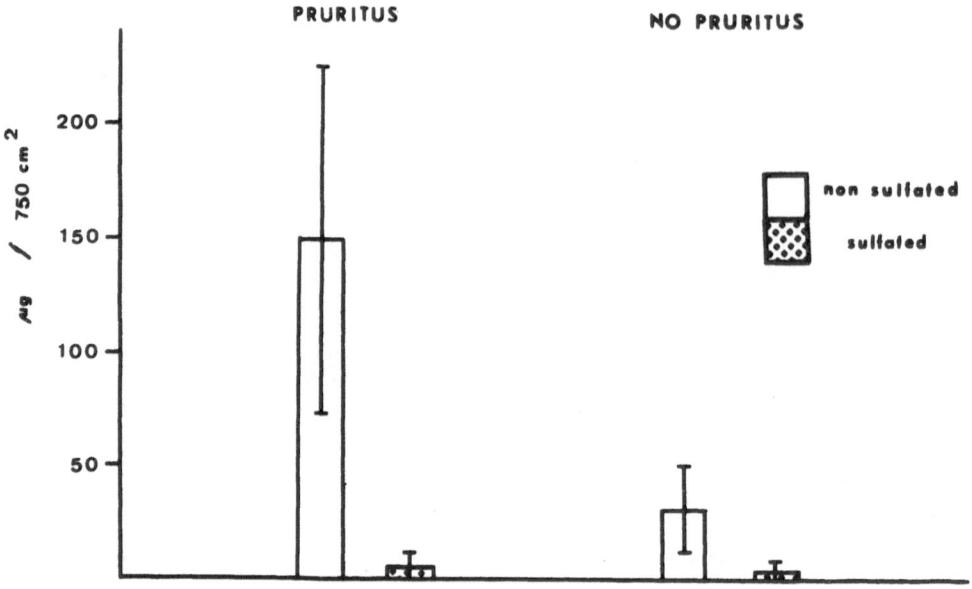

Fig.7: Bile salts in the skin of patients with cholestasis.

of lithocholate has been shown to increase fron 27% to 75% of the total lithocholate (20). This extensive sulfation of lithocholate enhances the elimination of this possibly toxic bile salt in these patients.

Studies on the toxicity of lithocholate and lithocholate sulfate indicate that the sulfated molecules are less toxic. In JAVITT's experiments lithocholate led to a marked reduction of bile flow in bile fistula rats, but sulfated lithocholate or sulfated glycolithocholate did not reduce bile flow (21). In our experiments in perfused rat livers taurolithocholate also led to an almost complete stasis of bile flow, but sulfated

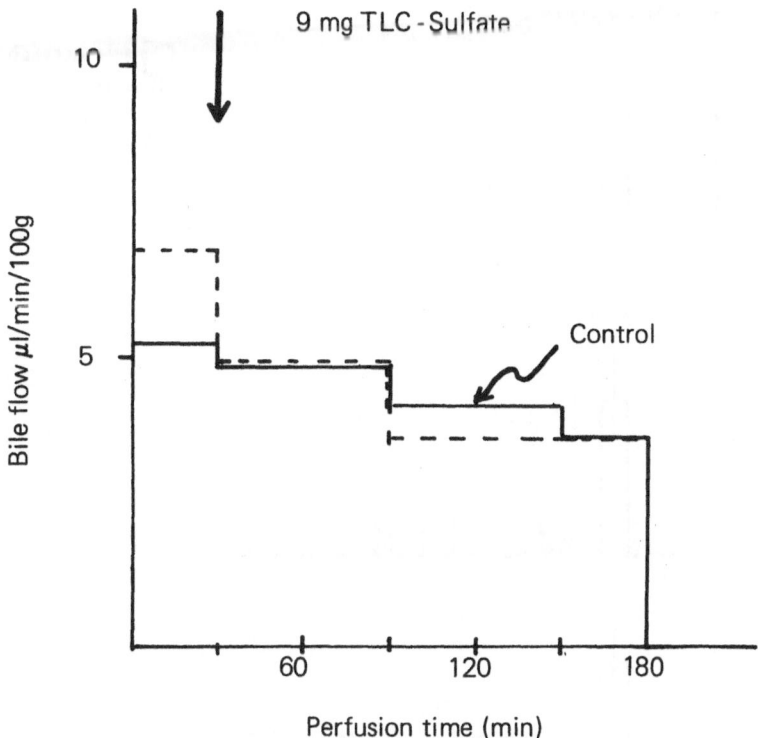

Fig.8:Bile flow of perfused rat livers after addition
of taurolithocholate sulfate. After a preperfusion
period of 30 minutes bile salts were added as a bolus.


taurolithocholate led only to a very small reduction
(fig.8) of bile flow. Lithocholate injections in rats
produced marked cholestasis with elevated levels of
serum bilirubin, SGOT and SGPT (fig.9). In contrast
sulfated lithocholate did not cause cholestasis and
although raised levels of SGOT and SGPT did occur, they
were significantly smaller (22).

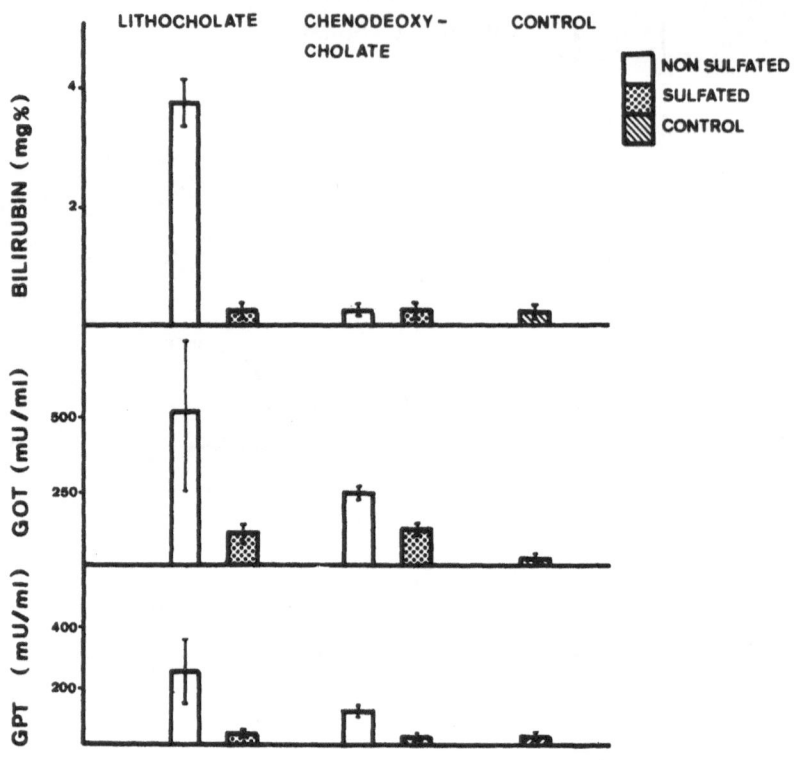

Fig.9: Serum bilirubin, SGOT, and SGPT in male rats
12 hours after bile salt injection (100mg/Kg).

The enzymatic reactions of the microsomal biotransformation system such as demethylation of aminopyrine
and hydroxylation of aniline are significantly less
inhibited by sulfated lithocholate than by non-sulfated
lithocholate (22). Light and electron microscopic
examinations of the rat livers revealed parenchymal
liver disease and cholestasis after injection of
lithocholate but not after injection of lithocholate
sulfate (23).

Elevated concentrations of mono- and dihydroxy bile
acids have hepatotoxic properties (24,25). In addition
monohydroxy bile acids such as lithocholate can cause
cholestasis. Sulfation of bile acids enhances their
fecal and urinary excretion and diminishes their toxicity.
Sulfation of lithocholate is an important metabolic
pathway in normal man. This pathway is especially effective
in patients who are treated with chenodeoxycholate in
whom increased amounts of lithocholate are formed by
bacterial degradation of chenodeoxycholate. Sulfation
of cholate, chenodeoxycholate, and deoxycholate become
important in patients with cholestasis in whom the
biliary excretion of bile acids is diminished and
enhanced urinary excretion is necessary.

References:
1. Palmer,R.H.: The formation of bile acid sulfates: a
   new pathway of bile acid metabolism in humans. Proc.
   Nat.Acad.Sci.,Wash., 58,1047 (1967).
2. Palmer,R.H.,Bolt,M.G.: Bile acid sulfates.I. Synthesis
   of lithocholic acid sulfates and their identification
   in human bile. J.Lipid Res. 12,671 (1971).
3. Palmer,R.H.: Bile acid sulfates.II. Formation,
   metabolism, and excretion of lithocholic acid sulfates
   in the rat. J.Lipid Res. 12,680 (1971).
4. Stiehl,A ,Thaler,M.M.,Admirand,W.H.: Formation and
   excretion of bile salt sulfates: an important metabolic
   pathway in cholestasis; in Greten,Levine,Pfeiffer,
   Renold: Lipid metabolism, obesity, and diabetes
   mellitus: impact upon atherosclerosis. International
   Symposium,1972, p.49 (Thieme,Stuttgart 1974).

5. Admirand,W.H.,Stiehl,A.,Thaler,M.M.: Sulfation of
   bile salts. An important metabolic pathway in
   cholestasis. Gastroenterology 62,190 (1972).

6. Stiehl,A.: Bile salt sulfates in intra- and extrahepatic cholestasis; in Back,Gerok: Bile acids in
   human diseases, p.73 (Schattauer,Stuttgart 1972).

7. Stiehl,A.,Earnest,D.,Admirand,W.H.: Urinary excretion
   of bile salt sulfates in patients with hepatic
   cirrhosis. Gastroenterology 68,534 (1975).

8. Back,P.,Sjövall,J.,Sjövall,K.: Monohydroxy bile acids
   in cholestasis of pregnancy. Identification of
   computerized gas chromatography-mass spectometry.
   Scand.J.clin.Lab.Invest.29,suppl.126, p.12 (1972).

9. Back,P.: Ausscheidung von Monohydroxy-Gallensäuren
   im Urin bei V rschlussikterus und akuter Hepatitis.
   Z.Gastroenterologie 11,477 (1973).

10.Makino,I.,Shinozaki,K.Nakagawa,S.: S lfated bile
   acid in urine of patients with hepatobiliary diseases.
   Lipids 8,47 (1973).

11.Stiehl,A :Bile salt sulfates in cholestasis. Europ.
   J.clin.Invest. 4,59 (1974).

12.Makino,I.,Shinozaki,K.Nakagawa,S.: Measurement of
   sulfated and non-sulfated bile acids in human serum
   and urine. J.Lipid Res. 15,132 (1974).

13.Norman,A.,Strandvik,B.: Metabolism of lithocholic
   acid-24-14C in extrahepatic biliary atresia. Acta
   Paediat.Scand. 63,92 (1974).

14.Makino,I.,Hashimoto,H.,Shinozaki,K., et al.: Sulfated
   and nonsulfated bile acids in urine, serum, and bile
   of patients with hepatobiliary diseases. Gastroenterology 68,545 (1975).

15.Makino,I.,Nakagawa,S.,Shinozaki,K.ψMashimo,K.:
   Sulfated and nonsulfated bile acid in human serum.
   Lipids 7,750 (1972).

16. Low-Beer,T.S.,Tyor,M.P.,Lack,L.: Effects of sulfation
    of taurolithocholic acids on their intestinal
    transport. Gastroenterology 56,721 (1969).

17. Cowen,A.E.,Korman,M.G.,Hofmann,A.F.,Cass,O.W.:
    Metabolism of lithocholate in healthy man.I.Biotrans-
    formation and biliary excretion of intravenously
    administered lithocholate, lithocholylglycine, and
    their sulfates. Gastroenterology,in press.

18. Cowen,A.E.,Korman,M.E.,Hofmann,A.F., et al.:
    Metabolism of lithocholate in healthy man. II.
    Enterohepatic circulation. Gastroenterology, in press.

19. Stiehl,A.: Gallensäuren und Gallensäurensulfate
    in der Haut von Patienten mit Cholestase. Z.
    gastroenterologie 12,121 (1974).

20. Stiehl,A.,Czygan,P.,Raedsch,H.: Increasing sulfation
    of lithocholate in patients during chenodeoxycholate
    treatment. 3rd.Int.Bile Acid Meeting, Freiburg,1974.

21. Javitt,N.B.: Excretion of monohydroxy bile acid
    ester sulfates in the rat; in Paumgartner,Preisig:
    The liver. Quantitative apects of structure and
    function, p.355 (Karger, Basel 1973).

22. Czygan,P.,Stiehl,A.: Bile salts versus bile salt
    sulfates: a comparison of the toxicity. Z.
    Gastroenterologie, 13,452 (1975).

23. Leuschner,U.,Czygan,P.,Stiehl,A.: Licht und elektro-
    nenmikroskopische Untersuchungen zur Toxizität
    sulfatierter und nicht sulfatierter Lithocholsäure.
    Verh.Dtsch.Ges.Inn.Med., in Druck.

24. Palmer,R.H.: Bile acids, liver injury, and liver
    disease. Arch.intern.Med. 130,606 (1972).

25. Greim,H.,Trülzsch,D.,Czygan,P., et al.: Bile acids
    in human livers with or without biliary obstruction.
    Gastroenterology 63,846 (1972).

DISCUSSION OF COMMENTARY BY A. STIEHL

Elliott:   It was not clear to me the exact chemical composition
of the sulphates of chenodeoxycholate and cholic which you prepared,
administered and recovered from your patients.   Were they fully
sulphated, di- and trisulphates in all cases?

Stiehl:   If you synthesize sulphate esters of bile salt like
chenodeoxycholate or cholate you always get a mixture of mono-,
di- and trisulphates.   These can be separated by a column of
Sephadex LH-20.   But in the experiments we did with lithocholate,
naturally this was a monosulphate ester.

Elliott:   What did you give the patients?   A mixture of chenodeoxycholate and cholate sulphates?

Stiehl:   This was a mixture of cholate sulphates.   We tested it
on thin-layer plate, and we do know that approximately 70 per cent
of the cholate was disulphate.

Elliott:   What was the nature of the product that you isolated
from the patient?

Stiehl:   In the urine 80 per cent was monosulphated, 18 per cent
disulphated and approximately 2 per cent trisulphated.

Ostrow:   This may seem a naive question, but has anyone looked to
see whether sulphated lithocholate forms micelles?

Stiehl:   No, not to my knowledge.

Murphy:   I was interested in the relationship you found between
pruritus and skin levels of nonsulphated bile acids.   A few years
ago we also looked at the correlation of pruritus with nonsulphated
serum bile acids.   We were unable to find any difference between
patients who had pruritus or not pruritus with respect to the
level of serum bile acids.   The data indicated that patients with
pruritus tended to have an increased proportion of taurine
conjugated bile acids.   So my first question would be:   did you
look at the conjugation pattern of those bile acids in the skin of
the patients?   And my second question is:   what proportion of

nonsulphated lithocholic acid do you find in duodenal fluid from normal subjects?

Stiehl:    In normal man we find that approximately one per cent of the total bile salts is lithocholic acid.   To answer your first question, it is quite clear that you do not get a correlation between the serum bile salt concentrations and pruritus in these patients.    There has been a recent study in which bile salts were injected in the skin.   The nonconjugated bile salts caused pruritus and not the conjugated ones.   We found small amounts of sulphates and we were interested in the question whether the sulphates perhaps would be of importance in the development of itching.

Bradley:    Did you notice any evidence of renal damage in association with the relatively rapid clearance of the sulphated bile acid loads?

Stiehl:    As judged by the ordinary clinical methods which are used to get information about kidney function, the patients with extra-hepatic obstruction, hepatitis and sclerosis had no kidney damage. So the clearance rates were normal.

Palmer:    Did you happen to look at the glycine to taurine ratios in your patients as they developed increased proportions of sulphation during the chenodeoxycholate administration?   The reason I ask this question is that Dr. Hofmann has shown that the glycine conjugated lithocholate is more apt to be sulphated than the taurine conjugated lithocholate.   One might expect that, as the chenodeoxycholate depletes the taurine pool, you would have increased sulphation of the glycolithocholate, which was becoming predominant.

Stiehl:    We did not study the ratio of taurine to glycine conjugated lithocholate, but we checked the conjugation and almost 98-99 per cent of the lithocholate in bile was conjugated with taurine or glycine.   But we did not check the ratio.

Taylor:    Could I go back to this question of the pruritus and the skin bile acids.   First of all a technical question:  how did you extract the bile acids from the skin?

Stiehl:    We used sponges with ethanol and just rubbed it off the skin.   This method has been used by others, and we were quite surprised that actually, by using this rough method, you get these striking differences in the concentrations.

Hofmann:    You alluded to urinary excretion of lithocholic sulphates. We have been carrying out a lot of measurements of lithocholic kinetics by isotope dilution in healthy patients and in patients ingesting chenodeoxycholic acid solution, and we have been astonished in finding really very little urinary excretion of radioactivity. Have you, in fact, observed much urinary excretion of lithocholic acid in health or in patients taking chenodeoxycholic acid?

Stiehl:   We have studied the urinary excretion of lithocholic acid in these patients by gas-liquid chromatography, and we found very small amounts of nonsulphated lithocholate. It was approximately 1-2 milligrams per 24 hours of sulphated lithocholate.

# THE ALLO BILE ACIDS

William H. Elliott

Department of Biochemistry
St. Louis University School of Medicine
St. Louis Missouri 63104, U.S.A.

Twelve years ago at the First NATO Advanced Study Institute on the Biliary System Professor Haslewood (1965) reported that a new bile acid, allocholic acid, was rather widely distributed in lower animals and a few mammals, including man. My colleague, Dr. Karavolas, described the identification of allocholic acid as a metabolite of cholestanol in the bile fistula rat (Karavolas and Elliott, 1965). The interest evidenced in allo bile acids at that meeting has flourished in several laboratories in an effort to ascertain the importance of these recently identified derivatives.

The allo bile acids are derivatives of $5\alpha$-cholanic acids, analogs of the common $5\beta$-bile acids discussed earlier. The $5\alpha$-hydrogen is <u>trans</u> to the C-19 methyl group, thus conferring a chair-chair conformation on Rings A and B resulting in a coplanar steroid nucleus, in striking contrast to the $5\beta$-bile acids where a <u>cis</u> relationship exists and Rings A and B are approximately at a right angle to each other. Fig. 1 shows this arrangement for allocholic and cholic acids.

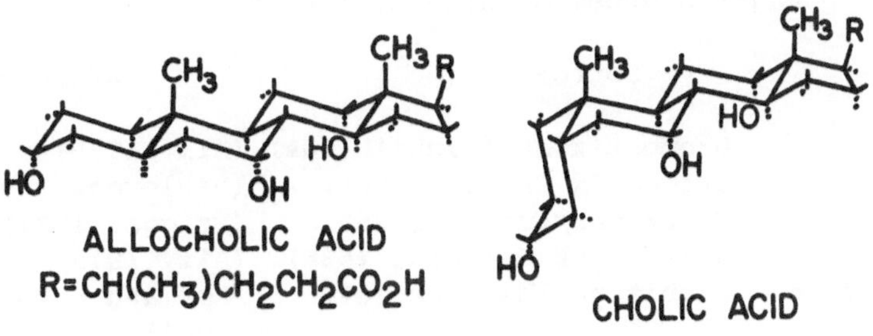

**ALLOCHOLIC ACID**
$R=CH(CH_3)CH_2CH_2CO_2H$

**CHOLIC ACID**

Figure 1

The prefix allo is retained by Chemical Abstracts to designate
the more thermodynamically stable of two geometric isomers, and
this prefix has been used to designate these trans 5α-derivatives.
Where the structure of the 5α-bile acid is otherwise identical to
a known 5β-bile acid, the 5α-derivative is frequently identified
by the trivial name of the 5β-analog with the prefix allo; i.e.,
allocholic acid (3α,7α,12α-trihydroxy-5α-cholanic acid) is the
5α-analog of cholic acid.  The prefix has been restricted to the
$C_{24}$ derivatives; the $C_{27}$ acids generally do not have trivial names,
and those of the 5α-series are 5α-cholestanoic acids, not allo-
cholestanoic acids.


## OCCURRENCE

From their early studies on the constitution of sterols and
bile acids, Wieland and Windaus were confronted with rationaliza-
tion of two isomeric acids, now known as the unsubstituted 5β- and
5α-cholanic acids.  Allocholanic acid was ultimately obtained in
pure form some 16 years after its initial isolation by Windaus
and Neukirchen (1919).  Of the naturally occurring allo acids all
are substituted at positions 3,6,7, and/or 12 and are isomeric
with the common 5β-bile acids.  Haslewood (1967) has tabulated
sources of allocholic acid including lizards, teleostean fishes,
snakes, birds and mammals.  The river carpsucker appears to be a
good source of this acid, but the best natural source is the bile
of the lizard, Uromastix, in which the solids represent about 90%
of allocholate as the tauro derivative.  Bile of Salamander necturus contains 53% allocholate as the tauro derivative (Table I).

Allodeoxycholate is a normal constituent of rabbit bile and
feces.  Glycoallodeoxycholate is a major constituent of gallstones
of the rabbit fed a diet containing 1% cholestanol.  Allodeoxycholate must be a secondary bile acid derived from allocholate by
bacterial removal of the 7α-hydroxyl group.


Table I

Major Sources of Allo Bile Acids

| Acid | Source | Reference |
|------|--------|-----------|
| Allocholate | Uromastix Hardwickii (90%) | (Ali, 1975) |
| | Uromastix Thomasi (90%) | (Haslewood, 1974) |
| | River Carpsucker (~25%) | (Briggs, 1972) |
| | Salamander Necturus (53%) | (Ali, 1975) |
| Allodeoxycholate | Rabbit gallbladder (6%) | (Hofmann & Mosbach, 1964) |
| Allochenodeoxycholate | Giant Salamander | (Hoshita et al., 1967) |

Allochenodeoxycholic acid is less well distributed in nature; it is a minor constituent in the bile of the giant salamander, but only traces were found in bile of Salamander Necturus. Like allocholic acid allochenodeoxycholic acid appears to be a primary bile acid derived from cholestanol in the rat.

Allolithocholic acid is rarely found in nature, but has been shown to be a metabolite of allochenodeoxycholate in the rat after intracecal administration, and is a product of reduction of 3-oxo-chol-4-enic acid in this species. The allo analog of hyodeoxy-cholate has been found as a minor metabolite of cholestanol in the rat; allohyocholate (the $3\alpha,6\alpha,7\alpha$-triol) has been identified as a minor metabolite of allochenodeoxycholate, but allomuricholates have not been found.

In lower animals the tauro derivatives apparently predominate. A preference for taurine or glycine can probably be predicted on the basis of the nature of the conjugates of the $5\beta$-analogs, although no comprehensive study has been made. The glyco and tauro derivatives of several of these allo acids have been prepared and characterized in our laboratory.

## SEPARATION AND PHYSICAL PROPERTIES

Because the allo derivatives are frequently found in nature in minor amounts in the presence of their $5\beta$-analogs, isolation and identification have been problems. Partial separation by repeated crystallization has been helpful for less polar allocholanates, but allocholate has not been successfully separated from cholate by this method. The coplanar ring system and the axial configuration of the $3\alpha$-ol of the commonest allo derivatives confer a small difference in mobility in some chromatographic systems. In acetic acid partition chromatography the $3\alpha$-hydroxy allo acids are eluted in fractions just preceding or with their $5\beta$-isomers. In thin layer chromatography on silica gel G methyl allocholate and methyl cholate show $R_f$ values of 0.17 and 0.23, respectively, in acetone-benzene/1:1; with Eneroth's system S-6 (cyclohexane-ethyl acetate-acetic acid/7:23:3) $R_f$'s of 0.26 and 0.33, respectively, are obtained by a second exposure to the solvent system. In gas liquid chromatography the methyl esters of allo acids are also generally retarded in elution from the columns; when the hydroxyl groups are derivatized as trimethylsilyl (TMS) ethers, trifluoracetates (TFA) or acetates (Ac), this behavior may change. Table I shows retention times of methyl cholate and methyl allocholate and a few such derivatives relative to methyl deoxycholate or the bis TMS ether of methyl deoxycholate, unless stated otherwise.

The combination of gas chromatography-mass spectrometry offers a positive means of identification of components of a mixture

## Table II

### Relative Retention Time on Several Columns

| Phase | OH | Cholate (TMS) | [TFA] | OH | Allocholate (TMS) | [TFA] |
|---|---|---|---|---|---|---|
| 3% QF-1 | 2.33 | (1.05) | -- | 2.68 | (1.00) | -- |
| 0.5-1% QF-1 | -- | -- | [1.30]² | -- | -- | [1.37]² |
| 3% OV-1 | 1.66 | (1.09) | -- | 1.77 | (1.05) | -- |
| 3% OV-17 | 2.26 | (0.90) | -- | 2.73 | (0.87) | -- |
| 0.5% HiEff-8BP | -- | (0.75)² | -- | -- | (0.61)² | -- |
| 0.5% SP525 | | (Ac)₂ = (1.62)³ | | | (Ac)₂ = (1.83)³ | |

1.  Elliott, W.H., Walsh, L.B., Mui, M.M., Thorne, M.A. and Sieg-
    fried, C.M. (1969) J. Chromatog. 452-464.
2.  Eneroth, P. and Sjovall, J. in Methods in Enzymology (R.B.
    Clayton, ed) Academic Press, New York (1969) XV, 262-266;
    relative to methyl deoxycholate [TFA]₂, or (TMS)₂.
3.  Szczepanik, P.A., Hachey, D.L. and Klein, P.D., personal com-
    munication; relative to methyl deoxycholate (Ac)₂.

separable by chromatography. Mass spectra of epimeric bile acid
derivatives are generally quite similar; positional isomers frequently provide significantly different spectra. Since gas chromatography ideally resolves the epimers, mass spectra of each may
be recorded. Although the mass spectra of methyl cholate and allocholate are very similar, the spectra of the TMS ethers of these
esters show a stronger fragment ion at m/e 261 for allocholate
(Sjövall et al., 1971). The fragment ion m/e 343 is consistently
stronger than m/e 253 for TMS derivatives of 5α-sterols and 5α-
cholanates; the reverse is true for the 5β-derivatives. Thus, the
3α-trimethylsilyl group is lost more easily in the 5β-series than
in the 5α-series. With the coupling of an on-line computor to the
mass spectrometer and the use of the procedure of mass fragmento-
graphy— the scanning of selected fragment ions rather than a complete mass spectrum— the sensitivity of this means of identification has moved into the nanogram range, and with forseable modifications the picogram range is readily at hand. Miyazaki et al.
(1974) have shown the value of internal standards labeled with
stable isotopes for the detection and identification of bile acids.
The method pioneered by Sjovall and Ryhage should become routine
within a short time.

Conjugated bile acids can be separated by high pressure liquid
chromatography (Shaw and Elliott, 1975). With a Waters Associate
Model ALC 201 Liquid Chromatograph equipped with a loop injector,
a differential refractrometer, and a series of five 1/8" x 2'
stainless steel columns packed with Corasil II and a flow rate of

2 ml/min, a mixture of glycocholate and glycoallocholate was resolved completely in four cycles (retention volumes 18.4 and 21.6
ml, respectively) with a solvent system of acetonitrile-acetic
acid-water/400:20:5. A mixture of taurocholate and tauroallocho-
late was completely resolved in six cycles with a solvent system
of 2-propanol-ethyl acetate-water-7N ammonium hydroxide/300:900:
100:0.5 (retention volumes, 19.6 and 21.2 ml, respectively). Although useful lower limits of detection of bile salts by this
method are only of the order of 20-30 μg, the procedures is worthy
of additional exploration. The role of sulphates in this procedures must yet be studied.

Allo acids and their conjugates are generally higher melting
solids than their 5β-analogs. Bile salts of the 5β- and 5α-
series have been compared in their ability to solubilize a hydrocarbon, [6-methyl-$^{14}$C]-3-methylcholanthrene after the method of
Norman (19). A plot of mmole of bile salt vs μmole of solubilized
$^{14}$C-hydrocarbon showed that the bile salts of the 5β-series were
generally better detergents than the 5α-series. These studies are
currently limited to the derivatives of the primary bile acids,
cholate, chenodeoxycholate, and their 5α-analogs, and support the
observation that glycodeoxycholate is a better detergent than glycoallodeoxycholate. NMR spectra of bile acids or their conjugates
show predictable differences in the 5β- and 5α-series with regard
to chemical shifts of the proton at C-3 and of the C-19 methyl
group as follows: 5β-C-3H, 3.47 (broad); 5α, 4.05 (sharp); 5β-C-
19-H, 0.93-0.95 (s); 5α, 0.81-83 (s). Haslewood (1967) has emphasized the importance of the absorption bands at 10.4 and 11.2 μ
in the infrared for the identification of allocholic acid. The
selective values of such procedures as molecular rotation and
column chromatography have been reviewed (Elliott, 1971) and will
not be treated here.

## PREPARATION OF ALLO ACIDS

Because of the paucity of these materials, generally, the
allo acids used for investigative work have been prepared largely
by synthesis. The methods used will be illustrated briefly for
the preparation of allocholate.

1. Anderson and Haslewood (1962) epimerized the C-5 hydrogen
of ethyl cholate by the sequence shown in Fig. 2. The bromoketone
(IV) was allomerized with alkali to the 5α-ketol (V) and the car-
bonyl group was removed via the action of Raney nickel on the
ethylene thioketal (VI) to provide the 7β-isomer of allocholate.
Selective oxidation and reduction at C-7 provided allocholate.
However, when the sequence was repeated to prepare allochenodeoxycholate, the product analogous to compound VII did not appear to
be allochenodeoxycholate. Subsequent studies showed that the

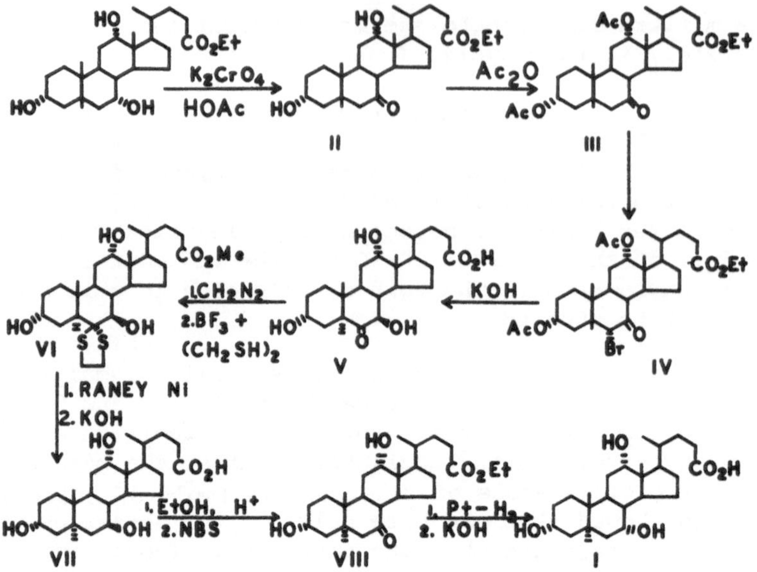

Fig. 2.  Synthesis of allocholate by Anderson and Haslewood (1962).

product was in fact methyl 3β,7β-dihydroxy-5α-cholanate, indicating
that Raney nickel in alcohol not only removed the thioketal but
also dehydrogenated at C-3, and then reduced the ketone to the
equatorial 3β-ol.

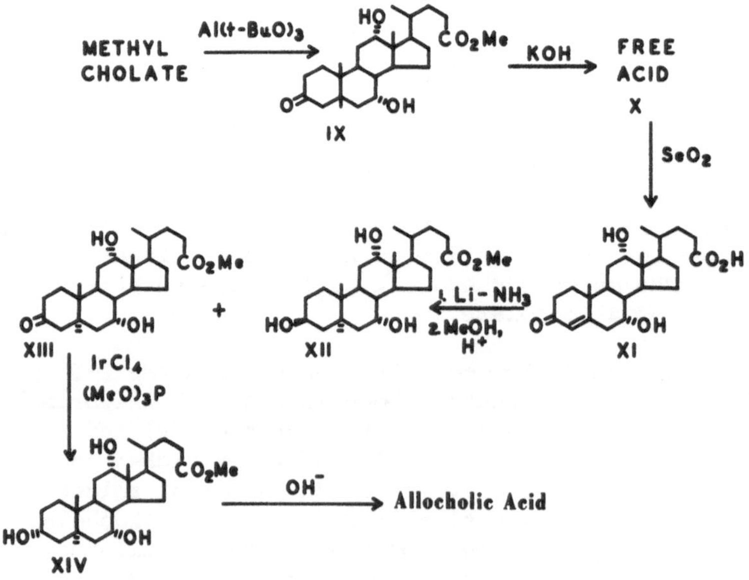

Fig. 3.  Synthesis of allocholate by Kallner (1967b).

2.  The method of Kallner (1967b) (Fig. 3) elicited conversion of methyl cholate to allocholate by attack in Ring A.  The
α,β-unsaturated ketone XI was reduced with lithium in liquid
ammonia to the 5α-derivatives XII and XIII.  Reduction of the ketone XIII with $IrCl_4$ and triphenyl phosphine afforded allocholate.

3.  The allomerization of the 5β-hydrogen to the 5α-configura-
tion with Raney nickel has been studied extensively in our laboratory (Elliott, 1971).  After refluxing methyl cholate in toluene
or p-cymene with freshly prepared W-2 Raney nickel, a mixture of
3-oxo derivatives was obtained, including the desired 3-oxo-5α-
product.  The reaction proceeds through the formation of an α,β-
unsaturated ketone via a mechanism proposed in Fig. 4.  Catalytic
reduction of the 3-oxo-5α-derivative provided a mixture of isomeric alcohols in which the 3α-ol generally predominates.  With
this method the overall yield of methyl allocholate from methyl
cholate was about 12%.  Clearly improved methods of synthesis are
badly needed.


BIOSYNTHESIS

Allo bile acids may be formed by any of three routes, either
via:  1.  cholestanol or cholesterol;  2.  other 5α-sterols;
other 5β-bile acids.

1.  A biosynthetic pathway for these acids stems from the report of Karavolas at this meeting twelve years ago in which we demonstrated that allocholic acid was the major metabolite of cholestanol in the rat.  Subsequent experiments by Ziller have shown
that allochenodeoxycholic acid is the second major metabolite;
small amounts of the 3β-epimers of the two primary allo bile acids,
and lesser amounts of isomeric 3,6-dihydroxy acids are also present in bile.  In the gerbil allocholic acid is the major biliary
metabolite of cholestanol.  As a result of experiments in Stockholm

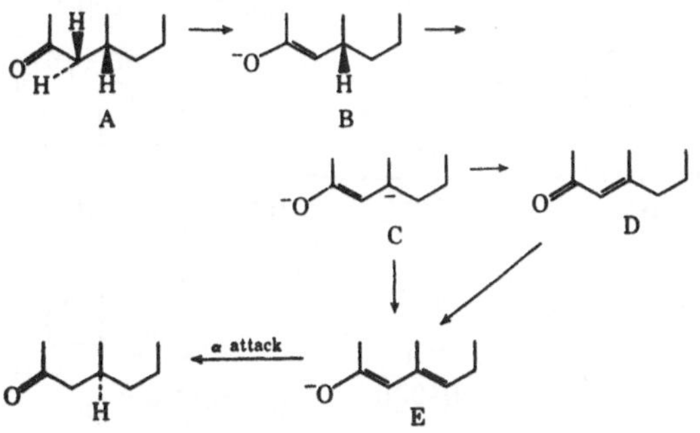

Fig. 4.  Mechanism for allomerization of methyl allocholate to
3-dehydrocholate (Mitra and Elliott, 1969).

and St. Louis a pathway of biosynthesis in the liver (Fig. 5) has been proposed. With certain exceptions this pathway is similar to that for the biosynthesis of the primary 5β-bile acids. Cholestanol undergoes 7α-hydroxylation by a hepatic microsomal enzyme fortified with NADPH, analogous to the formation of 7α-hydroxycholesterol. From a study of the specificity of this 7α-hydroxylase with 5α-cholestan-3-one and 5α-cholestan-3α-ol, the substrate of choice for this reaction was shown to be 5α-cholestan-3β-ol. The role of cytochrome $P_{450}$ in this reaction has not been studied, but the similarity to the reaction with cholesterol raises a strong possibility of similar involvement. Studies with rats with cannulated bile ducts given 5α-cholestan-3β,7α-diol, 5α-cholestane-3β, 7α,26-triol or 3β,7α-dihydroxy-5α-cholestan-26-oic acid showed that the major biliary products are the primary allo bile acids, allocholate and allochenodeoxycholate. In the latter case allochenodeoxycholate predominates. The question of the proper place in this pathway for epimerization of the 3β-ol to the 3α-ol was clarified by experiments of Björkhem and Gustafsson (1971) who found an efficient conversion of the 3β,7α-diol to 7α-hydroxy-5α-cholestan-

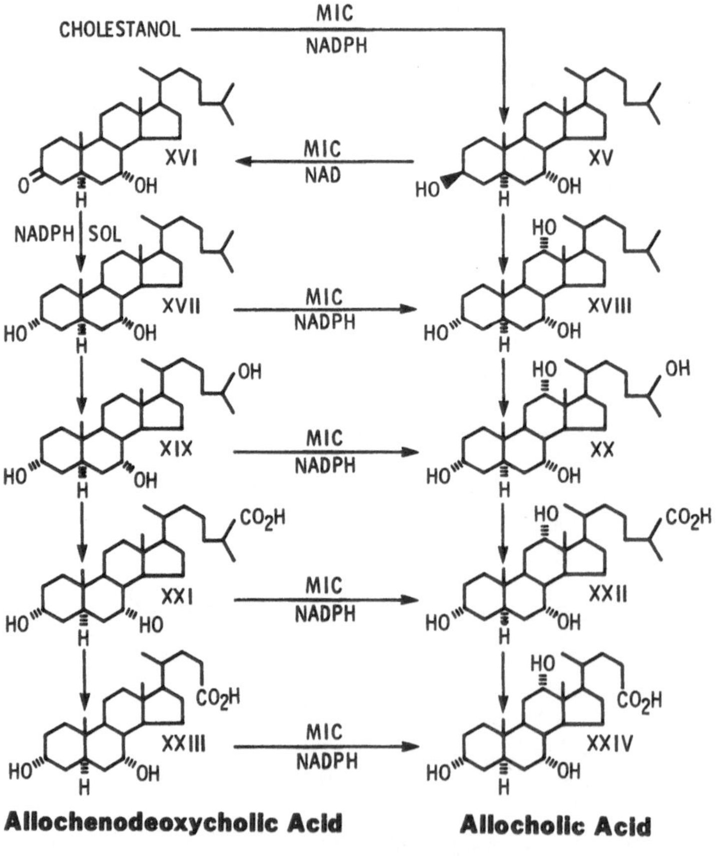

Fig. 5.  Biosynthesis of Allo Bile Acids from Cholestanol.

3-one with microsomes fortified with NAD. Incubation of this ketone with a soluble 3α-hydroxysteroid dehydrogenase fortified with
NADPH resulted in efficient conversion to 5α-cholestane-3α,7α-
diol, the key intermediate in the formation of either primary allo
bile acid. Finally, a microsomal 12α-hydroxylase supplemented with
NADPH promoted efficient conversion to 5α-cholestane-3α,7α,12α-
triol. The sequence of events in the conversion of 5α-cholestane-
3α,7α-diol to allochenodeoxycholate, or the 3α,7α,12α-triol to
allocholate — i.e. 26-hydroxylation, oxidation to the 26-oic acid,
and β-oxidation to the $C_{24}$ acids — may be similar to those in
formation of their 5β-analogs, but the details remain to be studied.

Since the rat metabolizes chenodeoxycholate to α- and β-
muricholates (the 3α,6β,7α- and 3α,6β,7β-trihydroxy-5β-cholanates,
respectively), allochenodeoxycholate was similarly studied in the
rat with a bile fistula. Most of the substrate was recovered unchanged, but about 4% was metabolized to allocholate, and about
0.5% to allohyocholate (3α,6α,7α-trihydroxy-5α-cholanate). This
example of 12α-hydroxylation of a $C_{24}$ bile acid was verified with
microsomes supplemented with NADPH from rat and from rabbit liver.
Since the $C_{24}$ acid served well as a substrate for 12α-hydroxyla-
tion, the reaction was investigated with $C_{27}$ sterols substituted
at C-26; 5α-cholestane-3α,7α,26-triol was more efficiently hydroxylated at the 12α-position than 5α-cholestane-3α,7α-diol. This
result is equally surprising, for the presence of a 26-hydroxyl or
a 26-carboxyl group in the analogous 5β-sterol virtually prevents
12α-hydroxylation and the formation of cholic acid. Certain of
these studies have been extended in the rabbit which produces
little or no chenodeoxycholate and presumably has an active 12α-
hydroxylase. As anticipated the yields of allocholate and 5α-
cholestane-3α,7α,12α-triol are markedly enhanced (Ali and Elliott,
1975).

The properties of the crude microsomal 12α-hydroxylase active
in cholic acid synthesis so resemble those involved in 12α-
hydroxylation of the 5α-$C_{27}$ sterols and the 5α-$C_{24}$ acid to suggest

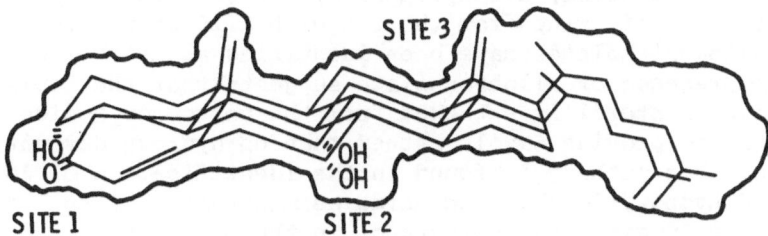

Fig. 6.   Recognition by 12α-Hydroxylase (Site 3) of 5α-cholestane-
          3α,7α-diol (upper structure) and 7α-hydroxycholest-4-en-
          3-one (lower structure).

that a single enzyme system is active on the several substrates
(Mui and Elliott, 1975).  Molecular models show (Fig. 6) that the
planar 5α-cholestane-3α,7α-diol is virtually superimposable upon
7α-hydroxycholest-4-en-3-one, the substrate for 12α-hydroxylation
in the synthesis of cholic acid.  The requirements for maximal
activity of the enzyme at Site 3 are the 3α-ol (Site 1) for the
5α-sterol and the 3-oxo group of the more planar Ring A containing
the 4,5-double bond, and the 7α-ol (Site 2).  Substitution of a
hydroxyl or a carboxyl group at C-26 of the 5α-sterol enhanced
the reaction, perhaps by tighter binding, whereas shortening the
side chain to the $C_{24}$ allo acid lessened the activity, but still
provided a substrate more active than the 3-oxo- or 3β-hydroxy-
5α-cholestane-7α-ol.  Studies with rabbit liver microsomes and the
two substrates shown in Fig. 6 support this proposal (Ali and
Elliott, 1975).  Additional experiments to test this hypothesis
are underway.

Further exposure of the substrates shown in Fig. 6 to microsomal enzymes of rabbit or rat liver provided products more polar
than the 12α-hydroxylated derivatives.  Investigation by gas
chromatography mass spectrometry of these products derived from
5α-cholestane-3α,7α-diol by rabbit microsomes showed that a mixture of polyols was formed by hydroxylation of the side chain; 5α-
cholestane-3α,7α,12α,25-tetrol was the major derivative with lesser
amounts of the 3α,7α,12α,24α-, 3α,7α,12α,24β-, and 3α,7α,12α,23-
tetrols.  No significant 26-hydroxylation occurred with this
species.  These results are comparable to those with 5β-cholestane-
3α,7α,12α-triol and microsomes from human liver, where hydroxylation at C-25 dominated, in contrast to studies with rat liver
microsomes in which 26-hydroxylation was predominate for 5β-
cholestane-3α,7α,12α-triol and for 5β-cholestane-3α,7α-diol.  They
are also of interest in relation to the nature of the 5β-cho-
lestane-polyols obtained from patients with cerebrotendinous
xanthomatosis, although no 5α-sterols have been reported as yet
from these patients.

A second metabolite derived from allochenodeoxycholate in the
rat with a bile fistula, allohyocholate, has been identified now
as a constituent of urine from the rat with a ligated bile duct.
Since no allomuricholates have been identified as metabolic products, the presence of allohyocholate suggests that the coplanar
5α-bile acid or sterol is attacked from the bottom or α-side of
the molecule to provide 6α-ols rather than 6β-hydroxy derivatives.
Support for this pathway is found in the identification of 3β,6α-
and 3α,6α-dihydroxy-5α-cholanic acids as minor metabolites of 5α-
cholestane-3β,26-diol and cholestanol in the bile fistula rat.
Thus, whereas chenodeoxycholic acid is metabolized extensively by
the rat through 6β-hydroxylation, the coplanar 5α-acid or sterol
undergoes 6α-hydroxylation, but to a very small extent.

Finally, the formation of cholestanol from cholesterol in the body is well documented. Small but significant amounts of cholest-4-en-3-one are formed from cholesterol by hepatic microsomal enzymes fortified with NAD. This reaction may be rate limiting in the formation of cholestanol, since microsomal 5α-steroid reductase and 3β-hydroxy-steroid reductase fortified with NADPH effectively provide cholestanol. Mitochondrial preparations have also been reported effective in this reduction of cholest-4-en-3-one. The activity of the above microsomal enzymes has been studied with 7α-hydroxycholest-4-en-3-one and 7α,12α-dihydroxy-cholest-4-en-3-one (Björkhem and Einarsson, 1970), and comparable reduction to the 3-oxo-5α-sterols was observed with rat liver microsomes fortified with NADPH; 3α-hydroxy-5α-sterols result from the action of a 3α-hydroxysteroid reductase in the soluble fraction. Since these 5α-sterols are converted to 5α-bile acids, the natural occurrence of allocholate in ox and carp bile (Yamasaki et al., 1972) and the appearance of allocholate after administration of 7α-hydroxycholesterol to the rat, rabbit or hen is quite reasonable. The efficient in vitro conversion of the unsaturated intermediates, 7α-hydroxycholest-4-en-3-one and 7α,12α-dihydroxy-cholest-4-en-3-one, to 5α-sterols, and their in vivo conversion to 5α-bile acids should be contrasted with the rather exclusive conversion of these unsaturated sterols to 5β-bile acids in the rat with a bile fistula. Clearly, the microsomal 3-oxo-$\Delta^4$-steroid 5α-reductase is inhibited or removed from the assembly of enzymes for the conversion of sterol to bile acid in vivo. In general, however, allo bile acids may be considered as metabolites of cholestanol, or cholesterol.

2. With this information pathways for the formation of allo bile acids from other 5α-sterols are easily visualized. 5α-Cyprinol (5α-cholestane-3α,7α,12α,26,27-pentol) is found frequently as a sulphate (and hence a bile salt) in lower animals, such as carp and salamander. In the latter species metabolites of this sterol have been identified as allocholic acid and an acid tentatively assigned the structure 3α,7α,12α,26-tetrahydroxy-5α-cholestanoic acid. In carp 5α-cyprinol is a major biliary sterol, which can be derived from cholesterol via some of the enzyme systems previously discussed; allocholic acid is a metabolite of this sterol. The antiatherogenic sterol, cholestane-3β,5α,6β-triol provides 3β,5α,6β-trihydroxycholanic acid as the major biliary metabolite. Other aspects of the metabolism of 5α-sterols to allo bile acids have been reviewed earlier (Elliott 1971).

3. The derivation of allo bile acids from their 5β-analogs was demonstrated by the conversion of deoxycholate by the rabbit to fecal allodeoxycholate. Kallner (1967a) showed that enzymes of the cecum promoted dehydrogenation of the 3α-hydroxy-5β-acid to a 3-oxo-5β- and then a 3-oxo-$\Delta^4$-acid which was reduced by a 5α-steroid reductase to the 3-oxo-5α-analog and thence to the 3α-

hydroxy allo acid.   This reduction of the $\alpha$,$\beta$-unsaturated oxo acid
was also shown to prevail in the liver with the formation of 5$\beta$-
and 5$\alpha$-bile acids.   These studies aid in explanation of the identification of all four isomeric 3-hydroxycholanic acids in bile of
the rat after administration of 3-oxo-chol-4-enic acid.   The
identification of cholate, allocholate and chenodeoxycholate after
administration of 3$\beta$,7$\alpha$-dihydroxychol-5-enoic acid to the carp may
also be explained by this mechanism; the failure to identify allochenodeoxycholate may be related to an active 12$\alpha$-hydroxylase.

### CONCLUSION

Allo bile acids are more prevalent in lower species.   The
relatively lower activity of hepatic microsomal 5$\alpha$-steroid reductase in mammals explains in part the presence of lower concentrations of these acids in these species.   Whether this difference is
evolutionary, or protective for mammals is not yet known.   Whether
allo bile acids can play a role in regulation or control of sterol
and/or bile acid synthesis remains to be ascertained.   Because of
the paucity of these acids, the question of their toxicity via
the diet, their role in induction or regulation of atherosclerosis,
large bowel cancer, cholelithiasis, or other diseases of mankind
remains before us.

### ACKNOWLEDGEMENT

Support for some of the studies reported here was provided by
Public Health Service Grants HL-07878 from the National Heart and
Lung Institute and Grant CA-16375 from the National Cancer Institute through the National Large Bowel Cancer Project.   This review constitutes Paper L in the series on Bile Acids.   The author
wishes to acknowledge the many contributions of his former and
present colleagues, particularly Drs. H.J. Karavolas, S.A. Ziller,
Jr., M.N. Mitra, S.Y. Kamat, M.I. Kelsey, B.W. Noll, M.M. Mui,
C.M. Siegfried, R.L. Blaskiewicz, G.J. O'Neil, Jr., Y. Shalon,
S.S. Ali, L.B. Walsh, R. Shaw and E.A. Doisy, Jr.   He is especially
pleased to extend grateful acknowledgement to Distinguished Service Professor Emeritus E.A. Doisy, Sr., for his patience, toler-
ance, advice, and encouragement during the early phases of
maturation of the author.

### REFERENCES

Ali, S.S. and Elliott, W.H. (1975) Biochim. Biophys. Acta, In Press.
Anderson, I.G. and Haslewood, G.A.D. (1962) Biochim. J. 85, 236.
Björkhem, I. and Einarsson, K. (1970) Eur. J. Biochem. 13, 174.
Björkhem, I. and Gustafsson, J. (1971) Eur. J. Biochem. 18, 207.

Elliott, W.H. (1971) in The Bile Acids (P.P. Nair and D. Krit-
chevsky, ed) Plenum Press, New York, Vol. 1, 47.
Haslewood, G.A.D. (1965) in The Biliary System (W. Taylor, ed)
F.A. Davis Co., Philadelphia, 107.
Haslewood, G.A.D. (1967) Bile Salts, Methuen and Co., London.
Kallner, A. (1967a) Acta Chem. Scand. 21, 315.
Kallner, A. (1967b) Acta Chem. Scand. 21, 322.
Karavolas, H.J. and Elliott, W.H. (1965) in The Biliary System
(W. Taylor, ed) F.A. Davis Co., Philadelphia, 175.
Miyazaki, H., Ishibashi, M., Inoue, M. and Itoh, M. (1974) J.
Chromatog. 99, 553.
Mui, M.M. and Elliott, W.H. (1975) Biochemistry 14, 2712.
Norman, A. (1960) Acta Chem. Scand. 14, 1295.
Shaw, R.G. and Elliott, W.H. (1975) Anal. Biochem., submitted.
Sjövall, J., Eneroth, P. and Ryhage, R. (1971) in The Bile Acids
(P.P. Nair and D. Kritchevsky, ed) Plenum Press, New York, Vol.
1, 209.
Windaus, A. and Neukirchen, K. (1919) Ber. 52, 1915.
Yamasaki, K., Ikawa, S., Ayaki, Y. and Yamamoto, Y. (1972) J.
Biochem. 12, 769, and reference therein.

DISCUSSION OF COMMENTARY BY W.H. ELLIOTT

Hofmann:    Have you done any binary phase studies with these allo
bile acids so that you can look at the size of the micellar zone
and the liquid crystal zone to compare these with results obtained
with 5-β acids?

Elliott:    No, we have not done this yet, but we intend to do it
as soon as we can, because I agree with you that we ought to look
at more complex systems.

Haslewood:    The question that Dr. Elliott raised about the
biological reason for mammals having 5-β bile acids is an
important one.    There is no doubt that the 5-α configuration
is the more primitive.    It occurs in the most primitive vertebrates, but even in quite primitive vertebrates there is a
considerable amount of 5-β acids.    There are quite a number of
amphibians which have about equal amounts of both 5-α and 5-β
alcohols conjugated with sulphate.    Therefore, any selective
process that has taken place has certainly been very slow.    One
is bound to conclude that some kind of biochemical advantage, not
necessarily in terms of detergent efficiency, resides in making
5-β rather than 5-α bile acids.    In view of the fact that we
are discovering more primitive bile acids in human patients with
liver disease, I think that this study is of great clinical
interest and importance.

Dam:    We might look at this problem in a different way.    The
allo bile acids have the great disadvantage in that when they are
conjugated with glycine and have only two hydroxyl groups, they
form insoluble calcium salts.    Therefore, in those species which
form considerable amounts of glycine conjugates it is important
that the bile acids should be of the normal and not the allo series.
To put it another way, there is a positive disadvantage with the
dihydroxy allo bile acids when they are conjugated with glycine.
Therefore, to argue teleologically, that is the reason why the
normal bile acids are predominant in man and mammals.

Elliott:    That is true with respect to glycoallodeoxycholate,
but we have not studied the other substances yet.    Professor
Haslewood's comment raised a point I did not have time to mention.

For some time I have been interested in the metabolism of
cholestane, which can be derived from cholesterol.    I am told
that chicken fat contains 20 per cent of cholesterol, and you may
be aware of how much fried chicken is consumed by many Americans.
So they may be ingesting a fair amount of cholestane, and so be
producing quite a lot of allo bile acids.    What the fate and
possible role of the allo acids are pose important questions for
us to solve.

Haslewood:    I would like to remind everyone that glycine conjugates are unknown in nature except in eutherian mammals, but there
are many normal and allo bile acids conjugated with taurine.

# DISSOLUTION OF GALLSTONES BY CHENODEOXYCHOLIC ACID

R. Hermon Dowling, Gerard M. Murphy and John Iser

Gastroenterology Unit, Department of Medicine

Guy's Hospital and Medical School, London, SE1 9RT

## INTRODUCTION

In another chapter in this volume, Dr. Hofmann has discussed in detail newer aspects of bile acid physiology and of the entero-hepatic circulation. The purpose of this chapter is to review the most important therapeutic advance in the bile acid field, namely the use of chenodeoxycholic acid (CDCA) in the treatment of gall-stones. Indeed, it was here in Scandinavia just five years ago, at the International Congress on the Biochemistry of Lipids(1), which took place in Lund, just across the Kategat in Sweden, that Dr. Hofmann told us about the results of studies by his colleagues at the Mayo Clinic(2,3) which showed that oral CDCA could reduce the saturation of bile with cholesterol, and following on from this, the first reports of successful gallstone dissolution with this agent appeared from the Mayo Clinic(4), and from our own Unit in 1972(5). Since then, approximately 1500 gallstone patients have been treated with chenodeoxycholic acid in at least eighteen different countries.*

The selection of these patients for treatment, their type of gallstones, the dose and duration of treatment and the preparations of chenodeoxycholic acid used have varied from country to country. For this reason, rather than attempting to summarise the world experience to date (which, as recently as January 1975, was collated at a Workshop on CDCA held in Frankfurt(6)) instead, this chapter discusses just a few aspects of this topic largely based on the ex-

*The addition of 3,000 patients from Italy brings this total to 4,500.

perience of our own Unit in treating 85 patients over the past 4
years (7).


SELECTION OF PATIENTS FOR TREATMENT - THE ETHICS OF THE PROBLEM

At present the selection of patients for CDCA treatment is
based on the clinical signs and symptoms, on radiology (which in
turn depends on the accuracy of clinical X-rays to assess gall-
bladder function and the size, number and type of gallstones) and,
in some cases, on analysis of bile-rich duodenal fluid.

The clinical criteria for accepting patients for treatment
varies from country to country and from physician to physician.  In
Britain, for example, the Committee on the Safety of Medicines has
recommended that CDCA should not be given to women capable of bearing children and that "chenotherapy" should not be combined with the
contraceptive pill.  Elsewhere CDCA is given to women in the child
bearing group only if accompanied by oral contraceptive agents.

There are sizeable ethical problems about the treatment of
asymptomatic gallstone patients with CDCA (although radiolucent
gallstones could only have been detected if there had been some
indication for contrast cholecystography in the first instance)
and indeed about the treatment of patients with symptoms when it
may take 6-36 months before gallstones dissolve, and subsequently,
even lifelong therapy may be necessary to prevent recurrence.  The
least controversial group of patients who might be considered for
"chenotherapy", is the group in whom surgery is either contra-
indicated, or for whom it constitutes a considerable risk.  But
even in this group, the number of patients who really need
surgery for their gallstones and who could not withstand modern
anaesthesia and surgery, is very small.

At present, the individual clinican must decide on arbitrary
grounds whether or not the frequency and severity of such symptoms
as biliary colic will or will not preclude prolonged medical treatment.  At present, since there is insufficient critical evidence
about the natural history of untreated cholelithiasis and the
relative merits and demerits of medical versus surgical treatment,
the problem is both emotive and controversial.  Furthermore, because
of the intangible nature of these problems and the lack of objective
scientific information, the ethics of CDCA treatment are seldom
discussed at scientific meetings.

In spite of these difficulties, valuable information is being
accumulated about many aspects of treatment with CDCA and the
introduction of this agent has been a potent stimulus in the
broader fields of bile lipid physiology and gallstone disease.

## THE EFFICACY OF CDCA IN DIFFERENT TYPES OF GALLSTONES

The pattern of results from many groups using CDCA is broadly similar and although the following conclusions are mainly based on the experience of our own Unit, they are, nonetheless, fairly representative of the results obtained by other workers in the field(6).

The numbers of patients studied in our Unit, together with some of the overall results, are summarised in Figure 1. Of a total of 85 patients, 6 had stones in the biliary tree and in 2 of these patients, the stones have disappeared. Seven patients initially had non-functioning gallbladders, but in none of these has there been any return of gallbladder function, and we no longer accept such patients for treatment. We have also failed to dissolve any stones in the 11 patients with radio-opaque gallstones: thus these patients represent therapeutic failures. There were, therefore, 61 patients who had radiolucent stones and functioning gallbladders. Thirteen of these patients had been treated for less than six months, and so had not yet had their first follow-up X-ray. One patient developed a non-functioning gallbladder during treatment, 6 failed to attend for follow-up and 10 have come to surgery. Since medical treatment failed both in the patients going to surgery and in those with radio-opaque stones, it seemed important to analyse the reasons for these failures, rather than to concentrate on the successes alone.

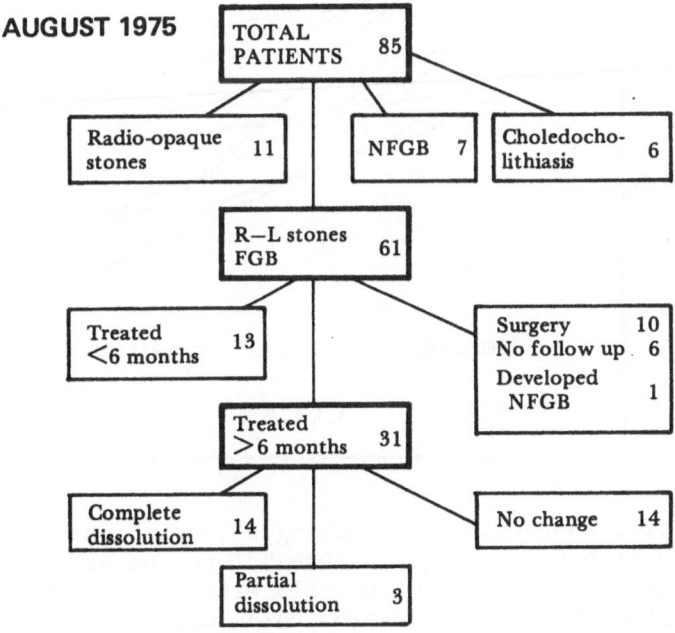

**Figure 1.** Numbers of patients studied and summary of the results of CDCA therapy in different treatment sub-groups.

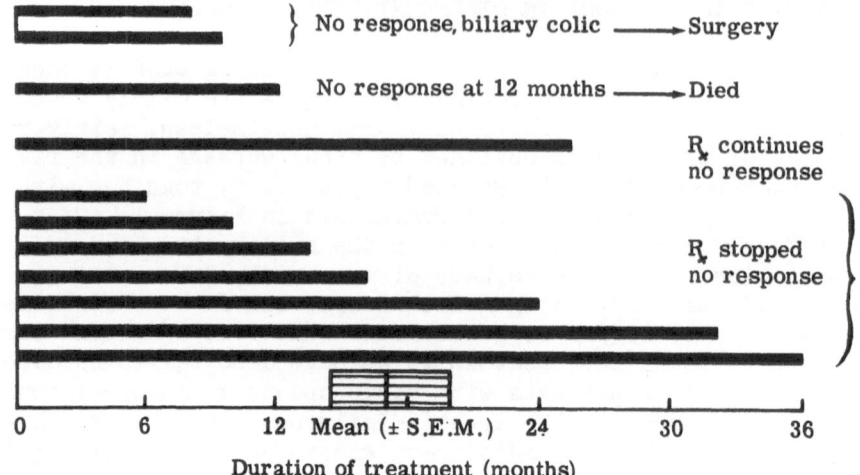

**Figure 2.** Duration of treatment in months and the outcome of CDCA therapy in 11 patients with radio-opaque gallstones.

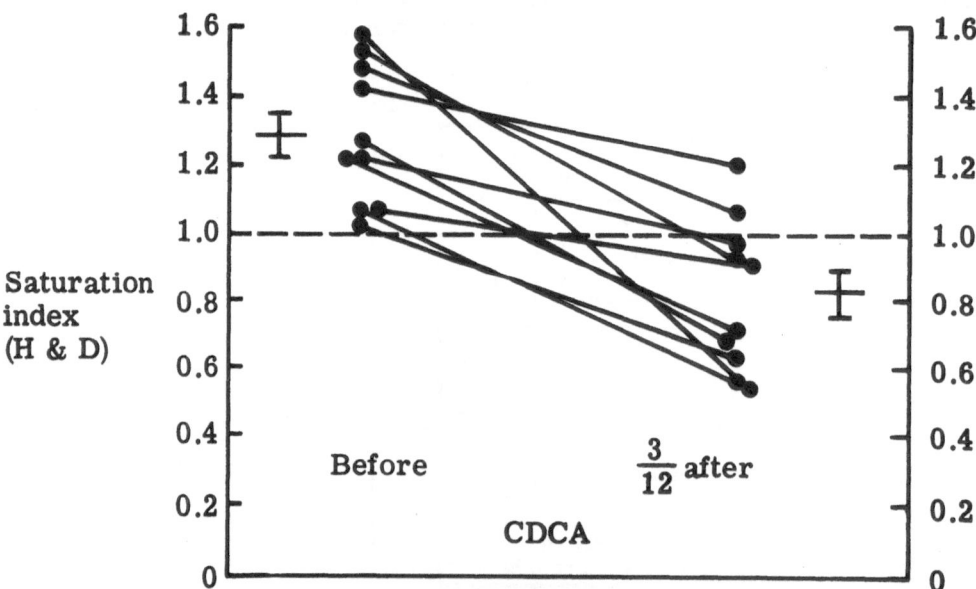

**Figure 3.** Lipid composition of fasting bile-rich duodenal-fluid from patients with radio-opaque stones before and after 3 months' CDCA treatment. The saturation of bile with cholesterol is expressed as the saturation index(8) calculated from the molar ratios of biliary bile salts, phospholipids and cholesterol, where values > 1 indicate supersaturated and < 1 unsaturated solutions as defined by Hegardt and Dam(9).

Patients with radio-opaque stones. The results of treatment in patients with radio-opaque stones are shown in Figures 2 and 3. In 2 of the 11 patients, there had been no radiological evidence of gallstone dissolution after 8 and 10 months' treatment, when frequent and severe attacks of biliary colic led to surgical referral. Another patient, who had been treated for 13 months, had shown no radiological response after one year's treatment and she died from unrelated causes. A further patient, who has mainly radiolucent stones with calcified nuclei, continues treatment, but after more than two years' therapy, her stones have shown no evidence of dissolution, while the remaining 7 patients, who have been treated for periods ranging from 6 months to 3 years (mean $17.0 \pm 2.6$ months) stopped CDCA because there had been no radiological response.

It seems that the failure to dissolve these radio-opaque gallstones was not due to any failure of CDCA treatment to change bile lipid composition. Figure 3 shows the lipid composition of bilerich duodenal fluid in 10 of the 11 patients, plotted as the saturation index(8) (SI) where 1 represents a solution saturated with cholesterol as defined by Hegardt and Dam(9), points greater than unity representing supersaturated and points less than unity undersaturated solutions. From the SI results measured before, and three months after treatment with chenodeoxycholic acid, 8 out of the 10 patients had an unsaturated bile after CDCA, in which cholesterol gallstones would have been expected to dissolve. (The significance of changes in bile lipid composition in response to CDCA is discussed later).

Patients coming to surgery during CDCA treatment. The clinical details in these 10 patients are summarised in Table I. All 10 patients had radiolucent stones in functioning gallbladders and again CDCA had satisfactorily reduced the saturation index from a mean of $1.26 \pm 0.09$ before treatment to $0.88 \pm 0.08$ after therapy. In most patients the duration of treatment had been adequate, ranging from 3-19 months with a mean of 10 ($\pm$ 2) months. The decision about surgery was a mutual one taken by both doctor and patient in 4 out of 10 cases, but 6 patients made the decision unilaterally. The principal reason for surgery was because of unacceptably severe and/or frequent biliary colic in half of the patients. Two of them had developed non-functioning gallbladders and in another patient, the gallbladder was removed as an elective procedure at the end of a full-term pregnancy and following the delivery of a normal child. One patient had multiple symptoms, probably unrelated to gallstones, one defaulted from treatment, while one patient, who had also had biliary colic, decided on surgery when her X-rays showed no evidence of dissolution after 12 months' treatment.

Patients with radiolucent stones and "functioning" gallbladders treated for at least 6 months. We were left, therefore, with 31 patients who had radiolucent stones in radiologically functioning

Table I.  Clinical details of patients with gallstones who underwent surgery during CDCA treatment.

Radiolucent stones + 'functioning' GB  -  10/10

Bile cholesterol satn. index (H. & D.)  -  before 1.26 ± 0.09 (n=10)
                                              after  0.88 ± 0.08 (n=8)

Duration of CDCA                        -  10 + 2 MONTHS
                                              (RANGE 3 - 19)

Decisions about surgery                 -  Doctor + patient 4/10
                                              Patient alone   6/10

Reasons for surgery - Biliary colic 5/10                Polysymptomatic 1/10
                      'non functioning' GB 2/10  Defaulted 1/10
                      Pregnancy 1/10                    Unchanged X-rays
                                                        (12 months $R_x$) 1/10

Table II.  Influence of stone size (the maximum stone diameter measured from cholecystogram films) and the duration of treatment in months on gallstone dissolution.  The upper number in each "fraction" shows the number of patients with partial or complete gallstone dissolution while the lower number indicates the total number of patients undergoing treatment at the different times periods.

| Stone size (mm) | Duration of treatment (months) | | | | |
|---|---|---|---|---|---|
|  | <6 | 6-12 | 12-24 | >24 | Total |
| Small < 5 | 4/4 | 2/3 | 3/3 | 0/1 | 9/11 |
| Medium 5-10 | 1/1 | 0/1 | 2/2 | 0/1 | 3/5 |
| Large > 10 | 0/0 | 0/5 | 3/6 | 2/4 | 5/15 |
| Total | 5/5 | 2/9 | 8/11 | 2/6 | 17/31 |

gallbladders who had been treated for 6 months or more, and of these
there has been partial or complete dissolution in 17, but no change
in gallstone size in the remaining 14 patients (Figure 1).

## ANALYSIS OF WHY TREATMENT SUCCESSFULLY DISSOLVES
## GALLSTONES IN SOME PATIENTS BUT NOT IN OTHERS

The influence of stone size and the duration of treatment on
gallstone dissolution. The influence of gallstone size, arbitrarily
defined as small (<5 mm), medium (5-10 mm) or large (>10 mm) when
measured from cholecystogram films, and the duration of treatment
in months, on gallstone dissolution is shown in Table 2. As might
be expected, small stones do well, 6 out of 7 dissolving in one
year, while 9 out of 10 showed evidence of dissolution in 2 years
(8 complete; 1 partial). In contrast, large stones seem to require
longer periods of treatment, and we had no successes in the first
year, but 5 out of 15 showed at least partial dissolution after
over two years' treatment. Taking patients with small, medium and
large stones together, we return to the total of 17 "responders"
and 14 "non-responders". The next question we considered was the
bile lipid response to CDCA treatment in these two groups.

The importance of bile lipid analysis and the response of bile
lipids to CDCA therapy. Figure 4 shows the saturation indices,
which were plotted in retrospect after the X-ray results were known,
for the "responders" and the "non-responders".

Before treatment, almost all patients had supersaturated bile.
After treatment, with the possible exception of one case, all
patients in the "responder" group had an unsaturated bile, the mean
value being $0.78 \pm 0.04$. By contrast, in the "non-responders",
although CDCA reduced the saturation of bile with cholesterol in
all patients, the mean value after therapy still indicated a
saturated solution ($1.00 \pm 0.06$). Five of the 14 "non-responders"
did have unsaturated bile following treatment, but in 4 of these
the stones were large and the patients had been treated for less
than 12 months which, as we have already seen, is probably too
early to assess gallstone dissolution (Table 2). It may well be,
therefore, that some of these 5 patients will, in time, belong
to the "responder" group, but even as the data stand, it does seem
that the bile lipid response to CDCA is a useful predictor of the
chances of successful gallstone dissolution.

But why was there a difference between these two groups? Were
there differences in the doses of CDCA or was the response to CDCA
variable in individual patients? In previous studies from our
Unit(10), we measured the saturation index before and after treatment with 0.25, 0.5, 0.75 and 1.0 gram of CDCA per day. In patients
given only 250 mg CDCA per day, there was an inconsistent response
and the mean saturation index after treatment was still greater than

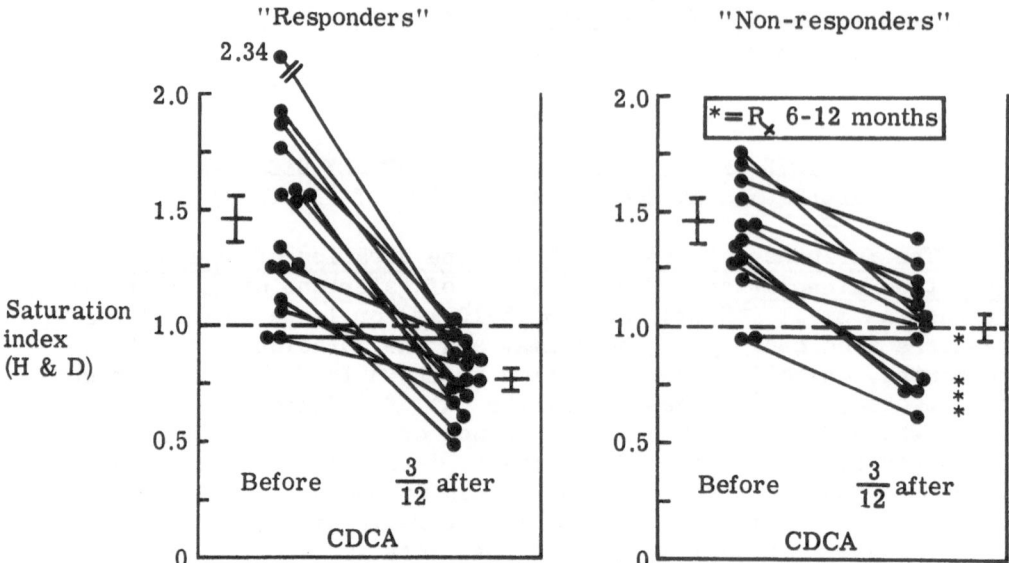

**Figure 4.** Bile lipid composition before and after treatment (see legend to Fig. 3) in patients whose gallstones showed evidence of partial or complete dissolution (the "responders" - left panel) and in those whose gallstone size remained unchanged ("non-responders" - right panel).


unity. In other words, after treatment the patients were, on average, still left with a supersaturated solution in which gallstones could not be expected to dissolve. With 500 mg CDCA/day, the mean SI was less than unity but 4 of the 7 patients had unsaturated bile but it was not until we reached higher doses (750-1000 mg/day) that there was a more consistent response.

These results were based on the absolute daily dose of CDCA, irrespective of body weight. But when the post-treatment saturation index was plotted against the dose of CDCA in mg per kg per day, in spite of a considerable scatter of results, there was nonetheless a significant correlation between the two variables, suggesting that the dose of CDCA should not be fixed, but should be based on body weight.

The absolute doses of CDCA, body weights and daily doses of CDCA/kgBW in the "responders" and "non-responders". The absolute daily dose of CDCA was roughly comparable in both groups of patients (824 mg $\pm$ 51 in the "responders" and 839 $\pm$ 82 in the "non-responders") but to our surprise, we found that there was, on average, a 12 kg difference in mean body weight between the two groups, and as a result, the dose of CDCA per kg body weight in the "non-responders" (11.5 $\pm$ 0.74) was significantly less than that in the patients whose stones showed signs of dissolving (14.2 $\pm$ 0.90) (t = 2.17; P < 0.05).

When the post-treatment saturation index was plotted against the dose of "cheno" in mg.kg$^{-1}$day$^{-1}$, there was an almost complete separation between the results for the two populations of patients. As already discussed, the "non-responders" were given a smaller dose of "cheno" per kg body weight, and were left with a supersaturated bile after treatment, whereas the patients whose stones dissolved had a mean post-treatment saturation index of about 0.8 and were given almost 15 mg.CDCA.kg$^{-1}$day$^{-1}$. However, in spite of these statistically valid general conclusions, there was nonetheless a considerable individual variation in the patients' response to treatment, and we would suggest that the response of bile lipids to CDCA should still be monitored in all patients, with the aim of achieving a post-treatment saturation index of not more than 0.8(7).

## CLINICAL SYMPTOMS AND SIDE-EFFECTS DURING CDCA THERAPY

Non-specific dyspepsia. The non-specific symptoms commonly associated with gallstones, such as flatulence, belching, heartburn and bloating, intolerance to dietary fat, etc., are well recognised. In our series, 53% of 45 patients complained of these non-specific symptoms before treatment and 16 of these 24 patients claimed a marked reduction in the frequency of their symptoms during therapy, only one patient, who had not previously had dyspepsia, developing symptoms during therapy. However, these are uncontrolled observations and may well represent a placebo effect for which, at present, we have no logical explanation. More important, however, is the frequency of biliary colic, since it has frequently been suggested that as stones dissolve they are more likely to migrate and cause biliary colic.

Biliary colic before and during CDCA treatment. Accurate records were available in 54 patients, of whom 47 (nearly 90%) had had attacks of biliary colic in the year before starting CDCA, and again half of these patients had a marked reduction in either the frequency or severity of attacks of colic during treatment. None of the patients who had been free of colic before therapy developed this symptom during treatment.

Side-effects and complications of CDCA.
(i)  Diarrhoea. When treatment began, it was predicted that patients might develop diarrhoea because of the cathartic effect of unabsorbed bile acids spilling into the colon, and indeed this dose-related complication occurs in about 40-50% of patients, usually during the first few weeks of therapy, but occasionally occurring sporadically throughout the period of treatment.

(ii) Hypercholesterolaemia. Hypercholesterolaemia was predicted because it was felt that exogenous chenodeoxycholic acid might block

the normal catabolism of cholesterol to bile acids, leading to a
stock-piling of cholesterol in the body, but none of the patients
treated so far has developed this complication(11,12), and in
recent studies from Aalborg, Dr. Pedersen and colleagues have
shown that cholesterol turnover is unaffected during the treatment
of gallstones(13).

(iii) <u>Liver dysfunction.</u>  More important, however, is the question
of hepatic dysfunction, either because of a direct toxic effect of
chenodeoxycholic acid on the liver itself, or as an indirect effect
of its bacterial metabolite, lithocholic acid, on the liver.  Our
own results in this respect (7,14) are comparable to those from
other Units(6).  For this reason, only a few representative results
are presented from the patients whose gallstones dissolved, thereby
setting the benefits of treatment against possible side-effects of
hepatotoxicity.

Figure 5 shows the serum transaminase and gamma glutamyl
transpeptide levels in the "responder" group, plotted over a 16-
month period of CDCA treatment.  The majority of patients had
normal values throughout, but about one-third showed occasional
"spikes" in enzyme activity, some half of which were associated
with clinical symptoms such as biliary colic, but in the remainder,
the transaminase values rose for no obvious reason.  It is largely
because of these occasional spikes of enzyme activity, to up to
twice the limit of normal, that we now find significant increases
in the mean transaminase levels before and after 6, 12, 18 and 24
months' treatment, although with the possible exception of the
results after 2 years' CDCA, the mean values were all within the
normal range(7).

The significance of these raised transaminase levels is
unknown, but needle biopsies of the liver before and after treatment from many centres(6,14) have shown that the histological
changes in the liver are, if anything, less frequent in patients
treated with "cheno" than in untreated cholelithiasis.  It seems,
therefore, that in the doses used, chenodeoxycholic acid is not
toxic in man, and recent evidence both from Germany and from the
United States suggests that this may be related to the capacity of
the human liver to sulphate lithocholic acid, and hence promote
its excretion from the body.


THE SPECIFICITY OF CHENODEOXYCHOLIC ACID

Dr. Mok in our group had started a double blind trial with
placebo, cholic acid and chenodeoxycholic acid.  When he measured
the saturation indices before and after three months' "treatment"
he found no response in patients given placebo or cholic acid but
3 of the 4 patients given CDCA showed unsaturated bile after therapy.

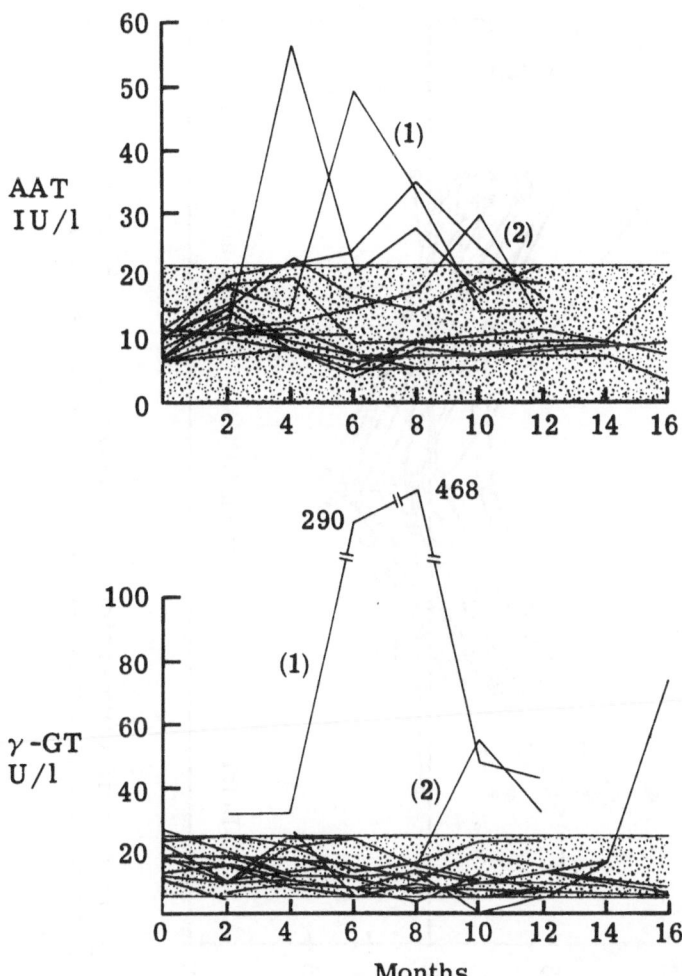

Figure 5. Serum transaminase (AAT or aspartate amino transferase) and γGT (gamma glutamyl transpeptidase) levels in the "responder" group measured monthly during the first 16 months of CDCA therapy. The normal laboratory range is shown by the shaded area: the results in patients (1) and (2) in the upper panel correspond to the results (1) and (2) in the lower panel.

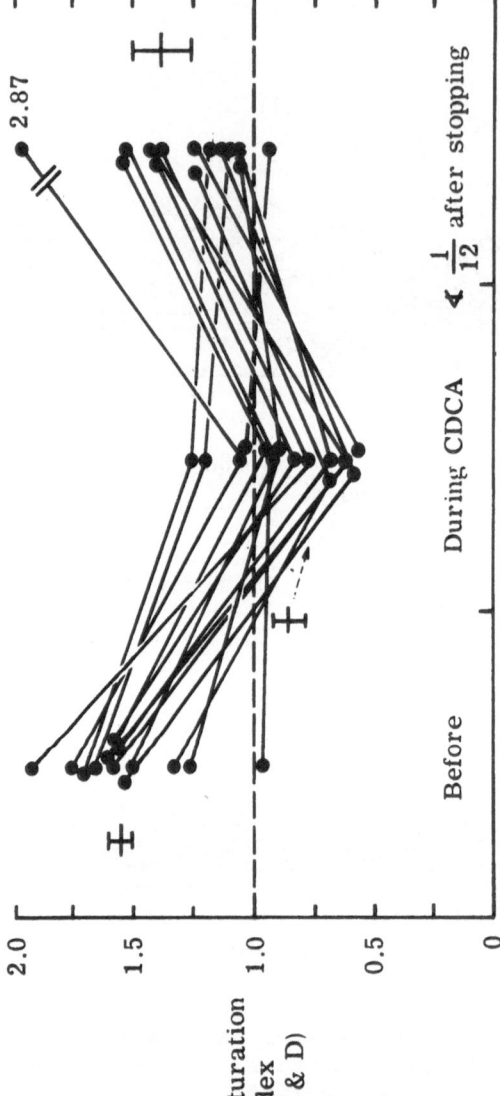

**Figure 6.** Bile lipid composition (see legend to **Fig.** 3) in patients with gallstones before, during and not less than one month after stopping CDCA.

At that time, trials in England were stopped because of CDCA hepatotoxicity in animals but fortunately at the same time, a comparable single blind trial with cholic acid, CDCA and placebo was in progress(15) at the Mayo Clinic.  After 6-12 months' therapy, they showed that none of 18 patients given placebo and none of 17 given cholic acid showed any change in gallstone size but more than half the patients treated with "cheno" showed evidence of gallstone dissolution.

Since the Bristol group have shown that deoxycholate <u>increases</u> the saturation of bile with cholesterol(16), it does seem <u>that CDCA</u> is almost unique in its beneficial effects - but how does it work?


### THE MECHANISM OF ACTION OF CDCA

In the past year, two studies, one from Rochester, Minnesota(17) and the other from Phoenix(18) have shown, by secretion-perfusion studies of the upper intestine that when biliary cholesterol secretion is plotted against bile acid output, before treatment, there is a linear relationship, and that during chenodeoxycholic acid therapy, the slope of this linear relationship becomes less steep so that for every given unit of bile acid produced, the amount of cholesterol secreted is markedly reduced.  Precisely how cholesterol secretion is depressed is, at present, uncertain but there is equivocal experimental evidence from animal studies(19) to suggest that different bile acids may have differing effects on the rate-limiting enzymes controlling cholesterol (HMG CoA reductase) and bile salt (cholesterol 7$\alpha$-hydroxylase) synthesis, but this is an area in which, for the moment, we have inadequate information in man.

Well, having dissolved our gallstones, what happens when treatment stops?  Does the bile revert to its supersaturated state, and if so, do gallstones re-form?


### EFFECTS OF WITHDRAWING CDCA

Figure 6 shows the bile lipid saturation indices before, during and not less than one month after stopping treatment.  The mean value of 1.56+ 0.05 before treatment fell to 0.86 ± 0.08 during therapy, but in almost every case, on withdrawing treatment the bile reverted to its supersaturated state.  It should be stressed, however, that supersaturated bile is not synonymous with gallstone formation, but to date two of our patients have had gallstone recurrence, while four recurrences have been recorded by the Mayo Group.  These disturbing results raise several important questions about the possible role of intermittent treatment and to see if this is feasible, Drs. Iser and Murphy in our Unit have been studying the problem.

### THE CHANGES IN BILE LIPIDS AND BILIARY BILE ACIDS
### AFTER STARTING AND STOPPING CDCA

In order to study the speed of improvement and persistence of effect of CDCA on bile lipids, gallstone patients were studied at frequent intervals during the first few weeks after either starting or stopping CDCA therapy(20).

Fasting bile-rich duodenal fluid was obtained from 6 patients with radiolucent gallstones starting CDCA therapy (13-15 mg.kg BW$^{-1}$day$^{-1}$) and from 6 other patients when treatment was stopped following gallstone dissolution after an average of 20 months' treatment. In both groups bile was collected on day 0 and approximately on days 4, 7, 14, 21, 28 and 35 after starting or stopping treatment respectively.

Before starting CDCA, all 6 patients had supersaturated bile (mean SI 1.49 $\pm$ SEM 0.17) but throughout the first month of therapy there was a variable pattern of response: in 3 patients bile became unsaturated within 4 days while in others it remained supersaturated for 3 weeks, but by 1 month all patients had unsaturated bile (mean 0.88 $\pm$ 0.10).

In the 6 patients whose treatment was stopped, the mean saturation index increased from 0.74 ($\pm$ SEM 0.10) during treatment to 1.17 $\pm$ 0.19 within 7 days and to 1.21 $\pm$ 0.17 by 3 weeks. These results, based on a small number of patients, suggest that, to maintain an unsaturated bile, it will be necessary to give continuous therapy and that intermittent treatment will probably not be adequate to dissolve stones.

To see if the change in SI was related to the proportion of CDCA in the biliary bile acids, the individual bile acid composition of each bile sample was measured by using thin layer chromatography, coupled with the 3$\alpha$- and 7$\alpha$-hydroxy steroid dehydrogenase enzyme reactions on non-solvolyzed material. In patients starting treatment, the proportion of CDCA increased from 27.7 $\pm$ 2.6% at Day 0, to 80.0 $\pm$ 6.5% within one month, while in patients whose stones had dissolved, the proportion of CDCA decreased from 71.7 $\pm$ 4.2 at Day 0 to 24.1 $\pm$ 3.5 within three weeks.

When the data from patients both starting and stopping treatment were considered together, there was a significant correlation between the percent CDCA and the SI ($y = 1.5 - 0.007\ x$, $n = 58$, $r = 0.49$, $t = 4.23$, $P < 0.001$). With few exceptions, bile was unsaturated in cholesterol when there was greater than 70% CDCA in the biliary bile acids.

## CONCLUSIONS

(i) <u>Summary.</u> We have seen that treatment should be confined to patients with radiolucent gallstones in functioning gallbladders, and that in these patients some 50-60% of radiolucent gallstones dissolve with chenodeoxycholic acid in a 6-24 month period, small stones usually showing evidence of dissolution within 1 year, although with larger stones, we may have to wait for two years or more before the response to treatment can be assessed. Both the bile lipid response to chenodeoxycholic acid and gallstone dissolution are related to the dose of chenodeoxycholic acid, based on body weight. A dose of 15 mg of chenodeoxycholic acid per kg body weight per day seems both effective and safe. However, because of the variable results in individual patients, we believe that the response of bile lipids to treatment should still be monitored with the aim of achieving a saturation index of not more than 0.8. Finally, continuous treatment seems to be necessary to maintain an unsaturated bile. However, there are many areas in which we remain ignorant.

(ii) <u>Future problems.</u> We know little about the bioavailability of different preparations of chenodeoxycholic acid and how this can be monitored. There is inadequate information about the suitability of "cheno" treatment in patients with stones in the biliary tree, and we know little about the precise intracellular mechanisms whereby chenodeoxycholic acid modifies cholesterol synthesis and secretion. If maintenance therapy is going to be necessary, we know nothing about the long-term effects of treatment carried on for more than three or four years, and since gallstones occur frequently in women of the child-bearing age group, we need to know something about the teratogenicity of this agent in man. We need further information about how often and when gallstones will recur after stopping treatment, and with this possibility in mind, we need to learn more about such alternative forms of treatment as ursodeoxycholic acid, which has recently been successfully used in Japan(21), the effects of bran-supplemented diets as advocated by the Bristol group(22) and the use of phospholipid precursors such as β-glycerophosphate, as advocated by Linscheer(23) and his colleagues.

## ACKNOWLEDGEMENTS

Dr. Iser is a Weddel Research Fellow. We are grateful to Messrs. Weddel Pharmaceuticals for their support, for supplies of CDCA. Some of the studies quoted include results obtained by our former colleagues, Drs. G.D. Bell and H.Y.I. Mok.

REFERENCES

1. Hofmann, A.F. (1970). Programme of the Fourteenth International Congress on the Biochemistry of Lipids, Lund,
Sweden, P.52 (Abstract).

2. Thistle, J.L. and Schoenfield, L.J. (1971). New Engl.J.Med.,
284: 177-181.

3. Thistle, J.L. and Schoenfield, L.J. (1971). Gastroenterology,
61: 488-496.

4. Danzinger, R.G., Hofmann, A.F., Thistle, J.L. and Schoenfield,
L.J. (1972). New Engl.J.Med., 286: 1-6.

5. Bell, G.D., Whitney, B. and Dowling, R.H. (1972). Lancet,
ii: 1213-1216.

6. Hofmann, A.F. and Paumgartner, G. (1975). Chenodeoxycholic
Acid Therapy of Gallstones,II. F.K. Schattauer Verlag,
Stuttgart, New York (in press).

7. Iser, J.H., Dowling, R.H., Mok, H.Y.I. and Bell, G.D. (1975).
New Engl.J.Med., 293: 378-383.

8. Thomas, P.J. and Hofmann, A.F. (1973). Gastroenterology, 65:
698-700.

9. Hegardt, F.G. and Dam, H. (1971). Z.Ernaehrungswiss., 10:
223-233.

10. Mok, H.Y.I., Bell, G.D. and Dowling, R.H. (1974). Lancet,
ii: 253-257.

11. Bell, G.D., Lewis, B., Petrie, A. and Dowling, R.H. (1973).
Brit.med.J. 3: 520-522.

12. Hoffman, N.E., Hofmann, A.F. and Thistle, J.L. (1974).
Mayo Clin.Proc. 49: 236-239.

13. Pedersen, L., Arnfred, T. and Thaysen, E.H. (1974).
Scand.J.Gastroenterol., 9: 787-791.

14. Bell, G.D., Mok, H.Y.I., Thwe, M., Murphy, G.M., Henry, K.
and Dowling, R.H. (1974). Gut, 15: 165-172.

15. Thistle, J.L. and Hofmann, A.F. (1973). New Engl.J.Med.,
289: 655-659.

16. Low-Beer, T.S. and Pomare, E.W. (1975).  Brit.med.J. 1: 438-440.

17. Northfield, T.C. and Hofmann, A.F. (1975).  Gut, 16: 12-17.

18. Adler, R.D., Bennion, L.J., Duane, W.C. and Grundy, S.M. (1975).  Gastroenterology, 66: 326-334.

19. Mosbach, E.H. (1972).  In "Bile Acids in Human Diseases", Ed. P.Back and W. Gerok, Pp. 89-96, F.K. Schattauer Verlag, Stuttgart, New York.

20. Iser, J.H., Murphy, G.M. and Dowling, R.H. (1975).  Gut, 16: (Abstract) (in press).

21. Makino, I. (1975).  Japanese Journal of Gastroenterology.

22. Pomare, E.W. and Heaton, K.W. (1973).  Brit.med.J. 4: 262-264.

23. Linscheer, W.G. and Raheja, K.L. (1974).  Lancet, ii: 551-553.

DISCUSSION OF COMMENTARY BY H. DOWLING

<u>Hofmann</u>:    There are two problems which Dr. Dowling and I are
thinking about.    One of them is whether we should monitor the
patients by measuring their biliary lipids to see if this might be
of some predictive value.    The second concerns dosage and gallstone response.    We have the problem of the prescribed dose, and
also the problem of compliance, because the patient may not take
what he is given.    These come under the heading of what I would
call "biological factors".    These factors give us the ingested
dose.    Then we have the second problem of bioavailability.    I
have neglected the question of drug purity, which is still a
problem which has not been perfectly sorted out yet.    One
preparation has a bioavailability of 100 per cent.    I am quite
sure about that.    But, to my knowledge, no other preparation has
been tested.    In <u>vitro</u> there are great differences in dissolution
kinetics with different preparations.    This gives us information
about the amount of the dose absorbed.    Then we come to the
problem of the desaturation response to produce unsaturated bile,
which is not linearly related to absorbed dose.    This is
particularly so in very obese patients who have a greater rate
of basal cholesterol secretion.    Then we have the problem of
dissolution kinetics which, <u>In vitro</u>, will vary according to the
bile acid:lecithin ratio because of interfacial barriers.    This
gives us the rate of cholesterol dissolution.    However, not all
of the cholesterol on the stone is available to the unsaturated
bile, because of calcium.    So we have the problem of accessibility
of cholesterol.    This will give us the rate of stone dissolution,
and also, as Dr. Dowling has shown, we have the problem of surface
to volume ratio being very different for large and small stones.
This, then gives us the X-ray response.

    Just to give an example of some of our data:    in one of our
patients treated for one year with (20 milligram per kilogram)
chenodeoxycholic acid, the gallstone is dissolving but the bile
is remaining saturated.    Obviously, in other patients, the bile
will become unsaturated but the gallstones do not dissolve because
they are not cholesterol stones.    With this problem of both
false "negatives" and false "positives", one wonders if we can
be very certain that we whould recomment "cholegrams" to correspond
to "haemograms" in all of our patients.    I think that we can say

that if 2 or 3 analyses show that bile remains very saturated during therapy, the gallstones are unlikely to dissolve. However, we need very much more information before we can come to a firm conclusion.

Ostrow:   I want to make a comment on the selection of patients based on the radio-opacity and radio-lucency of stones.   Our group has shown that a certain proportion of radio-lucent stones are actually pigment stones, and conversely, that some radio-opaque stones are cholesterol stones, although these tend to be rim opacities rather than diffuse opacity.   Have you had the chance to look at the patients who did not respond, and how many of these turned out to have non-cholesterol stones?

Dowling:   In our experience, about 20 per cent of radio-lucent stones are not predominantly of the cholesterol type, arbitrarily defined as containing less than 70 per cent of cholesterol.   So this is certainly a potential error.   Although we have not come up against this problem so far, I am sure it is only a matter of time before we do meet it.   We have to rely on radiology to indicate what type of gallstone we may be dealing with.   We have the combination of epidemiology, radiology and bile lipid analysis, with or without the presence of microcrystals, to work with.   By accumulating this information for a given patient, we can predict the sort of gallstone we are dealing with.   We plan to analyse the stones of patients who have been treated surgically.

Ostrow:   Have you tried to use duodenal drainage to look at micro-crystals to try to characterise the stones further, as an adjunct to the diagnostic approach?

Dowling:   Yes, we have, but we do not use this method routinely now.   In the early days we found cholesterol microcrystals in about 50 per cent of stones.   However, this method gives a high incidence of false positives and negatives.

Bouchier:   In a smaller sample than you have reported, we also find about the same percentage of patients responding to cheno-deoxycholic acid.   But in complete contrast to your data, we have not been able to use the saturation index in a predictive way.   Some patients show a trend, but others certainly dissolve their stones, but analysis of a spot sample of bile shows that the bile is still saturated.   A further point is that our initial optimism about treating stones in the common bile duct has not been sustained.   We have found that treating choledocolithiasis has led us into more trouble than it is worth.

Dowling:   Your point about bile saturation is related to what Dr. Hofmann said earlier: after all, how reliable can the analysis of

a spot sample of bile be?   We usually take samples after an overnight fast, and we know that this is the most pessimistic state
of bile lipid composition over a 24-hour period.   But it begs
the question of how reproducible this is in different patients
intubated on different days.   We think the results are reproducible in the individual case, and are closely representative of
the composition of gall-bladder bile.   I know that your data is
somewhat at variance with ours, but I have presented data as we
find it.   There is obviously a variation in saturation index
based simply on laboratory analysis of the bile lipid sample.   We
have calculated the maximum variation you can expect in the
saturation index given, say, a plus or minus 5 per cent variation
in the estimation of bile acids, phospholipids and cholesterol,
and given that the saturation is about 1.0.   In our hands, the
maximum variation is about 0.1 of a saturation index unit.   This
is very small, but it is enough to account for the very few false
negatives which we find in our responder group.

Fevery: With regard to biliary physiology, have you or Dr.
Hofmann looked at what happens to cholesterol output during cholic
acid treatment?

Hofmann: We have found that there is no change in cholesterol
secretion in gallstone patients when cholic acid is given over 6
weeks.   Also, deoxycholic acid causes no change in biliary
cholesterol secretion in normal subjects.

Fevery: Have you tried giving cholestyramine to patients with
diarrhoea?

Dowling: No, we have not.   I know that this has been suggested,
but it always concerns me a little bit that you are feeding bile
acids at one end and taking them out at the other end with
cholestyramine.   What we have done, occassionally, is to use
bowel-motility inhibitors such as codeine phosphate, and so on.
But this is very rarely necessary if you build up the dose of
chenodeoxycholate slowly.   We have had only one or two patients
who have been unable to tolerate the dose we use.

Paumgartner: It seems to me that there may be several reasons
why it is better to use a dose based on body weight.   One reason
may be is that obese patients excrete more cholesterol.   Now if
that is so, would it not be even better to give a dose based on
an estimate of the extent of "overweight"?

Dowling: Obese patients certainly secrete more cholesterol, and
it increases during a period of weight reduction.   This seems to
make these obese patients more vulnerable to gallstone formation.
We do not specifically ask our patients to try to lose weight or

to change their diet.    As for calculating the dose in terms of lean body mass or other criteria, I think that this would be too much of a refinement based on a rather crude clinical index.

Stiehl:   You yourself have shown that at higher doses of cheno-deoxycholate the serum transaminases are more elevated than when lower doses are used.   We have found a clear-cut correlation between serum chenodeoxycholate and transaminase levels.   It is my impression that the transaminase levels are raised by the chenodeoxycholate.

Dowling:   We have related peak transaminase levels to dose in absolute terms and we accept that there is such a relationship, but now that we have studied more patients we find that there is a plateau effect.   The changes in serum transaminases we observe are modest, and we have not found any histological changes in the liver to relate to this.   So I do not think we are concerned with a great deal of hepatotoxicity here.

Mayer:    I want to comment on the supposed mechanism for the dissolution of gallstones by chenodeoxycholic acid, because I am not very convinced by the theory.   In experiments with that bile acid we find that cholesterol $7\alpha$-hydroxylase is inhibited, but cholic acid also inhibits the enzyme.

Dowling:   I agree that the data in animals is conflicting, but as I understand it, we have no precise way of knowing whether the cholesterol which has been synthesized is destined for excretion into bile rather than for utilisation in other ways. We must keep an entirely open mind about the intracellular mechanisms involved.

Borgström:   There are indications that eating highly unsaturated fats will increase the biliary excretion of cholesterol and so increase the incidence of gallstones.   Have you taken into consideration the amounts of saturated or unsaturated fatty acids in the diets of your patients?   Might it help if you fed them on a diet containing more saturated fat?

Dowling:   No, we do not take this into account.

Dam:   First I would like to ask a technical question.   On how many samples or how many determinations are your figures based?

Dowling:   The patient is intubated after an overnight fast, and we take between 3 and 5 samples of 2-5 ml of bile-rich duodenal fluid.   We then select the two which are most concentrated on the basis of the degree of pigmentation.   So anything from one to three samples are analysed at any one time for bile lipid composition.

<u>Dam</u>:    Yes, that is, say, 3 analyses on virtually the same sample
of bile; but how many times is bile collected?

<u>Dowling</u>:    We have tried to validate this single intubation method
by intubating the same individual on different days, sometimes 8
or 9 times.    But, in general, these results are based on single
intubations.

<u>Dam</u>:    But it is well known that the values can change very much
without any treatment.

<u>Dowling</u>:    I have said that we validated the method by multiple
intubations.    There are minor variations in the position of the
point on the triangular co-ordinate phase diagram.    However, in
our experience, the molar ratio of cholesterol changes very little
in the same individual from day to day.

<u>Dam</u>:    The early publications from the Mayo Clinic showed that
quite large variations can occur.

<u>Dowling</u>:    All I can say is that this can occur, and one has to
be aware that this is a potential weakness of the single intubation
method.

<u>Popjak</u>:    My question is related to that asked by Professor
Borgström.    It is well known that people taking Atromid appear
to excrete more cholesterol in the bile, and many, in fact,
eventually develop gallstones.    Do you think it would be a good
idea to give chenodeoxycholic acid to patients being treated with
Atromid?

<u>Dowling</u>:    In fact, the highest cholesterol value we have ever
found was from a patient taking Clofibrate, and I think that there
is no doubt that this drug increases biliary cholesterol output
and produces a supersaturated bile.    I think what you have
suggested may already be on trial in such patients, and also in
obese patients who are losing weight.

<u>Boyer</u>:    With regard to hepatotoxicity, your results certainly are
encouraging.    However, bearing in mind the severe lesion which
the Rhesus monkey develops after chenodeoxycholate treatment, and
the fact that this monkey sulphates lithocholate very poorly, I
wonder if anyone has tried to correlate the percentage of lithocholate sulphate in bile with elevation in serum transaminase.
My reason for asking this is that we may find subgroups in the
population who have poor sulphation capacity, and these people
would be more prone to the hepatotoxic effects of lithocholate.

<u>Dowling</u>:    We have not studied this.

<u>Hofmann</u>:    We have measured serum sulphated and nonsulphated lithocholate by two usually specific radioimmuno-assay methods. Generally, there is a threefold increase in total lithocholate in fasting specimens of patients taking chenodeoxycholate. However, the percentage sulphated remains constant and there is no correlation between nonsulphated lithocholate and serum transaminase in our patients.

<u>Preisig</u>:    Dr. Dowling, if you were a member of a Drug Registration Board, would you issue this drug for clinical trials or would you even register it?

<u>Dowling</u>:    I was going to say thank you, but I can hardly thank you for a difficult question like that.    This is a philosophical question and I can only express a personal opinion.    At this stage, treatment ought to be confined to those centres which have the facilities for careful monitoring of the patients.    Yes, we should continue the studies, but caution is needed.

# GENERAL DISCUSSION OF SESSION 4A

<u>Haslewood</u>:   Shortly before this Institute began, I finished
making the 3-sulphates of the three common bile acids:   cholic,
chenodeoxycholic and deoxycholic.   It can be calculated that 39
sulphates of these common bile acids and their taurine and glycine
conjugates are possible.   As far as I know, the detailed chemistry
of these compounds is unknown.   Those working with sulphated bile
acids are working on a very insecure basis of chemistry.   I now
have crystalline samples of the disodium salts of these acids
available, and I should be delighted to present samples of these
to people who would like them.   These sulphates can easily be
made by protecting the free hydroxyl groups and removing the
protecting groups without affecting the sulphate group.   Therefore,
the sulphates can be obtained in high yield:   that from chenodeoxycholic acid is particularly easy to make and to crystallize as the
disodium salt.   I must tell you three very important things about
them.   First of all, they are less polar in thin-layer chromatography systems than the corresponding taurine conjugates.   The
difference is about the same as the difference produced by one
hydroxyl group in the molecule.   Secondly, the chenodeoxycholate
and cholate 3-sulphates, which have a free 7α-hydroxyl group, do
not react with the 7α-hydroxysteroid dehydrogenase.   Of course,
they do not react with the 3α-hydroxysteroid dehydrogenase either,
so their estimation by enzymatic methods creates a problem.   The
third, and most important point, is that the sulphate group comes
off very readily;   much more readily than in the many compounds
which have the sulphate group on the side chain.   I do not know
if this has anything to do with the 5β-configuration.   So you
have to be very careful not to lose the sulphate group.   However,
worse than that, I have not succeeded, even with very mild methods,
in solvolysing any of these sulphates without producing a large
number of artefacts.   In many instances, the corresponding bile
acid becomes a <u>minor</u> constituent.   Therefore, we need to be very
careful about drawing any biological conclusions about bile acid
sulphates without a lot more fundamental chemistry.

<u>Sjövall</u>:   Those were very wise words.   There is probably much
more to be learned about the biological role of bile acid sulphates
when we have good methods to study them.   I have some data on bile
acid sulphates to present.   We are interested in the effects of

steroid hormones on liver function, and decided to study changes
in biliary and urinary bile acids.   When we came to study these,
we found it was a very difficult problem.   When Dr. Taylor was
working with us for one year, we never got nearer than making an
attempt to analyse rat bile.   These are some of the results we
obtained.   Let us look at the taurine conjugates and monosulphates
in the fraction obtained in the first 12 hours after making the
bile fistula.   There is a marked sex difference in the sulphate
fraction, which is much more prominent in the female rat.
Quantitatively, it is a small fraction of the whole, but it
contains some interesting bile acids.   For example in the monosulphate fraction of male rat bile deoxycholic acid,and the 3β-
isomer of allodeoxycholic acid, which has not been described
before in this situation, are the two major components.   In the
bile of female rats allodeoxycholic, allochenodeoxycholic,
deoxycholic and chenodeoxycholic acids and the 3β-isomer of
allodeoxycholic acid are present.   Note that most of these are
allo bile acids.   Cholic and allocholic acids are also present.
We also found, but have not identified, unsaturated analogues of
the muricholic acids.

     If bile is collected for a further period the unsaturated
muricholate analogues disappear after 48 hours in the male rat.
In female rat bile, but not in male rat bile, allochenodeoxycholic
acid increases.   In the monosulphate fraction there are peaks
corresponding to allocholic, cholic, allochenodeoxycholic and
chenodeoxycholic acids.   That seems reasonable until you look
at the mass spectra and find that the cholic acid is not quite
cholic acid and the chenodeoxycholic is not quite chenodeoxycholic.
When these are oxidised, 80 per cent or more are allo bile acids.
So what appeared to be cholic acid was, presumably, the 3β-isomer
of allocholic acid;   and what seemed to be chenodeoxycholic acid
was the 3β-isomer of allochenodeoxycholic acid.

     This shows the complexity of bile acids in bile, but what is
really interesting is that allochenodeoxycholic acid is a prominent
compound in the female rat.   However, allocholic acid is found in
bile from both male and female rats.   This suggests that the allo
acids may be formed in different ways.

     The presence of so much allochenodeoxycholic acid in the
female rat may be related to the well-known sex difference in the
metabolism of steroids in the rat.

     Now let us look at the glycine-conjugated, nonsulphated bile
acids from human urine.   Here, of course, the picture is entirely
different.   One of the more common bile acids in human urine is
hyocholic acid;   allocholic acid also is always found.   A number
of tetrahydroxy bile acids have been found in human urine, and we

think that two of these have a 1-hydroxy group, but the synthesis of these is difficult.

Hofmann:   Things may not be so complex as you make them appear. We have been looking at the bile acids in bile of patients before and during chenodeoxycholic acid treatment.   It is my impression that about 97 per cent of the bile acids can be accounted for by known and expected compounds.   We have found about 25 bile acids so far, but these are present only in trace amounts.   Does that satisfy you?

Sjövall:   No, not if you analyse a variety of patients, some of whom produce considerable amounts of bile acids which have not yet been identified.

Hofmann:   What kind of patients were they?

Sjövall:   Intrahepatic cholestasis, cirrhotics, and so on.

Hofmann:   I agree with you that the problem really becomes complex in these cases.

Elliott:   Professor Sjövall, do you think that those 3β-allo compounds might be metabolites of cholestanol?

Sjövall:   Of course, direct side-chain cleavage could give rise to 3β-hydroxy-5-cholenoic acids or 7α-hydroxylated acids of that type.   For example, if one gives a 3-keto-delta-4 bile acid to the female rat, she will reduce this mainly to 5α-acids.

Danielsson:   Just a comment to Dr. Hofmann;   one can find conditions where there are a lot of peculiar bile acids.   Professor Sjövall mentioned an unsaturated muri-acid in rat bile.   In our work on biliary obstruction we found that this acid started to account for a sizeable amount of the bile acids produced by the rat after a day of biliary obstruction.   By a rough calculation this amounted to 10 per cent of the total bile acids.   What I am implying is that one has to bear in mind that in pathological conditions a variety of unusual bile acids may be produced.

Paumgartner:   Professor Sjövall, do you think that when using g.l.c. methods to study bile acids in patients it would not be wise to use hyodeoxycholic acid as an internal standard, since we and others do in fact do this?

Sjövall:   It would depend on what type of column you use.   I was showing chromatograms obtained with the polyester HiEff8BP and TMS-derivatives.   The closest compound to the hyodeoxycholic is this unsaturated acid I mentioned.   Of course hyodeoxycholic

is an unusual bile acid in man, but even β-muricholic has been
detected in human patients, so I suppose almost any bile acid
could occur in particular diseases.    Therefore it is necessary
to watch out for this.

Palmer:    I would like to follow up what Professor Haslewood said
about the artefacts which may be formed when solvolysing the
sulphate group.    When we studied the metabolism of lithocholate,
about 10-12 per cent of the total metabolites of this acid were
accounted for by an unsaturated compound.    I now think that this
is a metabolite of lithocholate produced by intestinal microorganisms.    If this kind of reaction does occur so readily with
sulphated compounds, I would be interested to know what kind of
artefacts may be formed in your isolation procedure.

Sjövall:    One can never guarantee against artefact formation.
The sort of compounds I have been talking about occur in different
fractions under different conditions, and they have not all been
treated in the same way.    Nevertheless, something happening in
a sulphate fraction could be an artefact.    However, I do not
think that the unsaturated acid I mentioned is an artefact of, say,
cholic or hyocholic acids.    If it were, you would expect to find
it every time you find the saturated acids, but this is not what
happens.    Of course, it could have an unknown precursor and so be
a secondary artefact.

Haslewood:    I wonder if it is appreciated just how easily these
sulphates are solvolysed.    They are more readily solvolysed than
the steroid sulphates.    Artefacts in high yield are formed even
by treatment with ammonium chloride in acetone at room temperature.

Sjövall:    Perhaps we ought to do experiments in vivo with labelled
urinary bile acids to see where they are.    Even so, when we analyse
urine we find that the monohydroxy acids are always in the sulphate
fraction.    So those at least are not solvolysed during our working
up procedure.

Low-Beer:    Does anyone know if sulphates are ever found in faeces?
This might be important for people using the dehydrogenase-enzyme
technique for analysing faecal bile acids.

Sjövall:    The steroids and sterols are hydrolysed by intestinal
bacteria, so one finds very little sulphated compounds of this
type in faeces.

Palmer:    We have tried several times to assay faecal homogenates
with the 3α-steroid dehydrogenase enzyme.    In the few patients
we have looked at, the yield can be increased 10-15 per cent by
doing a solvolysis first.    I take this to mean that small amounts

of sulphates are present.    When we gave glycolithocholate
sulphate to a rat, wo did find that some of the sulphate escaped
desulphation and could be found in the faeces.

Strandvik:    In infants with intrahepatic cholestasis we have
found lots of sulphates in the urine.    In some cases we have
done duodenal intubations, and we have found no sulphates in these
samples.

Hofmann:    I want to mention some experiments which show the
striking difference in properties of normal and allo bile acids.
That is the way they pack together with straight-chain lipids.
It has been known for many years that soaps have a critical
solution temperature above which they go into solution.    For
instance, sodium stearate goes into solution at about 80$^{\circ}$C, and
sodium octanoate at 15$^{\circ}$C.    If you make a one-to-one mixture of
these two, this goes into solution in between 15$^{\circ}$ and 80$^{\circ}$;    that
is about 50$^{\circ}$C.    Now if you mix sodium stearate either with
taurodeoxycholate or tauroallodeoxycholate, the difference in a
one-to-one mixture in terms of solution temperature is about 60$^{\circ}$C.
The stearate-tauroallodeoxycholate goes into solution at about
80$^{\circ}$C, whereas the stearate:taurodeoxycholate goes into solution
at about 20$^{\circ}$C.    So there is an enormous disordering effect of
the 5$\beta$-bile acid.

Taylor:    I have some data on bile acid sulphates which I present
with some hesitation after Professor Haslewood's comments.    I
have been studying bile acids in gall bladder bile of cats.    The
nonsulphated bile acids are not particularly unusual, except that
there is a sex difference in the total amounts of these acids in
the bile.    There is quite a lot of allocholic acid in this
fraction, presumably derived from cholestanol in the diet.    It
is interesting that allodeoxycholate, which is not present in the
nonsulphated fraction, is a prominent component of the sulphate
fraction.    Also, lithocholate, which was not present in the nonsulphate fraction, is present in the sulphate fraction.    There
are many other substances in the sulphate fraction in small amounts
which are not present in the nonsulphate fraction.    As in the rat,
as Professor Sjövall described, most of these sulphated compounds
are allo bile acids.    However the sex difference in the sulphate
fraction is the reverse of what we found in rats.    Male cat bile
has about 2.5 per cent of the total bile acids as sulphates,
whereas in female bile the sulphates account for only about 0.1
per cent.    It seems to me from these results that a system (or
systems) exists which can recognise that certain bile acids are
"abnormal", and these are sulphated under normal conditions.
When a cholestatic condition occurs the sulphating system becomes
saturated with bile acids, and the "normal" bile acids are also
sulphated to facilitate their excretion in urine.

# Bile Acids and Lipids II

# THE ENTEROHEPATIC CIRCULATION OF BILE ACIDS IN MAN

Alan F. Hofmann

Gastroenterology Unit, Mayo Clinic and Mayo Foundation

Rochester, Minnesota 55901, U.S.A.

## Abstract

Steady-state and dynamic descriptions of the enterohepatic circulation of bile acids in healthy man are given. Methods for characterizing the enterohepatic circulation of bile acids in health and disease are summarized.

## Introduction

Since the first NATO Advanced Study Institute on the Biliary System, substantial advances in our understanding of the enterohepatic circulation of bile acids in man have occurred. The major reasons for these advances may be summarized as follows: 1) development of improved analytical methods especially chromatography and radioimmunoassay; 2) commercial availability of labeled bile acids; 3) development of intestinal perfusion methodology permitting secretion into and absorption from the human intestine to be quantified; and 4) increasing awareness of the importance of bile acid metabolism in human disease leading to increased funding and research activity.

The enterohepatic circulation can now be conceptualized as an oscillating flux of detergent molecules, anatomically constrained by two chemical pumps--the liver and the terminal ileum. During fasting most of the bile acids are stored in the gallbladder; during digestion, most of the bile acids are secreted in the intestinal lumen. The mass present in portal blood or the liver parenchyma is always extremely small. Bile acids have multiple physiological actions: they induce the secretion of biliary lipids and solubilize them in mixed micelles; in the

517

intestinal lumen they solubilize the products of fat digestion
and fat-soluble vitamins, accelerating their diffusion through
the unstirred layer.  Bile acids also induce the secretion of
electrolytes and water from the small and large intestine.
The physiological significance of this effect in health is
unclear, but clinical syndromes of bile acid malabsorption, high
concentrations of bile acids, have been shown to be responsible
for diarrhea.


## Steady-state Description:  Steroid Moiety

Isotope dilution, as proposed and implemented by Lindstedt,
is the technique par excellence for the steady-state description
of the enterohepatic circulation.  The major bile acids, cholic
and chenodeoxycholic acids, and the major secondary bile acids,
deoxycholic and lithocholic acids, all exhibit first order
kinetics.  Using the isotope dilution technique, cholic acid
synthesis is about 400-600 mg/day (10 umoles/kg/day) and
chenodeoxycholic (chenic) acid synthesis is less--about 200-300
mg/day (5 umoles/kg/day).  (These values are higher than estimates based on gas chromatographic measurements of fecal bile
acids for unknown reasons.)  Since pool sizes of cholic acid and
chenic acid are similar, the lower synthesis rate of chenic acid
indicates a lower fractional turnover rate; this is most simply
explained by more efficient intestinal conservation of chenic
acid, which in turn is probably explained by considerable passive
jejunal absorption of chenylglycine.  When the isotope dilution
technique is applied to the secondary acids, one obtains a
figure for "input" which is the amount of newly formed secondary
bile acid entering the exchangeable bile acid pool daily.  Using
the isotope dilution technique, one finds that the input of
deoxycholic and lithocholic acid is about one-third to one-half
of the cholic and chenic acid synthesis respectively.  Therefore
if dehydroxylation of primary bile acids entering the colon is
complete, about one-third to one-half of the secondary bile
acids formed there are reabsorbed.  Accordingly, one can make a
simple compartmental model of the enterohepatic circulation of
the major primary bile acids (Fig. I).  One may define a simple
term $f_{dehydrox}$ which is equal to the input of a secondary
acid/synthesis of its primary bile acid precursor.  One can see
that $f_{dehydrox}$ for cholic and deoxycholic acid is equal to
$k_{43} \cdot chl/k_{31} \cdot chol$.

In the above model, the compartments represent the exchangeable steroid moiety, i.e. all the chemical species in isotopic
equilibrium for a given steroid moiety.  For cholate, for
example, most of the label will be present as the two conjugates
cholyltaurine and cholylglycine.  In the conventional Lindstedt
procedure, the bile acids are deconjugated before determination

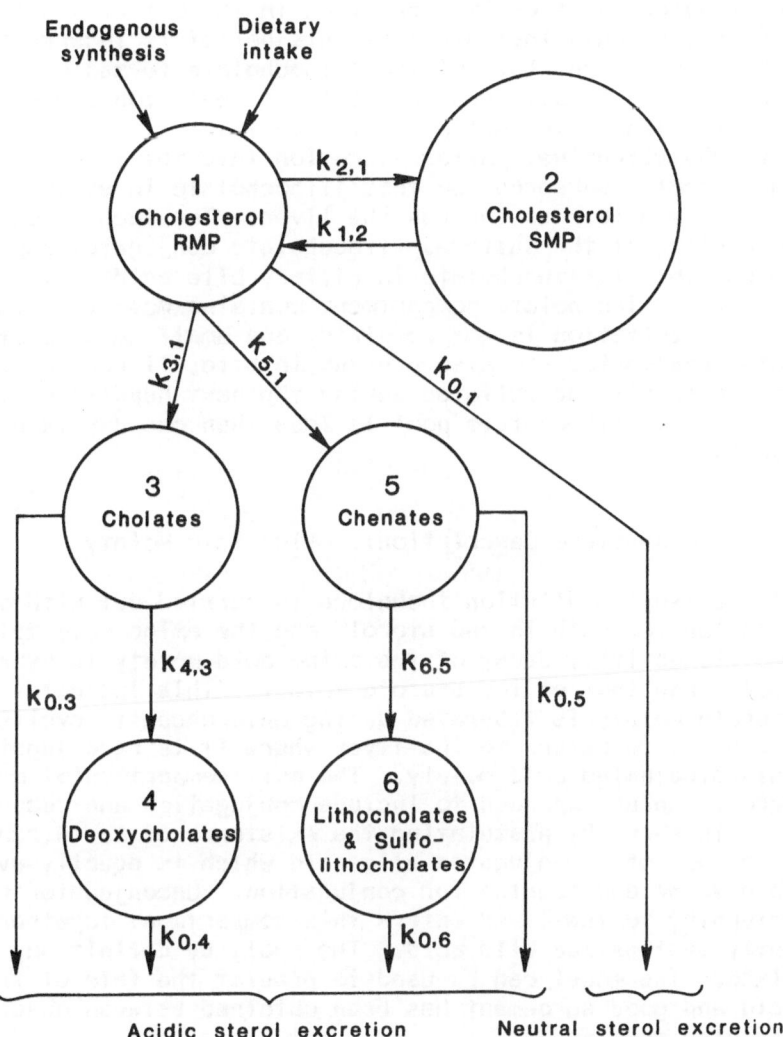

Fig. 1. Compartmental Model of Cholesterol and Bile Acid
Metabolism in Man

of specific activity so that the specific activity figure obtained
is actually a weighted average.

Because lithocholate is a minor constituent of biliary bile
acids, it has been assumed for some years that little lithocholate is absorbed after its formation in the colon. Isotope
dilution measurements indicate that this belief is incorrect.
About one-third to one-half of the lithocholate formed daily is
absorbed. During hepatic passage it is not only conjugated but
also mostly sulfated to form sulfolithocholylglycine and
sulfolithocholyltaurine. After secretion into the intestine,
these are poorly reabsorbed so that lithocholate in essence
makes only a single pass through the liver. The lack of enterohepatic cycling of the sulfated lithocholate conjugates explains
the low portion of lithocholate in biliary bile acids. In
Figure I, the lithocholate compartment contains mostly sulfated
conjugates. Sulfation is not complete, and small amounts of
unsulfated conjugates are also present in bile; if reabsorbed,
however, these will be sulfated during the next hepatic passage.
The $T_1/2$ of the lithocholate pool is less than one day in healthy
individuals.

## Steady-state Description: Amino Acid Moiety

If the isotope dilution technique is carried out with a
bile acid labeled both in the steroid and the amino acid moiety,
the specific activity decay of the amino acid moiety is usually
more rapid than that of the steroid moiety. This indicates that
some steroid moiety is liberated during enterohepatic cycling
and reabsorbed to return to the liver where it is reconjugated
with unlabeled amino acid moiety. The multicompartmental model
of Figure I can be expanded to include conjugation and reconjugation as is shown by postulating the existence of an intrahepatic
precursor pool of unconjugated bile acid which is equally available
to both glycine and taurine for conjugation. Unconjugated bile
acid returning to the liver enters this compartment together
with newly synthesized bile acid. The pool, by definition, is
well mixed. The model can be used to predict the fate of tracer
bile acid and good agreement has been obtained between observed
and predicted results.

Since the secondary bile acids are derived from primary
bile acids and are thought to enter the bile acid pool as the
unconjugated secondary bile acid, the model may be expanded
still further. Finally, for lithocholate, the sulfation biotransformation step may also be added. Thus, the complete
enterohepatic circulation of the steroid and amino acid moieties
of the major primary and secondary bile acids may be rationalized;
the model encompasses conjugation, deconjugation, and reconjugation.

It also includes sulfation, desulfation, and resulfation. Dehydroxylation is shown and rehydroxylation can be programmed easily. This model is useful conceptually but whether it will have practical value remains to be seen.

The fate of the amino acid moieties, glycine and taurine, have also been defined. Both are degraded completely to $CO_2$ and $NH_3$ and taurine is degraded to $SO_4^=$ in addition. The $CO_2$ is excreted in breath; the ammonia is absorbed to be converted to urea; and the sulfate is excreted in urine. Little of the amino acid moiety or its degradation products are lost by the fecal route.

## Dynamic Description

Secretion studies have confirmed the cyclical discharge of bile acids into the intestine with meal. During overnight fasting there is also a continuing secretion of bile acids into the intestine. Secretion studies have shown that bile acid secretion cannot be predicted from pool size measurements since there is a reciprocal relationship between pool size and recycling frequency. Secretion studies have also given information on phospholipid and cholesterol coupling to bile acid secretion. In man as in the primate, bile is supersaturated at low bile acid output rates. Patients ingesting chenic acid have been shown to secrete less cholesterol for a given rate of bile acid secretion than patients ingesting cholic acid or deoxycholic acid, providing a rationale for chenic acid therapy of cholesterol gallstones.

The site of absorption of individual bile acid conjugates has not been quantified as yet.

Using radioimmunoassay, there is a four- to eightfold increase in bile acid levels in peripheral blood after meals. Several lines of evidence suggest that this is related to spillover of absorbed bile acid. The fractional hepatic clearance remains constant--probably about 90% for cholyl conjugates and perhaps 70% for chenyl conjugates--during digestion, but with a greater load to the liver the absolute spillover is greater. Gas/liquid chromatography and radioimmunoassay analyses agree that the pattern of fasting-state serum bile acids is not identical to that of fasting-state biliary bile acids. Serum bile acids are relatively richer in chenyl conjugates which is probably attributable to more proximal absorption of these acids as well as their less efficient hepatic clearance.

Methodology for Characterizing the Enterohepatic Circulation

Hepatic uptake may be quantified by measuring the plasma disappearance of intravenously injected bile acids. Sufficient mass may be injected to follow plasma disappearance by chemical or immunochemical means; alternatively, a tracer dose may be used. The plasma disappearance rate of considerable mass (up to 10 umoles/kg) and tracer are identical in healthy subjects probably because the $V_{max}$ for hepatic uptake of bile acids is so vast. To date, delayed plasma disappearance of injected cholyl-glycine appears to be a very sensitive indicator of liver disease.

For quantifying hepatic secretion of bile acids into the intestine, marker perfusion techniques have been developed and partly validated. In the Mayo method, biliary lipid secretion is measured in response to 3 meals and an overnight fast. The method features a recovery marker and absorbable markers (labeled lecithin and cholesterol) to correct for absorption of secreted biliary lipids in the mixing segment. In the Grundy method, secretion is measured during steady-state digestion which is ob-tained by the continuous infusion of a liquid meal. Both methods give the proportionality constant for lecithin/bile acid and cholesterol/bile acid coupling, but the Mayo method gives measure-ments for a great range of bile acid outputs, whereas the Grundy method gives repeated estimates of lecithin and cholesterol output for only a single bile acid output.

For defining the overall efficiency of bile acid absorption, a variety of methods are available, some of which appear clinically useful. One may infer bile acid malabsorption by finding increased bile acid synthesis, which can be assessed by chemical measurement of fecal bile acids or by the isotope dilution technique. One may also show bile acid malabsorption by demonstrating increased fecal loss of a labeled bile acid; the specificity of the test is increased if a non-absorbable marker is administered simultaneously and the ratio of bile acid label to marker is defined. If a conjugated bile acid labeled in the amino acid moiety is given, one may demonstrate increased loss of the label in the feces or alternatively $^{14}CO_2$ may be assessed in breath using a simple technique for interval $^{14}CO_2$ specific activity measurements. Lastly, in patients with bile acid malabsorption, fasting-state levels of bile acids are lower than in health and the postprandial increase falls progressively during the day so that there is virtually no postprandial increase of bile acids after an evening meal.

## Bacterial Events

Increased deconjugation may be demonstrated by chromatography of small intestinal content or quantified by measuring the simultaneous turnover rate of the amino acid and steroid moiety of a conjugated bile acid such as cholylglycine. The simplest method for detecting increased bile acid deconjugation is to administer cholylglycine labeled in the carboxyl carbon of the glycine moiety and measure expiration of $^{14}CO_2$ in breath. Increased bile acid deconjugation means increased exposure of the bile acid pool to bacteria which in turn indicates bacterial proliferation in the small intestine or bile acid malabsorption or both.

The degree of dehydroxylation of colonic contents is assessed by gas/liquid chromatography. For unequivocal structural identification in feces or bile, mass spectrometry is mandatory. Increased input of secondary bile acids into the enterohepatic circulation can be inferred from biliary bile acid composition but only proved by measuring the input using isotope dilution. Ideally, one should determine simultaneously the input rates for both the primary and secondary bile acid of a given bile acid pair.

Certain bile acid measurments do not indicate any particular component of the enterohepatic circulation, but the results of both hepatic and intestinal events. Such measurements we have termed enterohepatic qualities. The most obvious of these is fasting-state serum bile acids which represent the balance between intestinal absorption and hepatic uptake. Biliary bile acid composition reflects the net interaction of hepatic synthesis of primary bile acids, input of secondary bile acids, intestinal conservation and in some instances further hepatic modification of secondary bile acids. The amino acid composition of biliary bile acids also reflects the interaction of hepatic conjugation and bacterial deconjugation.

## Perturbations of the Enterohepatic Circulation

The major perturbations of the enterohepatic circulation in man may be classified as follows: (See Table). A new disease has recently been identified. Chenic acid feeding to the non-human primate induces portal tract fibrosis which is caused by accumulation of lithocholate in the enterohepatic circulation. These species do not eliminate lithocholate rapidly like man since they are unable to sulfate it in the liver. Individuals with impaired sulfation have not as yet been identified.

Table 1.  Some Diseases of the Enterohepatic Circulation

| Disease | Pathogenesis | Consequence | Adaptive Mechanism | Diagnosis | Therapy |
|---|---|---|---|---|---|
| Cholestasis | Impaired hepatic transport; intra- or extrahepatic obstruction | Cholemia; pruritus | Bile acid sulfation; urinary excretion of bile acids as sulfates | Liver function tests; intravenous or retrograde cholangiography | Phenobarbital, cholestyramine Surgery |
| Cholesterol cholelithiasis | Relative excess of cholesterol secretion → Supersaturated bile in the gallbladder; nucleation; crystal retention | Cholecystitis | Increased recycling of bile acid pool in some patients | Cholecystography | Chenic acid Cholecystectomy |
| Stagnant loop syndrome | Intestinal stasis → Bacterial proliferation → Increased bile acid deconjugation → Bile acid precipitation | Decreased bile acid concentration Fat maldigestion Steatorrhea | Absorption of fat over larger anatomical area | Quantitative culture Breath test for bile acid deconjugation | Antibiotics Corrective surgery |
| Bile acid diarrhea | Ileal dysfunction → Bile acid malabsorption → Increased concentration of bile acids in colon → Decreased bacterial dehydroxylation → Increased concentration of chenic acid in solution | Induced secretion of electrolytes in water Diarrhea | Increased bile acid synthesis Absorption of fat over larger anatomical area | Balance studies Isotope dilution Excretion of labeled bile acids Breath test for bile acid deconjugation Postprandial serum bile acids | Cholestyramine |

## Conclusions

During the past five years, most of the components of the enterohepatic circulation of bile acids have been measured in healthy man. The challenge for the next ten years is to describe the enterohepatic circulation in disease and to determine whether such measurements provide important clinical information regarding diagnosis or therapy.

## References

Hofmann AF. _In_ Advances Internal Medicine, edited by G. Stollerman. Yearbook Publishers (in press)

Quarfordt SH and Greenfield MF. Estimation of cholesterol and bile acid turnover by kinetic analysis. J Clin Invest 52:1937, 1973.

Lindstedt S. The turnover of cholic acid in man: Bile Acids and Steroids 51. Acta Physiol Scand 40:1, 1953.

Vlahcevic ZR, Miller JR, Farrar JT, et al. Kinetics and pool size of primary bile acids in man. Gastroenterology 61:85, 1971.

Hoffman NE and Hofmann AF. Metabolism of steroid and amino acid moieties of conjugated bile acids in man. IV. Description of a multicompartmental model. Gastroenterology 67:887, 1974.

DISCUSSION OF LECTURE BY A.F. HOFMANN

Low-Beer:    You mentioned that there is disagreement about the
effects of deoxycholic acid, but I do not think that there is any
disagreement at all.    You were trying to compare pharmacological
effects between chenodeoxycholate and deoxycholate.    Our results
were obtained with very much smaller doses, where the total amount
of bile salt returning to the liver was probably not very
different.    Therefore, the smaller dose was probably much better
for uncovering a selective effect on cholesterol synthesis which
might not be evident at much larger doses.    Do you agree that
this is a possibility?

Hofmann:    I agree with your statement of the facts, but, as yet,
we have never seen any specificity in the feed-back inhibition.
My own belief is that there are still problems with the isotope-
dilution technique, and I will be happy only when we have repeated
our experiments with doses such as you have used.    We also need
to use sterol balance techniques.    All we can say at this moment
is that you and I have done different types of experiments and
have obtained different results.    The great problem is that
experimentation with human subjects involves a small number of
subjects and we have difficulty in showing a statistically
significant effect which may not be real, or missing an effect
because the number of observations is so small.

Popjak:    I think that your speculation about the possible
suppression of cholesterol biosynthesis by bile acids is incorrect.
It has been conclusively shown that increased cholesterol biosynthesis in bile fistula animals can be suppressed exclusively
by the reinjection of the cholesterol lost from the bile, but not
by purified bile acids.

Hofmann:    I am aware of that work, but I think there are other
experiments which could be interpreted in an alternative way.
In some of those experiments inadequate amounts of bile acids were
used.    In my opinion, this is still an open question.    For
example, patients with very small ileal resections and without
steatorrhoea, in whom there should be normal cholesterol absorption, show a marked increase in bile acid synthesis.

Popjak:    May I make a further point which concerns your nomenclature.    The term cholyl glycine may suggest to the uninitiated
that one of the hydroxyl groups of cholic acid is esterified with
glycine.    The suffix '-yl' in chemistry usually refers to an
alcohol which has a group esterified with an acid.    After all,
an amide linkage is present in the conjugated bile acid.    Could
you not call it a cholic amide?

Hofmann:    We say glycyl glycine, and an amide linkage is involved
in this and other peptides.

Taylor:    In all the discussions we have had so far, the lymphatic
system has not been mentioned.    This system may not be important
in normal subjects, but probably does play an important role in
patients with cholestasis.    When you talk about bile acids in
the blood compartment, do you include the whole lymphatic system
as part of the blood compartment?

Hofmann:    It is my belief that the intestinal lymphatic transport
is determined by the partition coefficient between the portal
blood and the chylomicron, and, of course, bile acids would have
a negligible partition coefficient.    There is experimental
evidence that in liver disease there is an increased concentration
of bile acids both in hepatic and intestinal lymph, reflecting,
presumably, albumin-bound bile acids.    I think that this is
partly artefactual, but certainly it is part of the enterohepatic
circulation.

# BILE PHOSPHOLIPIDS : ORIGIN AND FUNCTION

J.C. HAUTON

Lipid-Transport Research Group (INSERM-U130)
46 Chemin de la Gaye, 13009 Marseille, France

Hepatic bile is an aqueous medium containing, under normal conditions, 2-4 g of total solids per 100 ml. The main components are bile salts, phospholipids, cholesterol and electrolytes, with smaller amounts of bile pigments and proteins. The concentration of lipids in bile varies during the day, and wide species differences have also been reported. The gall bladder concentrates hepatic bile by reabsorbing sodium chloride and water in isotonic proportions (1). This process accounts for most of the differences between hepatic and gall bladder bile.

## Phospholipids in normal and infected bile

The concentration of phospholipids in human hepatic bile varies between 0.2-0.8 g per 100 ml. but the molar ratio of 3 between bile salts and phospholipids is usually maintained. The major bile phospholipids are phosphatidyl cholines (lecithins) (2-5), but small amounts of lysophosphatidyl cholines, phosphatidyl ethanolamines and traces of sphingomyelins are also present (6-8). We have studied the phospholipids in 6 samples of human gall-bladder bile using high pressure liquid chromatography with silicic acid columns (8). The results are shown in Table 1.

Table 1:  Phospholipids in human gall-bladder bile

The constituents are given as a percentage of the total biliary phospholipids (mean ±)

| | |
|---|---|
| Phosphatidyl cholines | 96.1 ± 0.6 |
| Lysophosphatidyl cholines | 3.0 ± 0.8 |
| Phosphatidyl ethanolamines | 0.8 ± 0.3 |

Only traces of other phospholipids, but no phosphatidic acids were found.

Since little information is available about phospho-derivatives in bile, we have investigated total bile phosphorus, and lipid and non-lipid phosphorus, using an automatic procedure which permits rapid determination of free orthophosphate in biological fluids (9). Data using this method on fresh, aseptic hepatic file from different species have been presented elsewhere (10), but the following points about the results shown in Table 2 should be noted.

Table 2:   Total phosphorus (P) and orthophosphate phosphorus
           ($PO_4$) in some species (mean ± S.D.)
           H.B. = hepatic bile;   G.B. = gall bladder bile.

| SPECIES | n | $PO_4$ (mg/100 mg) | Total P (mg/100 ml) | %$PO_4$ |
|---|---|---|---|---|
| Human (H.B.) | 10 | 0.1 - 2.5 (0.98±0.28) | 2.6 - 24.4 (10.55±1.82) | 9.35 |
| Human (G.B.) | 5 | 0.1 - 4.0 (1.72±0.76) | 71.0 - 193.0 (142.5±21.6) | 1.07 |
| Rabbit (H.B.) | 9 | 1.3 - 2.9 (2.0±0.23) | 7.2 - 10.2 (8.16±0.36) | 25.40 |
| Sheep (G.B.) | 10 | 1.6 - 13.2 (7.58±1.21) | 40.7 - 112.0 (67.55±7.69) | 11.2 |
| Pig (G.B.) | 10 | 2.6 - 6.0 (3.71±0.32) | 51.4 - 101.2 (77.52±5.77) | 4.8 |
| Ox (G.B.) | 4 | 1.0 - 4.7 2.00 | 21.0 - 52.3 40.30 | 5.0 |
| Rat | 6 | 0.1 - 0.9 0.35 | 2.6 - 11.4 9.60 | 4.0 |

a)   In aseptic hepatic bile, lipid P accounts for about 75-96% of the total phosphorus, with $PO_4$ accounting for the remaining 4-25%.

b)   Large species differences in $PO_4$ concentration are found.

c)   In a given species, $PO_4$ concentration varies considerably from one sample to another.

d)   There does not appear to be any positive correlation between total P and $PO_4$ in bile.

Total phosphorus and orthophosphate concentrations were studied in fresh, aseptic human hepatic and gall bladder bile (10).   The mean of the ratio $PO_4$/total P was about 0.1 in hepatic bile, but was considerably lower (0.01-0.02) in gall-bladder bile.   This indicates that orthophosphate is efficiently absorbed by the gall bladder while phospholipids are concentrated by a factor of about ten.   It follows from these results that the determination of total phosphorus in hepatic bile gives a 5-10% overestimation if used as a measure of phospholipid concentration.   On the other hand, the estimation of total phosphorus provides a more accurate value for phospholipids in fresh gall-bladder bile, the over-estimation being only 1-2%.

Certain data (11) indicates that in infected bile ducts, phosphatidyl choline may be degraded to such an extent as to yield orthophosphate.   In order to show that such degradation can occur in vivo and in vitro, it is necessary to isolate the intermediate phosphorylated compounds which may be produced, e.g. lysophosphatidyl choline, phosphatidic acids, glycerophosphoryl choline, phosphoryl choline, glycerophosphate and orthophosphate itself.   In order to investigate this problem we developed a high pressure column chromatographic technique using the anion-exchange resin Dowex 1-X4 (12), which permits separation of glycerophosphoryl choline, phosphoryl choline, glycerophosphate and orthophosphate from each other.   Experiments were carried out in vitro with infected bile, and the results obtained were as follows:

There was a) considerable decrease in phosphatidyl choline;
          b) moderate increase in lysophosphatidyl choline;
          c) considerable increase in orthophosphate;
          d) appearance of variable amounts of glycero-
             phosphate, and traces of glycerophosphoryl
             choline and phosphoryl choline.

Infected bile ducts are relatively common, and this condition results in an in vivo degradation of phosphatidyl cholines.   This degradation can be observed in freshly taken bile samples, and these contain abnormally large amounts of lysophosphatidyl choline and orthophosphate, and glycerophosphate is also present.   In such infected samples it is impossible to measure the initial concentration of phosphatidyl choline because the orthophosphate, and probably the other polar degradation products, will be absorbed from the gall bladder.   Since free fatty acids are efficiently absorbed by the gall bladder (13), this also precludes the measurement of the initial phosphatidyl choline in infected bile samples.

Conclusion:   It is not possible to determine phospholipids in infected bile with any degree of accuracy.

Fatty acid composition of phosphatidyl cholines

The fatty acid pattern of phosphatidyl choline in bile has
been determined by many investigators (6,14-19).   This pattern is
significantly different from that of phosphatidyl choline in plasma
and liver;  that from bile contains more palmitic and linoleic
acids and less stearic and polyunsaturated fatty acids than that
from plasma and liver.   The fatty acids in biliary phosphatidyl
choline may be produced by de novo synthesis in the liver, by
peripheral lipolysis or supplied in the diet.   Many factors can
affect the fatty acid pattern.   Dam et al. (20) studied the
influence of two different types of dietary fat (butter fat and a
special margarine containing almost 40 per cent linoleic acid) on
the fatty acid pattern of human biliary phosphatidyl choline.
The most clear-cut changes observed were a variation in the
percentage (from 20-35 per cent) of linoleic acid in relation to
the dietary fat intake.

It is known that carbohydrate feeding increases fatty acid
synthesis (21) and also the activity of enzymes which produce
unsaturated fatty acid (22,23).   An increased secretion of biliary
phosphatidyl choline containing palmitoyl and palmitoleoyl residues
has been reported in rats receiving ethanol together with glucose
or fructose (19).   When ethanol alone is given, the major part of
these acids is derived from the diet or peripheral lipolysis.
However, when fructose or glucose was added to the diet of the
ethanol-dosed rats, almost all of the palmitoyl residues in newly
synthesized biliary phosphatidyl choline were derived from de novo
synthesis in the liver of fructose-fed rats, while in animals
given glucose, only about half of the palmitoyl residues were
derived by such synthesis.

Conclusion:   The carbohydrate composition of the diet may
affect the origin and pattern of the fatty acids of bile phosphatidyl cholines.


Origin of biliary phosphatidyl cholines

Biliary phosphatidyl cholines are derived from the liver, and
bile and plasma phosphatidyl cholines are probably derived from a
common immediate precursor (24).   In the early stages after
administration of labelled phosphate to dogs, the specific activity
of biliary phosphatidyl cholines was higher than that of liver.
It has been suggested that the liver contains phosphatidyl cholines
which have a slow turnover rate, and these dilute the more active
phosphatidyl cholines from which biliary phosphatidyl cholines
appear to be derived (24).

The fatty acid composition of biliary and hepatic phosphatidyl cholines is different. Also, after injection of different precursors, the specific activity in totally or partially separated phosphatidyl cholines is higher in biliary than in hepatic phosphatidyl cholines. These facts have led some authors (25-28) to postulate the existence of a specific pool in the liver from which biliary phosphatidyl cholines are derived. Other studies (19) have produced a different conclusion. $[1-1-^2H_2]$ ethanol has been used to study de novo synthesis of phosphatidyl cholines in liver and bile of female Sprague-Dawley rats with a bile fistula. $[1-1-^2H_2]$ ethanol is used to obtain a constant flow of deuterium into pyridine nucleotide pools of the liver. During the oxidation of ethanol to acetaldehyde, the deuterium is transferred to $NAD^+$ to form NADH. The deuterium is transferred to different positions in glycerol-3-phosphate, which is then utilised for the synthesis of phosphatidyl cholines. Since ethanol produces only minor changes in the composition of biliary phosphatidyl cholines, the results obtained are likely to be equally valid when ethanol is not given. By this technique, it has been shown (19) that a specific pool of hepatic glycerol-3-phosphate is used for de novo synthesis of phosphatidyl cholines in bile, liver and plasma, and that the formation of this pool is closely coupled to ethanol oxidation. The triose phosphate involved is formed with malate via a gluconeogenetic pathway. Gas chromatography-mass spectrometry was used to identify pure molecular species of phosphatidyl cholines, and it was found that the liver contains a higher proportion of molecular species which have a longer half-life than those in bile (Fig.1). The half-lives for the corresponding species in liver and bile and the labelling of phosphatidyl cholines synthesized de novo were about equal, and the deuterium content of the glycerol moiety approached the same level for the corresponding molecular species in liver and bile. Therefore it was concluded that the major molecular species of biliary and hepatic phosphatidyl cholines are most probably synthesized in the same pool. Thus the different molecular species found in bile might be due to a selective step in biliary secretion of these compounds.

Gregory et al. (29) used the isolated, perfused rat liver to find the site of synthesis of these phospholipids in the liver. The experiments were done with or without adding taurocholate to the perfusion medium. The following precursors were tested: $[^{32}PO_4]$, $[^3H]$-choline, $[^3H]$-palmitate and $[^{14}C]$-linoleic acid. Isolated bile canalicular membranes and microsomes were studied at the conclusion of the perfusion. The following conclusions were drawn:

a)   Taurocholate significantly stimulates incorporation of orthophosphate, choline, palmitate and linoleate into biliary lecithins

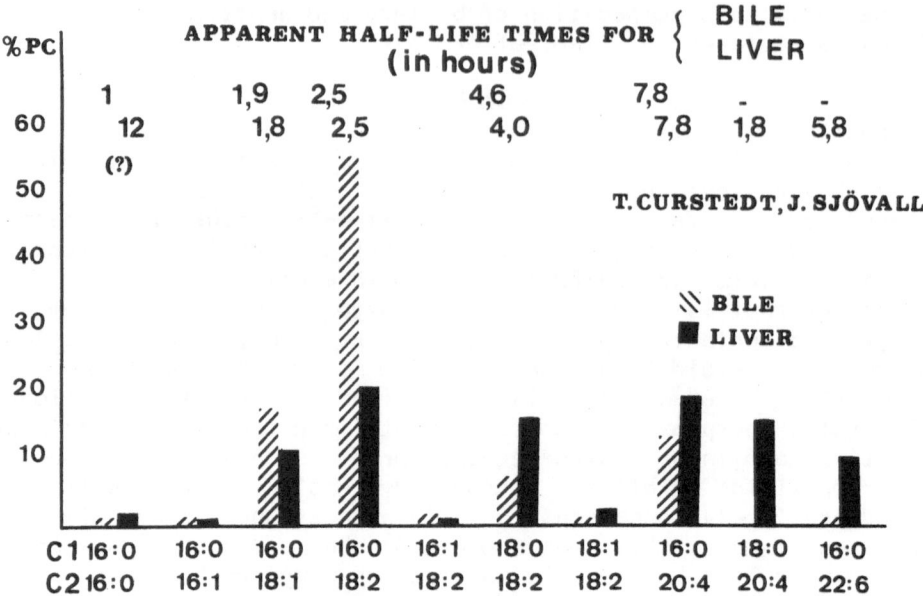

T. CURSTEDT, J. SJÖVALL

Fig.1: Percentage and half-life time of diverse molecular species of phosphatidyl cholines in bile
and liver (see text).  The half-life is similar
for a given species in liver and bile, except
for dipalmitoyl lecithin which has a much shorter
half-life in bile (one hour), but this molecular
species represent less than one per cent of bile
phosphatidyl cholines.

b)   The enzyme CDP-choline diglyceride transferase is not present
in the bile canaliculi, indicating that the canalicular
membrane is not involved in the synthesis of biliary lecithins

c)   The microsomes are probably the site of biosynthesis of bile
lecithins.  This is in agreement with the results of Wilgram
& Kennedy (30) that phosphatidyl cholines are synthesized in
the endoplasmic reticulum.  But it remains to be seen how
the lecithins are transported to and across the canalicular
membranes.

## Mechanism of secretion of lecithins in bile

It is known that biliary lipid excretion is regulated by the availability of bile salts returning to the liver in the entero-hepatic circulation (EHC) or of newly synthesized bile acids (31-34).   Moreover, it has been suggested that bile acids in the EHC are a determining factor in the synthesis of bile lecithins (29). In the light of the results of Curstedt & Sjövall (19), such a possibility seems to be extremely doubtful.   However, those results were obtained in a situation of complete diversion of the bile via the bile fistula, and it would be of interest to investigate this problem in animals with a normal enterohepatic circulation of bile acids.   Although a definite correlation exists between the secretion rate of biliary lecithins and of bile acids (34), this is not specifically related to bile acids.   Recent work has been carried out with some derivatives of sodium fusidate, a fungal steroid antibiotic (35) with physicochemical properties similar to those of bile acids (36).   Montet et al. (37) showed that 3-acetoxyl fusidate induces a significant secretion of biliary lipids in the rat.   Work in progress in our laboratory indicates that other derivatives of fusidic acid, such as glycodihydro-fusidate or taurofusidate, can also increase biliary lipid secretion.   The action of bile salts and these fusidate derivatives may be due to common physicochemical properties: e.g. detergency, affinity binding to membrane lipids and proteins.

Conclusion:   It is probable that the secretion of phospho-lipids in bile results from a physiological solubilization of some part of the endoplasmic reticulum induced by a high concentration of detergents (bile salts or other detergents) which are efficiently excreted in bile by the hepatocyte.

## Biliary lipid complex and synthetic mixed micelles

In bile, phosphatidyl cholines, cholesterol and bile salts form the biliary lipid complex with a molecular weight averaging 100,000.   However, little work has been done on the structure of this lipid complex, and there is no precise data on the actual molecular weight of the complex which, in fact, may be variable. The work of Small et al. (38-40) is well known and need not be extensively reviewed here.   The following lipid classification, developed by those workers, based on interactions with water is certainly the most convenient classification:

Non-polar lipids:   will not spread to form a monolayer. Insoluble in bulk.
   Polar lipids:
   1.   Insoluble non-swelling amphiphiles:  form a stable
      monolayer.  Insoluble in bulk.

II.    Insoluble swelling amphiphiles:  form a stable monolayer.
       Bulk phase = pure liquid crystals in pure water.

III.   Soluble amphiphiles (detergents):  form an unstable monolayer.
       Bulk phase = a micellar solution above CMC.

IIIA.  With lyotrophic mesomorphism.

IIIB.  Without lyotrophic mesomorphism.   (Lyotrophic mesomorphism:
       formation of a liquid crystalline phase in water;  lyotrophic
       because it occurs when water is added and mesomorphism
       because a change in physicochemical state results.)

        Cholesterol is an insoluble, non-swelling amphiphile;  phospha-
tidyl choline  is an insoluble swelling amphiphile while bile salts
are soluble amphiphiles without lyotrophic mesomorphism.    These
bile salts form Type C mixed micelles with the lecithins (type C
micelle is a mixed micelle formed by a soluble amphiphile and an
insoluble swelling amphiphile).    Such mixed micelles are able to
dissolve insoluble non-swelling amphiphiles such as cholesterol.
Thus, bile can be considered as an aqueous mixture of three
different lipid species, and Small and his colleagues have expressed
this inter-relationship between the three lipids in their well-
known phase diagram (38,39,40).    The average lipid composition
of bile is compatible with the concept of solubilisation of mixed
cholesterol-bile salt-lecithin micelles.    However, as Small &
Carey (40) have pointed out, little information is available about
the properties of complex micelles existing in bile and in
intestinal contents, and one can only extrapolate from the model
in vitro system.

        Conclusion:    While great progress has been made in our
understanding of the solubilisation of phosphatidyl cholines, some
points on bile are still obscure and require further study.


                Is there a polypeptide in the bile lipid complex?

        Investigations in our laboratory, not confirmed by others,
suggest that polypeptide components are involved in the structure
of the lipid complex of bile.   We have found that a polypeptide
fraction, consisting of one or more different polypeptides, moves
with biliary lipids into organic solvents such as butanol,
chloroform-methanol or glacial acetic acid (41-42).   The amino
acid pattern of this polypeptide fraction does not vary much from
species to species.   Its weight-percentage relative to lecithins
varies considerably between 0.5 and 4%.   However, it has not
been possible to prove the association of this polypeptide with
phospholipids under physiological conditions because of the
possibility that artefacts may be formed during the extraction
procedure, but recent results strongly suggest that the biliary

lipid complex may be a special type of lipoprotein complex and not
simply formed of mixed micelles, in the strict sense that a mixed
micelle is a protein-free association composed of more than a
single chemical species of lipid.

## Zonal centrifugation studies

(In the following part of this text, lecithins coming from
synthetic mixed micelles will be called micellar lecithins while
those coming from bile will be called biliary lecithins.)

Lairon et al. (43) compared the behaviour of synthetic bile
salt-lecithin-cholesterol mixed micelles, prepared as described
elsewhere (44), with the behaviour of the biliary lipid complex.
Ultracentrifugation was performed at $20^{\circ}$C and at 150,000 g for
24-64 hours in a zonal rotor.  A linear sucrose gradient of
1-15%(w/v) was used.  Mixed micelles do not penetrate appreciably
into the sucrose gradient, while the biliary lecithins are
stabilised in the zone with a density of 1.030.  A polypeptide
fraction can be extracted by butanol from this zone along with
lecithins.

## Gel filtration studies

Gel filtration on Agarose (BioGel A 5m. Biorad, Richmond,
Calif.) coupled with ultramicroscopic studies have been carried
out on mixed micelles and biliary lipid complex (45,46).  When
bile salt-lecithin-cholesterol mixed micelles are subjected to
gel filtration in the presence of bile salts (6 mM) in the eluting
medium, these lipids are eluted with 2.0 void volumes.  When bile
salts are not added to the eluting medium, most of the cholesterol
and lecithins are recovered almost immediately after the void
volume and the bile salts with 2.5 void volumes.  The pattern
obtained by subjecting bile to the same procedure is similar.

In conclusion, in columns equilibrated with bile salts,
micellar and biliary lecithins are eluted with the second void
volume, corresponding to a protein with a molecular weight of
80,000.  In columns not equilibrated with bile salts, micellar
and biliary lecithins are eluted with the first void volume,
while bile salts are eluted with 2.5 void volumes.  Although
one cannot assign a molecular weight based on a protein calibration,
the biliary lipid complex is obviously present as a complex of
moderate molecular weight in a bile salt rich medium, while in the
absence of bile salts, the biliary lipid complex is present as a
macromolecular aggregate.

## Electron microscopy studies

Electron microscope studies using a negative staining technique have also been carried out (45). Usually one cannot detect any structures by direct examination of samples of bile or synthetic mixed micelles. Structures are sometimes seen and these consist of cigar-shaped lamellar formations reminiscent of those also seen by Howell et al. (47). These discrete structures, which probably correspond to layers of lecithins and cholesterol spaced about 50-60 Å apart, may often be joined into a single unit by lateral extensions of the lamellar layer. The cigar-shaped aggregates, which are larger than 1000 Å, cannot correspond to the native state. We know that dehydration is a cause of the artefact, and by definition, a micellar state cannot exist without water. In addition, the increase in detergent concentration which occurs during dehydration must result in abnormal staining as well as structural abnormalities. Therefore, we think that no conclusions can be drawn from ultramicroscopic observations with the lecithins in the presence of a high concentration of bile salts.

Gel filtration, by separating the bile salts from the lecithin, makes it possible to eliminate the artefacts caused by detergents in negative staining. In columns not equilibrated with bile salts, gel filtration of synthetic mixed micelles gives rise to a dissociation phenomenon. Mixed micelles are broken up, the lecithins are eluted together with the cholesterol immediately after the void volume, and bile salts with 2.5 void volumes. The void volume micellar lecithins become organised into a classic myelinic phase with a spacing of 55 Å. Under the same conditions, biliary lecithins and cholesterol are also eluted immediately after the void volume, but totally different structures are seen. These are spherical formations 300-500 Å in size, or are more or less flat vesicular structures of much the same size, often in the form of stacks. These vesicular formations are similar to those seen by Hamilton et al. (48) with abnormal lipoprotein in cholestasis and in familial lecithin-cholesterol acyl-transferase deficiency (49). The appearance under the electron microscope seems correlated with a low percentage of esterified cholesterol.

The aspect of the vesicle is not specific for the presence of lipoprotein organisation. However, taken in conjunction with other data on the presence of polypeptide components in lipid extracts of bile and the results of zonal centrifugation studies, the electron microscopic data provide additional evidence in favour of the lipoprotein nature of the biliary lipid complex.

## Attempts to isolate polypeptides

Preliminary studies have been carried out on the biliary

phosphatidyl cholines eluted with the void volume with the
objective of isolating specific polypeptides.    The method of
Picard et al. (50) for the isolation of LP-X was used.    Ten
volumes of ether were added to the lecithin-containing fraction.
After 24 hours stirring at $4°C$, the lecithins were recovered
with a polypeptide fraction in the ether phase.    Evaporation
of the ether or addition of methanol, caused dissociation of the
polypeptide fraction, which can be recovered as an insoluble
residue.    The amino-acid pattern of this polypeptide is very
similar to that reported by Picard et al. (50).    Attempts to
analyse the polypeptide fraction are in progress,but great
difficulties are being experienced because of variable yields
and aggregation caused by the removal of the lipids.    The polypeptide fraction can be partly solubilised by using detergents
such as sodium dodecyl sulphate (SDS) or Nonidet P40, which
provides the opportunity to carry out immunological and electrophoretic studies.    SDS-polyacrylamide gel electrophoresis shows
the presence of many bands;  the major band corresponds to a
molecular weight of about 6000.    It is possible that the other
bands of higher molecular weight are produced by different states
of aggregation of the lighter band.    An antiserum against the
polypeptide corresponding to human biliary lecithins has been
produced in rabbits.    However, the production of an immunological
reaction between the polypeptide and the antiserum requires at
least partial solubilisation of the polypeptide fraction by
detergent.    These immunological studies are also complicated by
the fact that SDS causes non-specific precipitation when the
concentration of the detergent exceeds 0.1%.    In contrast,
Nonidet P40 appears to dissolve immunological precipitates when
used at too high a concentration.    Therefore, great caution
must be used when these detergents are employed in immunological
studies.    Bearing these precautions in mind, it has been found
that the antiserum reacts with the polypeptide fraction dissolved
in SDS solution and also with $\alpha$- and $\beta$-lipoproteins (private
communication, Picard).

Another relationship between the biliary lipid complex with
the abnormal plasma lipoprotein characteristic of obstructive
jaundice has also been observed.    Studies with the polypeptide
fraction dissolved in SDS (51), and also with specific antibodies
obtained after phospholipase $A_2$ treatment, revealed the presence
of apolipoprotein X on the surface and of albumin in the centre of
this abnormal lipoprotein.    We have found a positive response
against anti-albumin serum only after removal of the lecithins in
the fractions.    It is possible that some of the albumin in bile
may be trapped in vesicles during the aggregation process.

Conclusion:    It seems probable that the biliary lipid complex
is composed of lipoprotein subunits resulting from the physiological

detergent solubilisation of a part of the liver cell endoplasmic
reticulum in the vicinity of the bile canaliculi.

### Function of bile phosphatidyl cholines

Until recently no particular function could be ascribed to the
phosphatidyl cholines in bile, but investigations in the rat have
provided strong evidence that these phospholipids may play an
important role in fat absorption.   The work of Hofmann and
Borgström (52,53) has greatly clarified the mechanism of fat
absorption, emphasizing the primary importance of the detergent
properties of the bile salts in this process.   No particular
role has been ascribed by these authors to the biliary phosphatidyl
cholines, their fate in the intestine being apparently the same as
that of alimentary phospholipids.

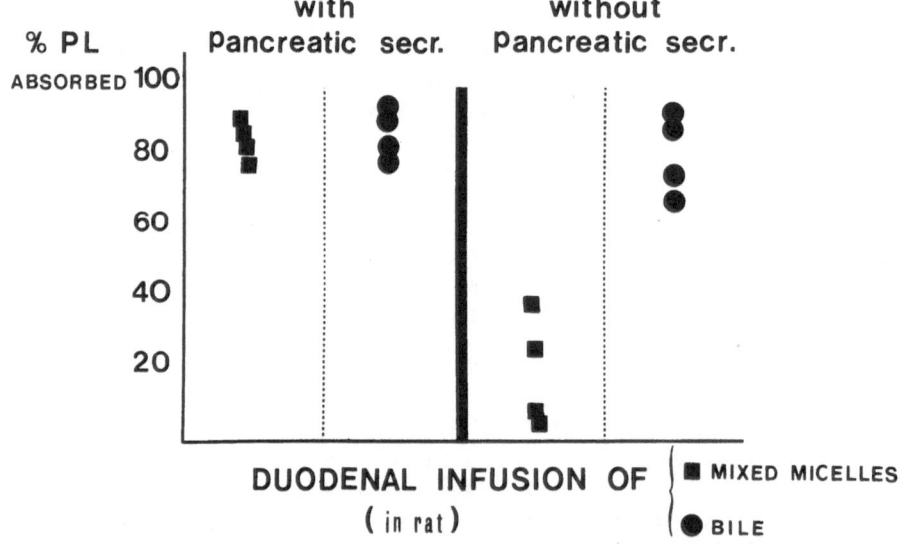

Fig. 2:   The disappearance rate of micellar and biliary
          lecithins are similar in the intestine of rat
          receiving pancreatic secretion.   If this secretion
          is diverted, micellar lecithins are poorly absorbed
          while the disappearance rate of biliary lecithins
          is not appreciably modified.

Nalbone (54) carried out in vivo experiments with rats to compare the behaviour in the intestine of phosphatidyl cholines of mixed synthetic bile salt-lecithin, cholesterol micelles and of bile itself.   Two groups of rats were studied.   In one group the bile was diverted from the intestine but pancreatic secretion to the intestine was preserved.   In the other group, both bile and pancreatic secretions were diverted from the intestine.   Synthetic mixed micelles or bile were then infused into the duodenum.   In the first group (pancreatic secretion intact) the disappearance of both the mixed micelles and of bile was similar (Fig.2).   However, in the second group (without pancreatic secretion), phosphatidyl cholines from mixed micelles were not absorbed, but those from infused bile were very efficiently absorbed.   Thus, it seems that biliary phosphatidyl cholines can be absorbed in the absence of pancreatic secretion, whereas those from synthetic micelles can not.

Boucrot and Clement (55,56) have reported some interesting properties of biliary phospholipids:

a)    in contrast to purified phospholipids, biliary phosphatidyl cholines are resistant to the hydrolytic action of pancreatic phospholipase

b)    some labelled biliary phospholipids are transported intact to the liver via the portal blood, in contrast to purified phospholipids which are recovered from the lymph

c)    some of the labelled biliary phospholipids can be recovered from bile after intestinal reabsorption.

The authors have postulated the existence of an enterohepatic circulation via the portal blood of at least part of the biliary phosphatidyl cholines.

We have investigated in vivo the behaviour of biliary phosphatidyl cholines in the lumen of the small intestine of the rat during fat digestion (57-59).   The experiments were carried out on Wistar rats which were fed on a balanced diet, but fasted before the start of the experiment.   A triolein-water emulsion, prepared by ultrasonication, was given by stomach tube.   At different time intervals the rats were killed, and the small intestine was ligated both at the pylorus and at the junction of the jejunum and ileum.   The intestinal contents were removed and filtered through glass wood to remove intestinal debris.   Gel filtration was carried out on 5m columns of BioGel A, previously equilibrated with bile salts.   The first observation made was the persistence of a high proportion (80%) of phosphatidyl cholines 1 hour after infusion of the triolein emulsion.   It was not possible to detect any signifi-

cant amounts of phosphatidyl-serines - ethanolamines or sphingomyelins.   In some experiments rats with a bile fistula were
given 1.0 ml of a 10 mM sodium taurocholate solution by duodenal
infusion after ingestion of triglycerides.   After 1 hour of
digestion, no significant amounts of phosphatidyl or lysophosphatidyl cholines were found.   This indicates that the lecithins
and lysolecithins found in the previous experiments were derived
from bile.   However, these lecithins appear to be particularly
resistant to enzymatic hydrolysis in the intestinal lumen.

Analyses of the intraluminal contents after different periods
of digestion led to the following conclusions:

a)   At the start of lipolysis, all the lecithins and cholesterol
     are eluted within the first void volume in highly opalescent
     fractions containing di- or tri-glycerides and small amounts
     of free fatty acids and monoglycerides.   These fractions
     contain all of the lipase and its cofactor, whereas under
     the same conditions pure rat lipase is eluted after 2.35
     void volumes

b)   As lipolysis proceeds, some of the biliary phosphatidyl
     cholines leave the emulsion together with the lipolysis
     products, resulting in the formation of a lipid complex
     eluted with 2.0 void volumes.   This complex has a much
     higher molecular weight than that formed in the absence of
     phosphatidyl cholines.   In the bile fistula rats receiving
     intraduodenal taurocholate solution in addition to the tri-
     glyceride emulsion, efficient lipolysis occurs.   Gel
     filtration of the intraluminal contents of these animals
     shows that di- and tri-glycerides emerge in the first
     void volume together with a very low percentage (1-2%) of
     free fatty acids and monoglycerides.   The later constituents
     are found almost totally in optically clear fractions eluted
     by 2.4 void volumes.   This elution volume corresponds to a
     protein of molecular weight of about 25,000.   In vitro
     mixing of triolein, bile salts and pancreatic juice gives
     similar results.   This soluble lipid complex eluted with
     2.4 void volumes corresponds to the bile salt-free acid-
     monoglyceride mixed micelles described by Hofmann and
     Borgström (52,53)

c)   Lipase and colipase are totally associated with the emulsion
     eluted with the void volume.

d)   Ultracentrifugation should be avoided in the study of
     intraluminal lipolysis because it causes (58):

     (i)  disappearance of the triglyceride/water interface and
          consequently of associations occurring at this interface

(ii)    partial sedimentation of biliary phosphatidyl cholines together with lipase.

In vitro experiments have been carried out to confirm these in vivo observations concerning the adsorption of bile lecithins on the triglyceride emulsion. Weakly polar interfaces strongly associate with biliary lecithins, such as triglyceride/water and silanized CPT-10/water interfaces (Fig. 3 and 4).

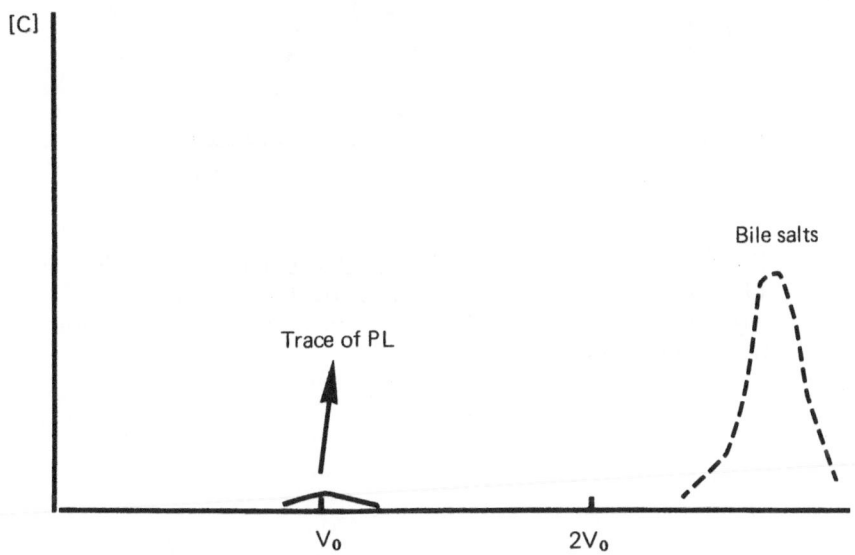

Fig. 3:  Schematic pattern of gel permeation chroma- tography of bile on silanized controlled-pore glass column (silanized CPG-10, Electro- nucleonics, Inc., Fairfield, N.J.). Eluant is NaCl 0.1 M. Bile lecithins are retained while bile salts are eluted with 2.5 void volumes.

In vitro studies of some properties of the biliary phospha- tidyl choline/water interface or the triglyceride-bile phosphatidyl choline/water interface have been carried out to ascertain the role of colipase, and the following conclusions were made:

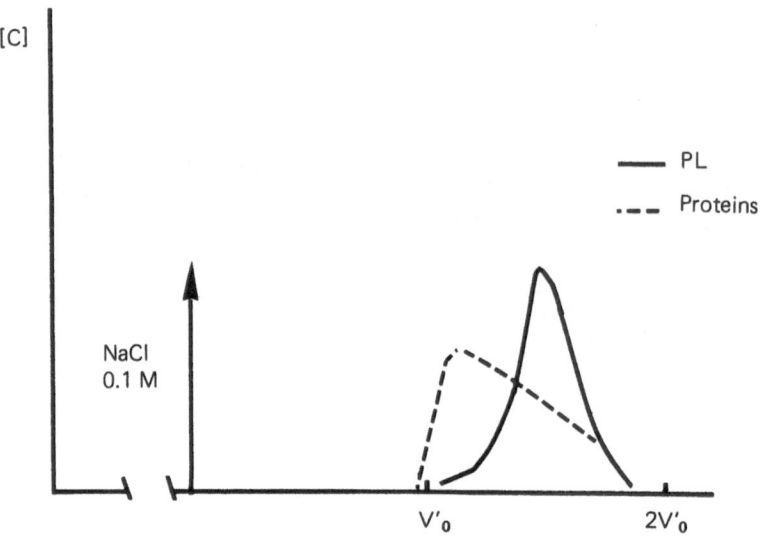

<u>Fig.4</u>:   Elution of the adsorbed lecithins on silanized
            CPG-10 by Ethanol 80%.   The lecithins are
            eluted immediately after the void volume together
            with some protein components.

a)    Pure colipase is almost totally absorbed on the phosphatidyl
      choline- or the triglyceride-phosphatidyl choline water
      interfaces.   The affinity of colipase for the biliary phos-
      phatidyl choline/water interface is much higher than that
      for the bile salt/water interface.

b)    Lipase alone is not appreciably associated with the biliary
      phosphatidyl choline/water interface nor the triglyceride-
      phosphatidyl choline/water interface.

c)    In the presence of colipase, lipase is almost completely
      associated with biliary phosphatidyl cholines or the tri-
      glyceride-phosphatidyl choline interface.

      These results suggest to us that, under physiological condi-
tions, colipase is adsorbed on the triglyceride-bile phosphatidyl
choline/water interface.   This adsorption induces a structural

conformational change of colipase rendering it more able to make lipase more strongly associated with its substrate (Fig.5). As lipolysis proceeds, the products together with bile phosphatidyl cholines are solubilised by bile salts. The presence of intact biliary phosphatidyl cholines in the soluble complexes containing the lipolysis products may be of importance during the intracellular steps of fat absorption.

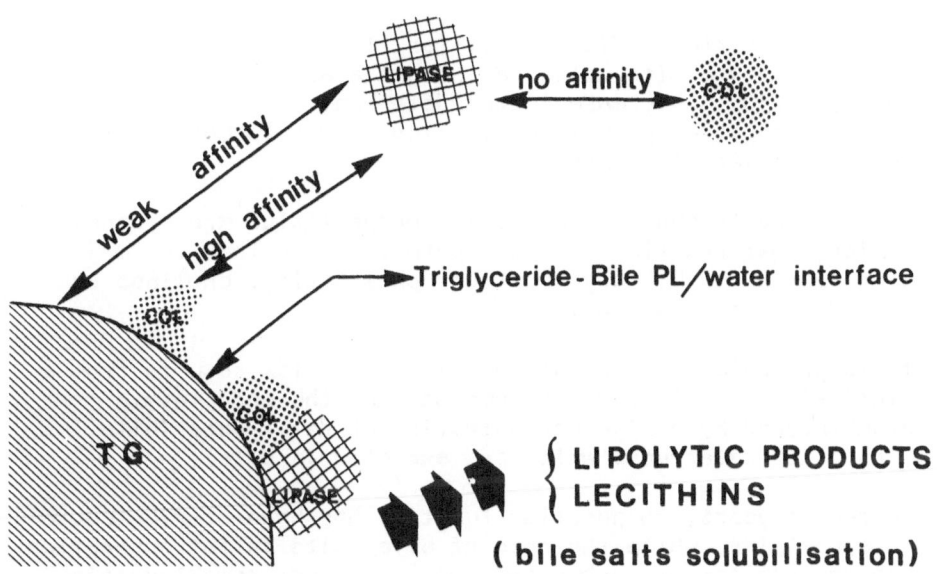

Fig.5:  Proposed physiological mechanism for the intra-
        luminal lipolysis in the rat:
        a) association of biliary lecithins to the tri-
           glycerides emulsion
        b) adsorption of colipase to the triglycerides-
           bile lecithins/water interface, inducing a
           structural conformational change which creates
           a high affinity for lipase
        c) binding of lipase to the adsorbed colipase.
        As the lipolysis proceeds, lipolytic products
        together with intact bile lecithins are transferred
        to the mucosa as water soluble complexes formed by
        bile salts.

GENERAL CONCLUSIONS AND SUMMARY

The lipids of bile consist chiefly of bile salts, non-
esterified cholesterol and phospholipids.  More than 90% of these
phospholipids are phosphatidyl cholines.  These lipids form a
complex (the biliary lipid complex) which is soluble in water.
Many characteristics of the biliary lipid complex are compatible
with a model of mixed micelles (bile salts-lecithins-cholesterol),
but studies using zonal ultracentrifugation, gel filtration,
ultramicroscopy, biochemical and immunological investigations
suggest a more complex structure, some proteins being associated
with phospholipids.

In detergent-rich media, the biliary lipid complex is present
in a monomeric state, its molecular weight averaging 100,000 and
its density 1.030.  Decrease in the detergent concentration
induces an aggregation phenomenon leading to the formation of
200-400 Å vesicular structures.

Recent results suggest that bile phospholipids are synthesized
in the microsomal fraction of the hepatocyte, and that the major
molecular species of biliary and liver phosphatidyl cholines are
synthesized in the same pool.

It is probable that the biliary lipid complex results from a
physiological solubilisation of some part of the endoplasmic
reticulum induced by a high concentration of detergents (bile
salts, or other detergents which are excreted in bile).

In recent years, no peculiar function has been attributed to
bile phospholipids, while the role of bile salts in fat absorption
has been the subject of much attention.  But now some investigations made in rats suggest that bile phospholipids have a
specific role during intraluminal fat digestion.

Triglyceride/water interfaces strongly associate with bile
phospholipids.  Colipase, which has a great affinity for bile
phospholipids, is associated with the triglyceride emulsion
"stabilized" by the biliary phospholipids.  The lipase is bound
to this triglyceride-bile phospholipid/water interface only in
the presence of colipase.  So it seems that a major role of
colipase is to bind lipase to its substrate.

As lipolysis proceeds, a water-soluble complex escapes from
the emulsion.  This complex is composed of bile salts, lipolytic
products, cholesterol and intact bile phosphatidyl cholines.

These results show, on the one hand, a direct participation
of bile phospholipids in the intraluminal digestion of tri-

glycerides, and on the other, suggest a possible role of these phospholipids during the intracellular steps of fat absorption.

## ACKNOWLEDGEMENTS

This work was supported by Institut National de la Santé et de la Recherche Médicale and by a Grant Number 73.7.1635 from the Délégation Générale à la Recherche Scientifique et Technique.

I wish to express my sincere gratitude to Dr. W. Taylor for the many hours he spent in preparing this paper from my very rough draft.

## REFERENCES

1.  Diamond J.M., "The concentrating activity of the gall bladder" The biliary system, Ed.W. Taylor, Blackwell Scientific Publ., Oxford 1965,495-514.
2.  Isaksson B., On the Lipid Constituents of Normal Bile. Ac. Med.Upsal.,(1951),56,177-195.
3.  Polonovski M. & Bourillon R., Les Phospholipides de la Bile. Bull.Soc.Chim.Biol., (1952),34,712-720.
4.  Blomstrand R., Analysis of Human Bile Lipids by Gas-liquid Chromatography. Acta Chem.Scand.,(1960),14,1006-1010.
5.  Phillips G.B., The Lipid Composition of Human Bile. Biochim. Biophys.Acta (1960),41,361.
6.  Adams E.P. and Heath T.J., The Phospholipids in ruminant bile. Biochim.Biophys.Acta, (1963),70,688-690.
7.  Spitzer H.L., Kyriakides E.C. and Balint J.A., Bile Phospholipids in Various Species. Nature, (1964),204,288.
8.  Montet J.C., Amic J. & Hauton J., Méthode Rapide de Séparation sous haute pression des Phospholipides sur Colonne d'Acide Silicique. Application à la bile Humaine. Bull.Soc. Chim.Biol.,(1970),52,831-840.
9.  Amic J., Lairon D. & Hauton J., Technique de dosage automatique de l'Orthophosphate de Grande Fiabilité. Clin.Chim.Acta, (1972),40,107-114.
10. Lairon D., Les phospholipides biliaires: dosage et Mode d'Organisation. Doctorate de Specialite de l'Universite de Provence, 31 Octobre 1972.
11. Amic J., Hauton J.C., Lafont H., Montet J.C. & Teissier N., Modifications du Comportement des Composés Phosphorés de la bile en relation avec le temps de Conservation. Ann.Biol. Clin.,(1969),27,177-180.
12. Lairon D., Amic J., Lafont H., Nalbone G., Domingo N. & Hauton J., High-pressure Chromatography separation of glycerophosphorylcholine, phosphorylcholine, glycerophosphate and

orthophosphate. J.Chromatog.,(L974),88,183-186.

13. Niederhiser D.H., Pineda F.M., Hejduk L.J. and Roth H.P.,
    Absorption of oleic acid by the guinea pig gallbladder.
    J.Lab.Clin.Med.,(1971),77,985-992.

14. Balint J.A., Kyriakides E.C., Spitzer H.L. and Morrison E.S.,
    Lecithin fatty acid composition in bile and plasma of man,
    dog, rats and oxen. J.Lipid Research,(1965),6,96-99.

15. Balint J.A., Beeler D.A., Treble D.H. and Spitzer H.L.,
    Studies in the biosynthesis of hepatic and biliary lecithins.
    J.Lipid Research,(1967),8,486-493.

16. Nakayama F. and Kawamura S., Composition of biliary lecithins.
    Clin.Chim.Acta,(1967),17,53-58.

17. Olsson O., Boucrot P. & Clement J., Obtention quantitative des
    Lipides biliaires; application à l'étude de deux du rat.
    Biochimie,(1973),55,491-496.

18. Alling C., Cahlin E. and Schersten T., Relationships between
    fatty acid patterns of serum, hepatic and biliary lecithins
    in man. Effect of sucrose feeding. Biochim.Biophys.Acta,(1973),
    296,518-526.

19. Curstedt T., Biosynthesis of molecular species of phosphatidyl
    cholines during metabolism of $(1,1-{}^2H_2)$ ethanol. Department
    of Chemistry, Karolinska Institutet, Stockholm 1974.

20. Dam H., Kruse I., Jensen M.K. and Kallehauge H.E. Studies on
    human bile. II.Influence of two different fats on the
    composition of human bile. Scand.J.Clin.Lab.Invest.,(1967),
    19,376-378.

21. Zakim D.(1973), in Progr.Biochem.Pharmacol.,(Paoletti R. &
    MacDonald I., eds.), vol.8, p.161, Karger, Basel.

22. Elovson J., Conversions in palmitic and stearic acid in the
    intact rat. Biochim.Biophys.Acta,(1965),106,291-303.

23. Elovson J. Immediate fate of albumin-bound $(1-{}^{14}C)$ stearic
    acid following its intraportal injection into carbohydrate
    refed rats. Early course of desaturation and esterification
    in the liver. Biochim.Biophys.Acta (1965),106,480-494.

24. Zilversmit D.B. and Van Handel E., The origin of bile
    lecithin and the use of bile to determine plasma lecithin
    turnover rates. Arch.Biochem.Biophys.(1958),73,224-232.

25. Balint, J.A., Beeler D.A., Treble D.H. and Spitzer H.L.
    Studies in the Biosynthesis of Hepatic and Biliary Lecithins.
    J.Lipid Research (1967),8,486-493.

26. Schersten T., Gottfries A., Nilsson S. and Samuelsson B.
    Incorporation of plasma free fatty acids into bile lipids
    in man. Life Sci. (1967),6,1775-1780.

27. Swell L., Bell C.C., Entenman C. Bile acid and Lipid
    metabolism. III.Influence of Bile acids on phospholipids
    in liver and bile of the isolated perfused dog liver.
    Biochim.Biophys.Acta,(1969),164,278-284.

28. Nilsson S. and Schersten T., Influence of bile acids on the
    synthesis of biliary phospholipids in man. Eur.J.Clin.Invest.
    (1970),1,109-111.

29.  Gregory D.H., Vlahcevic Z.R., Schatzki P. and Swell L.,
     Mechanism of secretion of biliary lipids. I.Role of bile
     canalicular and microsomal membranes in the synthesis and
     transport of biliary lecithin and cholesterol. J.Clin.Invest.
     (1975),55,105-114.

30.  Wilgram G.F. and Kennedy E.P., Intracellular distribution of
     some enzymes catalizing reactions in the biosynthesis of
     complex lipids. J.Biol.Chem. (1963),238,2615-2619.

31.  Thureborn E., Human hepatic bile - composition changes due
     to altered entero hepatic circulation. Acta Chir.Scand.
     (1962) Suppl.303.

32.  Swell L., Entenman C., Leong G.F. and Holloway R.J. Bile acids
     and lipid metabolism. IV.Influence of bile acids on biliary
     and liver organelle phospholipids and cholesterol. Am.J.
     Physiol.,(1968),215,1390-1396.

33.  Entenman C., Holloway R., Albright M.L. and Leong G. Bile
     acids and lipid metabolism. II.Essential role of bile acids
     in bile phospholipid excretion. Arch.Biochem.Biophys.(1969),
     130,253-256.

34.  Nilsson S. Synthesis and secretion of biliary phospholipids
     in man. An experimental study with special reference to the
     relevance for gallstone formation. Acta Chir.Scand.(1970),
     6, Suppl.405.

35.  Godtrredsen W.O. Fusidic acid and some related antibiotic.
     Aarhuus Stiftsboy Trykkerie, Copenhagen 1967.

36.  Carey M. and Small D. Micellar properties of sodium fusidate
     a steroid antibiotic structurally reassembling to bile salts.
     J.Lipid Research (1971),12,604-613.

37.  Montet J.C., Montet A.M., Gerolami A. and Hauton J.C. Effect
     of 3-acetoxy fusidate on the biliary secretion of lipids in
     the rat. Biol.Gastroent. (1975),8,53-62.

38.  Small D.M., Bourges M.C. and Dervichian D.G. The biophysics
     of lipidic associations. I.The ternary systems lecithin-bile
     salt-water. Biochim.Biophys.Acta (1966),125,563-580.

39.  Hofmann A.F. and Small D.M. Detergent properties of bile
     salts: correlation with physiological function. Ann.Rev.Med.
     (1967),18,333-376.

40.  Carey M.C. and Small D.M. The characteristics of mixed
     micellar solutions with particular reference to bile.  Am.J.
     Med. (1970),49,590-608.

41.  Hauton J.C., Laurent B., Gerolami Santandrea A., Greusard C.,
     Lafont H., Tessier N. and Sarles H. Etude préliminaire d'une
     fraction peptidique extraite avec les lipides biliaires et
     des lipides neutres du plasma. Clin.Chim.Acta (1967),17,
     171-182.

42.  Lafont H. and Hauton J. "Is a peptide fraction naturally
     associated with bile lipids?" Acta Helv.Med. (1973),
     37,137-141.

43.    Lairon D., Lafont H. and Hauton J.C. Lack of mixed micelles
       bile salt-lecithin-cholesterol in bile and presence of a
       lipoprotein complex. Biochimie (1972),54,529-530.
44.    Montet J.C. and Dervichian D.G. Solubilisation micellaire
       du cholesterol par les sels biliaires et les lecithines
       extraits de la bile humaine. Biochimie (1971),53,751-754.
45.    Nalbone G., Lafont H., Domingo N., Lairon D., Pautrat G.
       and Hauton J. Ultramicroscopic study of the bile lipoprotein
       complex. Biochimie (1973),55,1503-1506.
46.    Lafont H., Lairon D., Domingo N., Nalbone G. and Hauton, J.C.
       Does a lecithin-polypeptide association in bile originate
       from membrane structural subunits? Biochimie (1974),56,
       465-468.
47.    Howell J.I., Lucy J.A., Pirola R.C. and Bouchier I.A.D.
       Macromolecular assemblies of lipid in bile. Biochim.Biophys.
       Acta (1970),210,1-6.
48.    Hamilton R.L., Havel R.J., Kane J.P., Blaurock A.E. and
       Sata T. Cholestasis: labellar structure of the abnormal human
       serum lipoprotein. Science (1971),172,475-478.
49.    Forte T., Nichols A., Glomset J. and Norum K. The ultrastruc-
       ture of plasma lipoproteins in lecithin:cholesterol acyltrans-
       ferase deficiency. Scand.J.Clin.Lab.Invest. (1974),33,
       Suppl.137,121-132.
50.    Picard J., Veissiere D. et Voyer F. Identification de l'
       apolipoproteine des le oproteines sériques anormales de la
       cholostase. Clin.Chim.Acta (1972),37,483-489.
51.    Seidel D., Alaupovic P., Furman R.H. and McConathy W.J.
       A lipoprotein characterizing obstructuve jaundice. II.
       Isolation and partial characterization of the protein
       moieties of low density lipoproteins. J.Clin.Invest. (1970),
       49,2396-2407.
52.    Hofmann A.F. and Borgström B. The physico-chemical state of
       lipids in intestinal content during their digestion and
       absorption. Fed.Proc.(1962),21,43-50.
53.    Hofmann A.F. and Borgström B. The intraluminal phase of fat
       digestion in man: the lipid content of the micellar and oil
       phases of intestinal content obtained during fat digestion
       and absorption. J.Clin.Invest. (1964),43,247-257.
54.    Nalbone G. Les phospholipides biliaires: Etude ultramicro-
       scopique; comportement dans le contenu intraluminaire pendant
       le digestion des triglycerides chez le rat.   These de
       doctorat de spécialité de Chimie, Université de Provence
       (Aix-Marseille 1), 1974.
55.    Boucrot P. and Clement J. Resistance to the effect of phospho-
       lipase A2 of the biliary phospholipids.  Lipids (1971),6,
       652-656.
56.    Boucrot P. Is there an entero-hepatic circulation of the bile
       phospholipids? Lipids (1972),7,282-288.

57. Lairon D., Lafont H., Domingo N., Nalbone G. and Hauton J. On the state of lipids in the rat small intestine after a fatty meal. Biochimie (1973),55,1165-1166.

58. Nalbone G., Lairon D., Lafont H., Domingo N., Hauton J. and Sarda L. Behaviour of biliary phospholipids in intestinal lumen during fat digestion in rat. Lipids (1974),9,765-770.

59. Lairon D., Nalbone G., Domingo N., Lafont H., Hauton J., Julien R., Rathelot J., Canioni P. and Sarda L. In vitro studies on interaction of rat pancreatic lipase and colipase with biliary lipids. Lipids (1975),10,262-265.

DISCUSSION OF LECTURE BY J.C. HAUTON

<u>Haslewood</u>:    I think Dr. Hauton has done us a great service in
drawing our attention to the possibility of the existence in bile
of substances which may have an important effect in solubilizing,
but which are not one of the three well-recognised constituents.
I have handled a great many bile samples with the object of
isolating pure conjugates.    Usually we get the bile as fresh
and as pure as possible, the mucin is precipitated by ethanol and
the filtrate is evaporated to dryness.    The residue is extracted
with ether or petroleum ether to remove lipids, and then we try
to isolate the conjugates.    In some bile samples, no matter how
clean they appear to be, there are contaminants very closely
associated with the bile salts.    They do not show up on thin-
layer plates;  they interfere with infra-red and mass spectral
analysis, and they are similar to the bile salts in being water-
soluble.    I do not know what these contaminants are.

There is another completely unsolved problem associated with
bile salts prepared in this manner.    Some of them are extremely
hygroscopic and some are not.    To my knowledge, none of the
isolated bile salts are hygroscopic.    These contaminants are
certainly not phospholipids, since we have analysed them for
organic phosphate.    A preliminary investigation of the contaminants which occur in very large quantities in the bile of some
fish we are studying suggested that there was a high concentration
of small molecular weight hydroxy fatty acids.

So I do think that it is an oversimplification to explain the
solubility of cholesterol in bile only by the triangular
co-ordinate concept.    Therefore, we should keep an open mind
that there may be substances as yet unknown which have an important
effect in bile.

<u>Ostrow</u>:    Recently I have been trying to find out about the state
of bilirubin in bile, and I was interested to learn that when you
ultracentrifuge bile all the lipid components move together.    But
when the bile is applied to a Sephadex or Biorad column the bilirubin and bile salts are separated, while the cholesterol and
phospholipids come off in the void volume as vesicles.    I had
assumed that this was due to adsorption of the anionic components

to the column.    Your experiments with bile acid equilibrated
columns and polyamide-type gel clearly shows that anion adsorption
is not involved as I had thought.    It is probably due to the fact
that if you do not have monomers of bile acids on the columns then
the micelles break up.    So that part of your contribution has
certainly been valuable to me.

When you compare ultracentrifugation of bile and artificial
micelles, there are two technical points which might influence the
interpretation.    You centrifuged at 20°C whereas, of course, body
temperature is 37°C.    Would using this higher temperature affect
your results?    Secondly, what type of lecithins did you use:
were they identical to bile lecithins or was it egg-lecithin which
is so commonly used?

Hauton:    To answer your second question first:  sometimes we used
egg-lecithins and sometimes lecithins purified from bile, and the
results are the same.    I do not know what the results would be at
37°C.

Sjövall:    I want to add to what Professor Haslewood said.    The
presence of these unknown substances presents methodological
problems.    For example, many organic extracts which one wishes
to analyse for bile acids are run through anion-exchanges in
organic solvents, and one finds that they run through as neutral
compounds.    One can avoid this by running these extracts through
a cation-exchanger first to remove, presumably, cations.    We
therefore assume that there must be present some cations which
form very strong ion-pairs with bile acids so that the bile acids
behave as neutral compounds.    This is a little remote from Dr.
Hauton's topic, but these are associations which we do not usually
think of but which form artefacts which can complicate analyses.

BILIARY LIPIDS IN PREGNANCY

M.M. Fisher, V.M. Price and I.M. Yousef

University of Toronto

Toronto, Ontario, Canada

## I. Effect of pregnancy on the liver

Although there is remarkably little known about the effect of
pregnancy on the human liver and particularly about its effect on
the secretion and composition of bile there is evidence, much of
it indirect and some of it controversial, that there is a general
alteration in liver function during pregnancy (11,13,27,33,38,68,
69,71).   In the latter part of pregnancy one finds an increased
activity of serum alkaline phosphatase and leucine amino peptidase
which is not entirely attributable to placental contributions.
There is an increased activity of 5'-nucleotidase and there is a
general hyperlipemia (7,8,11,14,62,70).   This latter phenomenon,
first documented by Virchow in  1867, must involve the liver which
plays such a central role in lipid metabolism.   And it must
involve several different mechanisms.   Although the concentrations
of total triglycerides, cholesterol, phospholipids and free fatty
acids are all increased the relative increase of triglyceride is
greater than that of cholesterol which is in turn greater than
that of phospholipid.   In fact plasma lysolecithin is selectively
decreased and quite dramatically (70,76).   Numerous other metabolic
parameters are altered during pregnancy and while the pathogenetic
mechanisms remain unresolved, the impression has evolved that
these changes are in some way related to a cholestatic condition
which, although variable  in intensity, is common to all pregnancies
and which interferes with the biliary secretion and enterohepatic
circulation of certain steroids, bile acids and other compounds
(67,68,71).   BSP has provided an experimental mirror which reflects
this phenomenon (16,64,72).   These studies have documented a
marked increase in the uptake and storage of BSP, a marked increase
in the regurgitation of the dye from the liver back to plasma and

a marked reduction in the biliary secretion of the dye.   These
changes are not accounted for by increased uptake in extrahepatic
tissues, differences in plasma concentration, differences in
plasma protein binding, increased hepatic mass, increased intracellular binding, or major changes in the conjugation of BSP by
the liver.   Rather, they appear to be due to an increased capacity
of each hepatocellular unit and to cholestasis which is, presumably,
hormone mediated.

## II.   Effect of pregnancy on biliary lipids

The literature concerning the changes in biliary lipids during
pregnancy is well below the critical micellar concentration.   There
are no good data on biliary lipids in the pregnant human.

Following up observations during the early years of oral
cholecystography involving failure to visualise the gall bladder
of pregnant females (28), Riegel et al and Potter documented
gall bladder stasis and an increased concentration of cholesterol
and decreased concentration of bile acids in the thick tarry viscous
bile of patients undergoing delivery by Caesarian section (58,60,61).
Apart from inadequate methodology, these early studies featured a
complete lack of controls.   There was apparently no further
interest in the subject until 1960 when Large et al, using better
methods and some, if still inadequate, controls also studied
pregnancy bile obtained at Caesarian section (46).   In 28 subjects
they found no significant differences from normal in the cholesterol,
phospholipid and total cholic acid concentration of the bile.

Unable to take a sufficiently aggressive approach to the human
model, investigators turned to other animals.   Holzbach et al in
1971 demonstrated that the only significant change in biliary
lipids during pregnancy in the guinea pig was an increased concentration of bile acids (32).   And even this observation was significant
with a $\underline{P}$ value of only 0.05.

In another rodent study Johnson and Kalant found no significant
changes in the concentration of total bile acids, phospholipids and
cholesterol or in the bile acid composition of the gall bladder bile
of pregnant rabbits (34).

The influence of pregnancy on the biliary lipids of rats has
been studied in our laboratory.   Five groups of female rats were
studied: virgin Wistar rats; those pregnant 1-2 weeks; those
pregnant 2-3 weeks; those post-partum 1 week; and those post-
partum 2 weeks (Table 1).   There were at least 5 animals in each
group and although the pregnant rats were somewhat heavier the
variation in body weights between the 5 groups was not significant.
These animals were fasted overnight and their bile ducts cannulated
under ether anaesthesia.   Bile was collected for the 5 hours

TABLE 1

| | GROUP | | BODY WT g | BILE FLOW 0-5 h ml/hour |
|---|---|---|---|---|
| A | Virgin Females | 6 | 265 | 0.82 |
| B | Pregnant 1-2 wk | 6 | 308 | 0.85 |
| C | Pregnant 2-3 wk | 14 | 316 | 0.80 |
| D | Postpartum 1 wk | 8 | 295 | 0.75 |
| E | Postpartum 2 wk | 5 | 296 | 0.60* |

*$\underline{P} < 0.05$

following the creation of a biliary fistula and its lipid content analysed by standard methods (79).

When expressed on a concentration basis the data revealed a marked decrease in the total biliary lipids in the late partum and early postpartum groups, a decrease accounted for entirely by the decreased biliary secretion of bile acids conjugated with taurine, Table 2.

TABLE 2

BILIARY   LIPIDS

$\mu$mole/ml

| GROUP | A | B | C | D | E |
|---|---|---|---|---|---|
| Cholesterol | 0.23 | 0.24 | $0.35^1$ | 0.37 | $0.52^2$ |
| Phospholipids | 3.82 | 3.14 | 3.21 | 3.84 | 4.58 |
| Bile Acids | | | | | |
| Glycine | 2.04 | 1.63 | 2.67 | 2.08 | 2.04 |
| Taurine | 16.41 | 11.99 | $6.25^2$ | $9.47^1$ | 10.68 |
| Total Lipids | 22.55 | 17.00 | $12.48^2$ | $15.76^1$ | 17.82 |

$^1\underline{P} < 0.05$                    $^2\underline{P} < 0.001$

TABLE 3

BILIARY LIPIDS

molar %

| GROUP | A | B | C | D | E |
|-------|---|---|---|---|---|
| Cholesterol | 1 | 2 | $3^3$ | $5^1$ | $3^1$ |
| Phospholipids | 17 | 18 | $26^2$ | 22 | $26^2$ |
| Bile Acids | 82 | 80 | $71^3$ | $73^3$ | $71^3$ |

$^1\underline{p} < 0.01$　　　$^2\underline{p} < 0.002$　　　$^3\underline{p} < 0.001$

On a molar percent basis the biliary bile acids were significantly reduced in the later pregnant and both postpartum groups, Table 3. It appears therefore that pregnancy in the rat is associated with an absolute and relative reduction in biliary bile acids and specifically of taurine conjugated bile acids.

Table 4 presents the bile acid composition of the bile on a molar percent basis. Concentrating on the later pregnant group, it is clear that cholic acid, deoxycholic acid and β-muricholic acid are all reduced during pregnancy. Chenodeoxycholic acid and lithocholic acid are both increased. Keto bile acids, normally present only in trace amounts, are also increased during pregnancy. Based on experimental evidence from various sources, including our own with the intrahepatic cholestasis induced by lithocholic and chenodeoxycholic acids in the isolated perfused liver of the female rat, we think that this shift towards lithocholic and chenodeoxycholic acids favours the development of intrahepatic cholestasis (23,24,52).

The size of the bile acid pool was then studied. Twelve rats, 6 virgin and 6 pregnant 2-3 weeks, were fasted overnight and anaesthetised with diethyl ether. As much blood as possible was obtained by aortic puncture, and the liver, the entire gastrointestinal tract and the uterine contents of the pregnancy group, were harvested. The bile acids of the various tissues were extracted and the recovery of bile acids on the basis of the cholyl-[14]C-24-glycine internal standard added to the original homogenates was always over 90%.

TABLE 4

BILIARY  BILE  ACIDS

Molar %

| GROUP | A | B | C | D | E |
|-------|---|---|---|---|---|
| CA | 71 | 65 | $60^1$ | 64 | 69 |
| β–MURI | 2 | 2 | $1^1$ | $1^1$ | – |
| CDCA | 11 | $16^1$ | $18^2$ | $17^1$ | 11 |
| HYO–URSO | 5 | 4 | 5 | 6 | 9 |
| DOCA | 9 | 8 | $6^1$ | 7 | 7 |
| LCA | 1 | 2 | $4^2$ | 3 | 3 |
| KETO | 1 | $3^2$ | $6^2$ | $2^1$ | 1 |

$^1 \underline{p} < 0.05$          $^2 \underline{p} < 0.001$

Although there is a significant increase in that portion of
the bile acid pool which is in the blood and liver during pregnancy,
the reduced biliary secretion of bile acids is associated with a
very marked reduction in the total bile acid pool, Table 5.
The uterine contents did not contain a significant amount of bile
acid.

TABLE 5

BILE ACID POOLS OF FEMALE RATS

μmoles

|  | VIRGIN | PREGNANT (2–3 wk) |
|--|--------|-------------------|
| Blood (15ml/rat) | 0.45 | $0.72^1$ |
| Liver | 2.57 | $3.34^1$ |
| Intestinal Tract | 127.15 | $60.81^1$ |
| Total | 130.35 | $64.87^1$ |

$^1 \underline{p} < 0.001$          n = 6

TABLE   6

LIVER BILE ACIDS OF FEMALE RATS

nmoles/g wet wt

| | VIRGIN[1] | PREGNANT[1] (2-3 wk) |
|---|---|---|
| CA | 228 | $151^2$ |
| β-MURI | 8 | 4 |
| CDCA | 38 | $69^2$ |
| HYO-URSO | 22 | 38 |
| DOCA | 20 | 18 |
| LCA | 6 | $15^3$ |
| KETO | - | $12^2$ |
| TOTAL | 331 | 307 |

[1]$n = 6$    [2]$\underline{P} < 0.001$    [3]$\underline{P} < 0.02$

During pregnancy liver weight increases but this is not associated with any change in the total bile acid concentration, Table 6.    As in the case of the total pool the hepatic concentration of cholic acid is reduced while that of chenodeoxycholic acid, lithocholic acid and the keto bile acids is increased.

Pregnancy is also associated with hypervolemia but the concentration of total bile acids in the blood is actually increased in pregnancy, Table 7.

In summary, we found that pregnancy in the rat is associated with a reduced biliary secretion of lipids which is entirely due to a reduction in the biliary secretion of taurine conjugated bile acids and more specifically to the reduced biliary secretion of taurine conjugates of cholic, deoxycholic and β-muricholic acids.    The biliary secretion of the other bile acids is maintained or even increased.    This reduced biliary secretion of bile acids is associated with a marked reduction in the total bile acid pool, a reduction which is nevertheless associated with a normal concentration of total bile acids in the liver and an increased concentration of total bile acids in the blood.    It is of interest in this regard that Watanabe has recently reported that estradiol treatment of rats can result in decreased biliary secretion of bile acids.    At low doses only cholic acid secretion is reduced, that of chenodeoxycholic acid being actually increased (77).

TABLE 7

BLOOD BILE ACIDS OF FEMALE RATS

nmoles %

| | VIRGIN[1] | PREGNANT[1] (2-3 wk) |
|---|---|---|
| CA | 2060 | 2290 |
| β-MURI | 70 | 40 |
| CDCA | 340 | 1060[2] |
| HYO-URSO | 230 | 620[3] |
| DOCA | 270 | 350 |
| LCA | 50 | 250[3] |
| KETO | - | 180[2] |
| TOTAL | 2970 | 4780[3] |

[1] $n = 6$    [2] $\underline{P} < 0.001$    [3] $\underline{P} < 0.01$

Martin and his colleagues considered the effect of pregnancy on the biliary lipids of the Rhesus monkey, a species in which the plasma cholesterol, phospholipids and total lipids are actually decreased during pregnancy (48). In 4 animals they found no significant changes in the concentration of biliary cholesterol, phospholipids and total lipids during pregnancy.

On the other hand, another report from this same group concerned a Rhesus monkey who was subjected to seven laparotomies for bile samples in association with her first pregnancy and who was found to have eleven small "naturally occurring" gallstones when killed during the course of another experiment "several months later" (49). On a molar percent basis biliary cholesterol and phospholipids increased and bile acids decreased during the course of her pregnancy.

McSherry, Javitt et al reported that pregnant baboons have a significantly reduced concentration of bile acids in the gall bladder bile as the only change in the major lipid fractions of either gall bladder or hepatic bile (50). This same group also studied bile acid kinetics in the baboon (18). They found that pregnancy caused bile acid stasis with a reduced synthesis rate of both cholic and chenodeoxycholic acids and with a significant reduction in the chenodeoxycholic acid pool. In other words,

they found bile acid stasis and altered bile acid metabolism
during pregnancy in this species.

In summary, 5 groups of investigators have studied the changes
in biliary lipids during pregnancy in 5 different animals.    The
results are conflicting of course.    But changes in biliary lipids
do occur during pregnancy and these changes probably involve at
least a reduction in bile acid secretion.    Why do they occur?

## III.   Effect of female sex hormones on the liver

It is increasingly clear that cholestatic jaundice of pregnancy
merely represents one end of the spectrum of pregnancy - the overt
end - and that cholestasis is a feature of all pregnancies.
Furthermore it appears that this pregnancy-induced interference
with hepatic secretion is hormone and more specifically estrogen
mediated (36,37,38,71).

Although we don't really know what causes what, it is reasonable
to assume that the large quantities of estrogens and progestins
produced by the feto-placental unit and secreted into the maternal
circulation lead to altered hepatic function in the mother.

It is known that the ultimate source of the estrogen and
progesterone produced by the feto-placental unit is maternal
cholesterol (37).

It is known that large amounts of C-19 and C-21 neutral
steroids are secreted into the bile during pregnancy (43,44,57).
The concentration of these steroids, primarily sulphated
progesterone metabolites, ranges from 60-70 mg%.    Adlercreutz
and his associates have documented changes in the hepatic metabolism
of estrogens and a large increase in their biliary secretion during
pregnancy (2).

What is the evidence that leads one to believe that these
steroids are involved in the pathogenesis of the cholestasis which
is the hall-mark of the altered hepatic function in pregnancy?

It is known that in man estrogens lead to cholestatic phenomena,
with decreased clearance of bilirubin from plasma (53), increased
serum alkaline phosphatase (53) and increased hepatic storage and
reduced biliary secretion of BSP (38,40,53,55).    There have been
several studies in experimental animals documenting estrogen induced
cholestasis with reduced bile flow (39), reduced biliary bile acid
secretion rates (30,55,77), increased back diffusion of substrates
from the bile to plasma (26), etc.

Lynn et al demonstrated estrogen induced changes in the relative composition of the bile in primates (47). Using Rhesus monkeys they found that Estriol reduced bile volume, reduced bile acid secretion and produced marked changes in the lipid composition of the bile with increased cholesterol and phospholipids and decreased bile acids.

The above observations in the human have been reinforced by studies with oral contraceptives (9,68,69). All users of oral contraceptives have increased bromsulphthalein retention (9) and oral contraceptives have been shown repeatedly to be capable of reproducing the clinical and biochemical features of overt cholestasis of pregnancy in those subjects who have previously experienced this problem (20,29,41,59,68,69). One of these studies also provided information on the influence of oral contraceptives on biliary lipids in man (29). These authors studied the T-tube bile of a patient with a past history of overt cholestasis of pregnancy who underwent cholecystectomy and was thereafter given 0.5 mg of ethinyl estradiol twice daily. After 4 days of this treatment she developed clinical evidence of cholestasis with pruritus, increased serum bilirubin, SGOT and alkaline phosphatase, a reduction in bile flow and a delayed biliary excretion of BSP. In association with these changes, Glenn and McSherry found increased biliary concentrations of cholesterol, phospholipids, triglycerides and total lipids.

Another study in man has suggested that oral contraceptives cause a significant rise in biliary cholesterol concentration and a consistent decrease in the concentration, pool size and synthesis rates of bile acids (56,57). The subjects involved were in a post-cholecystectomy state and studied by means of a cystic duct catheter.

These observations have been complemented by studies documenting cholestasis and altered liver function induced by oral contraceptive steroids in experimental animals (22,31). It must be stated however that conflicting experimental data are easily come by. For example, McSherry et al reported that 10 mg of intravenously administered Premarin, a mixture of conjugated equine estrogens, failed to change bile volume or the biliary concentrations of cholesterol, phospholipids and bile acids over a 48-hour period of observation in 3 nonpregnant baboons (51).

And finally there have been the several studies documenting the marked fall in the biliary concentrations of all estrogens and progestins during the development of overt cholestasis of pregnancy (3,6,35,45). Altered metabolism of these steroids associated with the cholestasis has provided evidence that altered hepatocellular function is playing a role along with the obvious impairment of the enterohepatic circulation of the steroids (4,10, 43,65).

Conclusions

        Current evidence suggests that the female sex hormones act
on the liver cells of all subjects and that the underlying theme
of this action is cholestasis (68,69).   As part and parcel of
this cholestasis or as independent metabolic phenomena, the
estrogens, and possibly the less extensively studied progestins,
influence the synthesis and presumably the biliary secretion of
cholesterol, phospholipids and bile acids (7,15,17,19,54,73,74,
77,78).   Sex differences in the phospholipid concentration of the
hepatic bile of man have been established (75), and significant
sex differences in the bile acid concentration and composition
of gall bladder bile in the human have been documented (25).
Einarsson et al have reported sex differences in bile acid synthesis
in man (21).   Therefore, sex differences in biliary lipids in
the human do exist.   They are presumably hormone mediated and
they may well be exaggerated during pregnancy.

        It is likely therefore that the female sex hormones modify
the composition of bile.   But their relationship to the effects
of pregnancy on the liver still must be considered presumptive.
There are too many gaps in our knowledge, in our understanding
of hormone metabolism, of lipid metabolism and of the factors which
control the biliary secretion of lipids (12,63,66).   There is an
obvious but an obviously complex interaction  between female
sex hormones, bile acids, cholesterol, phospholipids and the liver,
Figure 1 (1,12,15,54,66,78).   How this interaction is involved
in the changes in biliary lipids during pregnancy in the human
has not yet been documented.

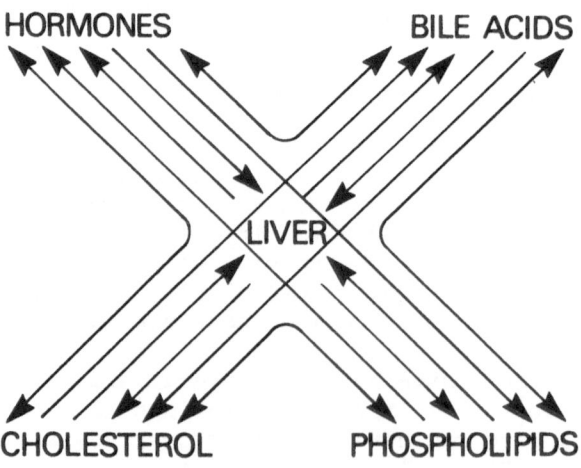

Figure 1

REFERENCES

1.  ADLERCREUTZ H:  Hepatic metabolism of estrogens in health
    and disease.  New Eng J Med 290:  1081-1083, 1974.

2.  ADLERCREUTZ H, ERVAST HS, TENHUNEN A, et al:  Gas chromato-
    graphic and mass spectrometric studies on oestrogens in
    bile:  Part I.  Pregnant women.  Acta Endocrinol 73:
    543-554,  1973.

3.  ADLERCREUTZ H, LUUKKAINEN T:  Biochemical and clinical aspects
    of the enterohepatic circulation of oestrogens.
    Acta Endocrinol, Suppl 124:  101-140,  1967.

4.  ADLERCREUTZ H, SVANBORG A, ANBERG A:  Recurrent jaundice in
    pregnancy.  II.  A study of the estrogens and their
    conjugation in late pregnancy.  Amer J Med 42:  341-347, 1967.

5.  ADLERCREUTZ H, TENHUNEN R:  Some aspects of the interaction
    between natural and synthetic female sex hormones and the
    liver.  Amer J Med 49:  630-648,  1970.

6.  ADLERCREUTZ H, TIKKANEN MJ, WICHMANN K, et al:  Recurrent
    jaundice in pregnancy.  IV.  Quantitative determination of
    urinary and biliary estrogens, including studies in
    pruritus gravidarum.  J Clin Endocrinol Metab 38: 51-57, 1974.

7.  ALFIN-SLATER RB, AFTERGOOD L:  Lipids and the pill.
    Lipids 6:  693-705,  1971.

8.  ALVAREZ RR, GAISER DF, SIMKINS DM, et al:  Serial studies
    of serum lipids in normal human pregnancy.  Amer J Obstet
    & Gynecol 77:  743-758,  1959.

9.  ARIAS IM:  Some effects of contraceptive steroids on hepatic
    function in normal women and in patients with acquired and
    inheritable defects in hepatic excretory function.
    In Metabolic effects of gonadal hormones and contraceptive
    steroids.  Eds HA Salhanick, DM Kipnis, RL Vande Wiele.
    Plenum Press, N.Y., 1969.  pp. 30-39.

10. BACK P, SJOVALL J, SJOVALL K:  Monohydroxy bile acids in
    plasma in intrahepatic cholestasis of pregnancy.  Identifica-
    tion by computerized gas chromatography - mass spectrometry.
    Medical Biology 52:  31-38,  1974.

11. BECKER H, BERLE P, WALLE A, et al:  Influence of late gestation
    and early puerperium on lipid and carbohydrate metabolism in
    normal females.  Acta Endocrinol 67:  570-576,  1971.

12. BEKERSKY I, MOSBACH EH:  Effect of hormones on bile acid
    metabolism.  In The Bile Acids, vol. 2.  Ed PP Nair,
    D Kritchevsky.  Plenum Press, N.Y., 1973. pp. 249-257.

13. BREWER DW, AUBRY RH:  The Physiology of Pregnancy.  Clinical
    pathologic correlations.  Part 2.  Postgrad Med 53:  221-226,
    1973.

14. BURT RL:  Plasma nonesterified fatty acids in normal pregnancy
    and the puerperium.  Obstet & Gynecol 15:  460-464, 1960.

15. CAHLIN E, JONSSON H, NILSSON S, et al:  Synthesis of phospho-
    lipids and triglycerides in human liver slices.  III.
    Influence of bile acids, choline and linoleic acid.
    Scand J Clin Lab Invest 29:  109-114,  1972.

16. COMBES B, SHIBATA H, ADAMS R, et al:  Alterations in sulfo-
    bromophthalein sodium - removal mechanisms from blood during
    normal pregnancy.  J Clin Invest 42:  1431-1442, 1963.

17. DEAN PD, WHITEHOUSE MW:  Inhibition of hepatic sterol
    oxidation by cholanic (bile) acids and their conjugates.
    Biochim Biophys Acta 137:  328-334, 1967.

18. DEITRICK JE, McSHERRY CK, JAVITT NB, et al:  Bile salt
    kinetics in the pregnant baboon:  a new model for the
    study of gallbladder function.  Gastroenterology 65:
    536,  1973.

19. DESPOPOULOS A:  Hepatic and renal excretory metabolism of
    bile salts:  a background for understanding steroid-
    induced cholestasis.  J Pharmacol Exp Therap 176:
    273-283,  1971.

20. DRILL VA:  Benign cholestatic jaundice of pregnancy and
    benign cholestatic jaundice from oral contraceptives.
    Amer J Obstet Gynecol 119:  165-174,  1974.

21. EINARSSON K, HELLSTROM K, KALLNER M:  Bile acid kinetics in
    relation to sex, serum lipids, body weights and gallbladder
    disease in patients with various types of hyperlipoprotein-
    emia.  J Clin Invest 54:  1301-1311, 1974.

22. FAHIM MS, HALL DG:  Effect of ovarian steroids on hepatic
    metabolism.  I. Progesterone.  Amer J Obstet & Gynecol 106:
    183-186,  1970.

23. FISHER MM, MAGNUSSON R, MIYAI K:  Bile acid metabolism in
    mammals. I. Bile acid-induced intrahepatic cholestasis.
    Lab Invest 25:  88-91, 1971.

24. FISHER MM, MAGNUSSON R, PHILLIPS MJ et al: Bile acid metabolism in mammals. IV. Sex difference in chenodeoxycholic acid metabolism in the rat. Lab Invest 27: 254-262, 1972.

25. FISHER MM, YOUSEF IM: Sex differences in the bile acid composition of human bile: studies in patients with and without gallstones. Can Med Assoc J 109: 190-193, 1973.

26. FORKER EL: The effect of estrogen on bile formation in the rat. J Clin Invest 48: 654-663, 1969.

27. GEALL MG, WEBB MJ: Liver disease in pregnancy. Med Clin NA 58: 817-822, 1974.

28. GERDES MM, BOYDEN EA: The rate of emptying of the human gall bladder in pregnancy. Surgery, Gynecol & Obstet 66: 145-156, 1938.

29. GLENN F, McSHERRY CK: Pregnancy, cholesterol metabolism and gallstones. Ann Surg 169: 712-723, 1969.

30. HARKAVY M, JAVITT NB: Effect of ethynyl estradiol on hepatic excretory function of the rat. In Metabolic effects of gonadal hormones and contraceptive steroids. Eds HA Salhanick, DM Kipnis, RL Vande Wiele. Plenum Press, N.Y.,1969. pp.11-18.

31. HEIKEL TA, LATHE GH: The effect of oral contraceptive steroids on bile secretion and bilirubin Tm in rats. Br J Pharmac 38: 593-601, 1970.

32. HOLZBACH RT, MARSH ME, HALLBERG MC: The effect of pregnancy on lipid composition of guinea pig gallbladder bile. Gastroenterology 60: 288-293, 1971.

33. HYTTEN FE, LEITCH I: The physiology of human pregnancy. Blackwell Scientific Publications, Oxford, London, Edinburgh, 1971. pp. 176-178.

34. JOHNSON J, KALANT N: Bile composition in the pregnant rabbit. Amer J Dig Dis 17: 1-5, 1972.

35. JOHNSON P: Studies in cholestasis of pregnancy with special reference to lipids and lipoproteins. Acta Obstet Gynecol Scand Suppl 27: 1-75, 1973.

36. KAPPAS A: Studies in endocrine pharmacology. Biologic actions of some natural steroids on the liver. New Eng J Med 278: 378-384, 1968.

37.  KELLIE AE:  The pharmacology of the estrogens.
     Ann Rev Pharmacol 11:  97-112,  1971.

38.  KREEK MJ:  Cholestasis of pregnancy and during ethinyl estradiol
     administration in the human and rat.  In Metabolic effects of
     gonadal hormones and contraceptive steroids.  Eds HA Salhanik,
     DM Kipnis, RL Vande Wiele.  Plenum Press, N.Y. 1969.  pp.40-58.

39.  KREEK MJ, PETERSON RE, SLEISENGER MH, et al:  Effects of
     ethinylestradiol-induced cholestasis on bile flow and biliary
     excretion of estradiol and estradiol glucuronide by the rat.
     Proc Soc Exp Biol Med 131:  646-650, 1969.

40.  KREEK MJ, SLEISENGER MH:  Estrogen induced cholestasis due to
     endogenous and exogenous hormones.  Scand J Gastroent Suppl 7:
     123-131,  1970.

41.  KREEK MJ, SLEISENGER MH, JEFFRIES GH:  Recurrent cholestatic
     jaundice of pregnancy with demonstrated estrogen sensitivity.
     Amer J Med 43:  795-803,  1967.

42.  KREEK MJ, WESER E, SLEISENGER MH, et al:  Idiopathic chole-
     stasis of pregnancy.  The response to challenge with the
     synthetic estrogen, ethinyl estradiol.  New Eng J Med 277:
     1391-1395,  1967.

43.  LAATIKAINEN T:  Excretion of neutral steroid hormones in
     human bile.  Ann Clin Res 2:  Suppl 5, 1-28, 1970.

44.  LAATIKAINEN T, KARJALAINEN O:  Excretion of conjugates of
     neutral steroids in human bile during late pregnancy.
     Acta Endocrinol 69:  775-788,  1972.

45.  LAATIKAINEN T, KARJALAINEN O, JANNE O:  Excretion of progest-
     erone metabolites in urine and bile of  pregnant women with
     intrahepatic cholestasis.  J Steroid Biochem 4:  641-648,
     1973.

46.  LARGE AM, JOHNSTON CG, KATSUKI T, et al:  Gallstones and
     pregnancy:  the composition of gallbladder bile in the
     pregnant woman at term.  Amer J Med Sci 239:  713-720, 1960.

47.  LYNN J, WILLIAMS L, O'BRIEN J, et al:  Effects of estrogen
     upon bile:  implications with respect to gallstone formation.
     Ann Surg 178:  514-524,  1973.

48.  MARTIN DE, WOLF RC, MEYER RK:  The effects of pregnancy on
     biliary lipids in Rhesus monkeys.  Proc Soc Exp Biol Med 139:
     115-117,  1972.

49.  MARTIN DE, WOLF RC, HOUSER WD: Naturally occurring cholelithiasis in a Rhesus monkey and its effects on plasma and biliary lipid concentrations. Am J Vet Res 34: 971-974, 1973.

50.  McSHERRY CK, JAVITT NB, CARVALHO JM, et al: Cholesterol gallstones and the chemical composition of bile in baboons. Ann Surg 173: 569-577, 1971.

51.  McSHERRY CK, MORRISSEY KP, JAVITT NB, et al: Role of hepatic bile composition in gallstone formation in baboons. Ann Surg 178: 669-675, 1973.

52.  MIYAI K, PRICE VM, FISHER MM: Bile acid metabolism in mammals. Ultrastructural studies on the intrahepatic cholestasis induced by lithocholic and chenodeoxycholic acids in the rat. Lab Invest 24: 292-302, 1971.

53.  MUELLER MN, KAPPAS A: Estrogen pharmacology. I. The influence of estradiol and estriol on hepatic disposal of sulfo-bromophthalein (BSP) in man. J Clin Invest 43: 1905-1914, 1964.

54.  NILSSON S: Synthesis and secretion of biliary phospholipids in man. Acta Chir Scand Suppl 405: 1-38, 1970.

55.  PALMER RH, GALLAGHER TF, MUELLER MN, et al: The effect of natural and synthetic estrogens on the excretion of BSP by the liver. In Metabolic effects of gonadal hormones and contraceptive steroids. Eds HA Salhanick, DM Kipnis, RL Vande Wiele. Plenum Press, NY, 1969. pp. 19-29.

56.  PERTSEMLIDIS D, PANVELIWALLA D, KIMBALL A: Effects of clofibrate and of oral contraceptives on biliary lipid composition and bile acid kinetics in man. Gastroenterology 64: 782, 1973.

57.  PERTSEMLIDIS D, PANVELIWALLA D, AHRENS EH: Effects of clofibrate and of an estrogen-progestin combination on fasting biliary lipids and cholic acid kinetics in man. Gastroenterology 66: 565-573, 1974.

58.  POTTER MG: Observations of the gallbladder and bile during pregnancy at term. J Amer Med Assoc 106: 1070-1074, 1936.

59.  RANNEVIK G, JEPPSSON S, KULLANDER S: Effect of oral contraceptives on the liver in women with recurrent cholestasis (hepatoses) during previous pregnancies. J Obstet Gynaecol Br Commonw 79: 1128-1136, 1972.

60.  RIEGEL C, RAVDIN IS, MORRISON PJ, et al:  Studies of gall-
     bladder function. XI. The composition of the gallbladder
     bile in pregnancy.  J Amer Med Assoc 105:  1343-1344, 1935.

61.  RIEGEL C, RAVDIN IS, JOHNSTON CG, et al:  Studies of gall-
     bladder function. XIII. The composition of the gallbladder
     bile and calculi in gallbladder disease.
     Surgery Gynecol & Obstet 62:  933-940,  1936.

62.  SAMSIOE G, JOHNSON P, GUSTAFSON A:  Aspects of the pathogenesis
     of cholestasis of pregnancy with reference to the serum lipid
     abnormalities.  Scand J Gastroent 10:  1-4,  1975.

63.  SCHERSTEN T:  Formation of lithogenic bile in man.
     Digestion 9:  540-553,  1973.

64.  SHAW HM, HEATH T:  Effect of pregnancy on the excretion of
     sulphobromophthalein in bile.  Aust J Biol Sci 25: 1101-1104,
     1972.

65.  SJOVALL J, SJOVALL K:  Steroid sulphates in plasma from
     pregnant women with pruritus and elevated plasma bile acid
     levels.  Ann Clin Res 2:  321-338,  1970.

66.  SMITH RL:  Biliary excretion and hepatotoxicity of contra-
     ceptive steroids.  Acta Endocrinol Suppl 185:  149-168, 1974.

67.  SOFFER LJ:  Bilirubin  excretion as a test for liver function
     during normal pregnancy.  Bull Johns Hopkins Hospital 52:
     365-375,  1933.

68.  SONG CS, KAPPAS A:  The influence of estrogens, progestins,
     and pregnancy on the liver.  Vitamins and Hormones 26:
     147-195,  1968.

69.  SONG CS, RIFKIND AB, GILLETTE PN, et al:  Hormones and the
     liver.  Am J Obstet & Gynecol 105:  813-847,  1969.

70.  SVANBORG A, VIKROT O:  Plasma lipid fractions, including
     individual phospholipids, at various stages of pregnancy.
     Acta Med Scand 178:  615-630,  1965.

71.  TAYLOR W:  The excretion  of steroid hormone metabolites in
     bile and feces.  Vitamins and Hormones 29:  201-285, 1971.

72.  TINDALL VR, BEAZLEY JM:  An assessment of changes in liver
     function during normal pregnancy - using a modified
     bromsulphthalein test. J Obstet Gynecol 72: 717-737,  1965.

73. UCHIDA K, NOMURA Y, KADOWAKI M, et al: Effects of estradiol, dietary cholesterol and 1-thyroxine on biliary bile acid composition and secretory rate, and on plasma, liver and bile cholesterol levels in rats. Endocrinol Japon 17: 107-121, 1970.

74. UCHIDA K, NOMURA Y, KADOWAKI M, et al: Stimulative and inhibitive effects of estrogen on cholesterol synthesis in rats. Endocrinol Japon 20: 129-134, 1973.

75. VAN DER LINDEN W, NORMAN A: Composition of human hepatic bile. Acta Chir Scand 133: 307-313, 1967.

76. VIKROT O: Quantitative determination of plasma phospholipids in pregnant and nonpregnant women, with special reference to lysolecithin. Acta Med Scand 175: 443, 1964.

77. WATANABE H: Effect of 17α-ethinylestradiol on biliary excretion of bile acids. Biochim Biophys Acta 399: 79-84, 1975.

78. YOUNG D: Estradiol- and testosterone-induced alterations in phosphatidylcholine and triglyceride synthesis in hepatic endoplasmic reticulum. J Lipid Res 12: 590-595, 1971.

79. YOUSEF IM, FISHER MM: Influence of pregnancy on the bile acid pool of rats. Clin Res 21: 1036, 1973.

80. YOUSEF IM, KAKIS G, FISHER MM: Bile acid metabolism in mammals. III. Sex difference in the bile acid composition of rat bile. Can J Biochem 50: 402-408, 1972.

DISCUSSION OF COMMENTARY BY M.M. FISHER

<u>Arias</u>:    This was an extraordinary and provocative presentation of
an area which has not been fully explored.    In our studies of
B.S.P. metabolism in normal women taking oestrogen-containing
oral contraceptives, we could not demonstrate that there is
normally a retention of B.S.P. in the plasma of these women, but
there was a significant reduction in the Tm.    The second comment
I have is perhaps more meaningful, and is concerned with the
nature of cholestasis as reflected by the model of the mechanism
whereby hormones may influence the cholestatic state.    Although
no data seems to be available on this, it would seem to be very
unlikely that oestrogens produce an effect analogous, let us say,
to the administration of taurolithocholate in the rat when there
is an immediate cessation of bile flow.    All the studies seem to
have been carried out on rats or women taking these agents over a
relatively prolonged period;    that is days rather than hours.
This raises the question of the multiple effects of oestrogens on
other aspects of the cell.    You mentioned protein synthesis.
However, it is important to bring into this context the question
of the plasma membrane of the liver cell, particularly the bile
canalicular component of that membrane.    What is the origin of
this membrane;    what is its composition and its control?    There
is very limited information about this.    Some years ago we
isolated this fraction from normal rat liver, from animals given
ethynyl oestradiol and from animals which had had their bile duct
ligated for a short time.    The composition of the membrane showed
minor changes in phospholipids measured by a rather crude method.
However, there were some interesting changes in the ATPase
concentrations in the membrane fraction, particularly the magnesium-
ATPase.    This decreased while the alkaline phosphate increased.

    Then we studied pulse-labelling with amino acids using a double
isotope technique, and we separated the proteins after solubilisation of the membranes.    We could not show any change in the overall
turnover rate of the pulse-labelled proteins.    More recently we
have put these protein fractions on electrophoretic gels and so
separated protein moieties more precisely than could be achieved
with columns containing detergent.    It is quite obvious that
there are quite dramatic changes in the pulse-labelling patterns
and the isotope ratios of different protein constituents of this

rather impure membrane fraction. It should be remembered that
the canalicular membrane contains proteins and lipids which are
in highly different states of differential turnover. The net
half-life for pulse-labelled protein in the rat plasma membrane
is of the order of 1.5 days, but there are enormous variations in
the half-lives of the individual protein components. The same
effect has been observed for the lipid moieties.

So we are dealing with a membrane which may look the same,
but has enormously different rates of incorporation and breakdown
of proteins and lipids. This produces a biological complexity
which I feel still defies explanation.

In experimental cholestasis, the differential relationships
of the proteins change very dramatically, but I am not at all
sure what this means. So my justification for making such a long
comment is to draw attention to the fact that what comes out into
the bile may be quite secondary to phenomena which are occurring
in the canalicular transport mechanism. Also I want to focus
attention on this problem, so that at our next conference there
may be a lot of information about the nature of the membrane, its
source and its control. It seems to me that the oestrogen-type
model offers a unique system for studying this problem.

Fisher: That was a very useful comment. We have not tried to
approach the basic mechanism by which oestrogen induces its effect,
but I suspect that oestrogens act in a much more subtle and
complicated way than other cholestatic agents.

Strandvik: I just want to draw attention to the fact that the
pregnant woman has another component which has been overlooked
here. I refer, of course, to the fetus itself. The maternal
hormones could act on the fetal liver, but I am not so sure that
fetal hormones could act on the maternal liver. We know very
little about the role of the human placenta in this respect.
However, we do know that the fetus produces bile very early in
pregnancy, and in this bile chenodeoxycholic acid is the most
prominent bile acid. Also, newborn and premature infants have
a lot of $3\beta$-hydroxy-5-cholenoic acid which we know is cholestatic.
This acid is also found in the mother, and I wonder if we can be
sure that this acid is not coming from the fetus during abnormal
conditions.

Fisher: As far as I know, we are not at all sure.

Sjövall: We have studied serum bile acid sulphates in pregnant
women with intrahepatic cholestasis. Normal pregnant women have
normal bile acid values. The $3\beta$-hydroxy-5-cholenoic acid and
lithocholate are found in the sulphate fraction. The interesting

thing in that study was that the highest value for lithocholate
sulphate was found in a normal pregnant woman with no sign of
intrahepatic cholestasis.    However, she delivered a child who
developed a very severe jaundice about two days after birth.

Popjak:    Dr. Fisher's review emphasised the need for studies in
comparative biochemistry, and also emphasised that data from one
species do not necessarily apply to another.    I would like to
emphasise this by giving two other examples.    People tend to
think that pregnancy is generally associated with hyperlipaemia,
because this is so in man.    But apart from the Rhesus monkey
there are two other species, the rabbit and the guinea pig, in
which there is an extraordinary degree of hypolipaemia.    In
rabbits, during the second half of pregnancy, something suddenly
happens which causes plasma lipids to be almost completely wiped
out;   for example, total plasma cholesterol may be reduced to 5
to 10 mg per cent.    At the same time, there is an incredible
reduction in the ability of the maternal liver to utilize acetate
for cholesterol synthesis.    I assume from this that the HMG CoA-
reductase is reduced to about one per cent of its normal value,
but the fetal liver is quite active at this time.    So the pregnant
rabbit and guinea pit would be well worth studying.

Low-beer:    I want to emphasise one practical aspect of the effect
of hormones on bile which concerns some of us here.    That is,
that there may be variations in bile composition during the
menstrual cycle, and we are looking at this at the moment.    Our
results are too few for us to comment on at the moment, but I
would stress that we should obtain bile from the same time in the
menstrual cycle when we are looking at the effects of various
agents on bile composition.

Popper:    The cholestatic effects of oestrogen- and androgen-like
steroids has many important aspects.    Many of the metabolites of
these steroids are excreted as organic anions and so could act as
competitive inhibitors for excretion.    Also, some of these
steroids have a very peculiar steric configuration, which may
vary from compound to compound.    It has been suggested that this
peculiar steric configuration could have an effect on biliary
secretion by actions on the plasma membrane.    So there are three
possible mechanisms:   the one Dr. Arias mentioned, the organic
anion effect and the steric configuration.

Fisher:    I do not know of any information about the possibility
that there is an organic anion, competitive inhibition effect.
There have been some studies with oestradiol and oestriol, but
the progestins seem to have been completely neglected.

Ostrow:    You referred to changes in lipids, but you did not

mention whether or not there is the increased frequency of
gallstones in pregnancy.    The only thing I recall is that
patients who have had recurrent jaundice of pregnancy have an
unusually high frequency of gallstones when followed up about
20 years later.    Do you have any new information on this?

Fisher:    I think that this is still a highly controversial area;
that is why I did not deal with it in any depth.

Sjövall:    I want to comment on the stereochemical factors which
may be involved.    In intrahepatic cholestasis of pregnancy there
are enormously elevated plasma levels of sulphates of pregnane
derivatives which are presumably progesterone metabolites.    This
is very stereospecific.    Compounds with the $3\beta$-$5\alpha$-configuration
are not elevated at all, whereas the $3\alpha,5\beta$-compounds are elevated.
This latter configuration may be the toxic one, as it is in the
bile acids:  but the steroids are sulphated so we cannot comment
too much about that.    The $3\alpha,5\alpha$-epimers are also elevated.
Several of these compounds also appear in bile.    However, there
is never any correlation between the elevated levels of these
steroids and the elevation of bile acid levels which you see at
the same time.    So these steroids are excreted unrelated to the
bile acids.    In one case that we studied the steroid changes
were found 6 weeks before there was any sign of cholestasis or
elevation of bile acids.

# GENERAL DISCUSSION OF SESSION 4B

Lucy:   Arising from some thoughts I have had during this meeting I would like to make some suggestions about the possible mechanism by which bile may be secreted.   The suggestions I am putting forward represent an attempt to answer some of the problems we have been considering during the past few days.   For instance, how is it that bile salts can be secreted across the canalicular membrane without causing damage to the membrane?   I suggest that, in fact, the passage of bile salts does damage the canalicular membrane, and that is why phospholipids occur in bile.   The second point I want to consider is why the major phospholipid in bile is lecithin, whereas the canalicular membrane contains a lot of phospholipids other than lecithin.   Another question is, where does the lyso-lecithin in bile come from, and finally, why are the fatty acids present in the biliary lecithin different from those in the canalicular membrane lecithin?   To take the last question first, there is a well-known biochemical pathway which involves the degradation of lecithin and other phospholipids by phospholipases. It is possible to remove one or other of the fatty acids from lecithin to yield lysolecithin.   This can occur by the action of membrane-bound phospholipases.   We also know that there are membrane-bound reacylating enzymes which can put back fatty acids as their coenzyme A derivatives.   So these fatty acids will be reacted with lysolecithin to put back a different fatty acid to reacylate the lysolecithin to produce lecithin with a different fatty acid composition from the original lecithin broken down.

The essence of the suggestion I would like to put forward for consideration is the figure shown overleaf, with a summary of what I think may be important events in biliary secretion.

Ostrow:   There are several points I would like to raise about your interesting hypothesis.   One does not have to postulate that bile acids passing through the membrane would do any damage at all. Indeed, Dr. Hauton has suggested that they are already packaged in micelles before they reach the membrane.   This is also related to what Dr. Hofmann told us about the effects of bile acids on the colon.   Many studies have shown that if bile acids are interacting with very small amounts of cholesterol or bilirubin or other components of bile, one mole per 2000 moles of bile acid would

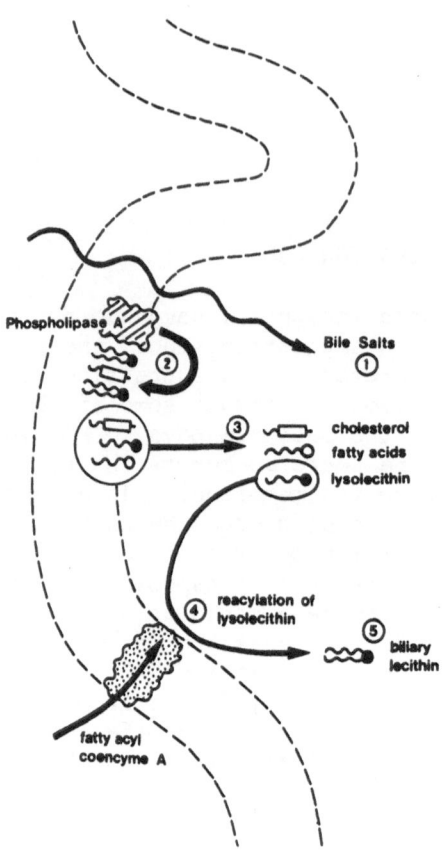

A diagrammatic illustration (not to scale) of possible mechanisms involved in the secretion of bile salts, cholesterol, fatty
acids, lecithin and lysolecithin into the biliary canaliculus.
During or following the secretion of bile salts (1), the structure
of the canalicular membrane is perturbed sufficiently to allow a
membrane-bound phospholipase A to degrade lecithin in the outer
half of the lipid bilayer to lysolecithin (2).   Lysolecithin
associated with membrane cholesterol, and fatty acids from the
degraded lecithin, leave the canalicular membrane and enter the
biliary canaliculus (3).   Most, but not all, of the released
lysolecithin is then reacylated to lecithin by a membrane-bound
enzyme, using fatty acids from the hepatocyte cytoplasm (differing
from those in the membrane) that are supplied as coenzyme A
derivatives and may traverse the canalicular membrane as esters of
carnitine (4).   The lecithin thus produced is released into the
canaliculus (5), where it is incorporated into mixed micelles with
bile salts and cholesterol.   (Thanks are due to Dr. U. Sleytr
for the preparation of this figure.)

produce an effect.   The damage produced is either markedly
decreased or completely abrogated.   In other words, if bile acids
are already tied up with phospholipids they are less likely to
attack phospholipids.   Therefore, one need not postulate any
damage if the micelles themselves could pass through the membrane.
So this is one alternative to your hypothesis.   The second point
is that the rate at which bile acids are secreted in bile is
extremely rapid, and I wonder if the turnover numbers of the
enzymes you mentioned are fast enough to account for the changes
that are seen in bile.   If your idea is correct one might expect
that the composition of the fatty acids in the lecithin might
change with the rate of bile acid excretion.   The third point is
that you indicated that lysolecithin is a good solubiliser of
cholesterol, but it is in fact less than half as effective as
lecithin in the presence of a 180 millimolar concentration of bile
acids in solubilising cholesterol.   However, if the fatty acids
are also included, the lysolecithin plus the released fatty acids
is as effective as lecithin itself as an amphiphile in the bile
acid-cholesterol micelle.

Lucy:   My reason for putting forward this hypothesis was in the
hope that it would stimulate more experimental work of the kind
you have mentioned.

Popper:   I think that the views of Professor Lucy and Dr. Ostrow
could be reconciled.   Under normal circumstances the plasma
membrane is always in a state of dynamic flux.   However, when
there is a trend towards the cholestatic situation, the process
which Professor Lucy has described could take place;  so that
process may possibly be in reserve to deal with the abnormal
situation.   There is some support for my suggestion.   Normally
we do not see any whirls, which we ascribe to phospholipids, in
the bile canaliculi, but one of the first signs of cholestasis is
the appearance of these membrane elements.   I assume that these
elements are present because the plasma membrane is being distorted.
So both views may be correct:  Dr. Ostrow's for the normal situation, and Professor Lucy's for the abnormal.

Haslewood:   It is an old story that there are a lot of fatty acids
in bile, but in fact analyses that we have done indicate that there
is very little fatty acid in bile.   This does not contradict
Professor Lucy's suggestion, but there is a more much serious
objection to his idea.   If he is right there should be some
relationship between the amount of bile salts and phospholipids
in bile.   But analyses of samples of human bile by others have
shown that this is not so.   In fact one sample contained 120 mg
per cent of cholesterol and plenty of bile salts, but no measurable
amount of phospholipid.

<u>Coleman</u>:   As I see it, the problem is this.   The bile salts have
to leave the cell either by moving down a concentration gradient
into the canaliculus, or, if they are going to end up in high
concentration in the canaliculus, they must be actively transported.
Available evidence suggests that active transport is involved.
This suggests that the bile salts are at a low concentration inside
the cell and are concentrated in the canaliculus.   If this concentration exceeds the critical micellar concentration the conditions
for mixed-micelle formation would now form.   I think that it is
at this stage that phospholipids might be withdrawn from the
canalicular membrane to enter the mixed micelle.   In support of
this concept I will say that we have presented micellar concentrations of bile salts to intact cells and to remove phospholipids
from their membranes without causing lysis.   These were model
experiments with erythrocytes.   A second piece of evidence is
that we have found in bile from five animal species plasma membrane
enzymes such as alkaline phosphatase and nucleotidase, as well as
leucine-β-naphthylamidase and alkaline phosphodiesterase I.   We
interpret this as an indication that there is a degree of membrane
damage during bile salt secretion.

        Does Professor Lucy know of any evidence that intracellularly
produced ATP and coenzyme A can be involved in the acylation of a
lyso-compound on the other side of the membrane?

<u>Lucy</u>:   It has been shown that if you provide intact red cells with
lysolecithin, reacylation does occur.   If you use lysed, ghost
cell preparations, then exogenous ATP must be provided.

<u>Elliott</u>:   Do we need to invoke the carnitine cycle to allow the
coenzyme A derivative to cross the membrane?

<u>Lucy</u>:   I did wonder about this, but it would make the model
extremely detailed, and it is speculative enough already.

<u>Hofmann</u>:   Many years ago it was shown that incubation of 2-mono-
glyceride and fatty acid with pancreatic lipase resulted in the
net generation of ester bonds without the formation of any coenzyme
A derivatives.   Therefore, is there a precedent for micelles
containing lysolecithin and fatty acid to form phosphatidyl choline
with known enzymes, or has anyone tried to add fatty acid and
lysolecithin to bile to see if reacylation does occur?

<u>Lucy</u>:   The precedents to which I refer concern work done with red
cells, but I have no idea about similar work with bile.

<u>Popper</u>:   There seems to be a good chance that, under entirely
normal circumstances, the phospholipids of bile are derived from
the endoplasmic reticulum membrane, or more probably from the

canalicular membrane, or from both.   Several times during our
present discussion reference has been made to "damage" in the
sense that these phospholipids are released by bile acids during
the active transport of bile acids through the membrane.   I want
to emphasize that what we have been calling "damage" could be a
perfectly normal physiological process.   So this clearly represents
the spectrum of the normal to the abnormal situation.   In pathological situations this "damage" could be real, but in the normal
situation what we call "damage" is really just normal turnover.

Slater:   I want to make some comments on biliary micelles relevant
to Dr. Hauton's presentation.   This is a brief report on some work
we have done on the great stabilising influence of micelles on
certain molecules which are otherwise very chemically reactive.
We were investigating the redox level of liver cells in relation
to bile flow and composition.   We injected rats, with cannulated
bile ducts, with phenazenemethosulphate and followed consequent
changes in the bile of the treated animals.   Phenazenemethosulphate is a well-known chemical oxidant which reacts very quickly
and non-enzymically with NADH and NADPH, and we thought that we
might observe changes in redox-couples after injecting this
substance into the animals.   To our surprise within a few minutes
of intraperitoneal injection of the oxidant, the bile began to
change colour to a pale red which darkened to a very deep mauve.
This mauve stage lasted for 2 to 2.5 hours, and gradually the
bile returned to its original yellowish colour.   The colour of
the bile suggested that what we were seeing was a free radical form
of phenazenemethosulphate, because the anionic, free radical forms
of these phenazine compounds are highly coloured.   We diluted
some of these bile samples, and by E.S.R. analysis, we found a
strong free radical signal.   The interesting feature is not that
a free radical is produced and excreted into bile, but that the
free radical form is exceedingly stable, even after storage of
the bile for several days at room temperature.   Yet it is well
known, from purely chemical studies, that the phenazine radical
in pure solution has a very short half-life.   Our interpretation
of this is that, in bile, the radical is trapped in an unreactive
environment in a micellar form.   This suggests that highly
reactive substances can be excreted in bile but are prevented
from damaging neighbouring structures by being trapped in micelles.

Popper:   Do you assume that the micelle is formed in the bile, or
that the free radical passes through the canalicular membrane
already trapped in a protective micelle?

Slater:   This obviously is important, and we are waiting for
electron micrographs of livers of treated animals to see whether
there is any canalicular damage.   One would think that if such
reactive substances were formed in the neighbourhood of the

membrane they might produce some serious damage unless they were
to be trapped.

Fisher:    Are you sure that the free radical is free and in a
micellar form?   Could it be protein-bound, for instance?

Slater:    Free radical was rather a loose expression:   I should
have said trapped radical.   However, the basic chemical structure
is that it has an unpaired electron as demonstrated by the E.S.R.
analysis.

Popjak:    Do you get formation of the free radical if you mix the
methosulphate with bile, or does it have to go through the liver
first?   The reaction may be photoactivated.

Slater:    That is a searching and interesting question.   If you
simply mix phenazenemethosulphate with bile in the dark there is
no detectable free radical formation.   However, if you mix bilirubin with the compound at a slightly higher pH than occurs in
bile, say pH 8.5, you do in fact get free radical formation.   We
are trying to study the chemistry of this, and it does seem to
involve an interaction with bilirubin.   As for the point about
photoactivation, this is difficult because phenazine salts are
themselves photoactive and readily decompose, especially in the
presence of oxygen.

Taylor:    I would like to make some comments about Dr. Fisher's
paper.   First, a comment about what Dr. Strandvik said about the
role of the fetus.   I had the idea that the fetus might be
involved, so I analysed some normal samples of amniotic fluid
for bile acids, but I could not find even a trace of these
substances.   Then I want to add a note of caution before a lot
of over-enthusiastic investigations are carried out on the effect
of sex hormones on biliary secretion.   Most of the work done so
far has involved giving animals large doses of ethynyl oestradiol,
which we know produces a marked cholestasis.   I would like to
digress to another part of the gastrointestinal tract and mention
the stomach.   We have done some work on the old problem about
the supposed protection from peptic ulceration afforded by sex
hormones.   The experiments were done on conscious cats fitted
with a chronic gastric fistula.   We gave male and female animals
mg doses of ethynyl oestradiol and found no effect on the secretion
of acid or pepsin or on serum gastrin levels.   We then treated
another batch of animals with mg doses of a synthetic progestin and
again found no effects.   Then we gave the cats a commercial oral
contraceptive which contains only 50 µg of ethynyl oestradiol plus
a synthetic progestin.   This combination of oestrogen plus
progestin caused a significant decrease in acid and pepsin output,
and also of serum gastrin.   The point I wish to make from these

experiments is that those people who wish to study the effects of sex hormones on biliary secretion should bear in mind that the pregnant woman produces a lot of oestrogen but also a lot of progesterone.   As Professor Sjövall mentioned earlier, the role of progesterone metabolites may be important in intrahepatic cholestatic jaundice of pregnancy, but we have tended to neglect the possible role of progesterone in affecting biliary secretion and, even more so, the possible synergistic effects of oestrogens and progestins.

Strandvik:   I thought Dr. Taylor's data on amniotic fluid was interesting, but I want to suggest that this does not exclude the possibility that high concentrations of bile acids could come from the fetus.   They could be so rapidly cleared by the placenta that they would not be detected in amniotic fluid.

Sjövall:   I just want to confuse the issue a little further.   The big sex difference in steroid metabolism in rat liver is due to the hypophysis.   If you remove the hypophysis of female rats the hepatic steroid metabolism takes on a male pattern.

Bouchier:   Does testosterone have any actions comparable to those which have been found for oestrogens?

Popper:   We assume that the cholestasis produced under the circumstances we have been discussing is probably very similar to that produced by the anabolic steroids, which are synthetic analogues of testosterone.   So I think the effects may be due to steric factors which I mentioned earlier.   The 17-substituted testosterones seem to produce the same type of lesion, at least as judged by electron microscopy.   Then, I would also like to complicate the problem further.   There is an impression that, as far as jaundice production is concerned, the effect of the contraceptive steroids increases with age.   I remember the time when these contraceptive pills were being used as "beauty" pills by menopausal women.   When we talk about pathological effects of sex steroids on the liver one definite and one problematic lesion have to be mentioned.   The definite lesion is a focal vasodilatation, which has been well established for both the contraceptive pill and for androgenic steroids.   We know that this may lead to marked widening of the vascular channels, and there is a similarity with the lithocholate lesion.   There is little doubt that there is an effect on the lining of the vasculature of the liver, and only in the liver.   This cannot be explained by haemodynamic factors because of the localisation of the lesion in an irregular way through the lobar acinar structures.   It is of major interest in many other areas because the same lesion can be produced by substances which eventually end up by producing angiosarcomas of the liver:   such substances are vinyl chloride, thorotrast and certain arsenicals.

I now want to mention a very mysterious pregnancy lesion, in contrast to recurrent jaundice of pregnancy. This is benign, familial, non-recurrent jaundice, which develops late in the trimester, associated with steatosis, which was previously called "pernicious", because most of the women died. Now we know that they probably die mainly because of renal failure. I know of one woman who survived and had a second successful pregnancy, so it is not related to the recurrent type of cholestasis. This is a mysterious, rare lesion which is frequently fatal. I would like to give Dr. Fisher a chance to comment on this.

Fisher: As far as I can tell from the literature, studies with oral contraceptives in menopausal women have produced results which do not differ from women in younger age groups. I am not convinced that there is an age-related effect. As for the effects on the vasculature, I cannot comment on this except to say that Dr. Bradley has observed substantial haemodynamic effects in dogs treated with oestrogens. However, I accept Dr. Popper's comments on the localisation of these effects within the liver. I suppose we have all seen a few cases of acute fatty liver of pregnancy. There does not seem to be anything in the oestrogen literature that would connect the two.

Bouchier: Dr. Popper, one occasionally sees a woman on oral contraceptives who develops the Budd-Chiari syndrome. One assumes that this is due to increased sludging related to increased viscosity of the blood and red cell hyperplasia. Do you think it may be related to a vascular lesion?

Popper: Definitely no. We have now seen a fair number of women with this condition. Originally we thought that this was a type of Budd-Chiari syndrome which should not be operated upon because the lesion is usually not in a location that the surgeon can reach. We thought it had a good prognosis, but, unfortunately, we have now lost quite a few of these women in our hospital. I have looked very carefully for venous endothelial lesions in this rather peculiar vasodilatation, and I am sure it is not due to a thrombotic effect.

Taylor: Can I complicate the situation even further? We have been talking a lot about oestrogens, but nobody has as yet mentioned stilboestrol. Dr. Popper mentioned the tendency of some menopausal American women to try to remain youthful by using the contraceptive pill. It is my impression that stilboestrol has been used, or rather abused, to achieve the same ends. I wonder if there is any information about the cholestatic effects of stilboestrol administered over a long period?

Fisher:   This is, of course, a non-steroidal oestrogen, and as
far as I can tell it has not been associated with cholestasis.

Popper:   There are reports of oestrogens causing necrotising
liver damage, but I am a little sceptical about this.   However,
I remember perhaps two cases in which necrosis but not cholestasis
was reported.

Taylor:   Dr. Fisher's answer merely emphasised the point I was
trying to make, which was that it is probably not the classical
oestrogenic effect, but the actual steroidal structure itself
which might be causing the liver lesion.

Bradley:   I want to refer to some remarks which Dr. Fisher
attributed to me.   Those of us who work with the liver tend to
forget that it has an environment, and I wanted to stress that
the liver and kidney, and the other organs in the body live in
an environment which is provided by the cardiovascular system.
In pregnancy that system is grossly disturbed and modified in all
parts of the body, including the liver.   One wonders if hyper-
aemia and hypervolaemia in the liver might play a part in inducing
changes that we should think of as primary changes.   Nobody denies
that metabolic changes occur, but these could be secondary to
cardiovascular changes.   Relatively small changes in pressure
and blood flow in the hepatic vein cause large decrease in bile
output, whereas changes in arterial pressures do not affect bile
flow.   Therefore, the effect on bile was not due to a change in
total blood flow.

Low-Beer:   Is it true that secondary bile salts are found in the
meconium of the fetus, and if so, is not this reasonably good
evidence that there is passage of maternal bile salts across the
placenta?

Strandvik:   Lithocholic acid has been found in the meconium of
full-term and premature babies.   The question then is, does this
come from the mother or is it formed by the fetus by, for instance,
the minor pathway to chenodeoxycholic acid?   The problem with the
question of placental transfer of bile acids is that deoxycholic
acid has never been found in the fetus.

Ostrow:   Based on the effect of oestrogens on rats, Forker has
suggested that the mechanism of oestrogen cholestasis is due to
an effect on the permeability of the tight-junction so that
substances could leak out of the bile after it has been secreted.
What bothers me about that idea is that Dr. Fisher showed us that
the biliary concentration of bile acid increases while that of
other components decreases.   This is hard to explain on the
basis of an effect on the tight-junction.

<u>Bradley</u>:   We have been studying this problem, using sucrose and
ferricyanide simultaneously as markers, and injecting these
against the methoxy- and carboxy-inulins.   In rats ethynyl
oestradiol treated, there was always a reduction in bile flow,
due to a decrease in the bile salt independent bile flow, with
only equivocal changes in bile salt associated flow.   There was
reduction in taurocholate transport, in B.S.P. clearance, but a
marked increase in the clearance of the sucrose, ferricyanide and
of the inulin derivatives, which are much larger molecules.   We
assume that there is increased permeability to these substances
to permit their movement into bile while bile flow is reduced.
This tells us nothing about back-diffusion.   So we conclude
that the canalicular membrane is damaged in such a way that it
permits passage of larger molecules, although at the same time
the total area is reduced and this limits the passage of small
molecules.

<u>Ostrow</u>:   But it has been shown that fluorescein can pass through
the tight junctions into the intercellular clefts.

<u>Bradley</u>:   Fluorescein and B.S.P. transport are directly inter-
related because they are virtually the same molecule.   Fluorescence microscopy has shown that movement of these fluorescent
substances from the hepatocytes to the bile is very mysterious.
When bile canaliculi are exposed to ultraviolet radiation for a
long time they develop irregular dilatations, which, as far as I
know, have not yet been studied by electron microscopy.   But the
point is that the use of ultraviolet light and fluorescent microscopy ought to make us very cautious about interpreting data
obtained by this technique.

<u>Hofmann</u>:   Dr. Fisher has found differences in the biliary bile
acid composition of men and women, but not everyone has found that.
Can he explain this?   Secondly, has anyone any information on the
biliary bile acid composition of the fetal rabbit?   The adult
rabbit secretes predominantly secondary bile acids, so I wonder
if the fetus is different.

<u>Fisher</u>:   I cannot explain the differences between our results and
those of others.   There is a considerable overlap in the results
from men and women, but there is a difference on a statistical
basis.

<u>Bouchier</u>:   Dr. Hofmann, you have studied bile acids in the germ-
free rabbit.   Might the results not be the same in the fetal
rabbit?

<u>Hofmann</u>:   In the normal rabbit the composition of the biliary
bile acids was about 90 per cent deoxycholate, 8 per cent cholate,

3 per cent allodeoxycholate and about one per cent allocholate. In the germ-free animals it was mostly cholate with a little chenodeoxycholate and some allocholate. My guess is that the fetal rabbit would be somewhere in between the two.

Taylor: I should like to draw Dr. Strandvik's attention to what was said earlier. As I understood it, the point was that some of the cholestatic effects observed in the mother could be due to bile acids produced by the fetus. Now we hear that the major, if not the only, bile acid in the meconium is lithocholic acid. This is not surprising because there are many biochemical reactions which are not triggered off until some hours or even days after birth, depending on the species. So I would suggest that the hydroxylases in the fetus have not reached a stage of development at which they can produce polyhydroxylated bile acids.

Strandvik: Perhaps I did not express myself clearly. Lithocholate is not the most prominent bile acid in the fetus until the 28th week. Before that time, chenodeoxycholate predominates, and at the end of pregnancy cholate is the predominant bile acid.

Taylor: This suggests that some change is taking place in bile acid biosynthesis during fetal growth.

Bouchier: What happens to the components of the biliary micelle when it enters the intestine?

Borgström: The micelle is completely rearranged mainly due to the effect of phospholipase which will be breaking up the lecithin. So the bile salt-cholesterol-lecithin micelle probably changes very rapidly into a bile salt - lysolecithin-monoglyceride micelle.

Murphy: In cystic fibrosis there is failure to hydrolyse triglyceride in the intestinal lumen, and there have been reports that patients with this disease excrete large amounts of bile acids in the faeces. Can anyone explain this?

Borgström: One possible explanation is that in this disease there will be no pancreatic phospholipase so the lecithin will not be split up. Therefore there will be mixed micelles all the way down the intestine, and they will carry the bile salts with them, so there will be a decrease in free bile acids resulting in lowered absorption of bile acids. Protein-binding of bile acids may also be an important factor.

Hofmann: I think it most reasonable to explain this by adsorption to undigested protein, since cystic fibrotics have solid residues in the distal end of the intestine.

_Dianzani_:    There has been very little comment about the presence
of lysosomal enzymes in bile, although Professor Slater has shown
that these enzymes are present in bile.    I think we should pay
more attention to these enzymes in bile in pathological conditions.

_Popper_:    It has been shown in our laboratory that the type of
lysosomal enzymes of various kinds are present in the bile;
there was no relation to the types of enzymes found in the serum,
but they were closely related to those in the liver cell.    I was
surprised that Dr. Billing did not raise the very important
question about the possible regurgitation of lysosomal enzymes or
of whole lysosomes into the blood stream in cholestasis.    Such
release could cause hydrolysis of bilirubin conjugates in blood.

_Low-Beer_:    Dr. Hofmann, when you give 2,4-tritium-labelled bile
salt, its behaviour is the same as $^{14}$C-labelled bile salt in the
enterohepatic circulation, but a large amount of tritium appears
in the urine.    You interpret this by suggesting that the
tritium is removed at a point in the colon beyond which bile
acids are normally adsorbed.    This suggests that the proximal
colon is a site where passive, non-ionic diffusion of bile acids
occurs, but that this cannot occur in the distal colon even
though the colonic contents remain for a longer time in the
distal colon.    Why do you think that this occurs, and how can
this important phenomenon be studied?

_Hofmann_:    We observed a 20 per cent loss of the tritium label
from cholic acid, and the loss of the label was especially
pronounced in the deoxycholic acid.    Therefore, we think that
this is a bacterial dehydrogenation which occurs in the caecum.
We examined 50 strains of bacteria,and found one strain which
could carry out this very rapid hydrogenation _in vitro_.    The
significance of this biotransformation is that it provides a
route from 5β- to 5α- bile acids.

# Cholestasis

# INTRAHEPATIC CHOLESTASIS

H. Thaler

Wilhelminenspital, Fourth Dept. of Medicine

Montleartstrasse 37, A-1171 Vienna, Austria

From a functional point of view, cholestasis is a biliary secretory failure of liver cells (11). The cause of the secretory handicap may be located at any point along the complex pathway the secretory products have to follow from the source of their production, inside the liver cell, down to the duodenal lumen. The histopathologist describes cholestasis as a microscopically visible accumulation of bile pigment in the liver tissue (2).

## Nomenclature

The distinction between intrahepatic and extrahepatic cholestasis is of paramount importance since it separates medical from surgical cases. Extrahepatic cholestasis is due to partial or complete obstruction of the biliary tree from the bifurcation of the common hepatic duct to the Ampulla of Vater, resulting generally from tumours, stones, strictures or malformations.

Intrahepatic cholestasis is caused by a lesion located within the anatomical confines of the liver. It would be an oversimplification to designate intrahepatic cholestasis metabolic, in contrast to the obstructive pathogenesis of extrahepatic cholestasis. In reality, intrahepatic cholestasis is a pot into which are packed many different metabolic and obstructive lesions. A clearer separation may be made between preductular cholestasis, covering the metabolic

disturbances of the hepatocytes and the bile canaliculi, and a ductular-post ductular cholestasis,
comprising obstructive lesions of the biliary tract,
from the small ductules to the Papilla of Vater.


Table 1

MORPHOLOGIC CHANGES FAVORING EXTRAHEPATIC CHOLESTASIS

Pathognomonic

Bile extravasation in portal tracts
Large bile infarcts


Highly Suggestive

Dilatation of interlobular ducts with flattened
epithelium
Bile plugs in interlobular ducts
Cholangitis with infiltration by neutrophil
leucocytes
Periductal laminar fibrosis
Bile lakes


Moderately Suggestive

Oedema of portal tracts
Predominantly polymorphonuclear portal infiltra-
tion
Marginal bile duct proliferation
Pseudoxanthoma cells
Severe degree of cholestasis
Feathery degeneration


The Morphologic Differential Diagnosis Between
Intrahepatic and Extrahepatic
Cholestasis

A clinician, performing a liver biopsy in a
patient with cholestasis, wants the histopathologist
to establish whether the cholestasis is intrahepatic or
extrahepatic in origin.  That the clinician is frequently disappointed, is not necessarily the fault of
the histopathologist.  In many cases a histological
differentiation between extrahepatic and intrahepatic
cholestasis is difficult or even impossible.  However,

some changes are more often found in extrahepatic
cholestasis and a few of these are considered to be
pathognomonic (tab.1).  On the other hand there are
only scanty and ill-defined features which point to
intrahepatic cholestasis.  The following morphologic
features are suggestive of extrahepatic cholestasis or
of mechanical obstruction to large bile ducts within
the liver:  oedema of the portal tract which often
causes a rounding of the portal triad, a predominantly
polymorphonuclear infiltration of the portal area, most
pronounced in its periphery and a marginal proliferation of bile ducts, more or less parallel to the border
of the portal tract.  Marginal bile duct proliferation
should not be confused with diffuse or plexiform ductular proliferation.  Oedema and marginal proliferation
occur during the first week of bile duct obstruction.
Polymorphonuclear infiltration needs more time to
develop.  These portal alterations are not pathognomonic but significantly associated with extrahepatic
cholestases (tab.2) (8).

     The presence of bile plugs in interlobular ducts,
their dilatation, and flattening or local hyperplasia
of their epithelium are widely considered to be signs
of extrahepatic obstruction, occurring about three
weeks after the first symptoms.

     The alterations, however, may also be found in
cases of intrahepatic cholestasis, e.g. in protracted
or necrotizing viral hepatitis (10, 12).  Cholangitis,
the infiltration of ductal epithelium and lumens by
polymorphonuclear leucocytes, is more reliable.
Cholangitis should not be confused with cholangiolitis,
characterized by a granulocytic infiltration of proli-
ferating ductules, being a frequent change in cholestasis of intrahepatic origin also.  Laminar periductal fibrosis is a typical finding after recurrent
attacks of biliary obstruction.  Pseudoxanthoma cells,
situated in the portal fields or in the periportal
areas, are usually but not invariably seen in extrahepatic cholestasis.

     Some additional help in differential diagnosis is
offered by cholestatic changes within the parenchyma.
Generally cholestasis is more pronounced in complete
extrahepatic obstruction than in intrahepatic cholestasis, but this finding is time-dependent and,
therefore, rather unreliable in the individual case.
Extreme widening of bile canaliculi to bile lakes is
usually observed in extrahepatic cholestasis.  It is

Table 2

FREQUENCY OF PORTAL CHANGES

| Group | Histological and Surgical Findings | | Number of Cases | Total of Portal Tracts | Portal Tracts with | | |
| --- | --- | --- | --- | --- | --- | --- | --- |
| | Cholestasis | Extra-hepatic obstruction | | | Marginal bile duct proliferation | Oedema | Neutrophil leucocytes |
| I | + | + | 39 | 1270 | 1036* (82%) | 432** (37%) | 623** (49%) |
| II | Ø | + | 33 | 792 | 398* (50%) | 13 ( 2%) | 12 ( 2%) |
| III | + | Ø | 9 | 168 | 17 (10%) | 12 ( 7%) | 12 ( 7%) |
| IV | Ø | Ø | 32 | 707 | 149 (21%) | Ø ( 0%) | Ø ( 0%) |

* significantly greater than in groups III and IV (p < 0.01)
** significantly greater than in groups II, III, and IV (p < 0.001)

(After Poulsen and Christoffersen (8))

often combined with a rearrangement of liver-cell-
plates into acinar structures around the central bile
plug.  Feathery degeneration, a brown reticulation of
liver-cell cytoplasm, caused by an increase of smooth
endoplasmic reticulum, by cytoplasmic vacuolisation
and an accumulation of bile constituents, is again a
sign of longstanding cholestasis, more often found in
cases of mechanical obstruction.  Siderosis in liver
cells of the periphery of the lobules has been
described as another sign of extrahepatic cholestasis
(3).  However, its value must be questioned:  extrahepatic obstruction of the biliary tract usually occurs
in the older age groups, in which periportal siderosis
is frequent.

    Evaluating the signs of extrahepatic cholestasis
critically, only two findings are of absolute diagnostic value:  large so-called bile infarcts and bile
extravasates.  Bile infarcts are accumulations of
pseudoxanthoma cells or degenerated hepatocytes,
generally located at the margins of portal fields.  In
time, their centres may become necrotic and filled with
bile.  Portal bile extravasates, caused by infarcts or
degenerated and ruptured bile ducts, are the second
pathognomonic feature.  Unfortunately these findings
are of late occurrence, and are apt to be observed in
autopsy material rather than in biopsy specimens.  In
the list of differentiating features intrahepatic
cholestasis has nothing to contribute except a portal
infiltration with eosinophils, sometimes observed in
drug-induced cholestasis but rarely also in extrahepatic obstruction.  As a substantial help in diagnosis additional features related to the cause of
intrahepatic cholestasis are of utmost importance.  A
few examples are the changes of viral hepatitis, fatty
liver or alpha-1-antitrypsin deficiency.

    Histochemistry may facilitate the differentiation
between extrahepatic and intrahepatic cholestasis to a
moderate extent.  Canalicular adenosine triphosphatase
disappears in cholestasis of a few days  duration.
Some authors have noted a more rapid disappearance in
intrahepatic cholestasis, obviously due to mild liver
cell damage.  Alkaline phosphatase-activity shows a
strong increase in both intrahepatic and extrahepatic
cholestasis.  It has been claimed that application of
extensive series of enzyme histochemical techniques on
the same liver biopsy specimen may allow differentiation between the metabolic type of intrahepatic cholestasis, characterized by the loss of numerous enzymes,

and obstructive cholestasis, in which the same enzymes
persist at least for some time (2, 6).

The organelle pathology of cholestasis will be
discussed separately.  Electron microscopy contributes
much to our understanding of the pathogenesis of
cholestasis but little or nothing to the differential
diagnosis of its various types.

Summarizing the possibilities of histopathology
in the differentiation of extrahepatic from intrahepatic cholestasis, we may conclude that, in the average
liver biopsy, a reliable single sign permitting differential diagnosis does not exist.  In mild cases of pure
cholestasis or of cholestasis with moderate inflammatory reaction, differentiation is especially difficult.
When, however, tentative diagnoses prove to be correct
in the majority of specimens even without knowledge of
clinical data (1), this can be achieved when an
experienced histopathologist carefully analyzes the
degree of the various cholestatic features on the one
hand and the accompanying phenomena due to the cause
of intrahepatic cholestasis on the other.  The accuracy
of the histologic diagnosis is certainly improved when
the patient's history and clinical findings are known.
Even under these ideal circumstances, however, biopsy
histology does not always provide the final piece in
the diagnostic puzzle.  In assessing the type or the
site of biliary obstruction endoscopic retrograde
choledochography and peritoneoscopic transhepatic
cholangiography are unquestionably superior.

The Primary Lesion in Intrahepatic Cholestasis

The classification of the various forms of intrahepatic cholestasis would be easy if the sites of the
primary lesion were known.  This lesion may be located
at different levels of the intrahepatic secretory
pathway:  the hepatocyte itself, the canaliculi, the
portal ductules, the interlobular ducts and larger
segmental bile ducts (2).  While disturbances within
the intrahepatic bile duct system are not too difficult
to prove, either by histopathology or by special
techniques of cholangiography, the site of hepatocellular or canalicular disorder remains hypothetical
or unknown.

The old concept of a direct open communication
between canaliculus and sinusoid has proved to be
wrong, exdept in instances of hepatocellular necrosis

Table 3

CAUSES OF INTRAHEPATIC CHOLESTASIS

A.  Obstructive
    1.  Atresia or hypoplasia of intrahepatic bile
        ducts
    2.  Congenital hepatic fibrosis
    3.  Congenital dilatation of segmental intrahepatic
        bile ducts (Caroli's disease)
    4.  Biliary mucoviscidosis
    5.  Nonsuppurative destructive chronic cholangitis
    6.  Intrahepatic primary sclerosing cholangitis
    7.  Parasitic disease of bile ducts
    8.  Intrahepatic cholangiocarcinoma
    9.  Intrahepatic stricture of bile ducts
   10.  Intrahepatic compression of bile ducts
        (tumour, cysts)

B.  Metabolic
    I.  Pure Cholestasis
        1.  Intermittent intrahepatic cholestasis
            (Summerskill-Tygstrup's disease)
        2.  Recurrent intrahepatic cholestasis of
            pregnancy
        3.  Benign postoperative intrahepatic
            cholestasis
        4.  Cholestatic drug-induced jaundice (e.g.
            anabolic steroids)
        5.  Inspissated bile syndrome
    II.  Cholestasis with inflammation and liver-cell
         damage
        1.  Cholestatic drug-induced jaundice (e.g.
            chlorpromazine)

C.  Intrahepatic Cholestasis as an Accompanying
    Feature in:
    1.  Acute viral hepatitis
    2.  Chronic aggressive hepatitis
    3.  Toxic (drug-induced) hepatitis
    4.  Alcoholic hepatitis
    5.  Fatty liver
    6.  Cirrhosis

or canalicular rupture.  These occurrences cannot play
an important role in the pathogenesis of cholestatic
jaundice, as they arise late, after exhaustion of the
cell's secretory activity.  The ductular reabsorption
of bile components has been convincingly confirmed but
seems to be of minor importance.

The major problems still centre around the hepatocyte itself and its intercellular junctions.  The
canalicular tight junctions might be or might become
permeable to water, electrolytes, and other small
molecules, allowing an escape of bile solutes from the
canaliculi toward the blood.  The extent of this intercellular escape remains to be established (2).

Transhepatocytic regurgitation offers further
possibilities.  Retrograde injection of peroxidase
into the bile duct suggest that a retrograde transport
from the canaliculus to the sinusoidal cell border may
occur (7).  However, this concept is difficult to
confirm.  So far, there is only little possibility of
distinguishing retained from regurgitated bile components (9).  A second possibility is a reverse over-
flow through the cytoplasm of the liver cell, from the
canaliculus to the sinusoid, as suggested by Hanzon's
study with fluorescent tracers (4).  Finally, there is
some evidence that bile pigmented organelles in the
form of autophagic vacuoles or secondary lysosomes are
discharged into the space of Disse.  This cellular
defaecation (5) may contribute to the regurgitation of
bile (2).

Causes of Intrahepatic Cholestasis

In table 3 the attempt is made to show the causes
of some intrahepatic cholestases and of some liver
diseases with intrahepatic cholestasis as an
accompanying feature.

# BIBLIOGRAPHY

1.  Baggenstoss, A.:  Morphologic and etiologic
    diagnosis from hepatic biopsies without clinical
    data.  Medicine (Baltimore) 45, 435 - 443 (1966).
2.  Desmet, V.J.:  Morphologic and histochemical
    aspects of cholestasis.  In Popper H. and F.
    Schaffner (editors):  Progress in Liver Diseases,
    Vol. IV, Grune and Stratton, New York 1972,
    pp. 97 - 132.
3.  Gardiol, D. et P. Loup:  Criteres histologiques de
    la cholestase extrahepatique.  Acta hepatosplenol.
    (Stuttgart) 18, 253 - 261 (1971).
4.  Hanzon, V.:  Liver cell secretion under normal and
    pathological conditions studied by fluorescence
    microscopy in living rats.  Acta Physiol. Scand.
    28, 1 - 168 (1952).
5.  Kerr, J.:  Liver cell defecation:  An electron
    microscope study of the discharge of lysosomal
    residual bodies into the intercellular space.
    J. Path. 100, 99 - 103 (1970).
6.  Lageron A., G. Theodoropoulos and J. Caroli:
    Extra and intrahepatic cholestasis in man.
    Histology and enzymology.  Presse Med. 79,
    2099 - 2102 (1971).
7.  Matter, A., L. Orci and C. Rouiller:  A study on
    the permeability barriers between Disse's space
    and the bile canaliculus.  J. Ultrastruct. Res.
    Suppl. 11, 1 - 71 (1969).
8.  Poulsen, H. and P. Christoffersen:  Histological
    changes in liver biopsies from patients with
    surgical bile duct disorders.  Acta Path. Micro-
    biol. Scand. Section A, 78, 571 - 579 (1970).
9.  Raia, S.:  Histochemical separation of conjugated
    and unconjugated bilirubin and its assessment by
    thin layer chromatography.  J. Histochem. 18,
    153 (1970).
10. Schmid, M. and B. Cueni:  Portal lesions in viral
    hepatitis with submassive hepatic necrosis.  Human
    Path. 3, 209 - 216 (1972).
11. Sherlock, S.:  Diseases of the liver and biliary
    system.  Blackwell, Oxford 1968, pp. 277 - 316.
12. Thaler, H.:  Ueber cholestatische und cholangio-
    litische Varianten der Virushepatitis.  Wien.
    klin. Wschr. 74, 326 - 329 (1962).

DISCUSSION OF LECTURE BY H. THALER

Popper: I would like to add two factual rather than controversial comments. Bile infarcts, which previously we have always considered to be an absolute indication of a mechanical obstruction of large bile ducts may need not be so under certain specific circumstances. In the later stages of massive necrotic hepatitis with transition to cirrhosis, bile infarcts may appear only occasionally, and I must confess that I do not understand this.

My second comment deals with Professor Thaler's Table. Recently there have been two interesting developments concerned with the "congenital" or "neonatal" type of cholestasis. There should be another type added to that Table: this is neonatal, giant-cell hepatitis which is also often associated with cholestatic manifestations. This used to be thought to be a congenital disorder, but it is now thought that it occurs because of a viral infection in utero.

We could consider the different types of neonatal disease as one unit: neonatal, obstructive cholangiopathy. We would include under this heading: biliary atresia which is a type of biliary cirrhosis of childhood; congenital hepatic fibrosis; congenital dilatation of the segmental intrahepatic ducts. We know that these lesions occur together. I wish to bring to your attention the fact that the most common cause of neonatal "obstructive" jaundice, which usually becomes apparent 3-4 weeks after birth is associated with $\alpha_1$-antitrypsin deficiency. Something like 40-50 per cent of cases of jaundice appearing within one month of birth are due to this $\alpha_1$-antitrypsin deficiency. We cannot demonstrate the presence of $\alpha_1$-antitrypsin in the liver in such cases. If the children are operated on, even for exploratory purposes, they die, so I suggest that no surgery should be done in these circumstances. The vast majority recover, but about 10 per cent develop non-icteric cirrhosis, which can develop to the stage of hepatic failure with jaundice. A small percentage of such cases may develop emphysema and the cirrhosis does not appear until about 5-6 years of age.

So we can say that the sort of Table which Professor Thaler has drawn up is very comprehensive, but it may not be complete even now.

Thaler:    I have also seen a case of biliary infarction associated
with intrahepatic cholestasis.    I did not list the giant-cell
hepatitis of neonates, because this group can be included under
viral hepatitis.

Popper:    I apologise for a major error.    When I spoke of "viral",
I did not mean virus A or B:  I meant the adeno-type viruses, so I
was referring to types of hepatitis caused by viruses other than
virus A or B.

Erlinger:    I have always been puzzled by the mechanism of the
cholestasis observed in congenital hepatic fibrosis.    You listed
that under "obstructive".    What is the evidence for, and the
possible mechanism of, such "obstruction"?

Thaler:    The evidence is questionable, but in congenital hepatic
fibrosis within the strands of fibrous tissue you do see dilated
ductules filled with bile or some other material.    Therefore,
under light microscopy it has the appearance of some type of
hepatic obstruction.    However, I cannot really be positive:  it
may be a metabolic disturbance.

Popper:    I think that the bile precipitates which you see have
nothing to do with the obstruction because they are in side
channels, in which the bile is just stagnating.    Most of the
colour is reported in cholangitis, and I think the classification
for Dr. Erlinger's laboratory is one of the best available.

Dowling:    What is the mechanism of the bile duct hyperplasia in
extrahepatic cholestasis?

Thaler:    There are two types of bile canalicular proliferation:
one is a proliferation in length, and so when sections are made
at different levels you get the impression that there is more
than one canaliculus.    The other possibility is a true spreading
of canaliculi, but this usually shows a plexiform picture.    This
is best seen when the connection between the parenchyma and the
biliary tree become mixed up, for example in portal necrosis.

Popper:    We are dealing with two different processes here.    One
is purely mechanical, and we discussed this after Dr. Palmer's
paper:  biliary obstruction is a tremendous stimulus for DNA
synthesis.    The second process is stimulation by an irritant
which we assume to be of intraluminal origin, and some of us
believe that bile acids are involved here.    Obviously lithocholate
is a classical example, but other bile acids may be involved.

Boyer:    We have sometimes seen patients with viral or drug-induced
hepatitis who develop histological evidence of severe cholestasis

associated with bile infarcts.   You suggested that these infarcts were characteristic of extrahepatic obstruction, but we have no evidence for this in our patients.   The interesting thing about most of these patients is that there are two related phenomena. Firstly, there is usually a severe impairment of renal function, so urinary excretion of bilirubin is impaired;   secondly, they very often have had multiple blood transfusions so that the bilirubin load in terms of total daily turnover is greatly increased. I have always interpreted that as a sort of human experiment of nature which supports the view that the cholestatic liver continues to put out organic anions such as bilirubin, but for some reason this bilirubin cannot flow out normally into the major ducts and so goes back into the hepatocytes.   Therefore, one has to postulate that there must be obstruction further down the biliary tree, but I know of no good evidence for that.   Would you care to comment on that, and also would you care to speculate about why we generally see mild cholestasis centrally located?

Thaler:    I do not have the slightest idea why this should be so, except that in viral hepatitis it is certainly a metabolic type of cholestasis.    In addition to the type of patients you mentioned, it has to be said that in very, very rare cases hepatitis B produces pure cholestasis without any other sign of viral hepatitis.

Hofmann:    It seems to me that in acute obstruction or acute intrahepatic cholestasis one has desynchronisation of the enterohepatic circulation, so one might expect a continued input of secondary bile acids, such as lithocholate, for 2 or 3 days, after which this should stop.   These bile acids could go to the liver for a short time before being excreted in urine.   This might be a clue to the cause of the bile duct hyperplasia.   What is the physicochemical way by which cholestasis regresses:   do the plugs go into the hepatocytes locally or does bile go round these plugs and dissolve them?   This is relevant to developing a therapeutic approach to cholestasis.

Thaler:    I really do not know how cholestasis regresses, but it happens very quickly.

Popper:    I think the plugs disappear by two mechanisms.   The first is by phagocytosis by macrophages, since one can see these macrophages in the bile ducts.   As for the second mechanism, bile plugs do not cause obstruction, but we have to consider what causes the intracellular bile pigment to disappear.   This I think is brought about by the lysosomes.

Bradley:    Are there any diseases associated with intrahepatic cholestasis which aggravate it or minimise it?   For example, is

it worse or better in diabetics, because I am thinking that
glucagon may have an effect on the liver here.   There may be
other hormonal disturbances which may have an effect.

Thaler:   Diabetes is a good example of the type of condition
which might influence cholestasis.   However, cholestasis is not
affected one way or the other by diabetes.   Cholestasis may be
an accompanying feature of some extrahepatic, metabolic disorders,
but the mechanisms are unknown.

# MOLECULAR PATHOLOGY OF CHOLESTASIS

Hans Popper, Fenton Schaffner, and Helmut Denk

Stratton Laboratory for the Study of Liver Diseases,
Mount Sinai School of Medicine of the City University of
New York, New York, U.S., and Pathologisch-Anatomisches
Institut der Universitaet Wien, Vienna, Austria

Cholestasis will remain a key problem in liver disease as far
as differential diagnosis, prognosis and therapy are concerned
until its pathogenesis is resolved. It thus challenges the
clinician, both gastroenterologist and surgeon; the morphologist;
and the physiologist, each of whom uses his own definition, varying
from 'piling up of biliary substances in the blood' to 'visible
stagnation of bile in the liver' to 'inhibition of hepatocellular
bile secretion' (1).

Cholestasis localized in the center of the lobule, or the
zone III of the acinus of Rappaport, in the early stage has been
considered to result from mechanical processes within the biliary
tract, obvious in extrahepatic obstruction and less clear in
mechanical obstruction of the intrahepatic biliary tract such as
biliary atresia or sclerosing and other types of cholangitis. In
the absence of anatomically demonstrable obstruction, a mechanical
interference with flow in the bile ductules by inflammation was
originally postulated because of the functional similarity to
established mechanical obstruction: "cholangiolitis" (2). Some
twenty years ago, when a lack of correlation between portal inflammation and bile flow stagnation in this disorder was established, we coined the term 'intrahepatic cholestasis' (3). Subsequently, transmission electron microscopy (4, 5, 6) demonstrated
the identical lesion of the area of the bile canaliculus in the
hepatocytes in both this unexplained intrahepatic cholestasis and
in biliary obstruction. This localized the lesion, now also
visualized by scanning electron microscopy (7), into a group of
pericanalicular hepatocytic organelles (the bile secretory apparatus) (8) as the structural basis of at least early cholestasis,
even in the absence of bile thrombi.

Specifically, an irregular dilatation of the bile canaliculus
with swollen, stunted or missing microvilli is accompanied by a
widening of the pericanalicular zone or ectoplasm, a hyperplastic
Golgi zone sometimes containing electron-opaque material, and an
increase of smooth endoplasmic reticulum (SER) and of the pericanalicular lysosomes.  Branching canaliculi with short lateral
branches (like diverticuli) and small holes in their walls, best
visualized by scanning electron microscopy (9), are also accentuated
in cholestasis.  The central location of early bile stagnation in
the mechanical form, far distant from the point of obstruction,
indicates that pressure alone does not explain the lesion, but a
hepatocellular alteration accentuated by the lower oxygen tension
in the lobular center does (10).  In not obviously obstructive
intrahepatic cholestasis metabolic or molecular abnormalities, i.
e. biochemical processes, are incriminated.

These electron-microscopic findings thus shifted the interest
from physical processes in the biliary passages to alterations of
the organelles of the bile-secretory apparatus, just as recently
the emphasis moved from mechanical processes in the biliary passages to alterations of hepatocytic secretion in the pathogenesis
of cholesterol gallstone disease.  Cholestasis is the only manifestation, not only in early mechanical obstruction  but also in
the lesions just listed by Thaler (11, see also 1).  Far more frequently, however, cholestasis is encountered in the common types
of hepatitis and cirrhosis, when the alteration of the bile-
secretory apparatus is associated with injury of the other hepatocytic organelles.

The recent success in localizing biliary obstruction, both of
extrahepatic and large intrahepatic ducts, by radiologic ("macrophysical") techniques contrasts with our ignorance about the pathogenesis of chemically induced cholestasis.  The localization in
the hepatocytes by organelle pathology raised the hope that the
initial event might be identified, for instance, whether and when
it is an alteration of the postprandial bile acid-dependent or the
basal bile acid-independent hepatocellular secretion or of the
ductular secretion of bicarbonate-rich fluid, all three of which
have been demonstrated in man (12, 13).  Just as in many other
areas, organelle pathology  by identifying but not solving a
problem raised more questions than it answered, particularly since
it can only suggest but not establish hydrodynamic processes in
and around hepatocytes and ductules as a "microphysical" component
of cholestasis.  This review, including observations just presented,
should also contribute to the understanding of the elusive mechanism
of bile secretion by looking at cholestasis as an experiment of
nature, thereby also correcting previous hypotheses of investigators, including ourselves.

As in all functional/morphological correlations, the question

arises as to whether an observed structural alteration is the basis
or the result of the functional defect. Morphometrically the canalicular dilatation in man correlates with the elevation of the serum
activities of enzymes increased in cholestasis, particularly leucine
aminopeptidase (14). However, the dilatation, which is present
throughout the entire lobule and not only in the zone of visible
bile retention, is not uniform. Even in severe cholestasis, normal
bile canaliculi may be adjacent to abnormal ones (1). Bile canaliculi or their diverticuli may newly develop in biliary obstruction of
rats since their appearance resembles the stages identified in the
neonatal liver (15). Adjacent hepatocytes vary in the amount of
bile deposition. The different degrees of cholestasis in neighboring
hepatocytes suggest variation of bile-secretory activity throughout
the liver, comparable to the variable cellular accumulation of proteins such as albumin, fibrinogen and alpha-1-antitrypsin (16).

## CHOLESTASIS, MICROSOMAL TRANSFORMATION AND BILE ACID METABOLISM

A disturbance of the bile acid metabolism was one of the first
chemical explanations of the structural alterations when functional
and structural cholestasis were produced in rodents by the monohydroxy lithocholate (17, 18). Shortly after its intravenous administration, reduced biliary secretion was accompanied by cholestatic
alterations of the bile canaliculi and widening of the pericanalicular zone. Since bile salts are in bile as polyionic aggregates or
micelles, together with cholesterol and phospholipids, excess of
lithocholate, which is a poor micelle former, was considered to cause
cholestasis by disturbing micelle formation. Moreover, the multi-
lamellar folding of the microvilli after acute administration results
from the focally accentuated precipitation of lithocholate in and
around the bile canaliculus (1). Simultaneous administration of taurocholic acid counteracts the cholestatic effect (20). This implies
disturbance of the bile acid-dependent fraction, but small doses of
lithocholate inhibit also the active transport of inorganic ions,
i.e. the bile acid-independent secretion (21); there is, however, no
evidence so far that this is associated with recognizable changes of
the bile-secretory apparatus. An excess of monohydroxylated bile
acids may be formed in the liver, either lithocholate or 3-beta-
hydroxy-5-cholenate (22), which has been identified in the meconium
in normal fetus and in the urine in neonatal biliary atresia (23) and
subsequently in adult liver disease (24). Hepatic synthesis of monohydroxy bile acids (25) implies a failure of both 7 and 12 alpha bile
acid hydroxylation in the SER, which, however, appears hypertrophic
in cholestasis of both man and experimental animals (26, 27), giving
rise to the concept of a hypoactive hypertrophic SER (28). Study by
various groups of the biotransformation system in mechanical, (29,
30, 31, 32) and chemical induced cholestasis (norethandrolone and
alpha-naphthyl isothiocyanate) (33, 34), also in man (35), demonstrated indeed a nonparallel decrease of the activities of several

microsomal enzymes, and especially in mechanical obstruction, a
significant reduction of the cytochrome P-450 content of the microsomal proteins.  Recent studies (36) after common-duct ligation in
rats demonstrated a significant increase in total microsomal protein without change of the protein/phospholipid ratio of the microsomal membranes and of the proportion of smooth to rough  ER.  The
activity of cytochrome P-450 reductase (NADPH cytochrome C reductase) was slightly reduced, but particularly the cytochrome
P-450 concentration, more in the rough than in the smooth ER, while
cytochrome b-5 was less diminished (Fig. 1).  Although in adult
rats total hepatic cytochrome P-450 was reduced, in the more adap-
table young animals this was compensated for by the increase in
total microsomal proteins.  The activity of P-448-dependent benzpyrene hydroxylase was greatly diminished in a noncompetitive
manner, far more than that of aminopyrine demethylase and aniline
hydroxylase (28) and not related to reduced reductase, supporting
a previously demonstrated qualitative change in the membranes
(Fig. 2).  This glucose-6-phosphatase activity was significantly
decreased, but not as result of lipid peroxidation, while the
concentration in the microsomal proteins of glucuronyl transferase remained unchanged and thus its total hepatic activity was
increased.  This enzyme is located in the deeper layer of the SER
(37), and its increased activity in cholestasis, also found in
man (35), indicates loosening of the membrane.  Turnover studies
of the heme proteins by two groups (31, 38) indicated normal rates
of degradation, with the rate of synthesis found normal by one (38)
and reduced by the other (31).  Morphometric studies (39) demonstrated an increased surface density of both the rough and smooth
ER three and six days after common duct ligation while the volume
density was not significantly altered.  This indicates that newly
formed enzymatic nonfunctioning membranes seem to account for the
reduction of the cytochrome P-450 concentration by dilution, thus
creating relative hypoactivity of the microsomal system sometimes,
but not necessarily decreasing the total hepatic content.

The qualitative and quantitative alteration of the P-450-
dependent biotransformation in the SER could account for alteration of the bile acid metabolism in cholestasis.  Various steps
of cholesterol conversion to bile acids occur in SER and some of
them are cytochrome P-450-dependent and CO-sensitive (40).  The
rate-limiting step is 7-alpha-hydroxylation, but its P-450 dependence is argued (41), particularly since it is not induced by phenobarbital and the best evidence available today indicates that if
it is P-450-dependent, the species of the hemoprotein may be
different.

Attractive as our theory of initiation of cholestasis by hypoactive SER may be (42), it is not confirmed and time curves after
experimental common duct ligation (26) suggest that the alteration
of the SER is secondary to cholestasis but not the primary event,

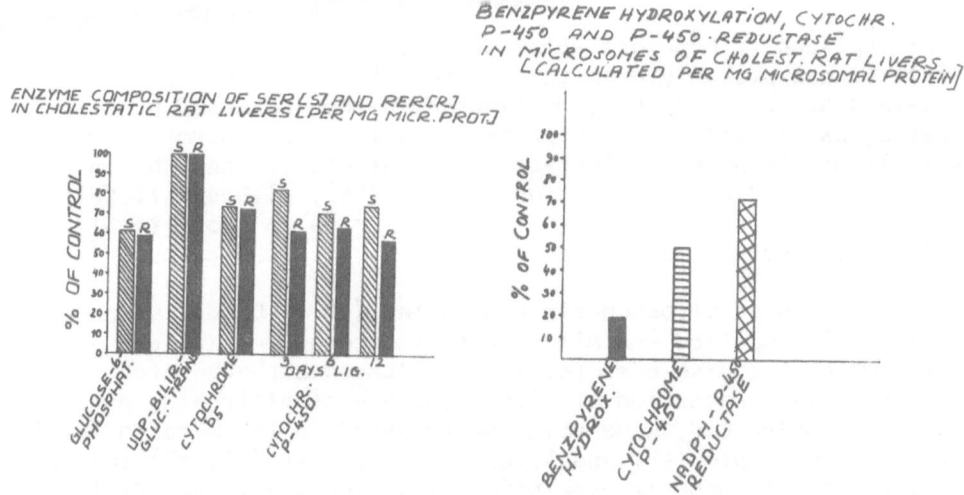

Figures 1 and 2

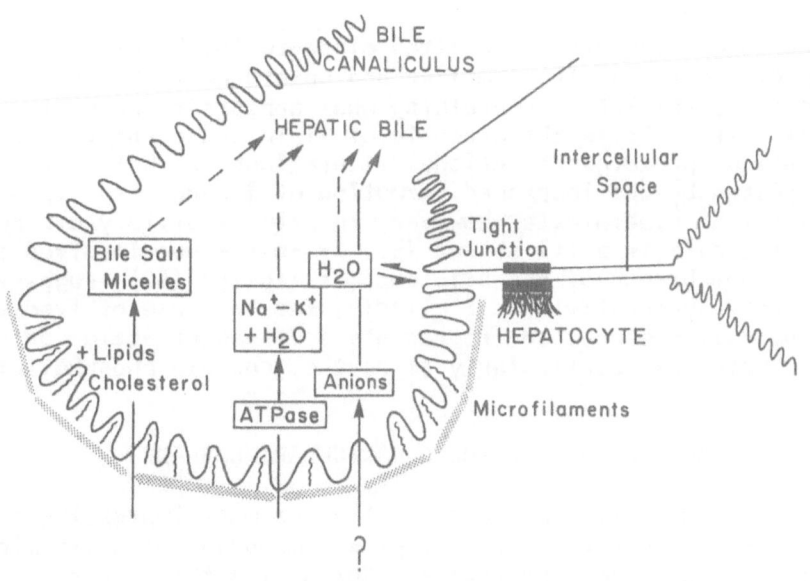

Figure 3.   Transport sites at the bile canaliculus

although it may accentuate existing cholestasis.

Alterations of hepatocellular organelles other than SER in cholestasis are probably even more so sequelae than that of SER. Involvement of the rough ER is reflected in the increased protein synthesis, particularly of lipoproteins (43). The abnormal low-density lipoprotein LPX is increased in cholestasis, and this has even been ascribed diagnostic significance (44), although it fails to identify the type of cholestasis. It is rich in cholesterol, the microsomal synthesis of which is excessive in cholestasis (45).

The cristae of mitochondria are curled (46). Oxidative phosphorylation is impaired and mitochondrial cytochromes are decreased, which has also been related to altered carbohydrate metabolism (47). Retention of bile acids and of bilirubin, particularly unconjugated, have been incriminated in the mitochondrial alterations. Cholate (48) and lithocholate excess (17, 19) lead to curling of mitochondria even before jaundice develops. Bilirubin in experimental animals (49) and in severe hemolysis in man (50) aggravates cholestasis. With bilirubin concentrations found in cholestasis, decreased oxygen uptake by hepatic mitochondria is associated with uncoupling of oxidative phosphorylation (43). Since, however, interference with the energy provision may occur under many clinical and experimental circumstances in the absence of cholestasis, its initiation by primary mitochondrial injury is improbable.

The Golgi apparatus, localized close to the bile canaliculus, reveals dilatation of its lamellae and enlargement of its vesicles and vacuoles, the latter containing what appears to be biliary material. Its role is the assembly of lipid and carbohydrate components of proteins; functional alterations in cholestasis are suggested by the increased formation of low-density lipoprotein. The Golgi zone hyperplasia, however, in primary biliary cirrhosis when cholestasis is still absent (51) or in the non-involved liver when only one branch of the bile duct is ligated (52), suggests a compensatory hyperactivity. Similarly, the increase of lysosomes marked by acid phosphatase represents a scavenger action on excess retained material, particularly since they contain phospholipid crystals.

## ALTERATIONS OF THE CANALICULAR MEMBRANE

Both structurally and functionally the most impressive alteration in cholestasis concerns the plasma membrane with its microvilli lining the bile canaliculus. Normally a thin, hazy layer of glycocalyx, rich in carbohydrates, covers a denser membranous layer in presumably the deeper portion of which ATPase is demonstrated histochemically. This membrane covers the ectoplasm, which is widened in cholestasis but free of vacuoles. It is rich in

filaments extending into the microvilli and, as was discussed here
(53), these filaments are along the entire canalicular membrane
but aggregated at the junction of neighboring hepatocytes (53, 54)
and are less numerous around the rest of the cell membrane. They
are altered by phalloidin (54). Reaction with heavy meromyosine
identifies some fibrils as containing actin. That cytochalasin B
indeed induces typical cholestasis (53) represents a major progress
in the understanding of cholestasis. Interference with a third
type of these proteins, the microtubules, is excluded in cholestasis because of the lack of effect of colchicine on biliary
secretion while it inhibits microtubular blood-directed secretion
(55). Weakening of the canalicular membrane is well illustrated
by scanning electron-microscopic pictures (7, 20, 63) which show
the tortuous, irregular and often angular widening of the canaliculi
with formation of diverticuli in obstruction, lithocholate and
steroid induced cholestasis. In isolated perfused rat livers,
ultrastructural features of cholestasis are produced by sporidesmin,
possibly reacting with contractile proteins, and by icterogenin,
which is supposed to affect $Mg^{2+}$-activated $Na^{+}$-$K^{+}$ ATPase (56), the
energy source of the mechanism pumping sodium into the canaliculus.
This points, in addition to the physical effect on the structural
level, to a chemical alteration. A variable reduction of the
histochemical reaction product of membrane-associated enzymes,
particularly ATPase and 5'-nucleotidase and appearance of that of
alkaline phosphatase (57), develops more rapidly in chemically induced than in obstructive cholestasis. Gamma-glutamyl transpeptidase appears earlier in the canalicular membrane, while in
extrahepatic cholestasis it is visualized there after it had accumulated in ductular cells (58). All this suggests a primary
hepatocellular injury in the chemical form. The most convincing
information is available about chemical alterations in isolated
membrane fractions in both chemically and mechanically induced
cholestasis. Activities of 5'-nucleotidase and ATPase are reduced,
not depending on bile salt exposure, while that of alkaline phosphatase is increased. Sialic acid content is raised while synthesis and degradation rates of protein, cholesterol, phospholipids
and neutral sugars are unchanged (59).


## THE ROLE OF THE TIGHT JUNCTION

Older concepts of the pathogenesis of jaundice assumed regurgitation of bile into tissue fluid and blood either through the
hepatocytes or between the damaged liver cells. Fine-structural
studies indicated the integrity of the tight junction even in
severe cholestasis when almost all microvilli seem to have disappeared, and the junction seems to open only when the liver cell
dies. Nevertheless, flow from the canalicular lumen to the peri-
sinusoidal recesses has been suggested (60). Recent studies also
reported here indicate flow of water and small molecular substances

through "leaky" junctions (61), possibly in either direction.
Clearance studies with various agents (62, 63) strongly suggest
such a permeability. Correlation of morphological features with
the forces governing flux across the tight junction still requires
clarification. Mitochondria appear attached to either side of the
desmosomal part of the tight junction, indicating energy supply
(64).

The three-dimensional view of the bile canaliculi made possible by scanning electron microscopy illustrates the distribution
of the junctions and microvilli. After fracturing prefixed specimens, the lateral surfaces of the hepatocytes are exposed (65).
The microvilli appear "clearly concentrated at their lateral margin
where adjacent hepatocytes adjoin" (65) in rows along the tight
junctions. They point to transport activity in this area presumably of bile water into the bile canaliculus. The lateral
intercellular cleft surfaces of the hepatocytes are almost smooth
except for some pits and protrusions with some species variations.
These narrow spaces are like tissue spaces anywhere else filled
with glycoproteins and proteoglycans which by themselves vary in
fluidity, thus influencing water flow. In cholestasis the microvilli around the tight junction seem to persist to a greater degree
than those on the roof of the canaliculi, which tend to disappear,
suggesting that the former have a special function. Moreover, the
intercellular cleft becomes shortened by extension of the peri-
sinusoidal recess with its more irregular perisinusoidal microvilli and by dilatation of the bile canaliculi. This might facilitate flow through the tight junction. However, even normally the
cleft may be as short as $0.1\mu$ (7). This fine-structural arrangement suggests a system of fluxes in either direction which is influenced by humoral, hydrodynamic and ionic factors and may be
subject to change under circumstances related to cholestasis (Fig.
3). Together with the ion delivery into the canalicular lumen,
it may account for variations in the bile acid-independent fraction
and by suppression of the flow-generating system may suffice to
initiate cholestasis.

## THE PRIMARY EVENT IN CANALICULAR CHOLESTASIS

The bile acid-independent flow may be inhibited by various
factors, for instance, dyes, sex and anabolic steroids and small
doses of bile acids. These may compete with anion secretion into
the bile canaliculus as they compete with each other for uptake by
hepatocytes (66) (Fig. 4). The inhibition is reflected in impaired
secretion of cations, especially sodium, in part by the $Na^+-K^+$
ATPase pump and in part along with bile salts. Reduction in the
bile water may be related to inspissation and precipitation of bile
salts and this event is apparently reflected in the alteration of
canalicular microvilli, initially on the canalicular roof, that

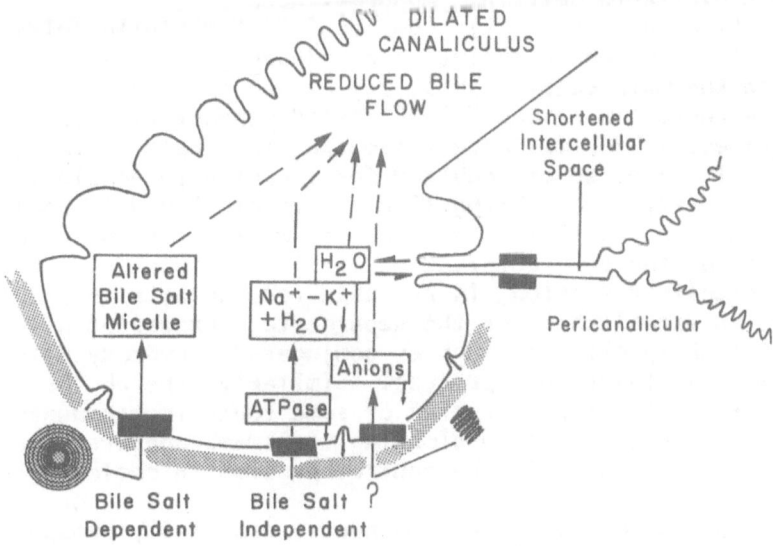

**Figure 4.   Blocks in canalicular transport sites in cholestasis**

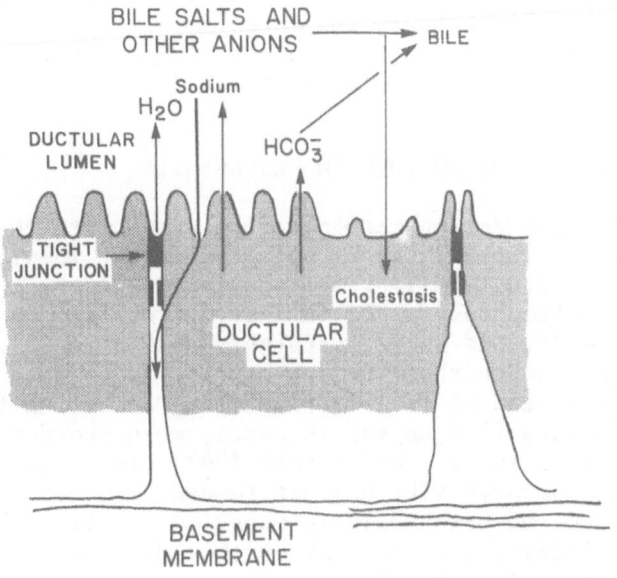

**Figure 5.   Transport sites in the ductule**

means now cholestasis sets in. Abnormal back flow from the canaliculi has been suggested (62). Depression of the bile acid-
dependent flow, for which cholate, chenodeoxycholate and deoxycholate are the main determinants, may either be associated with
conspicuous reduction of the bile salt-independent flow or may be
the initial event, for instance following disturbance of micelle
formation. It seems to be required for jaundice to develop.
Whether precipitates resembling liquid crystals found in cholestasis in the hepatocellular cytoplasm as well as in the bile
thrombi are related to precipitation of biliary substances because
of faulty micelle formation, is probable for the bile thrombus and
remains to be established for the hepatocyte. Excess of bile acids
solubilizing phospholipids, such as conjugated dihydroxy bile acids
(see below), may favor this process. Similarly, the cholestatic
steroids - anabolic, contraceptive or some found in pregnancy -
may have steric configuration blocking transmembrane transport,
the disturbance of which is the central process in cholestasis.

Participation of membrane components, especially phospholipids,
has been postulated in biliary secretion and appears enhanced in
cholestasis, possibly because of increased solubilization by bile
acids. This last phenomenon is probably also responsible for some
visible membranous components identified in the serum (67), particularly in cholestasis (68). Transport of organic anions other
than bile acids,like bilirubin and dyes, may also be altered,
although the disturbance of clearance of these in Dubin-Johnson
syndrome (69) suggests an additional process governing their
secretion. Impaired cholate transport and sodium secretion are
indeed linked (70), possibly because the intraluminal cations
required for initiation of bile acid-dependent flow may have to be
delivered there first by bile acids (72).

## THE ROLE OF THE DUCTULE IN CHOLESTASIS

The bile ductules connecting terminal bile ducts with the bile
canaliculi,located in the portal tracts but also on the lobular
periphery, differ ultrastructurally from the hepatocytes by the
smaller size of their mitochondria and luminal microvilli, by an
abundance of tonofilaments and by a straight basal layer placed
on a basement membrane, which thus forms a barrier to free exchange with tissue fluid and blood (72, 73). They occasionally
have cilia and their microvilli appear in ducts, more crowded in
longitudinal rows similar to bile canaliculi (74). The ductules
differ also from the hepatocytes by a great tendency to pathologic
variations in structure and presumably in function. Bile-ductular
cells multiply in cholestasis, as seen after thymidine administration to rats. Increased bile pressure lengthens them to tortuous
structures lined by cuboidal epithelium. Sprouting of greatly
varying epithelial cells reflects an irritation, often associated

with reabsorption of bile.  It is in early stages associated with periductular inflammation and subsequent fibrosis (bile-ductular reaction) (73).  The irritating factor may be luminal and excreted in the biliary tract, because upon parenteral lithocholate administration the bile ductules reveal irregularly shaped microvilli and increased cytoplasmic vesicles when the canalicular changes have disappeared (17).  Feeding of lithocholate produces a bile-ductular reaction progressing to fibrosis (75).  Severe ductular damage also follows the canalicular injury produced by alpha-naphthyl isothiocyanate.  The functional variation associated with this ductular lesion (76) is also reflected in ultrastructural loss of microvilli as well as in signs of both increased secretion as well as reabsorption in man of bile-pigmented phospholipid-containing material, eventually followed by duplication of the basement membranes (77) (Fig. 5).  The ductule contributes to the constitution of bile by secreting a bicarbonate-rich fluid under the control of gastro-intestinal hormones, like secretin, and by reabsorbing a sodium-rich fluid.  Glucose is reabsorbed in a "biliohepatic" circulation (78).

While, as mentioned, periductular inflammation is simply correlated with the degree of cholestasis, some observations suggest that ductular alterations may contribute to, or even initiate, mechanical features of cholestasis, whether they are primary or reactive.

1.  While ductal changes in chronic aggressive hepatitis favoring transition to cirrhosis need not be accompanied by cholestasis, in rare cholestatic forms of viral, drug (chlorpropamide) induced and cryptogenic hepatitis severe cholestasis seems to be associated with an acute ductular and periductular inflammation, also reflected in extremely high serum activities of alkaline phosphatase.  The pathogenesis of this process, which is usually protracted but self-limited, although sometimes progressive, is not clear (79).

2.  In chronic fibrosing portal lesions an obstructive element is readily recognized by compression of bile ducts and ductules and eventually by their disappearance after prolonged obstruction of large bile ducts (secondary biliary cirrhosis) (1).

3.  Three-dimensional reconstructions of the ductules carried out repeatedly have suggested mechanical disturbance of bile flow in the complex system of the proliferated ductules (1).

4.  The proximity of the bile ducts and ductules to portal capillaries, with which they may share the basement membrane (77), suggests the possibility of hydrodynamic effects by the blood flow. The movement of protein from portal capillaries (80) to portal bile passages suggests that an edema of the portal tracts from disturbed macromolecular transport might disturb portal bile flow in acute hepatitis (81).

## CONSEQUENCES AND EVOLUTION OF CHOLESTASIS

In correlating structural and functional features of cholestasis, the difficulty in separating cause and consequences was
stressed.  Fine-structural evidence indicates cellular retention
of the main biliary substances.  That of phospholipid is reflected
in whorl-shaped deposits resembling liquid crystals, usually surrounded by a membrane, but this is more a morphologic marker than
deleterious to the surrounding cytoplasm.  The same holds for
cholesterol clefts in hepatocytic cytoplasm (51).  Bilirubin
deposits, dense amorphous material usually not surrounded by a
membrane, might have a damaging effect primarily on mitochondria,
especially if unconjugated.  While so far no method exists to
morphologically demonstrate intracellular bile acids, their effect
is probably the most significant on the basis of several observations.

1.  The cholestatic effect of lithocholate and possibly other
monohydroxy bile acids was already mentioned and also their ability
to produce portal inflammation, fibrosis and possibly cirrhosis
(75).  This led to the incrimination of lithocholate in various
hepatic injuries, like those associated with inflammatory bowel
diseases, or after intestinal bypass operations for obesity and in
progressive familial intrahepatic cholestasis and cirrhosis (82).
In the therapy of cholesterol gallstones with chenodeoxycholic
acid, increased formation of lithocholate is at least under consideration as possible cause of liver injury.

2.  Competitive binding of bile acids to microsomal preparations
following Michaelis-Menten kinetics has been demonstrated in vitro
(83), explaining the reduction of microsomal biotransformation of
drugs and xenobiotics in cholestasis.  Bile acids or their metabolic intermediates may serve as physiologic regulators of some
functions of the microsomal biotransformation system as has, for
instance, been suggested for the porphyrin heme pathway (84).

3.  The primary bile acids exhibit a dose-dependent effect in
vitro on microsomes which undergo a gradual disintegration with
reduction of P-450, inhibition of its reductase, destruction of
the lipoprotein-binding site of P-450, which becomes inactive
P-420 (83, 85).  Dihydroxy bile acids are more effective than trihydroxy ones and the nonconjugated bile acids are more detergent
than conjugated ones.  The lesions in livers perfused with chenodeoxycholic acid may thus be explained (86).  Whether detergent
levels are reached in the liver is not certain since determination
of bile acids in liver tissue does not reveal their actual distribution among cytoplasm and its organelles, blood and bile.
Determination of hepatic concentration in rats with extrahepatic
biliary obstruction (87) and intrahepatic cholestasis (33) show
that only concentrations permitting competitive binding are reached,
whereas in human livers after prolonged biliary obstruction detergent levels of dihydroxy bile acids were found (88).  Study of
the distribution in the hepatocyte indicate that normally the bulk

of bile acids is bound to the microsomes (89), but after prolonged
cholestasis it is in the cytoplasm (90).

The detrimental effects of bile acid retention upon tissues
may be mitigated by some protective and in part alternate metabolic
pathways. Lithocholic acid can be metabolized by the liver (91).
Sulfation with resulting urinary excretion has been described in
cholestasis (92, 93). Excess cholate formation, in preference to
the more detergent chenodeoxycholic acid, may present a protective
mechanism in man (88). In rodents, ursodeoxycholic and
particularly beta-muricholic acid are formed preferentially,
reducing the concentration of detergent chenodeoxycholate (87).
However, formation of ursodeoxycholic acid from chenodeoxycholic
acid was also found in man (92). The most effective protection of
the liver cell against excess detergent action is an inhibition of
bile acid formation in the damaged liver (94), especially by inhibition of the rate-limiting 7-alpha-hydroxylation of either the
precursors (94) or deoxycholic acid (93). Interestingly, phenobarbital may restore activity of the system reduced by common bile
duct ligation in rats (27, 95).

## HEPATOCELLULAR INJURY PROGRESSING TO NECROSIS

Successful detergent action upon the hepatocytes results in
proliferation of hepatocytes and in an accumulation of phospholipid
whorls in hepatocytic vacuoles which, if present in excess, convey
to the rarified cytoplasm a brown color, a lesion designated as
feathery degeneration, the extent of which parallels the hepatic
concentration of dihydroxycholates in man (89). This lesion involves scattered hepatocytes in the lobular center and continuous
layers on the lobular periphery. The identical light- and electron-
microscopic appearance of the hepatocytes may be observed without
bile pigment retention and hyperbilirubinemia. Until the presence
of bile acids can be demonstrated by histochemical techniques, this
picture can only tentatively be designated as "cholate stasis".
Such hepatocytes are frequent in various forms of chronic hepatitis.
Around them, connective tissue fibers accumulate, suggesting that
these cells stimulate progressive hepatic fibrosis. Moreover, in
prolonged cholestasis and in primary biliary cirrhosis, hepatocytes
on the lobular periphery may contain deposits of Mallory's hyalin,
conventionally associated with alcohol abuse (96). This lesion in
prolonged cholestasis shows the electron-microscopic characteristics of the deposits in alcoholics which now have been identified
as altered contractile proteins (97), which otherwise are responsible, as mentioned, for the stability of the cell membrane as well
as for uptake, transport and secretion (98). Therefore, hepatocellular necrosis in cholestasis may result from a weakening of the
contractile protein system. The pathogenesis of alcoholic hyalin
is still problematic, however, recently evidence was offered (99)

that hepatic accumulation of export protein in alcoholic steatosis
may be induced by a disturbance of tubulin, one of the contractile
proteins.  Typical hyalin has been produced in mice by administration of griseofulvin following cholestasis as well as morphologically similar porphyrin stasis (100).

The cholestatic hepatocellular injury within the lobular
parenchyma elicits inflammation.  This cholestatic hepatitis (1)
may create difficulty in differential diagnosis from independent
hepatitis, although it is restricted to the cholestatic zone.  It
is followed by portal inflammation associated with ductular alteration  and proliferation and with fibrosis.  This is the lesion
which may persist after subsidence of cholestasis and represents
the interval alteration, e.g. between episodes of recurrent benign
cholestasis (1).  Periductular fibrosis, secondary to intralobular
cholestasis, if severe enough, may interfere with ductular transport and create a mechanical intrahepatic component secondary to
the preexisting cholestasis.  This accounts for persisting disturbance of the bile flow after prolonged extrahepatic mechanical
obstruction which has been corrected surgically.  Interference with
hepatic circulation develops, as seen after long-term obstruction
in rats (101), and is clinically reflected in portal hypertension.
The end result is progressive destruction of the ductal and ductular
system by continued inflammation and fibrosis creating secondary
biliary cirrhosis in prolonged mechanical obstruction and eventually even in intrahepatic cholestasis when it persists for years.

## THOUGHTS IN PATHOGENESIS OF CHOLESTASIS

Intraluminal pressure from obstruction in extrahepatic and
large intrahepatic bile ducts produces initial lesions of centrolobular hepatocytes, with early impairment of bile acid-dependent
flow.  This "macrophysical" large duct obstruction is joined by
mechanical "microphysical" factors in ductules and canaliculi
operating in both chemical and mechanical cholestasis.  Whether
the biliary precipitates in the form of bile thrombi retard bile
flow, is doubtful since even in severe obstruction the noninvolved
canaliculi probably serve as a bypass.  The centrolobular localization of the thrombi results from the effective flushing of the
lobular periphery when even in complete mechanical obstruction of
the large bile ducts a hepatoductular circulation permits better
flow than in the lobular center.  Only when, in prolonged obstruction, the fibrotic process, particularly in smaller portal
tracts, interferes with this circulation, peripheral cholestasis
with peripheral bile thrombi ensues.  In intrahepatic cholestasis
few initiating mechanisms can be postulated, most of which concern
experimental rather than clinical conditions (Table 1).  That
damage of the organelles outside the biliary pole of the hepatocytes (mitochondria and ER) leads to injury of the bile-secretory

TABLE I:   ESTABLISHED OR STRONGLY SUGGESTED INITIATING FACTORS
IN INTRAHEPATIC CHOLESTASIS

| FACTOR | SITE |
|---|---|
| LITHOCHOLATE | 1. PRECIPITATION IN AND AROUND CANALICULI<br>2. INHIBITION OF MICELLE FORMATION |
| BILIRUBIN | 1. OVERLOAD<br>2. COMPETITION WITH OTHER ANION SECRETION |
| ANABOLIC CONTRACEPTIVES &<br>"PREGNANCY" STEROIDS | 1. MEMBRANE ALTERATION BY STERIC<br>    CONFIGURATION<br>2. COMPETITION WITH ANION SECRETION<br>3. INHIBITION OF ATPase PUMP? |
| CHLORPROMAZINE AND OTHER DRUGS | 1. PRECIPITATION IN PERICANALICULAR SPACE<br>2. DISTURBANCE OF MICELLE FORMATION |
| CYTOCHALASIN B | ALTERATION OF CONTRACTILE PROTEINS<br>   WEAKENING CANALICULAR MEMBRANE<br>   (AND INHIBITING SECRETION?) |
| INJURY TO HEPATOCYTIC ORGANELLES | SECONDARY INJURY OF "BILE SECRETORY<br>   APPARATUS" |
| ALTERATIONS OF DUCTULAR<br>   EPITHELIUM? | SECONDARY TO LUMINAL FACTORS |

apparatus, is illustrated by the common occurrence of cholestatic jaundice in almost all severe liver diseases. Experimentally, carbon tetrachloride inhibits both bile acid-dependent and -independent flow (102).

Organelle pathologic findings correlated with functional observations suggest that in cholestasis, in addition to the inter-reaction between bile acid-dependent and -independent flow, two vicious circles operate (103) causing retention of both bilirubin and bile salts (Fig. 6). The latter are the most important effectors in both circles,their retention even producing identical lesions in organelles of renal tubules (104). In one of the circles molecular or organelle actions reinforce each other, whether the initial target is the ER, mitochondria or components of the canaliculus. The erratic results of treatment with pheno-barbital or other inducers upon the cholestatic manifestations (105, 106) may be accounted for by primary involvement of different organelles. Similarly, in the second circle,with two circular pathways, cellular and hydrodynamic processes follow in different sequences; hepatocellular necrosis, biliary epithelium lesions, inflammation and fibrosis being main links. But the "cholangio-litis", years ago assumed to be the primary event in intrahepatic cholestasis, is now usually considered a reaction.

## CONJUGATED HYPERBILIRUBINEMIA WITHOUT CHOLESTASIS

In several clinical conditions with elevated direct reacting bilirubin, cholestasis as defined structurally is absent. One is the Dubin-Johnson syndrome and related disorders not necessarily associated with abnormal pigment metabolism (Rotor syndrome). They represent disturbances in the hepatocellular secretion of organic anions including bilirubin but not bile acids (69) the blood level of which is not altered. This lesion is not involved in the vicious circles. In the early stage of primary biliary cirrhosis all biliary substances pile up in the blood, not because of cholestasis but presumably by regurgitation of biliary sub-stances through damaged bile ducts in which the contractile fibrillar system is also altered (107). Since this lesion causes bile acid retention, it enters the circles, as reflected in the early alterations of hepatocellular mitochondria and the Golgi zone (51, 107). Indeed, in later stages mechanical peripheral cholestasis may dominate the picture, while in early stages centro-lobular cholestasis can be provoked more readily than in healthy persons by administration of potentially cholestatic drugs. Possibly a third condition without primary cholestasis enters the vicious circles (possibly by ductular injury), namely, inter-ference with the uptake of bile acids by the hepatocytes for which specific receptors have been demonstrated (66). It has been suggested that such a mechanism may initiate recurrent benign cholestasis (108).

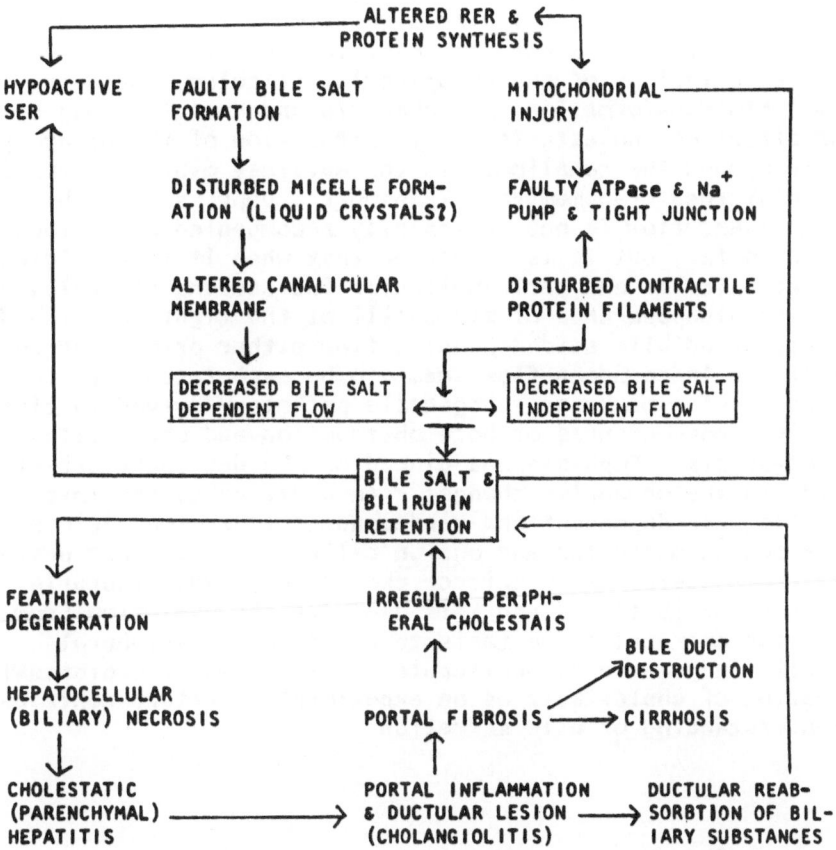

Figure 6.  Vicious circles operative in cholestasis; the one in the upper half is at the molecular organelle level while the one in the left lower portion is at the lobular hydromechanic level.  (Redrawn from reference 103)

## SUMMARY

Investigation of organelle alterations in cholestasis established a lesion in the pericanalicular region of the hepatocytes
initiated by pressure in mechanical obstruction of extrahepatic and
large intrahepatic bile ducts, while without evidence of obstruction, chemical processes are incriminated. Although organelle
pathology shifted concern from primary mechanical processes in the
biliary passages to hepatocellular alterations, it has failed to
identify the initiating event, at least in most clinical conditions.
Characteristic lesions of the endoplasmic reticulum, including
microsomal biotransformation, mitochondria and ductules may be
cause or effect of cholestasis, while alteration of the hepatocytic
organelles around the canaliculi is the earliest manifestation indicating disturbed transmembrane transport. Depression of bile
acid-independent flow is not necessarily accompanied by lesions
visualized so far, but it is suggested that when it is sufficiently
reduced, canalicular and pericanalicular indications of cholestasis
appear, with disappearance of microvilli at the tight junction delayed. Disturbed bile acid-dependent flow either primary or related
to that of the independent flow seems to be associated with changes
in the canalicular membrane. Organelle pathology served to clarify
the identical consequences of both obstruction and chemically induced cholestasis. Emphasis was placed on the detergent effect of
bile acids in the organelle changes. In addition to the interaction
between bile acid-dependent and -independent flow, two vicious
circles - one on molecular and one on cellular level - are postulated in cholestasis. They enforce the process, multifactorial in
nature, wherever it starts and this explains the evolution from
centrolobular chemical cholestasis to a secondary peripheral
mechanically induced form, applicable to all forms of cholestasis.
Investigation of cholestasis as an experiment of nature contributes
to the understanding of bile secretion.

## REFERENCES

1. Popper, H., and Schaffner, F.: Pathophysiology of cholestasis. Hum Pathol 1:1-24, 1970

2. Watson, C.J., and Hoffbauer, F.W.: Problem of prolonged hepatitis with particular reference to cholangiolitic type and to development of cholangiolitic cirrhosis of liver. Ann Intern Med 25:195-227, 1946

3. Popper, H., and Schaffner, F.: Laboratory diagnosis of liver disease. Coordinated use of histological and biochemical observations. JAMA 150:1367-1372, 1952

4. Rouiller, C.: Les canalicules biliares. Étude au microscope électronique. Acta Anat (Basel) 26:94-109, 1956

5. Schaffner, F., and Popper, H.: Morphologic studies of cholestasis. Gastroenterology 37:565-573, 1959

6. Steiner, J.W., Jezequel, A.M., Phillips, M.J., et al: Some aspects of the ultrastructural pathology of the liver. In: Progress in Liver Diseases, Vol II. H. Popper and F. Schaffner, editors. New York, Grune & Stratton, 1965. pp 303-372

7. Compagno, J., and Grisham, J.W.: Scanning electron microscopy of extrahepatic biliary obstruction. Arch Pathol 97:348-351, 1974

8. Popper, H.: Cholestasis. Ann Rev Med 19:39-56, 1968

9. Motta, P., and Fumagalli, G.: Structure of rat bile canaliculi as revealed by scanning electron microscopy. Anat Res 182: 499-514, 1975

10. Dubin, I.N., and Peterson, L.H.: An explanation for the centro-lobular localization of intrahepatic bile stasis in acute liver diseases. Am J Med Sci 236:45-52, 1958

11. Thaler, H. This volume

12. Boyer, J.L., and Bloomer, J.R.: Canalicular bile secretion in man. Studies utilizing the biliary clearance of [$^{14}$C] mannitol. J Clin Invest 54:773-781, 1974

13. Prandi, D., Erlinger, S., Glasinovic, J.-C., and Dumont, M.: Canalicular bile production in man. Europ J Clin Invest 5: 1-6, 1975

14. Roessner, A., van Husen, N., Pauls, E., Gerlach, U., and Themann, H.: Feinstrukturell-morphometrische Untersuchungen an Leberbiopsien von Patienten mit intrahepatischer Cholestase. I. Korrelation zwischen den morphometrischen Parametern der Gallencapillaren und den serochemischen Cholestasemessgroessen. Virchows Arch A Pathol Anat Histol 367:15-26, 1975

15. De Vos, R., De Wolf-Peeters, C., Desmet, V., Bianchi, L., and Rohr, H.P.: Significance of liver canalicular changes after experimental bile duct ligation. Exper Molec Pathol 23:12-34, 1975

16. Guillouzo, A., and Feldmann, G.: Localization of albumin in hepatocytes during postnatal development of the rat. Digestion 11:436-463, 1974

17. Schaffner, F., and Javitt, N.B.:  Morphologic changes in hamster liver during intrahepatic cholestasis induced by taurolithocholate.  Lab Invest 15:1783-1792, 1966
18. Javitt, N.B., and Emerman, S.:  Effect of sodium taurolitho-cholate on bile flow and bile acid excretion.  J Clin Invest 47:1002-1014, 1968
19. Miyai, K., Mayr, W.W., and Richardson, A.L.:  Acute cholestasis induced by lithocholic acid in the rat.  A freeze-fracture replica and thin section study.  Lab Invest 32:527-535, 1975
20. Miyai, K., Price, V.M., and Fisher, M.M.:  Bile acid metabolism in mammals.  Ultrastructural studies on the intrahepatic cholestasis induced by lithocholic and chenodeoxycholic acids in the rat.  Lab Invest 24:292-302, 1971
21. King, J.E., and Schoenfield, L.J.:  Cholestasis induced by sodium taurolithocholate in isolated hamster liver.  J Clin Invest 50:2305-2312, 1971
22. Javitt, N.B.:  Current status of cholestasis induced by mono-hydroxy bile acids.  In:  Hepatology - Research and Clinical Issues - Volume 2.  Jaundice.  C.A. Goresky and M.M. Fisher, editors.  New York and London, Plenum Press, 1975.  pp 401-409
23. Makino,I., Sjovall, J., Norman, A., and Standuik, B.:  Ex-cretion of 3-beta-hydroxy-5-cholenoic acid and 3-beta-hydroxy-5-alpha-cholanoic acids in urine of infants with biliary atresia.  FEBS Letters 15:161-164, 1971
24. Back, P.:  Identification and quantitative determination of urinary bile acids excreted in cholestasis.  Clin Chim Acta 44:199-207, 1973
25. Back, P.:  Die primaere hepatische Synthese von Mono-Hydroxy-Gallensaeuren bei extrahepatischer Gallengangsatresie.  Klin Wschr 51:926-932, 1973
26. Schaffner, F., Bacchin, P.G., Hutterer, F., et al:  Mechanism of cholestasis.  IV.  Structural and biochemical changes in the liver and serum in rats after bile duct ligation.  Gastro-enterology 60:888-897, 1971
27. Solymoss, B., and Zsigmond, G.:  Effect of microsomal enzyme inducers on the liver changes produced by common bile-duct ligature.  Proc Soc Exper Biol Med 147:430-433, 1974
28. Hutterer, F., Klion, F.M., Wengraf, A., et al:  Hepatocellular adaptation and injury.  Structural and biochemical changes following dieldrin and methyl butter yellow.  Lab Invest 20:455-464, 1969
29. McLuen, E.F., and Fouts, J.R.:  The effect of obstructive jaundice on drug metabolism in rabbits.  J Pharmacol Exper Ther 131:7-11, 1961
30. Hutterer, F., Bacchin, P.G., Raisfeld, I.H., et al:  Alteration of microsomal biotransformation in the liver in cholestasis.  Proc Soc Exper Biol Med 133:702-706, 1970
31. Mackinnon, A.M., and Simon, F.R.:  Reduced synthesis of hepatic microsomal cytochrome P-450 in the bile duct ligated rat.  Biochem Biophys Res Commun 56:437-443, 1974

32. Schaffner, F., Scharnbeck, H.H., Hutterer, F., et al: Mechanism of cholestasis. VII. Alpha-naphthyl isothiocyanate induced jaundice. Lab Invest 28:321-331, 1973

33. Czygan, P., Greim, H., Hutterer, F., Schaffner, F., and Popper, H.: Comparison of two types of intrahepatic jaundice in rats with bile duct ligation. Acta Hepato-Gastroenterol 681: 339-345, 1974

34. Gigon,P.L.: Influence of extrahepatic cholestasis on metabolism and biliary excretion of imipramine. Arch Internat Pharmacodyn Ther 213:211-221, 1975

35. Hietanen, E., Auranen, A., and Savvakis, C.: The rate of drug biotransformation reactions and cellular viability in the livers of patients with biliary diseases. Acta Hepato-Gastroenterol 22:170-175, 1975

36. Denk, H., Eckerstorfer, R., and Rohr, H.P.: Further studies of structure and enzyme composition of rat liver endoplasmic reticulum in experimental mechanical cholestasis. I. Biochemical findings. In preparation

37. Vainio, H.: Action of chaotropic agents on drug metabolizing enzymes in hepatic microsomes. Biochim Biophys Acta 307: 152-161, 1973

38. Denk, H., Greim, H., Hutterer, F., et al: Turnover of hepatic cytochrome P-450 in experimental cholestasis. Exper Molec Pathol 19:241-247, 1973

39. Rohr, H.P., and Denk, H. (Personal communication)

40. Björkhem, I., and Danielsson, H.: Hydroxylations in biosynthesis and metabolism of bile acids. Molec Cellul Biochem 4:79-95, 1974

41. Brown, M.J.G., and Boyd, G.S.: The specificity of the rat-liver cholesterol 7-alpha-hydroxylase. Europ J Biochem 44: 37-47, 1974

42. Schaffner, F., and Popper, H.: Hypothesis: Cholestasis is the result of hypoactive hypertrophic smooth endoplasmic reticulum in the hepatocyte. Lancet 2:355-359, 1969

43. Stakeberg, H., Lundborg, H., and Schersten, T.: Rate of in vitro incorporation of precursors into hepatic lipids and proteins in patients with extrahepatic cholestasis. Europ J Clin Invest 4:399-403, 1974

44. Seidel, D., Alaupovic, P., and Furman, R.H.: A lipoprotein characterizing obstructive jaundice. I. Method for quantitative separation and identification of lipoproteins in jaundiced subjects. J Clin Invest 48:1211-1223, 1969

45. Harry, D.S., Dini, M., and McIntyre, N.: Effect of cholesterol feeding and biliary obstruction on hepatic cholesterol biosynthesis in the rat. Biochim Biophys Acta 296:209-220, 1973

46. Carruthers, J. S., and Steiner, J.W.: Experimental extrahepatic biliary obstruction: Fine structural changes of liver cell mitochondria. Gastroenterology 42:419-430, 1962

47. Yamada, T., Ida, T., Yamaoka, Y., Ozawa, K., Takasan, H., and Honjo, I.: Two distinct patterns of glucose intolerance in

icteric rats and rabbits. Relationship to impaired liver mitochondria functions. J Lab Clin Med 86:38-45, 1975

48. Witzleben, C.L.: Hepatic ultrastructural effects of cholic acid overload. Exper Molec Pathol 16:47-53, 1972

49. Boyce, W., and Witzleben, C.L.: Bilirubin as a cholestatic agent. II. Effect of variable doses of bilirubin on the severity of manganese-bilirubin cholestasis. Am J Pathol 72: 427-431, 1973

50. Fulop, M., Katz, S., and Lawrence, C.: Extreme hyper-bilirubinemia. Arch Int Med 127:254-258, 1974

51. Klion, F.M., and Schaffner, F.: Electron microscopic observations in primary biliary cirrhosis. Arch Pathol (Chicago) 81:152-161, 1966

52. Cooper, A.D., Jones, A.L., Koldinger, R., and Ockner, R.K.: Selective biliary obstruction: A model for the study of lipid metabolism in cholestasis. Gastroenterology 66:574-585, 1974

53. Phillips, M.J., Oda, M., Mak, E., Fisher, M.M., and Jeejeebhoy, K.N.: Microfilament dysfunction as a possible cause of intrahepatic cholestasis. Gastroenterology 69:48-58, 1975

54. Agostini, B., and Govindan, V.M.: Morphological changes induced by phalloidin in the rat liver: Electron microscopic, immuno-fluorescence and in vitro studies. In: IV. Workshop on Experimental Liver Injury. Pathogenesis and Mechanism of Liver Necrosis. D. Keppler, editor. Lancaster, The Medical and Technical Publishing Co. Ltd., in press

55. Stein, O., Sanger, L., and Stein, Y.: Colchicine-induced inhibition of lipoprotein and protein secretion into the serum and lack of interference with secretion of biliary phospholipids and cholesterol by rat liver in vivo. J Cell Biol 62:90-103, 1974

56. Bullock, G., Eakins, M.N., Sawyer, B.D., and Slater, T.F.: Studies on bile secretion with the aid of the isolated perfused rat liver. I. Inhibitory action of sporidesmin and icterogenin. Proc R Soc Lond B 186:333-356, 1974

57. Desmet, V.J.: Morphologic and histochemical aspects of cholestasis. In: Progress in Liver Diseases, Vol. IV. H. Popper and F. Schaffner, editors. New York and London, Grune & Stratton, 1972. pp 97-132

58. Ronchi,G., and Desmet, V.J.: Histochemical study of gamma-glutamyl transpeptidase (GGT) in experimental intrahepatic and extrahepatic cholestasis. Beitr Pathol 150:316-321, 1973

59. Simon, F.R., and Arias, I.M.: Alteration of bile canalicular enzymes in cholestasis. A possible cause of bile secretory failure. J Clin Invest 52:765-775, 1973

60. Schatzki, P.F.: Bile canaliculus and space of Disse. Electron microscopic relationship as delineated by Lanthanum. Lab Invest 20:87-93, 1969

61. Diamond, J.M.: Tight and leaky junctions of epithelia: A perspective on kisses in the dark. Fed Proc 33:2220-2224, 1974

62. Forker, E.L.: Canalicular anion transport, pathogenetic mechanisms and a steady state distributed model for measuring

kinetics. In: Hepatology - Research and Clinical Issues -
Vol. 2. Jaundice. C.A. Goresky and M.M. Fisher, editors. New
York and London., Plenum Press, 1975

63. Bradley, S., Morris, A., and Baker, K.J.: Mechanism of proteo-
bilia. Clin Res 22:558A, 1974

64. Sternlieb, I.: Mitochondrion-desmosome complexes in human
hepatocytes. Z Zellforsch 93:249-253, 1969

65. Grisham, J.W., Nopanitaya, W., and Compagno, J.: Scanning
electron microscopy of the liver: A review of methods and
results. In: Progress in Liver Diseases, Vol. V. H. Popper
and F. Schaffner, editors. New York, Grune & Stratton, in press

66. Glasinovic, J.-C., Dumont, M., Duval, M., and Erlinger, S.:
Hepatocellular uptake of taurocholate in the dog. J Clin Invest
55:419-426, 1975

67. Holdsworth,G., and Coleman, R.: Enzyme profiles of mammalian
bile. Biochim Biophys Acta 389:47-50, 1975

68. De Broe, M.E., Borgers, M., and Wieme, R.J.: The separation and
characterization of liver plasma membrane fragments circulating
in the blood of patients with cholestasis. Clin Acta 59:369-372,
1975

69. Alpert,S., Mosher, M., Shanske, A., et al: Multiplicity of
hepatic excretory mechanisms for organic anions. J Gen Physiol
53:238-247, 1969

70. Erlinger, S., Dhumeaux, D.: Mechanisms and control of secretion
of bile water and electrolytes. Gastroenterology 66:281-304,
1974

71. Schaffner, F.: Morphologic features of cholestasis. In: Drugs
and the Liver. K.Sickinger and W. Gerok, editors. Stuttgart,
F.K. Schattauer, in press

72. Schaffner, F., and Popper, H.: Electron microscopic studies of
normal and proliferated bile ductules. Am J Pathol 38:393-410,
1961

73. Steiner, J.W., Carruthers, J.S., and Kalifat, S.R.: The ductular
cell reaction of rat liver in extrahepatic cholestasis. I.
Proliferated biliary epithelial cells. Exp Mol Pathol 1:162-
185, 1962

74. Grisham, J.W., and Porta, E.A.: Ciliated cells in altered
murine and human bile ducts. Exp Cell Res 31:190-193, 1963

75. Carey, J.B., Jr., Wilson, I.D., Zaki, F.G., and Hanson, R.F.:
The metabolism of bile acids with special reference to liver
injury. Medicine 45:461-470, 1966

76. Goldfarb, S., Singer, E.J., and Popper, H.: Biliary ductules
and bile secretion. J Lab Clin Med 62:608, 1963

77. Sasaki, H., Schaffner, F., and Popper, H.: Bile ductules in
cholestasis. Morphologic evidence for secretion and absorption
in man. Lab Invest 16:84-95, 1967

78. Guzelian, P., and Boyer, J.L.: Glucose reabsorption from bile.
Evidence for a biliohepatic circulation. J Clin Invest 53:
526-534, 1974

79. Popper, H., and Schaffner, F.: Chronic hepatitis. Taxonomic,

etiologic and therapeutic problems. In: Progress in Liver
Diseases, Vol. V. H. Popper and F. Schaffner, editors. New
York, Grune & Stratton, in press

80. Dive, C., and Heremans, J.F.: Nature and origin of the proteins
of bile. I. A comparative analysis of serum and bile proteins
in man. Europ J Clin Invest 4:235-239, 1974

81. Preisig, R., Rankin, J.G., Sweeting, J., and Bradley, S.E.:
Hepatic hemodynamics during viral hepatitis in man. Circulation 34:188-197, 1966

82. Williams, C.N., Kayser, R., Baker, L., Hurwitz, R., and Senior,
J.R.: Progressive familial cholestatic cirrhosis and bile acid
metabolism. J Pediat St. Louis 81:493-500, 1972

83. Hutterer, F., Denk, H., Bacchin, P.G., et al: Mechanism of
cholestasis. I. Effect of bile acids on microsomal cytochrome
P-450 dependent biotransformation system in vitro. Life Sci 9:
877-887, 1970

84. Javitt, N.B., Rifkind, A., and Kappas, A.: Porphyrin-heme
pathway: Regulation by intermediates in bile acid synthesis.
Science 182:841-842, 1973

85. Denk, H., Schenkman, J.B., Bacchin, P.G., Hutterer, F.,
Schaffner, F., and Popper, H.: Mechanism of cholestasis. III.
Interaction of synthetic detergents with the microsomal cytochrome P-450 dependent biotransformation system in vitro. A
comparison between the effects of detergents, the effects of
bile acids, and the findings in bile duct ligated rats. Exp
Molec Pathol 14:263-276, 1971

86. Fisher,M.M., Magnusson, R., and Miyai, K.: Bile acid metabolism
in mammals. I. Bile acid-induced intrahepatic cholestasis.
Lab Invest 25:88-91, 1971

87. Greim, H., Trulzsch, D., Roboz, J., et al: Mechanism of cholestasis. V. Bile acids in normal rat livers and in those after
bile duct ligation. Gastroenterology 63:837-845, 1972

88. Greim, H., Trulzsch, D., Czygan, P., Rudick, J., Hutterer, F.,
Schaffner, F., and Popper, H.: Mechanism of cholestasis. 6.
Bile acids in human livers with or without biliary obstruction.
Gastroenterology 63:846-850, 1972

89. Leuschner, U., Alfurayh, A., Uhlmann, W., Wildgrube, H.J., and
Erb, W.: Untersuchungen zur Lokalisation von Gallensaeuren in
der Leberzelle. Z Gastroenterol 12:95-102, 1974

90. Leuschner, U., Kurtz, W., Alfurayh, A., and Erb, W.: Die Ver-
teilung von Gallensaeuren in der Leberzelle bei extrahepatischer Cholostase. Z Gastroenterol 12:163-168, 1974

91. Björkhem, I., Einarsson, K., and Hellers, G.: Metabolism of
mono- and dihydroxylated bile acids in preparations of human
liver. Europ J Clin Invest 3:459-465, 1973

92. Czygan, P., and Stiehl, A.: Untersuchungen zur Toxizitaet
sulfatierter und nicht sulfatierter Gallensaeuren. Z Gastroenterol 4:468, 1975

93. Jensen, R., Davis, R., and Kern, F., Jr.: Increased sulfation

and decreased 7-alpha-hydroxylation of deoxycholic acid (DCA) in ethinyl estradiol (EE) induced cholestasis in rats. Gastroenterology 68:210, 1975

94. McCormick, W.C., III, Bell, C.C., Jr., Swell, L., and Vlahcevic, Z.R.: Cholic acid synthesis as an index of the severity of liver disease in man. Gut 14:895-902, 1973

95. Mackinnon, M., and Simon, F.: Pharmacological reversal of cholestasis-associated decrease in hepatic cytochrome P-450. Biochem Pharmacol 24:748-749, 1975

96. Gerber, M.A., Orr, W., Denk, H., Schaffner, F., and Popper, H.: Hepatocellular hyalin in cholestasis and cirrhosis. Its diagnostic significance. Gastroenterology 64:89-98, 1973

97. Nenci, I.: Identification of actin-like proteins in alcoholic hyaline by immunofluorescence. Lab Invest 32:257-260, 1975

98. French, S.W., and Davies, P.L.: Ulsrastructural localization of acin-like filaments in rat hepatocytes. Gastroenterology 68: 765-774, 1975

99. Lieber C. Personal communication

100. Denk, H., Gschnait, F., and Wolff, K.: Hepatocellular hyalin (Mallory bodies) in long term griseofulvin-treated mice. A new experimental model for the study of hyalin formation. Lab Invest 32; No. 6, 1975

101. Sheung -To, C. (Chou, S.T.) and Gibson, J.B.: A histochemical study of the bile ducts in long-term biliary obstruction in the rat. J Pathol 103:163-175, 1971

102. Chenderovitch, J., Raizman, A., and Infante, R.: Effect of phenobarbital and carbon tetrachloride on dehydrocholate induced choleresis in the guinea pig. Biol Gastroenterol 7: 171-178, 1974

103. Schaffner, F., and Popper, H.: Causation and consequences of cholestasis. An overview. In: Hepatology - Research and Clinical Issues - Vol. 2. Jaundice. C.A. Goresky and M.M. Fisher, editors. New York and London, Plenum Press, 1975

104. De Vos, R., De Wolf-Peeters, C., and Desmet,V.: Electron microscopy of the tubule cells of rat kidney after experimental bile duct ligation. Exp Molec Pathol 16:353-361, 1972

105. Bloomer, J.R., and Boyer, J.L.: Phenobarbital effects in cholestatic liver disease. Ann Intern Med 82:310-317, 1975

106. Stiehl, A., Thaler, M., and Admirand, W.H.: The effects of phenobarbital on bile salts and bilirubin in patients with intrahepatic and extrahepatic cholestasis. New Eng J Med 1: 858-861, 1972

107. Chedid, A., Spellberg, M.A., and DeBeer, A.: Ultrastructural aspects of primary biliary cirrhosis and other types of cholestatic liver disease. Gastroenterology 67:858-869, 1974

108. Van Berge Henegouwen, G.P., and De Pagter, A.G.F.: Is an cute disturbance in hepatic transport of bile-acids the primary cause of cholestasis in benign recurrent intrahepatic cholestasis? Lancet 1:1249-1251, 1974

# LIST OF PARTICIPANTS

## AUSTRALIA

Iser, J.
Present address: Gastroenterology Unit, Dept. of Medicine, Guy's Hospital, Medical School, London SE1 9RT.

## AUSTRIA

Graf, J.
Dept. of General and Experimental Pathology, University of Vienna, Währinger Strasse 13, A 1090 Vienna.

Thaler, H.
4 Interne Abteilung, Wilhelminenspital, 16 Montlearstrasse 37, A-1171 Vienna.

## BELGIUM

Fevery, J.
Academish Ziekenhuis, Sint-Rafaël, 3000 Leuven.

Heirwegh, K.P.M.
Laboratory of Liver Physiopathology, Rega Institute, 3000 Leuven.

## CANADA

Fisher, M.M.
Dept. of Pathology, University of Toronto, 100 College Street,
Toronto M5G 1LB.

Phillips, M.J.
Pathology Dept., University of Toronto, 100 College Street,
Toronto M5G 1LB.

Steiner, J.W.
Medical Sciences Building, University of Toronto, Toronto,
Ontario M5S 1A8.

Yousef, I.M.
Pathology Dept., University of Toronto, 100 College Street,
Toronto M5G 1LB.


## DENMARK

Bruusgaard, A.
Medical Dept. B., Frederisksberg Hospital, 2000 Copenhagen.

Dam, H.
Danmarks Tekniske Højskole, Østervoldgade 10L, 1350 Copenhagen K.

Krag, E.
Københavns Amts Sygehus i Gentofte, 2900 Hellerup.

Pedersen, L.
Medical Dept. 1, Aalborg Sygehus Nord, 9000 Aalborg.

Thaysen, E.H.
Dept. of Medical Gastroenterology, Aalborg Sygehus Nord,
9000 Aalborg.

Tygstrup, N.
Devision of Hepatology, Medical Dept. A, Rigshospitalet,
University of Copenhagen, 2100 Copenhagen.

Ussing, H.H.
Universitetets Institut for Biologisk Kemi A, Universitetsparken 13, 2100 Copenhagen Ø.

Winkler, K.
Dept. of Clinical Physiology, Kommunehospitalet, Øster
Farimagsgade 5, 1399 Copenhagen K.

## FRANCE

Chenderovitch, J.
INSERM, 184 Rue du Faubourg, St. Antoine, 75 Paris U-9.

Erlinger, S.
Unite de Recherches de Physiopathologie Hepatique, Hospital
Beaujon, 100 bd. Gl. Leclerc, 92110 Clichy.

Gerolami, A.
Hopital Sainte-Marguerite, 270 bd. St.-Marguerite, 13274
Marseille Cedex 2.

Hauton, J.C.
INSERM, Group de Recherches sur la Transport des Lipides,
46 Chemin de la Gaye, 13009 Marseille.

Infante, R.
Liver Research Unit, INSERM, 184 Rue du Faubourg, St. Antoine,
75012 Paris.

## GERMANY

Altmann, H.W.
Director of University Pathological Institute,
Josef-Schneider-Strasse 2, 8700 Würzburg.

Falk, H.
Dr. Falk GmbH & Co., Pharmaz. Präparate KG, Habsburger Strasse 79,
78 Freiburg i. Br.

Martini, G.A.
Medizinische Klinik der Universität, Mannkopffstrasse 1, 355
Marburg/Lahn.

Matern, S.
Medizinische Universitäts Klinik, Hugstetterstrasse 55,
Freiburg i. Brsg. D-78.

Mayer, D.
Dept. of Chemical Physiology, The University, Hannover.

Schwarz, L.
Institut für Toxikologie, der Universität Tübingen,
Wilhelmstrasse 56, Tübingen 74.

Stiehl, A.
Med. Univ. Klinik, Bergheimstrasse 58, 69 Heidelberg.

ITALY

Dianzani, M.U.
Institute of General Pathology, Corso Raffaello 30, Turin.

Jezequel, Anne-M.
Division of Gastroenterology, Ospedale Regionale CP538,
60100 Ancona.

Koch, M.
Pharmacology Department, Division of Gastroenterology,
Ospedale Regionale CP538, 60100 Ancona.

Orlandi, F.
Pharmacology Dept., Division of Gastroenterology, Ospedale
Regionale CP538, 60100 Ancona.


NORWAY

Bergan, A.
Surgery Dept. B., University Clinic, Rikshospitalet, Oslo 1.

Fausa, O.
Section of Gastroenterology, Medical Dept. A, University Hospital,
Rikshospitalet, Oslo 1.

Ritland, S.
Medical Dept. A, University Hospital, Rikshospitalet, Oslo 1.


PORTUGAL

Correia, J.P.
Dept. Patologia Medica, Hospital Escolar St. Maria, Lisbon 4.

Dias, Maria-Terese S.
Instituto de Quimica Fisiologia, Faculty of Medicine, Lisbon 4.


SWEDEN

Danielsson, H.
Uppsala Universitets Biomedicinska Centrum, 751 23 Uppsala.

Sjövall, J.
Kemiska Institutionen, Karolinska Institutet, 104 01 Stockholm 60.

Strandvik, Birgitta
Huddinge Hospital, Karolinska Institutet, Stockholm.

## SWITZERLAND

Kuenzle, C.C.
Institut für Pharmakologie und Biochemie der Vet. Med. Fakultät, Winterthurerstrasse 260, 8057 Zürich.

Paumgartner, G.
Dept. of Clinical Pharmacology, University of Berne,
Friedbuhlstrasse 49, 3010 Berne.

Preisig, R.
Dept. of Clinical Pharmacology, University of Berne,
Friedbuhlstrasse 49, 3010 Berne.

## UNITED KINGDOM

Billing, B.
Academic Dept. of Medicine, Royal Free Hospital, Pond Street,
London NW3 2QG.

Bouchier, I.A.D.
Dept. of Medicine, Ninewells Hospital, University of Dundee,
Dundee DD1 9SY, Scotland.

Coleman, R.
Biochemistry Department, University of Birmingham, P.O. Box 363,
Birmingham B15 2TT.

Dowling, R.H.
Gastroenterology Unit, Dept. of Medicine, Guy's Hospital,
Medical School, London Bridge SE1 9RT.

Eakins, M.N.
Dept. of Biochemistry, Brunel University, Kingston Lane,
Uxbridge, Middlesex.

Haslewood, G.A.D.
Dept. of Biochemistry and Chemistry, Guy's Hospital, Medical
School, London S.E.1.

Low-Beer, T.S.
Dept. of Medicine, University of Bristol, Southmead Hospital,
Bristol BS10 5NB.

Lucy, J.A.
Dept. of Biochemistry and Chemistry, Royal Free Hospital,
School of Medicine, 8 Hunter Street, London WCIN IBP.

Millburn, P.
Dept. of Biochemistry, St. Mary's Hospital, Medical School,
London W2 IPG.

Mitropoulos, K.
MRC Lipid Metabolism Unit, Hammersmith Hospital, Ducane Road,
London W12 OHS.

Murphy, G.
Gastroenterology Unit, Dept. of Medicine, Guy's Hospital,
Medical School, London Bridge SE1 9RT.

Slater, T.F.
Dept. of Biochemistry, Brunel University, Kingston Lane,
Uxbridge, Middlesex.

Taylor, W.
Physiology Dept., The Medical School, The University,
Newcastle upon Tyne NE1 7RU.


U.S.A.

Arias, I.W.
Albert Einstein College of Medicine, Yeshiva University,
1300 Morris Park Avenue, Bronx N.Y. 10461.

Barnhart, J.L.
Dept. of Internal Medicine, Southwestern Medical School,
Dallas, Texas 75235.

Berk, P.D.
Digestive Diseases Branch NIAMDD, National Institute of Health,
Bethesda, Maryland 20014.

Boyer, J.L.
The Pritzker School of Medicine, Dept. of Medicine, 950 East
59th Street, Chicago Ill. 60637.

Bradley, S.E.
College of Physicians & Surgeons, Columbia University, Dept.
of Medicine, 630 West 168th Street, New York N.Y. 10032.

Brooks, F.
Dept. of Medicine, University of Pennsylvania, Philadelphia PA,
19104.

Combes, B.
Dept. of Internal Medicine, Southwestern Medical School, Dallas,
Texas 75235.

Elliot, W.H.
Dept. of Biochemistry, St. Louis University, School of Medicine,
1402 South Grand Bd., St. Louis Mo. 63104.

Forker, E.L.
University of Iowa Hospitals and Clinics, Department of Internal
Medicine, Iowa City, Iowa 42242.

Hofmann, A.F.
Mayo Medical School & Mayo Foundation, Rochester, Minnesota
55901.

Javitt, N.B.
The New York Hospital, Cornell Medical Center, 525 East 68th
Street, New York N.Y. 10021.

Klaassen, C.D.
Clinical Pharmacology-Toxicology Center, University of Kansas,
Medical Center, Rainbow Boulevard at 39th, Kansas City,
66103 Kansas.

Ostrow, J.D.
Veterans Administration Hospital, University and Woodland
Avenues, Philadelphia Pa 19104.

Palmer, R.H.
The Rockefeller University, New York N.Y. 10021.

Popjak, G.
Mental Retardation Center, Neuropsychiatric Unit, UCLA School
of Medicine, Los Angeles, California 90024.

Popper, H.
Mt. Sinai School of Medicine, Fifth Ave & 100th St., New York
N.Y. 10029.

Vlahcevic, Z.R.
Gastroenterology Section, Veterans Administration Hospital,
Richmond, Virginia 23249.


## OCCASIONAL PARTICIPANTS


### DENMARK

Faergeman, O.
Rigshospitalet, Medical Dept. B, Blegdamsvej 9, Copenhagen.

Bremmelgaard, A.
Rigshospitalet, Medical Dept. A, Copenhagen.

Arnfred, T.
Central Laboratory, Aalborg Sygehus Nord, 9000 Aalborg.

Krarup, N.
Institute of Physiology, University of Aarhus, 8000 Aarhus C.

Larsen, J.A.
Institute of Physiology, University of Aarhus, 8000 Aarhus C.


### SWEDEN

Borgström, B.
Department of Physiological Chemistry, University of Lund, Lund.


### UNITED KINGDOM

Case, R.M.
Physiology Dept., The Medical School, The University,
Newcastle upon Tyne NE1 7RU.

APPENDIX I

Recommendations on Bile Salt Nomenclature

Members of the Committee: Professor G.A.D. Haslewood
Professor Henry Danielsson
Professor Jan Sjövall
Dr. Alan Hofmann
Dr. Hermon Dowling
Dr. Thomas Low-Beer (Secretary)

The ad hoc Committee met on August 26th, 1975, to draft recommendations on the naming of bile acids and salts. We hope that general acceptance of a standard set of names and definitions will clarify communication.

1.  **Bile salt, bile acid**

It was agreed that the term "Bile salt" should be used in the context of a physiological product of the liver concerned in fat digestion and absorption. "Bile acid" then implies that the substance is largely in its protonated form. For instance, "glycocholic acid" specifically implies glycocholate at a pH below its pK.

2.  The ending "ate" was recommended as a blanket trivial name for the individual bile salts, e.g. cholate, glycochenodeoxycholate.

3.  The term "free bile acid" should be discarded as it is ambiguous. It has usually been used to mean an unconjugated bile acid or salt and this is the way in which bile acids without conjugation should be described.

4.  **Trivial names** It was not thought wise to recommend any new trivial names. Thus the name "chenodeoxycholic acid", though clumsy, is the traditional name and should be retained. Any alternatives, such as "cheno" or "chenic acid" are to be thought of as conversational terms requiring prior definition.

5.   <u>Conjugated bile salts</u>

        Glycocholate - Cholyl glycine
        Taurochenodeoxycholate - Chenodeoxycholyl taurine

    Both these ways of describing glyco-3α, 7α, 12α-trihydroxy-
5β-cholan-24-oate and tauro-3α, 7α-dihydroxy-5β-cholan-24-oate in
the systematic IUPAC nomenclature*, were thought correct.   The
first is, of course, the traditional trivial name in each case.

6.   <u>Sulphation</u>

    Sulphation at the 3α position should be described, for example,
as follows: chenodeoxycholate 3-sulphate.   When there is only one
hydroxyl group, as in lithocholic acid, it is sufficient to say
lithocholate sulphate, or sulphated lithocholate.

7.   <u>Cholanoic vs. cholanic</u>

    Cholanoic acid is the more nearly correct term for what is
properly cholan-24-oic acid.

8.   <u>5α-cholanoates</u>

    These can be described by "allo-" prefixed to the trivial name
of the 5β-stereoisomer, e.g. glycoallodeoxycholate when referring
to glyco-3α, 12α-dihydroxy- 5α-cholan-24-oate.

9.   <u>Primary and secondary bile salts</u>

    Primary bile salts should be defined as those formed from
cholesterol.

    Secondary bile salts result from alteration of the steroid
nucleus of the primary bile salt, an alteration usually initiated
by bacteria and sometimes continued by the liver.   Deconjugation
and reconjugation without alteration of the steroid nucleus does
not lead to the formation of a "secondary" bile salt.

10.  <u>Abbreviations</u>

    The following were recommended.   Any substance not on the
list can easily be abbreviated to conform with this system.

*   <u>IUPAC = International Union of Pure and Applied Chemistry</u>
    The IUPAC Commission on the Nomenclature of Organic Chemistry
    and the IUPAC-IUB Commission on Biochemical Nomenclature issue
    "Revised Tentative Rules" for the nomenclature of steroids from
    time to time, e.g. Biochemical Journal (1969) <u>113</u>, 5.

| Trivial name | Abbrev-iation | IUPAC name |
|---|---|---|
| Cholate | C | 3α, 7α, 12α-trihydroxy-5β-cholan-24-oate |
| Deoxycholate | DC | 3α, 12α-dihydroxy-5β-cholan-24-oate |
| Chenodeoxycholate | CDC | 3α, 7α-dihydroxy-5β-cholan-24-oate |
| Lithocholate | LC | 3α-hydroxy-5β-cholan-24-oate |
| Ursodeoxycholate | UDC | 3α, 7β-dihydroxy-5β-cholan-24-oate |
| Hyodeoxycholate | HDC | 3α, 6α-dihydroxy-5β-cholan-24-oate |
| α-Muricholate | α-MC | 3α, 6β, 7α-trihydroxy-5β-cholan-24-oate |
| β-Muricholate | β-MC | 3α, 6β, 7β-trihydroxy-5β-cholan-24-oate |
| Allocholate | 5α-C | 3α, 7α, 12α-trihydroxy-5α-cholan-24-oate |

Conjugates with glycine or taurine have G or T in front,
e.g. GC, TC, GCDC, etc.

The sulphates:  e.g. GLC sulphate,
  TCDC 3-sulphate

The same abbreviations may be used irrespective of whether the
acid or salt is implied.

Enterohepatic circulation can be abbreviated to EHC.

11. Other

"Iso" as a prefix, as isolithocholate to describe 3β-hydroxy
5β-cholan-24-oate should not be used.

Deoxy- is correct and desoxy is incorrect (IUPAC).

12. In general, communication would be best served by defining any
trivial names in terms of the IUPAC nomenclature, referring either
to a footnote or to a publication where this is done.

# INDEX OF SPEAKERS AND PARTICIPANTS
## IN DISCUSSIONS

(The page number of the speaker's main contribution is underlined)

# SUBJECT INDEX